Tumor Board Review

Tumor Board Review

Guideline and Case Reviews in Oncology

Editors

Robert F. Todd III, MD, PhD
Margaret M. Alkek Distinguished Chair of Medicine
The Margaret M. and Albert B. Alkek Department of Medicine
Professor of Medicine
Baylor College of Medicine
Houston, Texas

Kathleen A. Cooney, MD
Frances and Victor Ginsberg Professor of Hematology/Oncology
Professor of Internal Medicine and Urology
Chief, Division of Hematology/Oncology
Associate Director for Faculty Affairs, UMCCC
Director, U of M Prostate Cancer Genetics Project
University of Michigan Medical School
Ann Arbor, Michigan

Teresa G. Hayes, MD, PhD
Associate Professor of Medicine
Director, Section of Hematology/Oncology Fellowship Program
Baylor College of Medicine
Chief, Hematology/Oncology Service Michael E. DeBakey V.A. Medical Center
Houston, Texas

Martha Pritchett Mims, MD, PhD
Associate Professor of Medicine
Chief, Section of Hematology/Oncology
Dan L. Duncan Professor
Director, Clinical Trials Support Unit
Dan L. Duncan Cancer Center
Baylor College of Medicine
Houston, Texas

Francis P. Worden, MD
Associate Professor of Internal Medicine
Director, Division of Hematology/Oncology Fellowship Program
University of Michigan Medical School
Ann Arbor, Michigan

demosMEDICAL
New York

Visit our website at www.demosmedpub.com

ISBN: 978-1-936287-17-8
E-book ISBN: 978-1-617050-46-6

Acquisitions Editor: Rich Winters
Production Editor: Dana Bigelow
Compositor: Newgen Imaging

Library of Congress Cataloging-in-Publication Data
Tumor board reviews : guidelines and case reviews in oncology / editors,
Robert F. Todd III ... [et al.].
p. ; cm.
Includes bibliographical references and index.
ISBN 978-1-936287-17-8 (alk. paper) — ISBN 978-1-617050-46-6 (e-book)
I. Todd, Robert F.
[DNLM: 1. Neoplasms—Case Reports. 2. Neoplasms—Practice Guideline.
3.Evidence-Based Medicine—Case Reports. 4. Evidence-Based Medicine—Practice
Guideline. QZ 200]
616.99'4--dc23
2011036095

Printed in the United States of America at Bradford & Bigelow.
11 12 13 14 / 5 4 3 2 1

Contents

Preface

As physicians, we generally practice medicine one patient at a time, focusing our knowledge base on the specific problems of each individual. As trainees, we are urged to learn as much as we can from each patient who provides a case-specific context for applying the broader body of information derived from textbooks, lectures, and other didactic materials. In the academic practice of oncology, we encourage our trainees to attend tumor boards which, by applying the knowledge and expertise of relevant oncology specialists to the problems of individual patients, serve as a wonderful venue for learning the practice of oncology. The tumor board as a venue for learning was the concept we applied to the design of *Tumor Board Review: Guideline and Case Reviews in Oncology*. Each of the thirty-two chapters follows a uniform format: a concise summary of the epidemiology, risk factors, natural history, and pathology of each major organ-specific tumor type; an abbreviated display of the relevant staging (generally based on the *American Joint Commission on Cancer [AJCC] Staging, 7th edition*); and several "tumor board-style" illustrative patient case summaries (representative of major stage categories of each tumor), each followed by an evidence-based case discussion which reviews the current guidelines and rationale for the diagnostic and therapeutic steps taken. Clearly, it was our intention to make the case summaries and accompanying evidence-based discussion (the latter including helpful management algorithms) the dominant focal point of the book. The authors of each chapter have endeavored to provide the most up-to-date evidence upon which treatment decisions are based, including the latest advances in targeted cancer therapy.

We are hopeful that several categories of readers will find *Tumor Board Review* particularly useful, including oncology subspecialty trainees and practitioners who are preparing for subspecialty certification or recertification, respectively; trainees at all levels (e.g., medical students, residents, and subspecialty fellows) who are seeking a readable, case-based review of the relevant oncology literature; and oncologists in practice who are looking for a concise opportunity to refresh their knowledge across the broad field of medical oncology.

The development of *Tumor Board Review* was made possible by the combined efforts of selected subspecialty fellows and expert faculty of two academic institutions, the Baylor College of Medicine (Houston, TX) and the University of Michigan Medical School (Ann Arbor, MI). The editors gratefully acknowledge the dedicated participation of our trainee and faculty authors, and the support staff of both academic centers, the latter including the invaluable editorial support of Ms. Leneva Moore at Baylor. The successful completion this project was made possible by the editorial and publishing staff of Demos Medical Publishing, especially Richard Winters, Executive Editor (who originated the tumor board concept), and Dana Bigelow, Production Editor.

Robert F. Todd III, MD, PhD
Kathleen A. Cooney, MD
Teresa G. Hayes, MD, PhD
Martha Pritchett Mims, MD, PhD
Francis P. Worden, MD

Contributors

Matthew L. Anderson, MD, PhD
Assistant Professor of Obstetrics and Gynecology
Director, Clinical & Translational Cancer Research
Baylor College of Medicine

Mohsen Arani, MD, FACP
Fellow, Section of Hematology/Oncology
Baylor College of Medicine

Dawit Aregawi, MD
Fellow, Division of Hematology/Oncology
University of Michigan Medical School

Ahmed Awais, MD
Fellow, Section of Hematology/Oncology
Baylor College of Medicine

Diego Bedoya, MD
Fellow, Section of Hematology/Oncology
Baylor College of Medicine

Kathleen E. Bickel, MD, MPhil
Fellow, Division of Hematology/Oncology
University of Michigan Medical School

Dale Bixby, MD, PhD
Assistant Professor of Internal Medicine
Division of Hematology/Oncology
University of Michigan Medical School

Mariela Blum, MD
Fellow, Section of Hematology/Oncology
Baylor College of Medicine

Catherine M. Bollard, MD, FRACP, FRCPA
Associate Professor of Medicine
Center for Cell and Gene Therapy
Baylor College of Medicine

Ronald J. Buckanovich, MD, PhD
Assistant Professor of Internal Medicine
Division of Hematology/Oncology
Assistant Professor of Obstetrics and Gynecology
University of Michigan Medical School

Michelina M. Cairo, MD
Fellow, Section of Hematology/Oncology
Baylor College of Medicine

Elizabeth Yu Chiao, MD, MPH
Assistant Professor of Medicine
Sections of Infectious Diseases and Health Services Research
Baylor College of Medicine

Rashmi Chugh, MD
Assistant Professor of Internal Medicine
Division of Hematology/Oncology
University of Michigan Medical School

Kathleen A. Cooney, MD
Frances and Victor Ginsberg Professor of Hematology/Oncology
Professor of Internal Medicine and Urology
Chief, Division of Hematology/Oncology
University of Michigan Medical School

Gerald S. Cyprus, MD
Professor of Medicine
Section of Hematology/Oncology
Baylor College of Medicine

Naval G. Daver, MBBS
Fellow, Section of Hematology/Oncology
Baylor College of Medicine

Concepcion R. Diaz-Arrastia, MD
Associate Professor of Obstetrics and Gynecology
Director, Division of Gynecologic Oncology
Baylor College of Medicine

Irina Y. Dobrosotskaya, MD, PhD
Fellow, Division of Hematology/Oncology
University of Michigan Medical School

Ahmed A. Eid, MD
Assistant Professor of Medicine
University of Texas M.D.
Anderson Cancer Center

Shan Guo, MD
Fellow, Section of Hematology/Oncology
Baylor College of Medicine

Megan R. Haymart, MD
Assistant Professor of Internal Medicine
Section of Hematology/Oncology
University of Michigan Medical School

Helen E. Heslop, MD
Professor of Medicine and Pediatrics
Dan L. Duncan Chair
Center for Cell and Gene Therapy
Baylor College of Medicine
The Methodist Hospital and Texas Children's Hospital

Collette M. Hodges, NP
Nurse Practitioner, Thoracic Oncology
Division of Hematology/Oncology
University of Michigan Medical School

Maha H. Hussain, MD
Professor of Internal Medicine and Urology
Division of Hematology/Oncology
University of Michigan Medical School

Andrzej J. Jakubowiak, MD, PhD
Associate Professor of Internal Medicine
Inpatient Service Director, Hematology/Oncology
Director, Myeloma Program, UMCCC
University of Michigan Medical School

Gregory P. Kalemkerian, MD
Professor of Internal Medicine
Division of Hematology/Oncology
Co-Director of Thoracic Oncology, UMCCC
University of Michigan Medical School

Rami Khoriaty, MD
Fellow, Division of Hematology/Oncology
University of Michigan Medical School

Stuart M. Knoepp, MD, PhD
Assistant Professor of Pathology
University of Michigan Medical School

Jenny J. Kim, MD
Clinical Lecturer, Division of Hematology/Oncology
University of Michigan Medical School

Christopher D. Lao, MD, MPH
Assistant Professor of Internal Medicine
Division of Hematology/Oncology
University of Michigan Medical School

Dongxin Liu, MD
Fellow, Section of Hematology/Oncology
Baylor College of Medicine

Garrett R. Lynch, MD
Professor of Medicine
Section of Hematology/Oncology
Baylor College of Medicine

John Magenau, MD
Bone Marrow Transplant Fellow
Clinical Lecturer
Division of Hematology/Oncology
University of Michigan Medical School

Sami N. Malek, MD
Assistant Professor of Internal Medicine
Division of Hematology/Oncology
University of Michigan Medical School

Atisha Manhas, MD
Fellow, Section of Hematology/Oncology
Baylor College of Medicine

Vera Maranci, MD
Fellow, Division of Hematology/Oncology
University of Michigan Medical School

Kevin McDonnell, MD, PhD
Fellow, Division of Hematology/Oncology
University of Michigan Medical School

Karen McLean, MD
Fellow, Division of Gynecologic Oncology
University of Michigan Medical School

Martha Pritchett Mims, MD, PhD
Dan L. Duncan Professor
Associate Professor of Medicine
Chief, Section of Hematology/Oncology
Baylor College of Medicine

Colin J. Mooney, MD
Fellow, Division of Hematology/Oncology
University of Michigan Medical School

Benjamin Musher, MD
Assistant Professor of Medicine
Section of Hematology/Oncology
Baylor College of Medicine

Pamela New, MD
Associate Professor
Clinical Neurological Surgery, Neuro-Oncology
Weill Cornell Medical College and Methodist Neurological Institute

Polly Niravath, MD
Fellow, Section of Hematology/Oncology
Baylor College of Medicine

Yuval Raizen, MD
Fellow, Section of Hematology/Oncology
Baylor College of Medicine

Nithya Ramnath, MBBS
Associate Professor of Internal Medicine
Division of Hematology/Oncology
University of Michigan Medical School

Bruce G. Redman, DO
Professor of Internal Medicine
Division of Hematology/Oncology
University of Michigan Medical School

Mothaffar F. Rimawi, MD
Assistant Professor of Medicine
Clinical Director, The Breast Center
Baylor College of Medicine

Igor I. Rybkin, MD, PhD
Fellow, Division of Hematology/Oncology
University of Michigan Medical School

Yvonne Sada, MD
Fellow, Section of Hematology and Oncology
Baylor College of Medicine

Eduardo Vilar Sanchez, MD, PhD
Fellow, Division of Hematology/Oncology
University of Michigan Medical School

Scott M. Schuetze, MD, PhD
Associate Professor of Internal Medicine
Division of Hematology/Oncology
University of Michigan Medical School

David Shepard, MD
Fellow, Division of Hematology/Oncology
University of Michigan Medical School

David C. Smith, MD
Professor of Internal Medicine and Urology
Medical Director, UMCCC Clinical Trials Office
University of Michigan Medical School

Baskaram Sundaram, MBBS, MRCP, FCRP
Assistant Professor of Radiology
University of Michigan Medical School

Moshe Talpaz, MD
Alexander J. Trotman Professorship in Leukemia Research
Professor of Internal Medicine
Associate Director of Translational Research, UMCCC
Associate Chief, Division of Hematology/Oncology
Director, Hematologic Malignancies
University of Michigan Medical School

Muhammad Anas Tarakji, MD
Fellow, Section of Hematology/Oncology
Baylor College of Medicine

Mark M. Udden, MD
Professor of Medicine
Section of Hematology/Oncology
Baylor College of Medicine

Susan Urba, MD
Professor of Internal Medicine
Division of Hematology/Oncology
University of Michigan Medical School

Janet Wang, MD
Fellow, Section of Hematology/Oncology
Baylor College of Medicine

Maria Yvette Williams-Brown, MD
Fellow, Gynecologic Oncology
University of Texas Medical Branch

Francis P. Worden, MD
Associate Professor of Internal Medicine
Director, Division of Hematology/Oncology Fellowship Program
University of Michigan Medical School

Sarvari V. Yellapragada, MD
Assistant Professor of Medicine
Section of Hematology/Oncology
Baylor College of Medicine

Aihua Edward Yen, MD
Fellow, Section of Hematology/Oncology
Baylor College of Medicine

Mark M. Zalupski, MD
Professor of Internal Medicine
Division of Hematology/Oncology
University of Michigan Medical School

Jingsong Zhang, MD, PhD
Fellow, Division of Hematology/Oncology
University of Michigan Medical School

Paul Zhang, MD, PhD
Assistant Professor of Medicine
Section of Hematology/Oncology
Baylor College of Medicine

1

Head and Neck Cancer

IRINA Y. DOBROSOTSKAYA AND FRANCIS P. WORDEN

EPIDEMIOLOGY, RISK FACTORS, NATURAL HISTORY, AND PATHOLOGY

Squamous cell cancer of the head and neck (SCCHN) accounts for about 3% of new cancers diagnosed in the United States each year, with a 3-fold higher incidence in men compared with women. The American Cancer Society estimated that about 50,000 Americans will be diagnosed with SCCHN in 2010, and approximately 11,000 patients will die of this disease in that year.

SCCHN is related to several environmental and lifestyle risk factors. Of them, tobacco exposure and alcohol consumption are the two main causes, and when combined, they increase the risk by about 100-fold compared to nonusers. Epstein-Barr virus (EBV) is present in a significant proportion of nasopharyngeal cancers, while carcinogenic strains of human papillomavirus (HPV) have been recognized as a major contributor to carcinogenesis, especially of oropharynx (about 70% of squamous cell cancer (SCC) of tonsils and base of tongue). HPV-related cancers of the head and neck are more prevalent in younger patients (aged 40–60), whereas traditional smoking- and alcohol-related SCCHNs are diagnosed more frequently in patients older than 60 years of age. HPV-associated oropharynx cancers have a better prognosis for reasons which are not completely understood. This may reflect a difference in tumor biology or simply more favorable host factors such as younger age and fewer comorbidities (and therefore better tolerance of treatments).

Significant advances in the treatment of SCCHN have been possible due to progressive improvement in surgical technique, radiation modalities, and chemotherapeutic regimens. The multimodality approach allows cure even in locally advanced, unresectable cancers. Furthermore, organ preservation is achievable in a considerable number of these patients. This is due to the good results that can be achieved with definitive chemoradiation in patients with locally advanced tumors. Patients with early-stage disease (stage I or II) without high-risk features are treated with a single-modality approach, either surgery or radiation, depending on which technique allows for better function preservation. Positive margins necessitate re-excision or radiation treatment in most cases. Adverse features such as extracapsular extension, vascular embolism, and perineural invasion should prompt consideration for adjuvant therapy.

Patients with locally advanced, curable disease are treated with surgery followed by radiation with or without chemotherapy or with definitive chemoradiation. The latter is used for inoperable tumors or for organ preservation purposes. Adjuvant chemoradiation is preferred over adjuvant radiation alone in patients with more than two positive lymph nodes (LNs), positive surgical margins, or nodal disease with extracapsular extension.

Induction chemotherapy followed by definitive locoregional treatment may be considered in a subset of patients with advanced nodal disease. Patients with metastatic or incurable, recurrent disease may benefit from palliative chemotherapy, depending on their functional status.

Because of the great heterogeneity amongst SCCHN, treatment is based on the primary site of origin (see Table 1.1). For example, oral cavity tumors are treated primarily with surgery since advances in reconstruction using microvascular techniques have led to improved functional outcomes. Locally advanced oropharynx and nasopharynx SCCs, on the other hand, are invariably treated with combined chemoradiotherapy, and locally advanced larynx and hypopharynx cancers can be treated either with organ preservation approaches or total laryngectomy followed by radiation with or without chemotherapy.

Table 1.1 Primary Sites of Origin for SCCHN

Area	Components
Oral cavity	Lips, alveolar ridge, hard palate, buccal mucosa, anterior 2/3 tongue, floor of mouth, retromolar trigone
Oropharynx	Palatine tonsils, posterior 1/3 tongue, vallecula, lingual tonsil, mid portion of posterior pharyngeal wall, inferior surface of soft palate, uvula
Nasal cavity	Nasal septum, mucosa of floor of nasal cavity, superior, middle, and inferior turbinates
Nasopharynx	Superior surface of soft palate, upper portion of posterior pharyngeal wall above the level of uvula
Hypopharynx	Postcricoid area, pyriform sinuses
Larynx	Epiglottis, true vocal folds, false vocal folds, aryepiglottic folds, arytenoids, anterior, and posterior commissures

SCCHN, squamous cell cancer of the head and neck.

STAGING

Overview of Staging

The most useful classification subdivides into early-stage (I–II), advanced but potentially curable (stage III–IVb) and incurable (stage IVc) disease, since the treatment differs significantly between these groups. Early-stage disease generally indicates primary tumor no more than 4 cm in size with no LN involvement. The exception is nasal cavity and ethmoid sinus (stage I or II allows invasion of some regional bony structures) and nasopharynx (stage II allows LN involvement). Advanced but potentially curable disease implies extensive local involvement and/or progressively more bulky LN disease. Incurable disease implies the presence of distant metastases.

Site-Specific Staging for SCCHN

Staging of head and neck cancers (HNCs) (derived from NCCN Clinical Practice Guidelines for Treatment of Head and Neck Cancers, v.2.2010).

Head and Neck Cancers

Oral Cavity	
Stage I	Tumor ≤2 cm, no LN involvement
Stage II	Tumor >2 cm but ≤4 cm, no LN involvement
Stage III	Tumor >4 cm with no LN involvement or such or smaller tumor with involvement of a single, ipsilateral LN ≤3 cm
Stage IVA	Tumor may invade skin of face, cortical bone of the face but not the skull, may invade extrinsic tongue muscles, maxillary sinus; LNs may be involved ipsi- or conrtalaterally but are ≤6 cm
Stage IVB	Either tumor invades very deep such as masticator space, pterygoid plates, base of skull, encases carotid artery, or LN metastases are >6 cm
Stage IVC	Distant metastases are present, irrespective of tumor size or LN involvement
Nasopharynx	
Stage I	Tumor is limited to nasopharynx, nasal cavity or oropharynx, no LN involvement
Stage II	Tumor may involve parapharyngeal space or be less extensive, unilateral involvement of cervical LN or uni- or bilateral involvement of retropharyngeal LNs ≤6 cm
Stage III	Tumor extends into base of skull or paranasal sinuses and/or there is bilateral involvement of cervical or retropharyngeal LNs ≤6 cm
Stage IVA	Tumor may involve intracranial structures, cranial nerves, orbit, infratemporal fossa, masticator space, or hypopharynx and there may be bilateral involvement of cervical or retropharyngeal LNs ≤6 cm
Stage IVB	Any tumor size as above with LN >6 cm or involvement of LNs in supraclavicular fossa
Stage IVC	Distant metastases are present, irrespective of tumor size or LN involvement
Oropharynx	
Stage I	Tumor ≤2 cm, no LN involvement
Stage II	Tumor >2 cm but ≤4 cm, no LN involvement
Stage III	Tumor >4 cm or involves lingual surface of epiglottis with no LN involvement or such or smaller tumor with involvement of a single, ipsilateral LN ≤3 cm
Stage IVA	Tumor may invade larynx, hard palate, mandible, medial pterygoid space or extrinsic tongue muscles; LN involvement may be unilateral or bilateral but does not exceed 6 cm
Stage IVB	Tumor may invade base of skull, pterygoid plates, lateral pterygoid muscle, extend to lateral nasopharynx or encase carotid arteries, and/or LN metastases are >6 cm
Stage IVC	Distant metastases are present, irrespective of tumor size or LN involvement
Hypopharynx	
Stage I	Tumor ≤2 cm and is limited to 1 subsite in hypopharynx, no LN involvement
Stage II	Tumor >2 cm but ≤4 cm and may extend to more than 1 subsite of hypopharynx, no LN involvement
Stage III	Tumor >4 cm or involves esophagus or causes fixation of hemilarynx with no LN involvement or such or smaller tumor with involvement of a single, ipsilateral LN ≤3 cm

Stage IVA	Tumor may involve laryngeal cartilage (thyroid, cricoid), hyoid bone, thyroid gland, prelaryngeal muscles and fat; LN involvement may be unilateral or bilateral but does not exceed 6 cm
Stage IVB	Tumor may encase carotid arteries, invade prevertebral fascia or involve mediastinal structures, and/or LN metastases are >6 cm
Stage IVC	Distant metastases are present, irrespective of tumor size or LN involvement
Larynx	
Stage I	Tumor is limited to the respective area of the larynx (supraglottis, glottis, or subglottis) with normal mobility of vocal cords, no LN involvement
Stage II	Tumor extends to the adjacent region: from supraglottis to glottis or to areas outside of supraglottis without fixation of larynx; from glottis to supra- or subglottis; from subglottis to glottis, no LN involvement
Stage III	Tumor is limited to larynx with vocal cord fixation or, for supraglottic or glottic tumors, may extend to paraglottic space, inner cortex of thyroid cartilage, or, for supraglottic tumors, may extend into postcricoid or preepiglottic space. There is no LN involvement with the tumor extent as above or such or smaller tumor with involvement of a single, ipsilateral LN ≤3 cm
Stage IVA	Tumor may invade through thyroid or cricoid cartilage, trachea, soft tissues of neck, thyroid, esophagus, deep extrinsic tongue muscles; LNs may be involved ipsi- or conrtalaterally but are ≤6 cm
Stage IVB	Either tumor spreads very deep such as prevertebral space, mediastinum, carotid artery encasement, or LN metastases are >6 cm
Stage IVC	Distant metastases are present, irrespective of tumor size or LN involvement
Nasal Cavity and Paranasal Sinuses	
Stage I	Tumor of maxillary sinus is limited to such with no involvement of bone; tumor of nasal cavity or ethmoid sinus is limited to such regardless of bone involvement, each site with no LN involvement
Stage II	Tumor of maxillary sinus involves bone except as below (see Stage III), tumor of nasal cavity and ethmoid sinus involves 2 subsites or an adjacent region regardless of bony invasion, each site with no LN involvement
Stage III	Tumor of maxillary sinus involves posterior or superior bony wall, medial orbital wall, pterygoid fossa, ethmoid sinus, or subcutaneous fat; tumor of nasal cavity or ethmoid sinus involves maxillary sinus, palate, cribriform plates or inferomedial area of orbit, each site with no LN involvement or such or smaller tumor with involvement of a single, ipsilateral LN ≤3 cm
Stage IVA	Tumor of maxillary sinus involves infratemporal fossa or cribriform plate, tumor of nasal cavity or ethmoid sinus involves skin of nose or minimally anterior cranial fossa; either tumor of maxillary sinus or nasal cavity or ethmoid sinus involves skin of cheek, anterior orbit, pterygoid plates, sphenoid or frontal sinus; LNs may be involved ipsi- or conrtalaterally but are ≤6 cm
Stage IVB	Tumor of either maxillary sinus or nasal cavity or ethmoid sinus involves clivus, middle cranial fossa, orbital apex, dura mater, brain, cranial nerves other than maxillary division of trigeminal nerve, or nasopharynx, or LN metastases are >6 cm
Stage IVC	Distant metastases are present, irrespective of tumor size or LN involvement

CASE SUMMARIES

Locoregionally Advanced Disease

J.S. is a 56-year-old man who initially presented to his primary care physician 3 months after noticing a small, pea-size right neck mass that subsequently started to grow. Treatment with antibiotics and steroids brought initial, short-lived relief, but then the neck mass further increased in size. He underwent fine needle aspiration of his neck mass, which revealed undifferentiated SCC. A CT scan of his neck demonstrated multiple enlarged, necrotic LNs in the right cervical chain. J.S. deferred further medical and surgical management and pursued alternative treatment with herbal medications. His neck mass remained stable until 5 months after his initial presentation when it increased in size. He sought medical care after developing dysarthria, difficulty chewing, and a sensation of airway narrowing. J.S. had no other medical problems and did not take any medications. He had a 60 pack-year smoking history and a history of excessive alcohol consumption. His family history was noncontributory.

On physical examination, there was a palpable 8-cm firm, fixed conglomerate of LNs at levels I through V in his right neck, which were adherent to the sternocleidomastoid muscle. The remainder of his physical examination was unremarkable.

On fiberoptic examination, the right tonsil was enlarged, and there was a 4.5 cm area of fullness in the right glossotonsillar sulcus, tonsillar fossa, and the tongue base. This was biopsied and revealed an invasive, poorly differentiated non-keratinizing SCC. A full body PET/CT and contrast CT scan of his neck revealed a 4 cm, FDG-avid mass emanating from the right glossotonsillar sulcus that invaded tongue muscles and encased the right carotid artery. Multiple, enlarged, FDG-avid right neck LNs forming a 7-cm conglomerate mass were also noted. There was no evidence of distant disease.

Evidence-Based Case Discussion

Combined Chemoradiotherapy

The aforementioned patient has T4b, N3, M0 (stage IVB) SCC of the right tonsil. Given the nature of its carotid involvement, the tumor is unresectable, but still may be curable in 10% to 15% of patients. The current standard of care for such a tumor is definitive, concurrent chemoradiation, which employs a platinum-containing regimen. There is stronger evidence supporting the use of cisplatin versus carboplatin, and cisplatin (100 mg/m^2) every 21 days with radiation is generally recommended. A carboplatin-based combination regimen (such as carboplatin-paclitaxel or carboplatin-fluorouracil) may be considered if toxicities of cisplatin are prohibitive. Cisplatin is more likely than carboplatin to cause neuropathy, hearing loss, and renal failure, whereas carboplatin has a higher risk of cytopenias, especially thrombocytopenia. Cisplatin is also more emetogenic when given in high doses (>80 mg/m^2). Unlike cisplatin, carboplatin is generally used in combination with other drugs in the setting of concurrent chemoradiation. The most efficacious combinations include carboplatin with 5-fluorouracil (5-FU) or carboplatin with a taxane. In patients who are not candidates for platinum-based therapies (i.e., poor renal function or severe sensory neuropathy), cetuximab alone may be given as a radiosensitizing agent, although the efficacy of this targeted agent has not been compared directly to cisplatin with radiotherapy. Recently, there has been a renewed interest in the addition of induction chemotherapy prior to definitive chemoradiotherapy in an effort to improve survival outcomes.

Induction Chemotherapy

The interest in induction chemotherapy for locally advanced HNC has undergone a revival. The rationale for its use is related to the possibility for better delivery of chemotherapy to the tumor tissue not yet affected by radiation and improved distant control. Historically, the treatment of such locally advanced SCCHN used to be confined to surgery and radiation therapy. Local control was difficult, and the pattern of recurrence was more frequently local than systemic. Furthermore, the site-specific differences in prognosis and treatment were not clear. More recently, better radiation techniques and surgical approaches improved local control and survival in such patients. However, there is still room for improvement in both local and distant disease control.

The earlier trials performed before 1990s included mostly laryngeal cancer patients and showed that induction chemotherapy, when added to local control measures (either surgery or radiation), did not adversely affect survival and allowed superior organ preservation outcomes by allowing to avoid extensive surgery (for example, Veterans Affairs Laryngeal Cancer Group study published in 1991). Similar results were seen in RTOG 91-11 trial published in 2003. Of note, at that time radiation therapy was not given concurrently with chemotherapy; this concept was introduced later. The earliest meta-analysis of the role of chemotherapy in HNC by MACH-NC group evaluated 63 trials, including 10,741 previously untreated patients with various head and neck SCC locations treated between 1965 and 1993 (1). It showed improved survival with the addition of chemotherapy to local treatment (surgery or radiation or both) with absolute benefit of 4% at 2 and 5 years. The analysis of timing of chemotherapy showed that overall survival (OS) was better with concomitant, but not neoadjuvant or adjuvant chemotherapy versus local therapy alone. Subgroup analysis showed better survival with chemotherapy in patients younger than 61 years of age, males, ECOG performance status 0 or 1, stage IV disease, with tumors of oral cavity, and marginally of hypopharynx. This contributed to the subsequent shift of paradigm from radiotherapy to chemoradiotherapy, both as a definitive treatment in inoperable patients as well as part of adjuvant chemoradiation treatment after surgery. The overall analysis of induction chemotherapy did not show a survival benefit, except for platinum and 5-FU-based regimens (hazard ratio (HR) 0.88, 0.79–0.97). An update to the aforementioned meta-analysis by MACH-NC group was recently published (2). It analyzed an additional 24 new trials, to bring the total number of trials to 87 and number of patients to 16,485. It included analysis of 31 induction chemotherapy trials including 5311 patients. There was no survival advantage to induction chemotherapy (HR of death 0.96, 0.9–1.02, P = .18), although the fluorouracil-platinum-based therapies once again proved to be better than other analyzed regimens (HR of death 0.9, 0.82–0.99), and there was significant benefit for prevention of distant metastases (HR 0.73, 0.61–0.88, P = .001). Subsequent phase III studies of advanced curable disease showed better survival with neoadjuvant cisplatin and 5-FU as well as improved locoregional control compared to local therapy alone (3–5). In a study by Paccagnella et al. (6), the induction chemotherapy group (n = 118) received four cycles of cisplatin plus 5-FU followed by locoregional treatment: surgery followed by radiation in operable patients or radiation alone in inoperable patients. The comparison group (n = 119) received locoregional treatment alone. There was a significantly lower rate of distant metastases in the induction chemo group for both operable and inoperable patients. However, the OS benefit from induction chemotherapy was limited to inoperable patients (at 3 years, OS was 24% vs. 10%, P = .04). In this study, the majority of patients had oropharyngeal cancer (54–59%); they were younger than 70 years of age, most had stage IVA or B disease (63–64%), and most patients were inoperable (71–73%). A later update by Zorat et al. (7) confirmed these findings:

the OS benefit was limited to inoperable patients (10-year survival 16% vs. 6%, $P = .04$). In a similar phase III study by Groupe d'Etude des Tumeurs de la Tête et du Cou (8), only younger patients (age 69 or younger) with curable oropharyngeal disease were included. The chemotherapy group ($n = 157$) received a similar induction chemotherapy with cisplatin and 5-FU, followed by surgery and/or radiation therapy. The nonchemotherapy group ($n = 161$) received only locoregional treatment. This study demonstrated an OS benefit, which was conferred by neoadjuvant chemotherapy in both resectable and unresectable patients (median survival 5.1 years vs. 3.3 years, $P = .03$).

TPF Induction Chemotherapy

In an effort to capitalize on the potential survival benefit of induction chemotherapy, taxanes have been added to platinum and 5-FU. The combination of cisplatin, 5-FU, and docetaxel (TPF) has recently emerged as the standard induction chemotherapy regimen if induction chemotherapy is to be considered. TPF was shown to improve OS when compared to treatment with neoadjuvant cisplatin and 5-FU followed by radiotherapy (3,9). These findings set the stage for the investigation of induction chemotherapy followed by chemoradiotherapy in locally advanced SCCHN. Posner and colleagues demonstrated an improvement in OS and progression-free survival (PFS) when TPF was compared to PF as induction chemotherapy followed by treatment with weekly carboplatin combined with radiotherapy (4).

Despite data from randomized trials suggesting that TPF is the new standard induction regimen for locally advanced HNCs, definitive data assessing the value of neoadjuvant TPF in combination with chemoradiation from large randomized phase III studies is still lacking. However, results from two recent randomized trials suggest that there may be a clinical benefit to the use of induction therapy prior to definitive chemoradiation for patients with locally advanced SCCHN that is not amenable to surgical resection. In one randomized phase II study by Paccagnella et al., patients received three cycles of TPF followed by two cycles of PF combined with radiotherapy (60–70 Gy) versus chemoradiotherapy alone utilizing the same PF-radiotherapy regimen (5). This trial showed improved rates of complete response in inoperable non-laryngeal HNC patients treated with neoadjuvant chemotherapy in addition to chemoradiation, and induction therapy did not comprise subsequent therapy. A second study presented at the 2009 American Society of Clinical Oncology Annual Meeting by Hitt et al. (10) reported the results of a phase III randomized trial in unresectable SCCHN patients treated with chemoradiation without ($n = 128$) or with induction chemotherapy with PF ($n = 156$) or TPF ($n = 155$). A significant number were oropharyngeal cancer patients (42–43%). Median follow-up was 37.6 months. The per-protocol analysis revealed an improved time to treatment failure in the induction chemotherapy group, but no OS difference was detected. The OS rates for chemoradiation alone, PF followed by chemoradiation, and TPF followed by chemoradiation group were 27.1 months, 33.6 months (HR 0.87, 0.62–1.24), and 37.2 months (HR 0.82, 0.57–1.18), respectively. Notably, no difference between PF and TPF was detected, contrary to prior trials (4,9). In this trial, an intention to treat analysis was not performed, suggesting that further confirmatory data are needed before sequential therapy (i.e., induction chemotherapy followed by chemoradiotherapy) is considered standard of care. Results from two randomized studies from the University of Chicago and the Dana Farber Cancer Institute with similar methodology are currently pending.

Overall, the toxicities generated by TPF induction chemotherapy are manageable. Colony stimulating factor prophylaxis is indicated since the risk for febrile neutropenia is higher when taxanes are administered with platinum and 5-FU. In addition, compliance with sequential therapy is approximately 50%, meaning that half of the patients do not complete the full course of intended treatment. This ultimately leads to a worse prognosis for such patients. With this in mind, sequential therapy with TPF followed by chemoradiotherapy should only be considered for select patients until confirmatory data are available (Figure 1.1). Patients for whom such treatment may be most beneficial

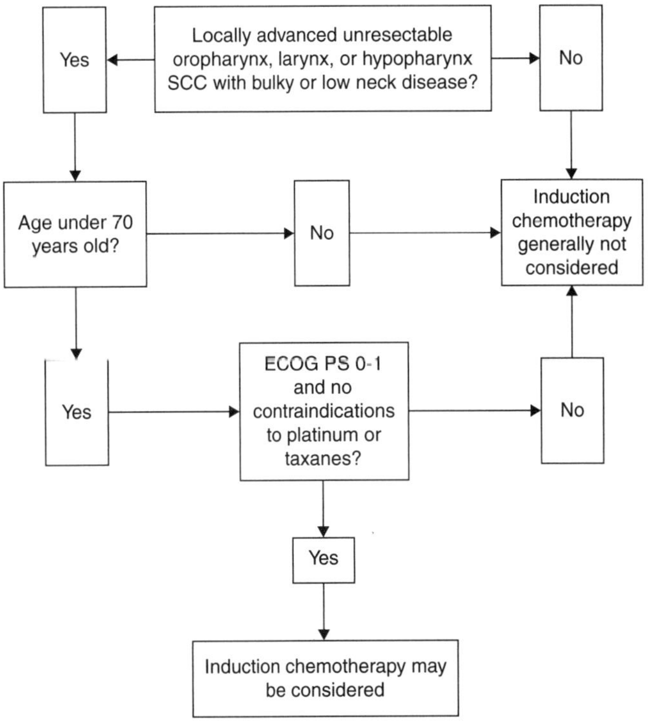

Figure 1.1

Induction chemotherapy for locoregionally advanced disease.

are younger individuals (generally those less than 70 years of age) with good performance statuses and whose locally advanced head and neck cancers are of large tumor burden (i.e., unresectable with bulky or low neck disease). In addition, TPF sequential regimens have only been studied in patients with SCC of the oropharynx, hypopharynx, or larynx. Further study is needed to determine if induction chemotherapy could benefit other head and neck tumor types.

Adjuvant Chemotherapy

Adjuvant chemotherapy is typically not given in HNC, except for nasopharyngeal carcinoma since this tumor type is exquisitely sensitive to the effects of chemotherapy as well as radiation. The evidence for this is largely represented by several studies conducted in late 1990-early 2000s. In the Intergroup Trial 0099, Al-Sarraf et al. compared radiotherapy alone versus chemoradiotherapy (including adjuvant chemotherapy) in 193 patients with advanced nasopharyngeal cancer (11). This study showed both a PFS and an OS advantage for patients in the chemoradiotherapy arm, which included three cycles of adjuvant cisplatin-fluorouracil. The 3-year PFS was 69% versus 24% in the chemoradiation versus radiation-alone groups, respectively ($P < .001$). The 3-year OS was 78% versus 47% ($P = .005$). A conceptually similar trial was reported by Wee et al. in 221 patients with stage III to IV nasopharyngeal carcinoma (12). Disease-free survival (DFS) was better in chemotherapy-treated patients versus radiation-alone (HR for DFS was 0.57, $P = .0093$). The OS was also better in this group: HR for OS was 0.51 ($P = .0061$). The question that remains unanswered is the timing of chemotherapy in this setting: whether concurrent chemoradiation confers the observed benefit or the adjuvant chemotherapy explains the difference in outcomes, or a combination of both. Indeed, Chan et al. reported a trial of 350 patients with various stages of nasopharyngeal carcinoma and showed a similar benefit of concurrent-only chemoradiation versus radiation therapy alone in patients with stage III to IV disease (13). Similarly, OS was improved to a comparable extent by concurrent chemoradiation as compared to radiation alone in another trial reported by Lin et al. (14).

Recurrent/Metastatic SCCHN

D.C. is a 63-year-old man who was diagnosed with a T2N2bM0 (stage IVA) SCC of the floor of mouth 1 year prior to presentation. At that time, he underwent surgical extirpation with a unilateral neck dissection. Surgical margins were negative, but extracapsular extension and perineural invasion were noted. He then received adjuvant chemoradiation. Seven months following definitive therapy, he developed cough. A CT scan of the chest revealed multiple, new pulmonary nodules. A biopsy was performed and confirmed SCC, consistent with metastatic disease.

D.C.'s medical history was otherwise positive for hypertension well controlled with lisinopril. He had developed mild neuropathy after treatment with cisplatin, manifesting as numbness in bilateral finger and toe tips. He had an 80 pack-year history of smoking and remote history of excessive drinking (he quit both 2 years prior to his initial diagnosis). His family history was noncontributory. His physical examination was unremarkable with the exception of the stigmata related to his previous surgery and radiotherapy.

Evidence-Based Case Discussion

Single-Agent Chemotherapy

The aforementioned patient has metastatic cancer of the oral cavity. The extracapsular extension in his neck nodes attests to the aggressive nature of his cancer, portending a poor prognosis, despite aggressive surgical and chemoradiotherapy. Survival in patients with recurrent or metastatic SCCHN (R/M SCCHN) is approximately 6 months. Median survival rates, however, can be extended to 9 to 11 months with systemic chemotherapy.

Single-agent chemotherapy has been studied in metastatic HNC, but response rates are low, generally on the order of 10% to 30%. Traditional cytotoxic agents, including cisplatin, carboplatin, 5-FU, low-dose methotrexate, paclitaxel, docetaxel, ifosfamide, and bleomycin, have been tested as single agents in this setting. Given the improved tolerability of single-agent chemotherapy, such regimens are best suited for patients with a marginal performance status (i.e., ECOG PS 2). Combination regimens, on the other hand, improve response rates and are usually reserved for patients with an ECOG PS of 0–1.

Targeted Therapies

Newer targeted therapies have also been tested as single-agent regimens for R/M SCCHN. Cetuximab is FDA approved as second-line therapy for patients with a platinum-refractory disease, with a toxicity profile that is more tolerable compared to conventional, cytotoxic chemotherapy drugs. Vermorken and colleagues noted a response rate of 13%, and a disease stabilization rate of 46% (15). Erlotinib has also been tested in this setting. In a phase II study, 115 patients with previously treated or untreated R/M SCCHN received 150 mg of erlotinib daily (16). Most patients (76%) had high epidermal growth factor receptor (EGFR) expression level. A small number (4.3%) had a partial response, whereas 38.3% achieved disease stabilization. The median OS was 6 months, whereas PFS was 9.6 weeks.

Gefitinib is another novel, oral tyrosine kinase inhibitor that has been investigated in the therapy of HNC. In a group of 52 patients with R/M HNC (half of them previously treated for their metastatic disease), the overall response rate to single-agent gefitinib was 10.6% with a disease control rate of 53% (17). This resulted in PFS of 3.4 months and OS of 8.1 months. Most importantly, gefitinib was well tolerated with few grade 3 or 4 toxic events reported. More recently, a phase III study by Stewart et al., which compared the efficacy of gefitinib versus weekly methotrexate, showed no differences in survival between the two study arms, although quality of life was better in gefitinib group (18).

Combination Chemotherapy

Combination chemotherapy for metastatic or recurrent HNC with a platinum-based regimen remains standard of care and provides higher response rates compared with single-agent chemotherapy. A SWOG trial compared outcomes with combinations of cisplatin or carboplatin with 5-FU versus single-agent methotrexate (19). The response rates were higher for the combination regimens (32% for cisplatin plus 5-FU, 21% for carboplatin plus 5-FU, and 10% for methotrexate). There was, however, no significant difference in survival amongst the three treatment arms. Jacobs et al. reported similar results when cisplatin and 5-FU were administered either together or as single agents (20). Again, the response rate was higher in the combination arm, but no OS benefit was noted. Cisplatin in combination with a taxane has been evaluated and does not appear superior to other combination regimens. A phase III trial evaluating cisplatin with 5-FU versus cisplatin and paclitaxel demonstrated no difference in OS, though the quality of life scores were higher in the paclitaxel arm (21). Three-drug combinations of conventional cytotoxic agents have also been tested. However, these are more toxic and offer no survival advantage over doublet combinations.

Recently, the introduction of targeted agents with combination chemotherapy regimens has proven to be advantageous in the treatment of recurrent or metastatic HNC. Cetuximab, a chimeric mouse-human monoclonal antibody against EGFR, was combined with either carboplatin plus 5-FU or cisplatin plus 5-FU in a large phase III trial (EXTREME trial) (22). The control group received a combination of either cisplatin or carboplatin with 5-FU. The patients in the cetuximab arm who attained stable disease continued to receive maintenance weekly cetuximab until disease progression or development of intolerable side effects. This study enrolled 442 previously untreated patients with recurrent or metastatic HNC. The addition of cetuximab increased the response rate from 20% to 36% ($P < .001$) and prolonged the median PFS from 3.3 to 5.6 months ($P < .001$) as well as OS (10.1 months vs. 7.4 months, HR of death 0.8, 0.64–0.99, $P = .04$). Quality of life was not adversely affected by the addition of cetuximab. The combination of platinum, 5-FU, and cetuximab is now considered an accepted, first-line, standard regimen for patients with R/M HNC. One remaining question, however, relates to the benefit of maintenance cetuximab therapy. Given its expense and potential for excessive toxicity, further evaluation of cetuximab in this setting is needed before such treatment is considered standard of care.

Cetuximab has also been combined with docetaxel in a regimen that may be promising for patients with platinum refractory metastatic and/or recurrent HNC. Knoedler and colleagues reported the results of a multicenter, phase II study of this combination in 84 patients (23). They noted a 12% partial response rate with a disease control rate (partial response plus stable disease) of 39%. The median OS was 7 months, with a satisfactory toxicity profile.

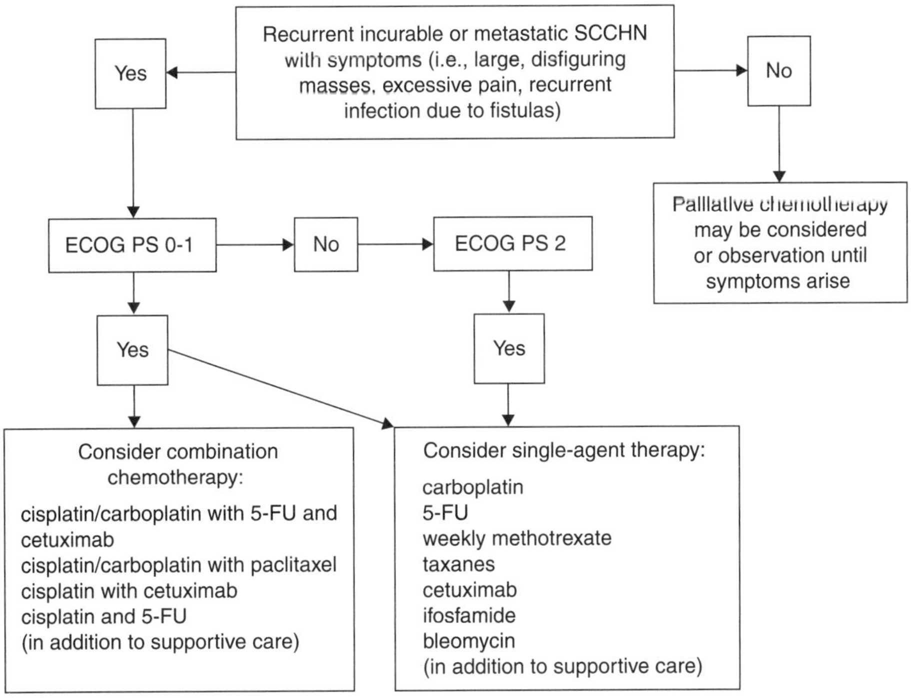

Figure 1.2

Palliative chemotherapy for recurrent/metastatic SCCHN. SCCHN, squamous cell cancer of the head and neck.

Erlotinib has also shown promising results when combined with cisplatin and docetaxel in a phase II trial in patients with untreated recurrent or metastatic HNC (24). The overall response rate for this study was 67% with a disease control rate of 95%. The median OS was 11 months and median PFS was 6 months.

Summary

As shown in Figure 1.2, combination chemotherapy consisting of platinum plus 5-FU with or without cetuximab, or platinum combined with a taxane, are considered standard of care for patients with recurrent or metastatic HNC. Combination regimens are best suited for patients with ECOG PS 0-1 who have large bulky, disfiguring tumors or who have distant metastatic disease. Disease that is asymptomatic can be treated with best supportive care until symptoms arise. Patients with a marginal or limited performance status (PS 2–3) are more likely to tolerate single-agent therapy.

REFERENCES

1. Pignon JP, Bourhis J, Domenge C, Designé L. Chemotherapy added to locoregional treatment for head and neck squamous-cell carcinoma: three meta-analyses of updated individual data. MACH-NC Collaborative Group. Meta-Analysis of Chemotherapy on Head and Neck Cancer. *Lancet.* 2000;355(9208):949–955.
2. Pignon JP, le Maître A, Maillard E, Bourhis J. Meta-analysis of chemotherapy in head and neck cancer (MACH-NC): an update on 93 randomised trials and 17,346 patients. *Radiother Oncol.* 2009;92(1):4–14.
3. Pointreau Y, Garaud P, Chapet S, et al. Randomized trial of induction chemotherapy with cisplatin and 5-fluorouracil with or without docetaxel for larynx preservation. *J Natl Cancer Inst.* 2009;101(7):498–506.
4. Posner MR, Hershock DM, Blajman CR, et al. Cisplatin and fluorouracil alone or with docetaxel in head and neck cancer. *N Engl J Med.* 2007;357(17):1705–1715.
5. Paccagnella A, Ghi MG, Loreggian L, et al. Concomitant chemoradiotherapy versus induction docetaxel, cisplatin and 5 fluorouracil (TPF) followed by concomitant chemoradiotherapy in locally advanced head and neck cancer: a phase II randomized study. *Ann Oncol.* 2010;21(7):1515–1522.
6. Paccagnella A, Orlando A, Marchiori C, et al. Phase III trial of initial chemotherapy in stage III or IV head and neck cancers: a study by the Gruppo di Studio sui Tumori della Testa e del Collo. *J Natl Cancer Inst.* 1994;86(4):265–272.
7. Zorat PL, Paccagnella A, Cavaniglia G, et al. Randomized phase III trial of neoadjuvant chemotherapy in head and neck cancer: 10-year follow-up. *J Natl Cancer Inst.* 2004;96(22):1714–1717.
8. Domenge C, Hill C, Lefebvre JL, et al. Randomized trial of neoadjuvant chemotherapy in oropharyngeal carcinoma. French Groupe d'Etude des Tumeurs de la Tête et du Cou (GETTEC). *Br J Cancer.* 2000;83(12):1594–1598.
9. Vermorken JB, Remenar E, van Herpen C, et al. Cisplatin, fluorouracil, and docetaxel in unresectable head and neck cancer. *N Engl J Med.* 2007;357(17):1695–1704.
10. Hitt R, Grau JJ, Lopez-Pousa A, et al. Final results of a randomized phase III trial comparing induction chemotherapy with cisplatin/5-FU or docetaxel/cisplatin/5-FU follow by chemoradiotherapy (CRT) versus CRT alone as first-line treatment of unresectable locally advanced head and neck cancer (LAHNC). *J Clin Oncol.* 2009;27:15s (suppl; abstr 6009).
11. Al-Sarraf M, LeBlanc M, Giri PG, et al. Chemoradiotherapy versus radiotherapy in patients with advanced nasopharyngeal cancer: phase III randomized Intergroup study 0099. *J Clin Oncol.* 1998;16(4):1310–1317.
12. Wee J, Tan EH, Tai BC, et al. Randomized trial of radiotherapy versus concurrent chemoradiotherapy followed by adjuvant chemotherapy in patients with American Joint Committee on Cancer/International Union against cancer stage III and IV nasopharyngeal cancer of the endemic variety. *J Clin Oncol.* 2005;23(27):6730–6738.
13. Chan AT, Leung SF, Ngan RK, et al. Overall survival after concurrent cisplatin-radiotherapy compared with radiotherapy alone in locoregionally advanced nasopharyngeal carcinoma. *J Natl Cancer Inst.* 2005;97(7):536–539.
14. Lin JC, Jan JS, Hsu CY, et al. Phase III study of concurrent chemoradiotherapy versus radiotherapy alone for advanced nasopharyngeal carcinoma: positive effect on overall and progression-free survival. *J Clin Oncol.* 2003;21(4):631–637.
15. Vermorken JB, Trigo J, Hitt R, et al. Open-label, uncontrolled, multicenter phase II study to evaluate the efficacy and toxicity of cetuximab as a single agent in patients with recurrent and/or metastatic squamous cell carcinoma of the head and neck who failed to respond to platinum-based therapy. *J Clin Oncol.* 2007;25(16):2171–2177.
16. Soulieres D, Senzer NN, Vokes EE, Hidalgo M, Agarwala SS, Siu LL. Multicenter phase II study of erlotinib, an oral epidermal growth factor receptor tyrosine kinase inhibitor, in patients with recurrent or metastatic squamous cell cancer of the head and neck. *J Clin Oncol.* 2004;22(1):77–85.
17. Cohen EE, Rosen F, Stadler WM, et al. Phase II trial of ZD1839 in recurrent or metastatic squamous cell carcinoma of the head and neck. *J Clin Oncol.* 2003;21(10):1980–1987.
18. Stewart JS, Cohen EE, Licitra L, et al. Phase III study of gefitinib compared with intravenous methotrexate for recurrent squamous cell carcinoma of the head and neck [corrected]. *J Clin Oncol.* 2009;27(11):1864–1871.
19. Forastiere AA, Metch B, Schuller DE, et al. Randomized comparison of cisplatin plus fluorouracil and carboplatin plus fluorouracil versus methotrexate in advanced squamous-cell carcinoma of the head and neck: a Southwest Oncology Group study. *J Clin Oncol.* 1992;10(8):1245–1251.
20. Jacobs C, Lyman G, Velez-García E, et al. A phase III randomized study comparing cisplatin and fluorouracil as single agents and in combination for advanced squamous cell carcinoma of the head and neck. *J Clin Oncol.* 1992;10(2):257–263.
21. Gibson MK, Li Y, Murphy B, et al. Randomized phase III evaluation of cisplatin plus fluorouracil versus cisplatin plus paclitaxel in advanced head and neck cancer (E1395): an intergroup trial of the Eastern Cooperative Oncology Group. *J Clin Oncol.* 2005;23(15):3562–3567.
22. Vermorken JB, Mesia R, Rivera F, et al. Platinum-based chemotherapy plus cetuximab in head and neck cancer. *N Engl J Med.* 2008;359(11):1116–1127.
23. Knoedler M, Gauler TC, Matzdorff A, et al. Phase II trial to evaluate efficacy and toxicity of cetuximab plus docetaxel in platinum pretreated patients with recurrent and/or metastatic head and neck cancer. *J Clin Oncol.* 2008;26:abstr 6066.
24. Kim ES, Kies MS, Glisson BS, et al. Final results of a phase II study of erlotinib, docetaxel and cisplatin in patients with recurrent/metastatic head and neck cancer. *J Clin Oncol.* 2007:6013.

2

Thyroid Cancer

KEVIN MCDONNELL AND MEGAN RIST HAYMART

EPIDEMIOLOGY, RISK FACTORS, NATURAL HISTORY, AND PATHOLOGY

The incidence of thyroid cancer is increasing at a rate surpassing that of all other malignancies (1–3). During the year 2010, there was estimated to be greater than 44,000 new cases of thyroid cancers diagnosed with a female:male ratio of 3:1. The median age at diagnosis for all thyroid cancers was 49 years. The majority (68%) of thyroid cancers present as localized disease at the time of diagnosis; regional lymph node disease and disseminated metastatic disease account for 24% and 5% of cases, respectively (2). The 5-year survival rate overall is 99.8%, 97.1%, and 58.1%, respectively, for localized, regional, and distant thyroid cancer (2). There are three primary histological subcategories of thyroid carcinoma: differentiated (comprising papillary, follicular, and Hürthle cell), medullary, and anaplastic.

Among the primary risk factors associated with the development of thyroid carcinoma are a family history of thyroid carcinoma, and a history of exposure to ionizing radiation, particularly during childhood. An additional risk factor is iodine deficiency, especially relating to the development of anaplastic and follicular thyroid carcinomas.

Differentiated Thyroid Carcinoma

Papillary Thyroid Cancer

Papillary thyroid cancer accounts for approximately 80% of all thyroid cancers. Papillary carcinomas may present clinically as an enlarged, palpable thyroid nodule; however, they frequently are incidentally discovered on imaging studies performed for other reasons. The incidence of papillary thyroid cancers peaks in the fourth or fifth decade of life, with a characteristic female predominance. The diagnosis of papillary thyroid cancer is typically made with an ultrasound-guided fine needle aspiration (FNA). Histological analysis of the papillary thyroid carcinoma reveals papillae comprising multiple layers of malignant cells. These structures are often cystic in nature, lack a capsule, are multifocal, and contain the cytologically distinguishing psamomma bodies, which are degraded papillary structures. The growth and proliferation of papillary thyroid carcinomas are driven by mutations in a variety of molecular pathways, including the mitogen-activated protein kinase, RAS, BRAF, RET/PTC, and neurotrophic tyrosine kinase receptor type 1 molecular pathways (4,5). Presence of the BRAF mutation is associated with a more aggressive phenotype and worse prognosis. Characteristically, papillary thyroid carcinomas respond to therapeutic intervention, with only a small percentage of patients dying secondary to the cancer. Uniquely, the staging of differentiated thyroid carcinomas includes age as part of the staging schema, with age greater than 45 years representing an independent risk factor associated with worse survival outcomes relative to younger patients (6).

Follicular Thyroid Carcinoma

Follicular thyroid carcinoma accounts for approximately 11% of thyroid cancers. Follicular thyroid cancer most often presents as a palpable nodule with peak incidence occurring in the fifth or sixth decade, later than papillary thyroid cancer. As with papillary cancer, there is a female predominance. Unlike papillary thyroid cancer, the diagnosis of follicular thyroid cancer cannot be achieved with an FNA. The FNA typically reveals a follicular neoplasm but growth beyond the tumor capsule and vascular penetration cannot be assessed. An excisional biopsy or lobectomy is required to identify these features. Eighty percent of follicular neoplasms are benign and 20% are malignant follicular cancer. Histologically, follicular thyroid carcinoma appears as an assembly of cuboidal cells circumscribing a follicle. Follicular thyroid carcinoma may present either as a less aggressive, minimally invasive variant characterized by limited angiogenic and tumor extension or as a more aggressive vascular and tumor invasive variant. On the molecular level, follicular thyroid carcinomas may express a PAX8 peroxisome proliferator-activated receptor gamma 1 (PPAR-γ1) fusion protein, which promotes cellular growth and prevents cellular differentiation. RAS mutations are also found not only in the papillary thyroid carcinoma but also in the follicular cell carcinomas. More than three fourths of follicular thyroid carcinomas have either a PAX8 or RAS mutation. Epigenetic alterations, for example, hypermethylation of tumor suppressor genes such as RASSF1A, are thought to play a role in the tumor progression of follicular thyroid carcinoma (7). Overall, follicular thyroid carcinomas have a worse prognosis relative to papillary thyroid carcinoma.

Hürthle Cell Carcinoma

Hürthle cell carcinoma constitutes nearly 3% of thyroid cancers. The Hürthle cell carcinoma often manifests as a palpable nodule. As with follicular carcinoma, an FNA specimen of a suspected Hürthle cell carcinoma is insufficient to establish a diagnosis; thus, as with follicular cell carcinoma, the definitive diagnosis of Hürthle cell carcinoma is made following pathological assessment of a surgical specimen. Histologically, Hürthle cell carcinoma is variously classified as a variant of follicular thyroid carcinoma or as a separate independent subtype of differentiated thyroid carcinoma. Microanatomically, the Hürthle cell carcinoma is a tumor comprising at least 75% Hürthle cells, which are large, eosinophilic, oxyphilic, thyroglobulin-producing cells designated "oncocytes." The Hürthle cell carcinoma may present with either a papillary or follicular growth pattern. Hürthle cells are distinguished by a pathological overabundance of mitochondria. Genetic mutations harbored by these mitochondria underlie their increased proliferation and malignancy-promoting physiological dysfunction. A significant percentage of Hürthle cell carcinomas demonstrate the *RET/PTC* gene rearrangement, which may also be found in papillary thyroid carcinomas. Hürthle cell carcinoma demonstrates an increased incidence of metastatic disease as compared to either papillary or follicular thyroid carcinoma, and accordingly, it is considered to be a more aggressive disease with a higher mortality.

Medullary Thyroid Carcinoma

Medullary thyroid carcinoma constitutes approximately 4% of cases of thyroid cancer and is typically detected as a solitary nodule. There is a great propensity for medullary thyroid carcinoma to metastasize, so that at the time of diagnosis the tumor has often spread to distant sites. Medullary thyroid carcinoma occurs with near equal frequency among men and women, and most often, patients are in their 40s or 50s at the time of their presentation. FNA of the solitary nodule provides sufficient pathological information to establish the diagnosis of medullary thyroid carcinoma. Medullary thyroid carcinoma, a type of neuroendocrine tumor, arises from the parafollicular C cell of the thyroid gland and characteristically produces calcitonin. Thus, at the time of diagnosis, the calcitonin levels are characteristically elevated. Histologically, medullary thyroid carcinoma demonstrates a glandular phenotype comprising malignant epithelial cells. Molecularly, mutations occur frequently in the RET proto-oncogene. Sporadic mutations in the RET proto-oncogene in medullary thyroid carcinoma represent the majority (>75%) of cases. Whereas most sporadic mutations are restricted to the tumor itself, the remainder of medullary thyroid cancers develop in the setting of an inherited germline mutation as part of an hereditary cancer syndrome: either multiple endocrine neoplasia (MEN), 2A or 2B, or familial medullary thyroid cancer (FMTC). MEN2A, MEN2B, and FMTC are inherited in an autosomal dominant fashion. MEN2A is associated with medullary thyroid carcinoma, pheochromocytoma, and parathyroid hyperplasia. MEN2B tends to manifest clinically as medullary thyroid carcinoma and pheochromocytoma. Frequently, in MEN2B, there are additional clinical manifestations, including Marfinoid features and the development of neuroganglioneuromas. With FMTC, hereditary medullary thyroid cancer occurs in the absence of other endocrine manifestations observed in the MEN syndromes. Because of the propensity of the medullary thyroid carcinoma to derive from a germline genetic mutation, patients who are diagnosed with medullary thyroid carcinoma should be routinely screened for the presence of pheochromocytomas, parathyroid hyperplasia, and a RET proto-oncogene mutation. Because of its greater propensity to metastasize and be associated with other comorbidities, the prognosis for medullary thyroid cancer is generally less favorable than either papillary or follicular thyroid cancers.

Anaplastic Thyroid Carcinoma

Anaplastic thyroid carcinoma, which constitutes around 2% of thyroid cancers, is an extremely aggressive, undifferentiated carcinoma arising from the thyroid follicular epithelium. It typically presents as an enlarging neck mass or lymphadenopathy and tends to occur in older age, in the seventh or greater decades of life. FNA of the cervical mass or lymph node allows diagnosis of the anaplastic thyroid cancer. Histologically, the presence of enlarged, spindle-shaped cells, often with multiple nuclei, typifies anaplastic thyroid carcinoma. It is estimated that half of anaplastic thyroid carcinomas transform from an antecedent or synchronous differentiated thyroid carcinoma. Genetic alterations associated with anaplastic thyroid carcinoma include BRAF and RAS mutations. These same mutations can also be found in differentiated thyroid carcinomas and so are believed to represent foundational mutational events in the development of anaplastic thyroid carcinoma. Subsequent secondary mutations include alterations in p53, β-catenin, and PIK3CA, which confer upon anaplastic carcinoma its highly aggressive and deadly phenotype. Anaplastic thyroid carcinoma is nearly 100% fatal.

STAGING

A summary of AJCC cancer staging (8) for thyroid carcinoma is below.

Staging Thyroid Carcinomas

Stage	Description
Staging Papillary and Follicular Thyroid Carcinomas	
Under 45 years of Age	
I	Primary tumor of any size with or without regional lymphatic spread (N0 or N1), but without distant metastases (M0)
II	Primary tumor of any size with or without regional lymphatic spread (N0 or N1), with distant metastases (M1)
Over 45 years of Age	
I	Primary tumor 2 cm or less in greatest dimension limited to the thyroid (T1), without regional lymphatic (N0) or distant metastatic spread (M0)
II	Primary tumor greater than 2 cm but not more than 4 cm in greatest dimension limited to the thyroid (T2), without regional lymphatic (N0) or distant metastatic spread (M0)
III	Primary tumor 4 cm or less in greatest dimension limited to the thyroid (T1, T2), with regional lymph node metastases to Level VI (pretracheal, paratracheal, and prelaryngeal/Delphian lymph nodes) (N1a) and without distant metastases (M0) Or Primary tumor greater than 4 cm in greatest dimension limited to the thyroid or any tumor with minimal extrathyroid extension (T3), with or without regional lymph node metastasis to Level VI (pretracheal, paratracheal and prelaryngeal/Delphian lymph nodes) (N0 or N1a) and without distant metastases (M0)
IVA	Primary tumor of any size limited to the thyroid or with minimal extrathyroid extension (T1, T2, or T3) with regional lymph node metastases to the unilateral, bilateral or contralateral cervical or superior mediastinal lymph nodes (N1b) and without distant metastases (M0) Or Primary tumor of any size extending beyond the thyroid capsule to invade subcutaneous soft tissues, larynx, trachea, esophagus or recurrent laryngeal nerve, with any regional lymph node metastasis (N0, N1a, or N1b) and without distant metastases
IVB	Primary tumor of any size invading the prevertebral fascia or encasing the carotid artery or mediastinal vessels (T4b), with or without regional lymphatic spread (N0 or N1), and without distant metastases (M0)
IVC	Primary tumor of any size with or without regional lymphatic spread (N0 or N1), and with distant metastases (M1)
Staging Medullary Thyroid Carcinoma	
I	Primary tumor 2 cm or less in greatest dimension limited to the thyroid (T1), without regional lymphatic (N0) or distant metastatic spread (M0)
II	Primary tumor greater than 2 cm, but not more than 4 cm in greatest dimension limited to the thyroid (T2), without regional lymphatic (N0) or distant metastatic spread (M0)
III	Primary tumor 4 cm or less in greatest dimension limited to the thyroid (T1, T2), with regional lymph metastases to Level VI (pretracheal, paratracheal, and prelaryngeal/Delphian lymph nodes) (N1a) and without distant metastases (M0) Or Primary tumor greater than 4 cm in greatest dimension limited to the thyroid or any tumor with minimal extrathyroid extension (T3), with or without regional lymph node metastasis to Level VI (pretracheal, paratracheal, and prelaryngeal/Delphian lymph nodes) (N0 or N1a) and without distant metastases (M0)
IVA	Primary tumor of any size limited to the thyroid or with minimal extrathyroid extension (T1, T2, or T3) with regional lymph node metastases to the unilateral, bilateral or contralateral cervical or superior mediastinal lymph nodes (N1b) and without distant metastases (M0) Or Primary tumor of any size extending beyond the thyroid capsule to invade subcutaneous soft tissues, larynx, trachea, esophagus or recurrent laryngeal nerve, with any regional lymph node metastases (N0, N1a, or N1b) and without distant metastases
IVB	Primary tumor of any size invading the prevertebral fascia or encasing the carotid artery or mediastinal vessels (T4b), with or without regional lymphatic spread (N0 or N1), and without distant metastases (M0)
IVC	Primary tumor of any size with or without regional lymphatic spread (N0 or N1), and with distant metastases (M1)
Staging Anaplastic Thyroid Carcinoma (All Anaplastic Thyroid Carcinomas Are Stage IV)	
IVA	Primary tumor is intrathyroidal and surgically resectable (T4a), with or without regional lymphatic spread (N0 or N1), and without distant metastases (M0)
IVB	Primary tumor is extrathyroidal and surgically unresectable (T4b), with or without regional lymphatic spread (N0 or N1), and without distant metastases (M0)
IVC	Primary tumor of any size with or without regional lymphatic spread (N0 or N1), and with distant metastases (M1)

CASE SUMMARIES

Early-Stage Papillary Thyroid Cancer: Stage I

A.M. is a 24-year-old woman who was involved in a low-speed motor vehicle accident. She developed neck pain for which she underwent a CT scan of the head and neck in the emergency department. These imaging studies did not demonstrate any acute pathology but did reveal, incidentally, a 2.5-cm solid mass in the right lobe of the thyroid. The emergency department physicians recommended that she have further evaluation as an outpatient, and the patient followed up with her primary care physician. She had no overt symptoms of a dysfunctional thyroid state and no compressive symptoms secondary to the nodule. There was no history of previous malignancy, prior irradiation, or family history of thyroid cancer. A thyroid-stimulating hormone (TSH) was obtained and was normal. The patient was directed to obtain a diagnostic ultrasound of the neck. The ultrasound confirmed the presence of a $2.3 \times 1.7\ cm^2$ solid mass in the right lobe of the thyroid. There were no other nodules and no suspicious cervical lymph nodes detected. Subsequently, an FNA of the nodule was performed, which revealed a well-differentiated papillary thyroid carcinoma.

Evidence-Based Case Discussion

This case illustrates the evaluation of an incidentally discovered thyroid nodule with the establishment of early-stage papillary thyroid carcinoma.

The clinical approach to this patient begins with evaluation of the thyroid nodule. Frequently, as with this case, the thyroid nodule is discovered incidentally. Unless there exists a heightened suspicion for the occurrence of malignancy, such as the presence of a concomitant lymphadenopathy, a family history of thyroid cancer, a personal history of radiation exposure, high-risk features on a thyroid ultrasound, or the patient possesses a number of additional risk factors, only thyroid nodules larger than 1 cm merit further evaluation. The history and physical examination initiate the evaluation of the thyroid nodule (see Figure 2.1) to assess for signs and symptoms consistent with the development of a thyroid cancer, including, dysphonia secondary to impairment of the vocal cords or enlarged lymph nodes. A cervical ultrasound examination is recommended to further assess the thyroid nodule and assess for any additional neck pathology associated with the thyroid gland (9). Measurement of TSH directs the further work up. With a high or normal TSH value, an FNA is indicated. With a low TSH value, thyroid

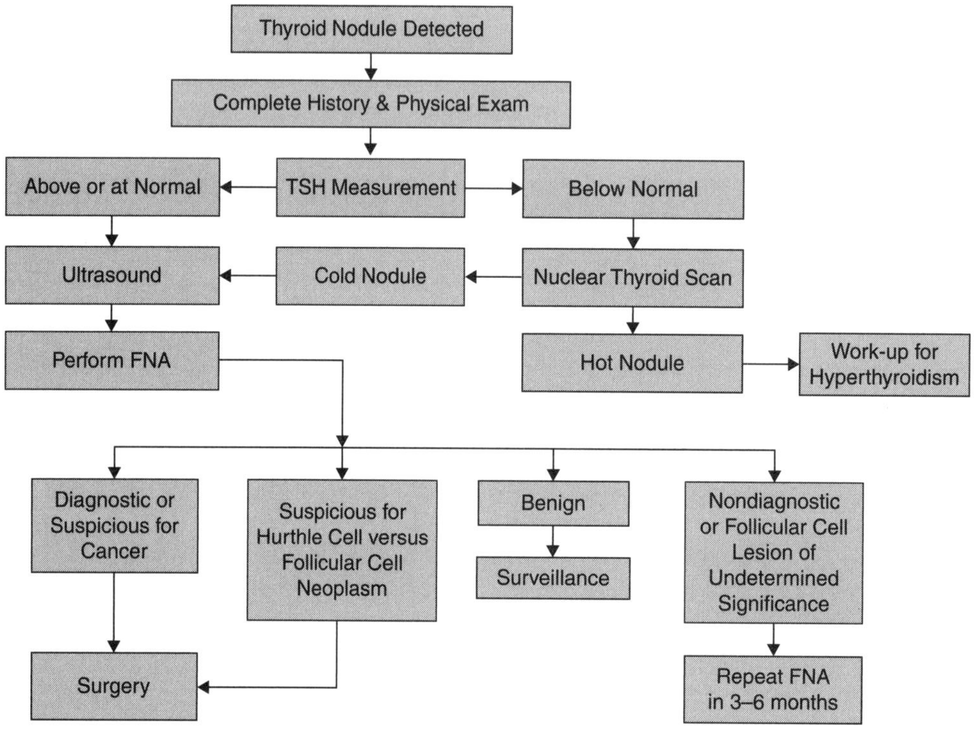

Figure 2.1

Algorithm: Evaluation of the thyroid nodule. Adapted from ATA Guidelines (9).

scintigraphy is recommended to determine whether the nodule shows avidity for radioactive iodine (RAI) and is therefore considered functioning, or does not incorporate the radiotracer and is nonfunctioning. The functioning thyroid nodule is rarely malignant, and in this case, no further evaluation for malignancy is required, though further clinical assessment for a hyperthyroid state would be indicated. With a nonfunctioning thyroid nodule, the suspicion for malignancy is increased and a tissue diagnosis by an FNA is indicated.

In the case of an FNA diagnosis of papillary thyroid carcinoma, management entails surgical resection of the nodule either as a total or hemithyroidectomy (Figure 2.2). Prior to surgical intervention, a neck ultrasound is recommended to assess more carefully for thyroid pathology and lymphadenopathy. If the patient demonstrates a thyroid nodule greater than 1.0 cm, has intermediate- or high-risk features, multifocal disease, a history of prior head or neck irradiation, or cervical lymph node metastases are observed on the presurgical evaluation, then a near total or total thyroidectomy is recommended. In the case of A.M., since her nodule was 2.3 cm and her FNA was diagnostic for papillary thyroid carcinoma, she proceeded to undergo a total thyroidectomy.

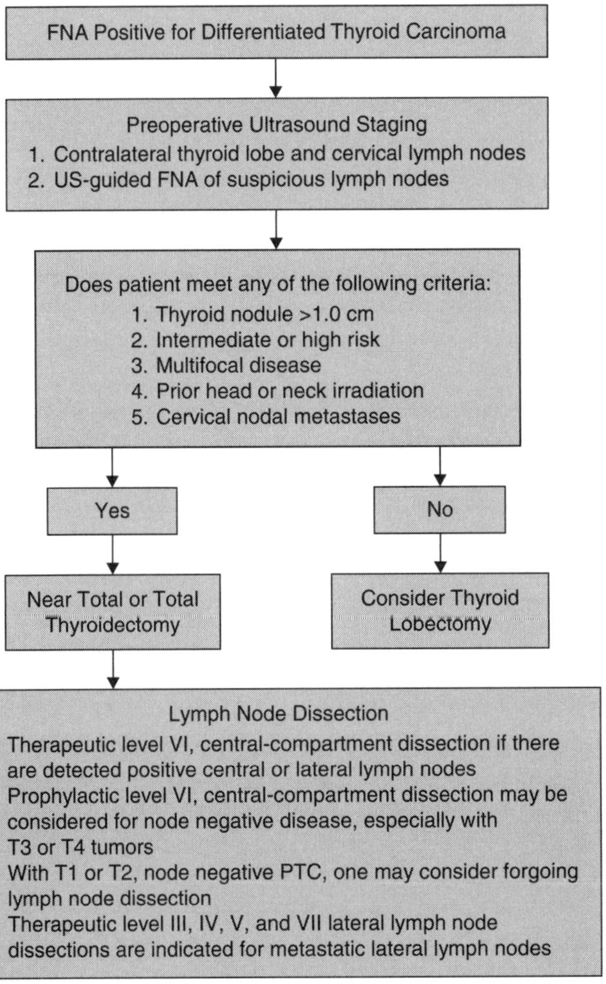

Figure 2.2

Algorithm: Surgical management to the thyroid nodule in differentiated thyroid carcinoma.

The question of whether a lymph node dissection is required depends on the presence of detectable lymph node disease as well as the size of the thyroid nodule. Where lymph node metastases are found, a therapeutic lymph node dissection is indicated. Prophylactic lymph node dissection is controversial but can be considered for T3 or T4 tumors. In the case of smaller T1 or T2 primaries without evidence of lymph node metastases, it is acceptable to forgo the prophylactic lymph node dissection. Accordingly, A.M. did not undergo lymph node dissection.

The present case highlights the impact that the patient's age has on clinical staging. Because A.M. is less than 45 years old, she is considered as having stage I disease. If she were older than 45 years, she would have stage II disease.

Postoperatively, the clinician must decide whether to utilize RAI ablation and to what extent the TSH should be suppressed. Recent clinical studies have provided conflicting evidence for the use of RAI, with some studies demonstrating clinical benefit, including decrease in disease recurrence and increase in survival, whereas other studies have not demonstrated these same benefits (9). In view of this conflicting information, the American Thyroid Association (ATA) has generated consensus guidelines for the postoperative use of RAI in differentiated thyroid cancer (9). The ATA recommends the use of RAI if there is distant metastatic disease, extrathyroidal tumor extension, or the tumor exceeds 4 cm in size. For thyroid nodules 1 to 4 cm in size, the ATA advocates the selective use of RAI ablation if there is lymph node metastases or other higher risk features for recurrence such as microscopic invasion into the perithyroidal soft tissues. The ATA does not recommend RAI ablation for patients with a single lesion <1 cm in size, unless there are also present high-risk features. However, there remains a large category of patients for whom the ATA leaves use of RAI up to provider discretion since the available data are unclear. In the case of A.M., although the patient did not meet the criteria for high-risk disease, she was treated with RAI because of both the patient's and provider's preferences.

With well-differentiated thyroid cancers, the TSH receptor molecular signaling cascade remains intact and responsive to TSH. Reduction of TSH levels inhibits the proliferation of well-differentiated thyroid cancer. Postoperatively, administration of suppressive doses of thyroxine acts in a negative feedback fashion to reduce TSH levels and can be used to decrease the growth and spread of remnant thyroid cancer. Clinical studies have demonstrated that in the postoperative setting an association exists between levels of TSH and the risk of thyroid cancer recurrence and mortality (10). The clinical benefit of thyroxine use to prevent thyroid cancer reduction must, however, be balanced against the risks associated with the induction of subclinical hyperthyroidism, which may lead to the development of osteoporosis and exacerbation of cardiovascular disease (11). One clinical study (12) has demonstrated that for patients with advanced stage III or IV differentiated thyroid cancer, postoperative suppression of TSH to undetectable levels, or for patients with stage II disease, suppression below normal levels results in increased overall survival. In this same study, patients with early stage I disease did not benefit from TSH suppression. Reflecting these clinical observations, the ATA recommends that for high-risk postoperative patients (who are defined as having macroscopic tumor extension, metastatic disease to distant sites, or incomplete primary tumor resection) or for intermediate-risk patients (which includes patients with microscopic extension of their tumor into neighboring tissue, cervical lymph node involvement, or tumors with vascular invasion or aggressive histology), the TSH should be suppressed to below 0.1 mU/L. In low-risk patients (identified as those patients with complete macroscopic resection of their tumor and without metastatic disease, locoregional tumor invasion, aggressive histology, or vascular invasion), the TSH should be suppressed in the range 0.1 to 0.5 mU/L, which is below the lower normal limit. In the long term, patients are later risk stratified based upon the presence or absence of residual disease and the TSH goal is adjusted appropriately. Other postoperative therapeutic modalities such as radiotherapy or chemotherapy are rarely if ever utilized in the postoperative setting to treat differentiated thyroid cancer. One exception involves the employment of palliative external beam radiation for inoperable localized disease.

In summary, in the present case A.M. presented with an early stage, differentiated papillary thyroid cancer. She was treated with total thyroidectomy followed by RAI and TSH suppression.

Differentiated Follicular Thyroid Cancer: Late-Stage Follicular Thyroid Cancer

A.C. is a 78-year-old man with a history of chronic, progressive back pain who underwent an MRI of his lower spine, which revealed a 5-cm expansile mass at the L1 vertebral body. Additional CT imaging was performed, demonstrating an 8-cm mass at the T7 vertebral body invading through the posterior wall with extension to the adjacent rib, with possible left neuroforaminal involvement. In addition, hypodense nodular lesions were seen in both lobes of the thyroid. The patient underwent a biopsy of the rib lesion, the pathology of which documented metastatic follicular thyroid cancer. A total thyroidectomy with a central compartment (level VI) neck dissection was subsequently performed with pathological analysis identifying a $2.1 \times 1.4\ cm^2$ follicular thyroid cancer.

Evidence-Based Case Discussion

This is a 78-year-old man discovered to have metastatic follicular thyroid cancer in bone. Given the metastatic spread of the cancer and the patient's age, this thyroid cancer is pathologically classified as stage IVC disease. As with the previous case of papillary thyroid cancer, the age of the patient is a significant variable in the pathological classification of this differentiated thyroid cancer. The current patient has stage IV disease but had he been younger than 45 years of age he would have been classified as having stage II disease.

Approximately 20% of patients with a diagnosis of follicular thyroid carcinoma develop distant metastatic disease. The initial therapeutic intervention for metastatic follicular thyroid cancer is RAI; however, this metastatic disease does not uniformly respond to this therapy. Important variables associated with response include whether the metastatic tumor takes up iodine (iodine-avid) and the anatomic locus and size of the tumor. Patients with non-iodine-avid metastatic tumors fare worse than patients with iodine-avid metastatic tumors, with overall 10-year survivals of 10% to 18% versus 30% to 55%, respectively (13). In addition, among patients with iodine-avid disease, micrometastatic pulmonary follicular thyroid cancer demonstrates an excellent response to RAI with a greater than 90% 10-year survival (14). For larger (>1 cm), iodine-avid pulmonary metastatic tumors, patients often demonstrate a response to RAI, though, survival is inferior to patients with micrometastatic disease. Similarly, patients with iodine-avid bone metastatic follicular thyroid cancer may respond to RAI but not as robustly as patients with pulmonary micrometastatic lesions (14).

A significant percentage of patients with metastatic follicular cancers are not iodine-avid, thus presenting the clinician with the task of how best to treat these patients. Standard chemotherapy, which includes doxorubicin-based modalities, has proven to be suboptimal (15). Laboratory investigations have revealed, however, that RAI-resistant differentiated thyroid cancers constitute a unique genetic subgroup comprising tumors with frequent mutations of the BRAF (in the case of papillary thyroid cancer), RAS, and AKT molecular pathways (16). This observation raised the possibility that RAI-resistant tumors may be susceptible to biologic agents targeting these molecular pathways, specifically the tyrosine kinase inhibitors (TKIs).

The clinical utility of sorafenib, a TKI that acts on a variety of molecular targets, including BRAF, KIT, and RET, has been assessed in multiple phase II clinical trials and shown to be an effective agent to treat RAI-resistant metastatic thyroid cancer of follicular origin with a greater than 10% partial response rate and a majority of patients achieving disease stability (17). Additional clinical reports have documented benefit in upward of 80% of patients with RAI-resistant metastatic follicular or papillary thyroid cancer treated with sorafenib (18). As with RAI therapy, treatment response with sorafenib is variable. Pulmonary metastases demonstrate increased responsiveness to sorafenib relative to other sites of disease, including bone and lymph nodes (18). In addition to sorafenib, a number of other TKIs have demonstrated clinical promise for the treatment of RAI-resistant metastatic follicular thyroid cancers, thereby expanding the therapeutic options for this clinically challenging subgroup of patients (19,20).

In the present case, A.C. underwent a total thyroidectomy with a central lymph node dissection to assess for and surgically eliminate any regional metastatic lymph node disease. Given his metastatic disease and high-risk categorization of his thyroid cancer, the patient thereafter underwent postoperative RAI with administration of suppressive thyroxine therapy; the patient's TSH levels were maintained below 0.1 mU/L. In addition, because of symptoms resulting from his metastases, he underwent palliative radiation therapy to the thoracic and vertebral lesions and received monthly zoledronic acid infusions. Should his disease progress, the patient is aware that TKI therapy remains an option.

Medullary Thyroid Cancer

W.E. is a 50-year-old woman who detected a slight discomfort on the right side of her throat. She underwent a physical examination, which revealed a discrete nodule in the right lobe of the thyroid. A TSH level was determined to be normal. An ultrasound was performed revealing a 2.7-cm nodule in the right lobe of the thyroid gland. The patient then underwent an FNA and the cytopathology was consistent with medullary thyroid carcinoma. There was no history of thyroid cancer in her family or any history of other malignancies. The calcium level was normal but the calcitonin and CEA levels were elevated. A RET mutational analysis from peripheral blood leukocytes was done, which identified an exon8 G533C activating RET germline mutation. A CT scan was performed of the neck, chest, and abdomen, which confirmed the mass in the right lobe of the thyroid, but otherwise revealed no pathology. Specifically, there were no adrenal masses to suggest the presence of a pheochromocytoma. The patient underwent a total thyroidectomy as well as a level VI compartment lymph node dissection. Pathological analysis documented a 2.7 × 2.1 cm^2 medullary thyroid carcinoma; the final pathological assessment was stage II disease.

Evidence-Based Case Discussion

This is a case of a patient with a thyroid nodule diagnosed as an early stage II medullary thyroid cancer. Imaging studies showed no evidence of metastatic spread or additional malignancies.

Because medullary thyroid cancer typically originates from an underlying RET mutation, genetic testing was performed. In this case, an exon8 G533C germline mutation was observed. A number of RET mutations have been identified and each of these is associated with a different mortality risk. The ATA has compiled a listing of the various RET mutations and their associated risk (21). In the present case, W.E.'s exon8 G533C mutation confers a relatively low risk.

Because medullary thyroid cancers are often associated with the MEN2 syndromes, patients diagnosed with medullary thyroid cancer are screened for the presence of other neoplastic disease, most notably pheochromocytoma. In the current case, screening did not reveal evidence of an additional malignancy. To assess for locoregional spread, the ATA also recommends neck ultrasound (see Figure 2.3) (21).

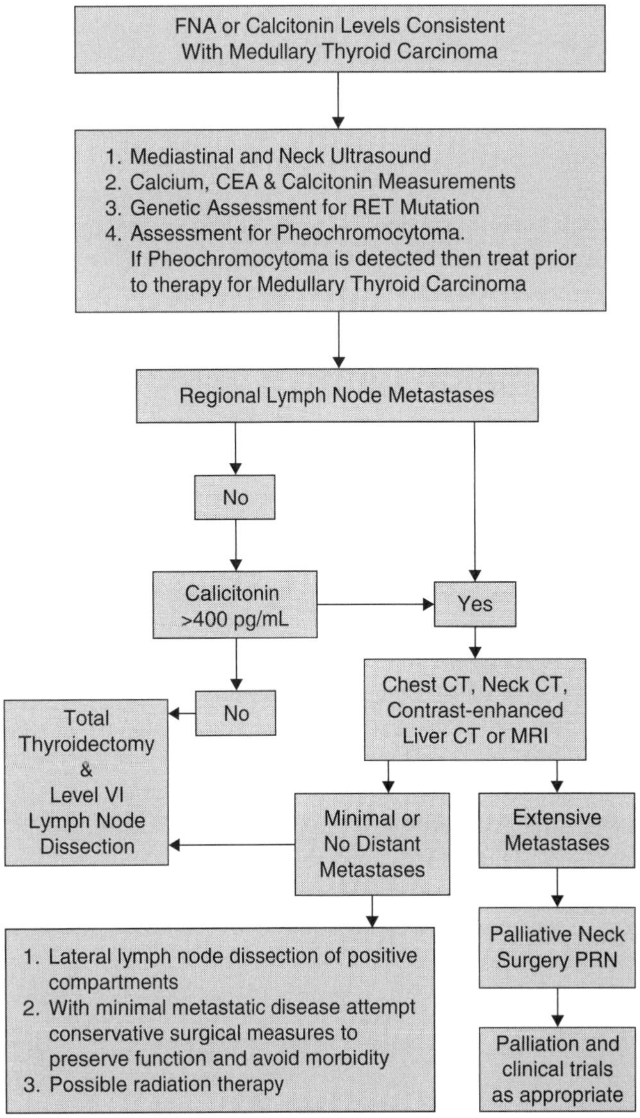

Figure 2.3

Diagnosis and management algorithm for medullary thyroid carcinoma. Adapted from ATA Guidelines (21).

Laboratory testing should include calcitonin, CEA, and calcium measurements. If there is no evidence of regional metastatic disease and the calcitonin is not grossly elevated, then thyroidectomy and a central compartment lymph node dissection is recommended. Where lymph node involvement is detected by ultrasound, further assessment for distant metastatic disease is suggested. A lateral compartment lymph node dissection is recommended if there is evidence of lateral neck disease or extensive central neck disease. More aggressive radiation therapy is sometimes considered in these instances. With extensive distant metastatic disease, palliative measures and possible enrollment in a clinical trial can be implemented.

In the case of W.E., because of the early stage with no evidence of regional or distant metastatic spread, she underwent a total thyroidectomy with central, level VI lymph node dissection.

Anaplastic Thyroid Cancer

T.M. is a 78-year-old woman who noted the rapid development of a mass on the right side of her throat. She also reported some recent dyspnea, fatigue, and hoarseness. A physical examination performed by her primary care physician demonstrated a firm nodule in the right lobe of the thyroid gland. Laboratory testing was performed. The thyrotropin was found to be below normal, while the free thyroxine, free triiodothyronine, and thyroglobulin were significantly elevated. An ultrasound of the thyroid was performed which demonstrated four discrete solid nodules in the right lobe of the thyroid, the largest measuring 3.5×2.0 cm^2. The remainder of the ultrasound examination did not demonstrate any abnormal findings on the left side; central and lateral compartment lymph nodes were assessed and were normal. An FNA biopsy was performed and demonstrated an undifferentiated malignancy consistent with anaplastic thyroid cancer. The patient proceeded to undergo a core biopsy of the mass, which confirmed the presence of the anaplastic thyroid cancer. Additional laboratory testing was accomplished including a CBC and serum calcium, both of which were normal. CT scans of the head, neck, chest, abdomen, and pelvis revealed multiple pulmonary metastatic lesions in the middle lobe of the right lung. The CT scan of the neck confirmed the presence of the four nodules in the right lobe of the thyroid; one of the nodules, it was noted, was impinging on the right recurrent laryngeal nerve. A bone scan was also performed, which did not demonstrate any evidence of bony metastases.

Evidence-Based Case Discussion

This patient is an older woman diagnosed with anaplastic thyroid carcinoma. All cases of anaplastic thyroid carcinoma are stage IV but in this case, because T.M. had distant pulmonary metastases, the anaplastic thyroid carcinoma is stage IVC.

Suspicion for anaplastic thyroid cancer on an FNA requires that a core or excisional biopsy be performed to confirm the diagnosis. Laboratory testing, including a CBC, TSH, and calcium levels, is recommended. Anaplastic thyroid cancer is a particularly aggressive neoplasm thought to arise from dedifferentiation of an antecedent differentiated thyroid carcinoma as a result of an accumulation of additional genetic mutations. Metastatic disease is common, with the vast majority of metastatic disease targeting the lungs. To assess for the extent of disease and to identify potential sites of metastatic disease, CT studies of the head, neck, chest, abdomen, and pelvis; PET imaging; and a bone scan are performed.

Since anaplastic thyroid carcinoma commonly extends beyond local control at the time of diagnosis, surgical resection is typically performed only when indicated for palliative relief of symptoms. In those infrequent clinical cases where the primary anaplastic thyroid carcinoma is amenable to local resection (stage IVA disease), thyroidectomy and resection of local and regional metastatic lymph node disease is indicated. Most typically, anaplastic thyroid cancer is stage IVB or IVC. At these late stages radiation may be employed with the aim of achieving local control (22). Radiation therapy may also be combined with doxorubicin employed as a sensitizing agent (23). There is some evidence that doxorubicin combined with cisplatin may be more effective than doxorubicin alone (15). The use of I^{131} as a therapeutic modality is not effective because the anaplastic carcinoma is dedifferentiated and remains incapable of iodine uptake or processing. Novel agents, including antiangiogenic agents, RET inhibitors, and peroxisome proliferator-activated receptor agonists, are currently being evaluated as therapeutic agents for anaplastic thyroid cancer (24). All patients should be encouraged to consider participation in a clinical trial. Optimization of current therapeutic modalities and investigational efforts notwithstanding anaplastic thyroid cancer has a dismal prognosis with the vast majority of patients succumbing to the disease in less than 12 months' time (25).

REFERENCES

1. Davies MA, Stemke-Hale K, Lin E, et al. Integrated Molecular and Clinical Analysis of AKT Activation in Metastatic Melanoma. *Clin Cancer Res.* 2009;15(24):7538–7546.
2. Altekruse SF, Krapcho M, Neyman N, et al. *SEER Cancer Statistics Review, 1975–2007.* Bethesda, MD: National Cancer Institute; 2010.
3. American Cancer Society. *Cancer Facts and Figures 2010.* Atlanta, GA: American Cancer Society; 2010.
4. Fagin JA, Mitsiades N. Molecular pathology of thyroid cancer: diagnostic and clinical implications. *Best Pract Res Clin Endocrinol Metab.* 2008;22(6):955–969.

5. Xing M. BRAF mutation in papillary thyroid microcarcinoma: the promise of better risk management. *Ann Surg Oncol.* 2009;16(4):801–803.
6. Haymart MR. Understanding the relationship between age and thyroid cancer. *Oncologist.* 2009;14(3):216–221.
7. Kondo T, Ezzat S, Asa SL. Pathogenetic mechanisms in thyroid follicular-cell neoplasia. *Nat Rev Cancer.* 2006;6(4):292–306.
8. American Joint Committee on Cancer (AJCC). Thyroid. In: Edge SB, Byrd DR, Compton CC, et al., eds. *AJCC Cancer Staging Manual.* 7th ed. New York: Springer; 2010:87–96.
9. Cooper DS, Doherty GM, Haugen BR, et al. Revised American Thyroid Association management guidelines for patients with thyroid nodules and differentiated thyroid cancer. *Thyroid.* 2009;19(11):1167–1214.
10. Hovens GC, Stokkel MP, Kievit J, et al. Associations of serum thyrotropin concentrations with recurrence and death in differentiated thyroid cancer. *J Clin Endocrinol Metab.* 2007;92(7):2610–2615.
11. Toft AD. Clinical practice. Subclinical hyperthyroidism. *N Engl J Med.* 2001;345(7):512–516.
12. Jonklaas J, Sarlis NJ, Litofsky D, et al. Outcomes of patients with differentiated thyroid carcinoma following initial therapy. *Thyroid.* 2006;16(12):1229–1242.
13. O'Neill CJ, Oucharek J, Learoyd D, Sidhu SB. Standard and emerging therapies for metastatic differentiated thyroid cancer. *Oncologist.* 2010;15(2):146–156.
14. Durante C, Haddy N, Baudin E, et al. Long-term outcome of 444 patients with distant metastases from papillary and follicular thyroid carcinoma: benefits and limits of radioiodine therapy. *J Clin Endocrinol Metab.* 2006;91(8):2892–2899.
15. Shimaoka K, Schoenfeld DA, DeWys WD, Creech RH, DeConti R. A randomized trial of doxorubicin versus doxorubicin plus cisplatin in patients with advanced thyroid carcinoma. *Cancer.* 1985;56(9):2155–2160.
16. Ricarte-Filho JC, Ryder M, Chitale DA, et al. Mutational profile of advanced primary and metastatic radioactive iodine-refractory thyroid cancers reveals distinct pathogenetic roles for BRAF, PIK3CA, and AKT1. *Cancer Res.* 2009;69(11):4885–4893.
17. Kloos RT, Ringel MD, Knopp MV, et al. Phase II trial of sorafenib in metastatic thyroid cancer. *J Clin Oncol.* 2009;27(10):1675–1684.
18. Cabanillas ME, Waguespack SG, Bronstein Y, et al. Treatment with tyrosine kinase inhibitors for patients with differentiated thyroid cancer: the M. D. Anderson experience. *J Clin Endocrinol Metab.* 2010;95(6):2588–2595.
19. Sherman SI, Wirth LJ, Droz JP, et al. Motesanib diphosphate in progressive differentiated thyroid cancer. *N Engl J Med.* 2008;359(1):31–42.
20. Cohen EE, Rosen LS, Vokes EE, et al. Axitinib is an active treatment for all histologic subtypes of advanced thyroid cancer: results from a phase II study. *J Clin Oncol.* 2008;26(29):4708–4713.
21. Kloos RT, Eng C, Evans DB, et al. Medullary thyroid cancer: management guidelines of the American Thyroid Association. *Thyroid.* 2009;19(6):565–612.
22. Wang Y, Tsang R, Asa S, Dickson B, Arenovich T, Brierley J. Clinical outcome of anaplastic thyroid carcinoma treated with radiotherapy of once- and twice-daily fractionation regimens. *Cancer.* 2006;107(8):1786–1792.
23. Kim JH, Leeper RD. Treatment of locally advanced thyroid carcinoma with combination doxorubicin and radiation therapy. *Cancer.* 1987;60(10):2372–2375.
24. Tuttle RM, Leboeuf R. Investigational therapies for metastatic thyroid carcinoma. *J Natl Compr Canc Netw.* 2007;5(6):641–646.
25. Neff RL, Farrar WB, Kloos RT, Burman KD. Anaplastic thyroid cancer. *Endocrinol Metab Clin North Am.* 2008;37(2):525–38, xi.

3

Non-Small Cell Lung Cancer

KATHLEEN E. BICKEL, BASKARAM SUNDARAM, STUART M. KNOEPP, COLLETTE M. HODGES, AND NITHYA RAMNATH

EPIDEMIOLOGY, RISK FACTORS, NATURAL HISTORY, AND PATHOLOGY

Lung cancer, including non-small cell lung cancer (NSCLC) and small cell lung cancer, is the leading cause of cancer death among men and women in the United States. In the year 2010, there were an estimated 222,520 new cases of lung cancer (116,750 men and 105,770 women) with an estimated 157,300 deaths due to lung cancer (86,220 men and 71,080 women). The 5-year survival rate for all lung cancers combined is 15%, with disease stage at diagnosis the most important prognostic indicator. Other poor prognostic factors include poor performance status, male gender, older age, and African American heritage. In the United States, as many men die from lung cancer as from prostate and colon cancer combined. Also, as many women die from lung cancer as from breast, ovarian, and uterine cancers combined. By 1986, lung cancer had surpassed breast cancer as the leading cause of death in Caucasian women in the United States, and the same occurred in African American women in 1990. The incidence has plateaued since 2003, but lung cancer death rate in women is still slowly increasing. In men, both the incidence and the death rates are slowly decreasing. The trends in incidence and mortality tend to parallel smoking rates, with a 20-year latency. The diverse smoking prevalence from state to state results in large variations in lung cancer incidence, with the lowest rate (per 100,000) in Utah (37.8 male and 23.0 female) and the highest rate in Kentucky (133.1 male and 76.9 female).

Most lung cancers are attributable to cigarette smoking (80–85%). Other risk factors include exposure to radon, radiation, asbestos, arsenic, chromium, nickel, chloromethyl ethers, and cadmium. Cigarette smoke contains more than 300 chemicals, 40 of which are known carcinogens. Two of the major carcinogens, N-nitrosamine ketones (NNK) and polycyclic aromatic hydrocarbons, cause DNA adduct formation, resulting in mutations. Nicotine and NNK also activate AKT signal transduction, causing apoptotic inhibition and increased cellular proliferation. Lung cancer risk increases with smoking duration and daily number of cigarettes smoked. The risk in smokers is about 20-fold more than in nonsmokers. Changing to cigarettes marked as "light," menthol, or improved filtering, does not decrease risk. Risk decreases with smoking cessation and approaches that of a nonsmoker after 15 to 20 years of abstinence. About 25% of lung cancers in nonsmokers may be related to passive smoke exposure.

Radon is a radioactive gas produced by uranium and radium decay, emitting alpha particles, which can damage cells. Uranium miners have the greatest occupational exposure, but residential exposure may cause up to 10% of NSCLC. There is a dose-response effect, and the risk is synergistic with smoking. Asbestos exposure is also synergistic with smoking due to impaired bronchial clearance of asbestos. For example, if the relative risk is 2 to 4 in a nonsmoker exposed to asbestos, it would be 40 to 100 in a smoker. After asbestos exposure, lung cancer incidence peaks 25 to 35 years later and is much higher than the mesothelioma incidence. Prior radiation treatments for breast cancer and lymphoma also increase lung cancer risk, especially in smokers. The latency is typically 5 to 10 years, and the tumors are often more aggressive.

Given the large high-risk population, there were several randomized, double-blinded, placebo-controlled lung cancer chemoprevention trials. However, supplementation with Vitamin A, beta-carotene, their derivatives, or selenium provided no benefit. Lung cancer risk was increased in smokers who were given extra beta-carotene. Smoking's confounding effect has made it difficult to elucidate any genetic hereditary factors. However, mutations in genes associated with DNA repair, cell cycle progression, or carcinogen metabolism may be involved. Genome-wide association studies have identified and verified lung cancer susceptibility loci at 15q25 and 5p15. The single nucleotide polymorphisms involved in the 5p15.33 region map to *TERT*, a telomerase extension reverse transcriptase. *TERT* is activated in many cancers and increases cellular proliferation through abnormal telomere maintenance. The 5p15 locus has an association with adenocarcinoma, regardless of smoking status. However, the 15q25 locus, which maps to the nicotinic acetylcholine receptor, appears to be only associated with smokers.

Most patients present with signs and symptoms related to the primary mass, locoregional spread, metastasis, or paraneoplastic syndromes (Table 3.1). About 10% of patients are asymptomatic, often diagnosed after a chest x-ray or CT scan obtained for other reasons.

Lung adenocarcinoma (AC) has surpassed squamous cell carcinoma (SCC) as the most common histologic subtype in the United States. These tumors tend to be peripherally located, and may not cause significant early symptoms. They also tend toward early lymph node metastasis, hematogenous spread, and appearance near old scars. Histologically, ACs exhibit glandular differentiation and evidence of mucin production, often with cytoplasmic vacuoles. There are four major types: acinar, papillary, solid with mucin formation, and bronchioalveolar (BAC). Nonmucinous BAC tends to be solitary with a better prognosis, while mucinous variants are multifocal and more aggressive. Since the 1999 WHO classification, BAC has been restricted to noninvasive tumors with lepidic spread. However, a recent update to pulmonary AC pathologic staging has removed the BAC classification (1). Although other NSCLC subtypes have a higher incidence in men, in BAC the ratio is 1:1. Activating mutations of the epidermal growth factor receptor (EGFR) are more common in BAC, especially in nonsmoking Asian women.

SCC currently accounts for about 25% of NSCLC in the United States and is exclusively related to tobacco smoke exposure. Typically, SCCs are larger and centrally located, forming in the segmental bronchi and extending to involve the lobar and main-stem bronchi. Central necrosis and cavitation are common. Histologically, SCCs are characterized by intercellular bridging, squamous pearl formation, and individual cell keratinization.

Table 3.1 Clinical Signs and Symptoms of Lung Cancer

Primary Central/Endobronchial Tumor	**Primary Peripheral Tumor**
Cough (+/- sputum production)	Cough
Hemoptysis	Pain—pleural or chest wall involvement
Dyspnea (related to obstruction)	Dyspnea (more restrictive basis)
Wheezing (often unilateral) or stridor	Pleural effusion
Post-obstructive pneumonia	Pneumonitis
Locally Advanced Disease (direct or metastatic spread)	
Hoarseness (recurrent laryngeal nerve paralysis)	
Phrenic nerve paralysis (elevated hemidiaphragm and dyspnea)	
Dysphagia (esophageal compression)	
Stridor (tracheal obstruction)	
Superior vena cava (SVC) syndrome	
Pancost/Horner's syndromes (apical tumor)	
Dyspnea (pleural effusions, trachea/bronchial obstruction, pericardial effusion, phrenic nerve palsey, SVC obstruction, lymphangitic spread)	
Metastatic Disease	
Brain (altered mental status, seizures, headache, nausea/emesis, motor or sensory deficits)	
Bone (pain, exacerbated by movement or weight bearing)	
Spine (extremity weakness, pain)	
Liver (right upper quadrant and/or epigastric pain, nausea/emesis, icterus)	
Paraneoplastic Syndromes *(more common in small cell lung cancer)*	
Hypercalcemia (most common in squamous cell)	
Pulmonary hypertrophic osteoarthropathy (clubbing, painful arthralgias)	
Trousseau's syndrome/hypercoagulability	
Syndrome of inappropriate secretion of antidiuretic hormone (SIADH)	
Cushing's syndrome—ectopic adrenocortiotropic hormone production	
Eaton-Lambert syndrome	
Dermatomyositis	

Note: Text in italics indicates findings more common in small cell lung cancer.

Large cell carcinomas account for about 10% of NSCLC and are clinically similar to ACs. Histologically, the cells are larger, with abundant, minimally differentiated cytoplasm. Some large cell carcinomas can have a partial neuroendocrine phenotype, staining positive for chromogranin A and/or synaptophysin. A poor prognosis is associated with a subtype showing increased mitotic figures and necrosis with neuroendocrine features. Large cell neuroendocrine carcinoma is a rarer subtype that also includes evidence of palisading or rosette-like morphology.

Lung cancer develops over time, through a series of genetic and epigenetic changes in bronchial epithelial cells. Three known premalignant morphologies, squamous dysplasia, atypical adenomatous hyperplasia, and diffuse idiopathic pulmonary neuroendocrine hyperplasia can develop into SCC, AC, and carcinoid tumors, respectively. Multiple chromosomal alterations occur during tumor pathogenesis, including loss of 3p, 4q, 9p, and 17p. Loss of one copy of 3p is an early event, found in 96% of lung tumors. Multiple tumor suppressor genes, including fragile histidine triad (FHIT), have mapped to 3p. Other alterations have been noted in oncogenes and tumor suppressor genes including mutations, amplification, loss of protein expression or overexpression, gene hypermethylation, and increased telomerase activity (Table 3.2).

Epidermal growth factor receptor (EGFR) is an epithelial cell surface transmembrane receptor of the ErbB family of tyrosine kinase receptors. When activated, the resulting signal transduction cascade leads to decreased apoptosis along with increased cellular proliferation, angiogenesis, and invasiveness. EGFR is overexpressed or aberrantly activated in approximately 50% to 90% of NSCLC. Two small molecule inhibitors of EGFR, erlotinib and gefitinib, and the monoclonal EGFR antibody, cetuximab, take advantage of this frequent NSCLC dependence on EGFR signaling and its downstream *RAS/RAF*, *PI3K/AKT*, and *STAT* pathways. However, despite examining EGFR protein expression by immunohistochemistry (IHC), fluorescent in situ hybridization (FISH), or gene copy number, the *EGFR* gene mutational status is most predictive of response to small molecule inhibitors. NSCLC *EGFR* mutations are most common (~40%) in never or light-smoking Asian women with adenocarcinoma, especially BAC. These mutations are seen in 10% or less of non-Asian populations and almost never in SCC. Located in the tyrosine kinase domain, the mutations cause constitutive receptor activation. The small molecule inhibitors bind to the tyrosine kinase domain, turning off the downstream signaling cascade. Although the inhibitors were designed against wild-type *EGFR* receptors, they more potently inhibit mutated receptors. About 45% of *EGFR* mutations are small in-frame deletions in exon 19 and another 40% to 45% are an exon 21 point mutation, L858R. A rare intrinsic or frequently acquired point mutation in exon 20, T790M confers resistance to erlotinib or gefitinib.

Ras family gene members encode cell membrane associated GTPases involved in cellular signal transduction. The most common *K*-ras mutation (90%) in NSCLC is a G→T transversion in codon 12 causing constitutive activation, but mutations can also occur in codons 13 and 61. When *K-ras* is mutated in nonsmokers, a G→A transition is more common. *K-ras* mutations are typically seen in AC and are associated with tobacco smoke exposure. They are mutually exclusive from *EGFR* mutations and the *EML4-ALK* fusion oncogene. There is no clear evidence of a difference in survival between patients with *K-ras* mutated

Table 3.2 Selected Molecular Alterations in NSCLC

Description	All NSCLC	Adenocarcinoma	Squamous Cell Carcinoma
Tumor Suppressor Genes			
Rb mutations (13q14)	20–40%		
Rb loss of protein expression	15–60%	23–57%	6–14%
p16/CDKN2A mutations (9p21)	10–40%		
p16/CDKN2A hypermethylation	15–41%	21–36%	24–33%
p53 mutations (17p13)	50–60%	50–70%	60–70%
Oncogenes			
EFGR mutations	20%	<10% (West) ~40% (Asia)	Rare
EFGR protein overexpression	50–90%	40–65%	60–85%
Her-2 protein overexpression	20–35%	16–38%	6–16%
K-ras mutation	10–30%	15–35%	<5%
B-raf mutation	1–3%		
Myc family gene amplication	8–22%		
EML4-ALK fusion oncogene	1–4%	1–4%	Rare
Bcl-2 protein overexpression	10–35%		

Source: Adapted from Ref. 2.

versus *K-ras* wild-type tumors, particularly if the tumors also have wild-type *EGFR*. Tumors with *K-ras* mutations are less likely than those with wild-type *K-ras* to respond to treatment with the small molecule inhibitors erlotinib or gefitinib, but this was not noted with the EGFR monoclonal antibody, cetuximab.

p53 is the most frequently mutated gene in human cancer. In NSCLC these mutations are smoking related. Again, G→T transversions are most common. Without functional p53, there is no G1 arrest in the cell cycle to allow for DNA repair. Instead, the cells continue to divide and propagate damaged DNA. Retrospectively, p53 overexpression in NSCLC has been related to poor prognosis and decreased overall survival (OS). However, prospectively, *p53* mutations only predicted decreased survival in surgically resected stage I tumors, not in stage II or III tumors.

Recently, it has been discovered that some NSCLCs contain a chromosome 2p inversion, Inv(2)(p21p32), forming the *EML4-ALK* fusion oncogene. The resulting protein has an N-terminus derived from echinoderm microtubule-associated protein like 4 (EML4) and a C-terminus with the tyrosine kinase domain of anaplastic lymphoma kinase (ALK). This fusion tends to be mutually exclusive from *EGFR* and *K-ras* mutations, occurs in about 4% of NSCLC, and is associated with AC in younger patients with little or no smoking history. Tumors with this alteration have a significant response to crizotinib (a small molecule inhibitor of c-MET and the ALK fusion protein) but do not respond to the small molecule EGFR inhibitors.

Additional molecular markers are also being examined as potential prognostic and/or predictive markers, such as ERCC1 (excision repair cross-complementing rodent repair deficiency group 1) and RRM1 (ribonucleotide reductase M1). ERCC1 contributes to a rate limiting step in the nucleotide excision repair pathway used to overcome the DNA cross-links formed by platinum agents. RRM1 is the regulatory unit of ribonucleotide reductase, needed for DNA synthesis and repair. Gemcitabine is a cytidine analog that inhibits RRM1 and thus DNA production. Mostly retrospective data suggest that in advanced NSCLC, a high ERCC1 level is associated with decreased survival and decreased tumor response to platinum-based therapies. Similarly, a high RRM1 level has been associated with decreased tumor response to gemcitabine. However, in stage I disease treated with surgical resection alone, high levels of RRM1 and ERCC1 correlate with improved survival. There is no clear consensus on the quantification method of these markers, for example, mRNA expression or IHC, and these markers can change in metastatic or previously treated disease. Thus, large-scale prospective studies are still needed to validate *RRM1*, *ERCC1*, *K-ras*, *p53*, and *EGFR*, or others as predictive or prognostic markers.

STAGING

The AJCC (Seventh Edition) staging for non-small cell lung cancer is shown below.

Non-Small Cell Lung Cancer Staging

Stage	Description
IA	Primary tumor (≤3 cm, T1a, T1b) surrounded by lung or visceral pleura, without bronchoscopic invasion to the main bronchus and no nodal or distant metastasis (N0M0) OR Uncommon superficial spreading tumor of any size, with invasive component limited to the bronchial wall, but may extend proximal to the main bronchus
IB	Primary tumor (≤5 cm, T2a) that may invade visceral pleura, involves the main bronchus (2 cm or more distal to the carina), or may be associated with atelectasis or obstructive pneumonitis extending to the hilar region, but not involving the entire lung, and N0M0
IIA	Primary tumor (≤5cm, T1a, T1b, T2a), but not involving the entire lung, AND metastasis in the ipsilateral peribronchial, ipsilateral hilar, and/or intrapulmonary lymph node(s), including by direct extension (N1), but no distant metastasis (M0) OR Primary tumor (>5 cm, ≤7 cm, T2b), but not involving the entire lung and N0M0
IIB	Primary tumor (>5 cm, ≤7 cm, T2b), AND N1 lymph node metastasis, but M0 OR Primary tumor (>7 cm, T3) *or* one that directly invades the chest wall (including superior sulcus tumors), diaphragm, phrenic nerve, mediastinal pleura, parietal pericardium, *or* tumor in the main bronchus < 2 cm distal to the carina without involving the carina, *or* tumor associated with atelectasis or obstructive pneumonitis of the entire lung, *or* separate tumor nodule(s) located in the same lobe as the primary tumor, but N0M0

IIIA	Primary tumor of any size (T4) that invades the mediastinum, heart, great vessels, trachea, recurrent laryngeal nerve, esophagus, vertebral body, or the carina, *or* separate tumor nodule(s) in the same or ipsalateral lobe to that of the primary, but N0M0 OR Primary tumor (>7 cm, T3, T4), AND N1 lymph node metastasis, but M0 OR Primary tumor (T1, T2, T3), AND metastasis in the ipsilateral mediastinal and/or subcarinal lymph nodes(s) (N2), but M0
IIIB	Primary tumor (T4), AND N2 lymph node metastasis, but M0 OR Primary tumor of any size or invasion, AND metastasis in the contralateral mediastinal, contralateral hilar, or scalene or supraclavicular lymph node(s) of either side (N3), but M0
IV	Primary tumor of any size and any invasion, with or without any lymph node metastasis AND evidence of pleural nodules *or* separate tumor nodule(s) in a contralateral lobe *or* a malignant pleural or pericardial effusion (M1a) OR any evidence of distant metastasis (M1b)

Source: AJCC Cancer Staging Handbook, 7th edtion.

CASE SUMMARIES

Early-Stage NSCLC

M.E. is a 68-year-old man with a 60-pack-year smoking history and a persistent cough, recently treated for community-acquired pneumonia, who was found to have a 3.2 × 2.4 cm^2 left lower lobe mass on CT scan. A CT-guided biopsy revealed SCC. He had a history of well-controlled hypertension and hyperlipidemia and is a retired construction worker. He is active and likes to go mountain climbing. A positron emission tomography (PET)-CT scan was negative for involvement of lymph nodes or distant metastases. He is enquiring about his treatment options.

Evidence-Based Case Discussion

Surgery Alone in Early-Stage NSCLC

In this otherwise healthy patient with a good performance status, surgical resection of a clinical stage I or stage II NSCLC provides the greatest chance of cure. The type of procedure depends on the extent of disease and the patient's cardiopulmonary reserve. On the basis of pulmonary function testing, a patient with a pre-resection forced expiratory volume in 1 second (FEV1) ≥ 2 L or 80% of predicted is able to tolerate pneumonectomy, and generally, an FEV1 of 1.5 L is required for lobectomy. If either the FEV1 or the diffusion lung capacity for carbon monoxide (DLCO) is less than 60% of predicted, then quantitative ventilation-perfusion scans can be used to predict the postoperative lung function. If the FEV1 and/or DLCO is less than 40% of predicted, then exercise testing is needed. Patients with a maximal oxygen consumption (Vo_{2max}) of 15 mL/kg/minute or greater can still be considered for resection.

Mediastinal lymph node evaluation is important in staging, as the treatment for stage IIIA disease and stage I disease differs. Traditionally, mediastinoscopy is the gold standard and is recommended for any enlarged (>1 cm) mediastinal lymph nodes on CT scan, regardless of the PET scan. In prospective studies, PET detected mediastinal lymph node metastases more accurately than CT alone, and PET or PET-CT is now frequently used to evaluate new lung nodules. However, PET is more costly, has limited availability, and cannot detect lesions smaller than 8 mm. Inflammatory processes can cause false-positive results, and some low metabolic tumors, such as BAC or carcinoid, can have false negative results. Therefore, PET positive lymph nodes still require tissue confirmation. Currently, there is no data to recommend transthoracic, transbronchial, or endoscopic ultrasound guided biopsies over mediastinoscopy. However, emerging data suggest that endobronchial ultrasound (EBUS) may be a safe alternative to cervical mediastinoscopy. Choice of diagnostic modality is based on nodal location, locally available resources, and practitioner experience. For example, paraesophageal and pulmonary ligament lymph nodes are accessible by esophageal endoscopic ultrasound, but not by mediastinoscopy. On the basis of the American College of Chest Physician (ACCP) guidelines (see Figure 3.1A), further preoperative mediastinal lymph node evaluation would not be necessary in our patient M.E., as he has nonenlarged, PET-negative mediastinal lymph nodes.

The extent of intraoperative lymph node sampling has been widely studied, but the results are unclear. A Cochrane meta-analysis concluded that systematic mediastinal nodal dissection in patients resected for stage I to IIIA NSCLC improved OS, compared using only lymph node sampling (hazard ratio [HR] 0.63, 95% CI 0.51–0.58, $P \leq .0001$) (4). However, a trial conducted by the American College of Surgeons Oncology Group, randomizing patients to mediastinal lymph node dissection, or to sampling only, showed no difference in OS or

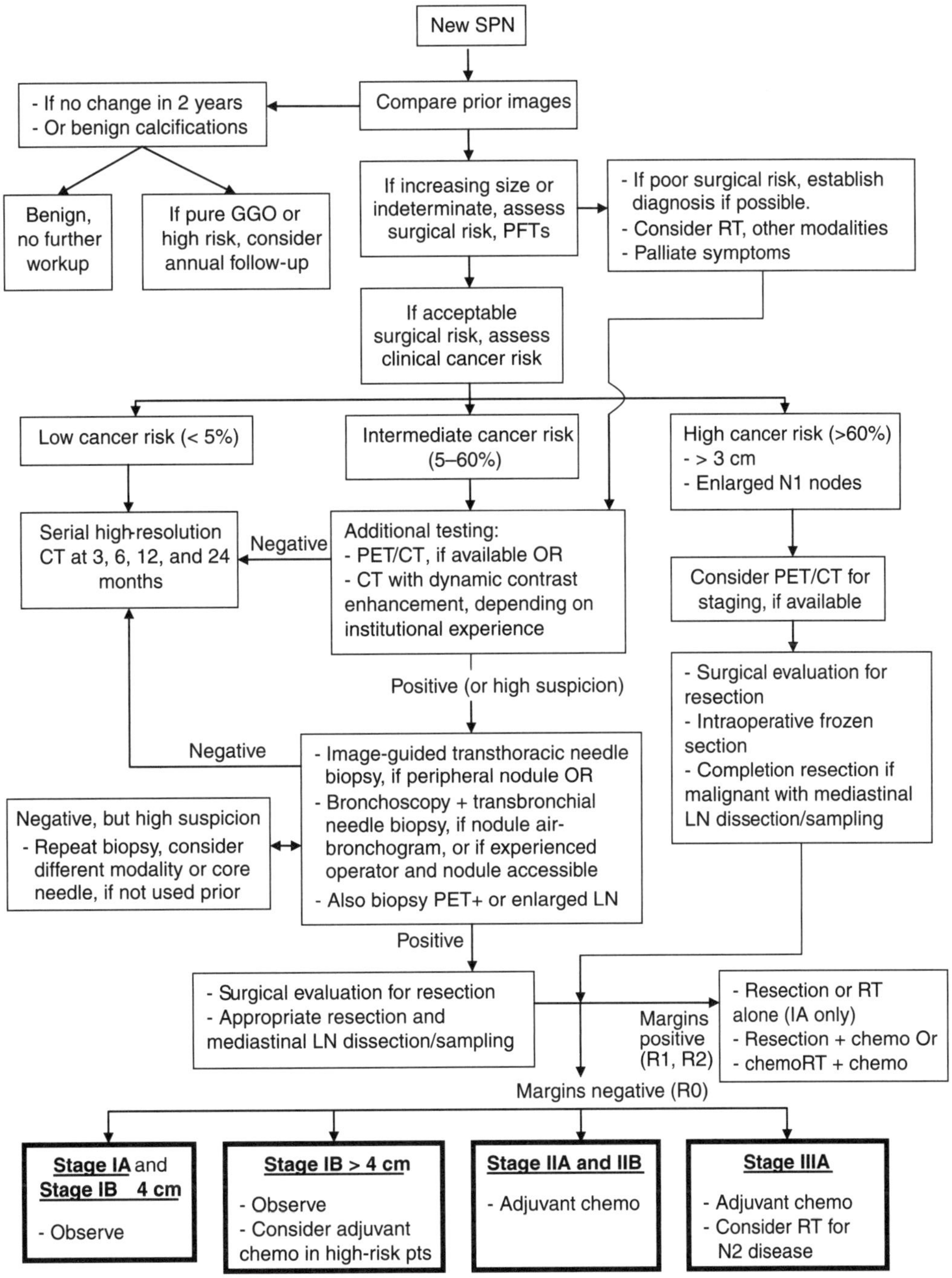

Figure 3.1A

Pathway for diagnosis and clinical decision making in early-stage non-small cell lung cancer. SPN, solitary pulmonary nodule; GGO, ground glass opacity; PFTs, pulmonary function tests; XRT, radiation therapy; LN, lymph node; RT, radiotherapy; chemo, chemotherapy; chemoRT, chemoradiotherapy; pts, patients; R0, no residual tumor; R1, microscopic residual tumor; R2, macroscopic residual tumor. Adapted from Gould et al. (3).

time to recurrence. Adequate mediastinal lymphadenectomy should include stations 2R, 4R, 7, 8, and 9 for right-sided cancers and stations 4L, 5, 6, 7, 8, and 9 for left-sided cancers.

Lobectomy, a single lobe surgical resection, became the standard treatment for early-stage NSCLC, on the basis of a Lung Cancer Study Group trial that randomized 276 stage T1N0 NSCLC patients to either lobectomy or to limited resection. In the limited resection arm, the overall recurrence rate increased by 75% ($P = .04$), and the local recurrence rate tripled ($P = .008$), with a trend toward increased overall and cancer-specific death rates. Since the study's tumor size limit was ≤3 cm, trials are now examining the same question with tumors ≤2 cm. In patients with decreased cardiopulmonary reserve and single tumors ≤ 2 to 3 cm, retrospective data suggest that surgical morbidity and mortality is similar or improved when receiving a sublobar resection versus a lobectomy, partly due to the smaller postoperative drop in pulmonary function.

Video-assisted thoracic surgery (VATS) has become an option in early-stage lung cancer, but there is not yet any definitive data that VATS delivers an equivalent oncologic resection to open lobectomy. Patients undergoing VATS have a similar operative mortality, but with a shorter hospital stay, fewer postoperative complications, and less pain-related issues than with open lobectomy. In more proximally located tumors, where lobectomy may not be an option, a lung-sparing sleeve resection is preferred over pneumonectomy, when possible. Although OS is fairly similar, sleeve lobectomy in stage-appropriate patients, can better preserve pulmonary function and avoids pneumonectomy-related complications. Meanwhile, T3 tumors invading the chest wall or mediastinum often require an en bloc resection for clear margins.

It is of note that given the size of M.E.'s tumor (>3 cm) and his smoking history, the suspicion of cancer is high enough that he could have proceeded directly to resection without a tissue diagnosis. The evidence is less clear for tumors < 3 cm. On the basis of the tumor size, pretest probability of malignancy, potential for surgical resection, available resources, and patient preferences, a useful algorithm has been suggested by the ACCP (see Figure 3.1A). When patients are not good surgical candidates, a tissue diagnosis prior to treatment is preferred. However, some patients may be averse to undergoing surgery without a definitive cancer diagnosis.

Options for patients with limited cardiopulmonary reserve include definitive thoracic radiation therapy (60 Gy in 30 daily fractions), continuous hyperfractionated accelerated radiotherapy (CHART, 1.5 Gy, 3 times a day for 12 days, total dose 54 Gy), stereotactic body radiation therapy (SBRT), radiofrequency ablation (RFA), and cryoablation. Radiation therapy alone for stage I-II NSCLC has a 10% to 25% survival rate at 5 years. The randomized phase III trial comparing CHART to conventional therapy had 169 (of 563 total) patients with stage I-IIA NSCLC. In this subset, the 2-year OS rate was 24% in the traditional arm versus 37% in the CHART arm, with 4-year OS rates of 12% and 18%, respectively. The data on SBRT, RFA, and cryoablation are currently limited to phase I or II studies, and no comparisons have been made between modalities or to surgical resection. Any option could be considered for a nonsurgical candidate with a peripheral tumor ≤ 3 cm. SBRT can be used for tumors up to 5 cm. A recent meta-analysis showed better 2-year and 5-year OS with SBRT than with conventional radiation therapy (CRT), but the CRT studies were older, and the SBRT studies had shorter follow-up.

Surgery and Adjuvant Chemotherapy in Early-Stage NSCLC

Despite adequate surgery, patients with stage II disease often recur, with a 5-year OS of about 30% to 40%. Thus, adjuvant treatment has been evaluated in stage I, II, and III disease. The most recent meta-analyses by the LACE (Lung Adjuvant Cisplatin Evaluation) and NSCLC collaborative groups indicate that adjuvant chemotherapy provides a 5-year OS benefit of about 4% to 5% in stage II-III disease. In the LACE study, the HR was 0.89 (95% CI 0.82–0.96, P = .005), corresponding to a 5-year survival benefit of 5.4% (5). In the NSCLC collaborative group meta-analysis, the HR was 0.86 (95% CI 0.81–0.92, P < .0001), corresponding to a 5-year survival benefit of 4%, increase from 60% to 64% overall (6). In a separate analysis of trials using adjuvant chemotherapy with/and radiation, the overall HR was 0.88 (95% CI 0.81–0.97, P = .009), corresponding to a 5-year survival benefit of 4%, increase from 29% to 33% overall. The patients in this second group were mostly men with a median age of 59, good performance status, and stage III disease. An exploratory analysis showed no difference between combination chemoradiotherapy and chemotherapy followed by radiation. Cisplatin plus vinorelbine showed slightly more benefit than other combinations, but the cisplatin doses were also higher. Although never compared head-to-head in the adjuvant setting, cisplatin plus either etoposide, gemcitabine, docetaxel, or pemetrexed are all acceptable adjuvant regimens, based on their relative equivalence in the advanced setting. If cisplatin cannot be used, carboplatin and paclitaxel is recommended but is not considered equivalent (7).

Although adjuvant chemotherapy for stage IA patients is not helpful, and may actually decrease OS, the data for stage IB patients is less clear. Nodal metastases and increased size are the biggest risk factors for relapse in early-stage disease. Visceral pleural invasion and vascular invasion are also independent prognostic factors. Until recently, the stage IB patient population was more heterogeneous, including primary N0 tumors > 5 cm, without direct invasion beyond the visceral pleura, and those ≤ 5 cm with N1 disease. The Cancer and Leukemia Group B (CALGB) 9663 trial, which specifically examined adjuvant chemotherapy in stage IB (old classification), only showed a survival benefit for patients with tumors ≥4 cm (HR 0.69, 95% CI 0.48–0.99, P = .043). However, this study was criticized for its use of carboplatin/paclitaxel instead of a cisplatin-doublet, early stopping due to initial positive results, and being underpowered to detect a small difference. The updated survival analysis of the JBR-10 adjuvant trial provides additional evidence, showing a trend toward benefit for tumors ^{3} 4 cm (HR 0.66, 95% CI 0.39–1.14, *P* = .13) and lack of benefit for tumors < 4 cm (HR 1.73, 95% CI 0.98–0.34, *P* = .06). As previously discussed, various molecular markers and gene expression profiles are being evaluated to determine which specific subgroups would benefit most from adjuvant chemotherapy, but this is not routine clinical practice. Given M.E.'s tumor location, he may have evidence of visceral pleural invasion at surgery, and thus may want to consider adjuvant chemotherapy, after an informed discussion about risks and benefits.

Adjuvant radiation has also been examined in early-stage lung cancer, but several meta-analyses indicate that postoperative radiation has an adverse effect on overall survival for N0 and N1 disease. The best evidence is for N2 disease (HR 0.855, 95% CI 0.762–0.959; *P* = .0077) (8). Therefore, unless this patient has pathologic N2 nodal involvement or positive margins, adjuvant radiation therapy would not be recommended (see Figure 3.1B).

Neoadjuvant Chemotherapy in Early-Stage NSCLC

Multiple smaller studies have suggested that chemotherapy can also be given neoadjuvantly. However, many studies were stopped early as the adjuvant data became available or because of slow accrual. A recent Cochrane meta-analysis revealed a benefit of platinum-based neoadjuvant chemotherapy over surgery alone with an HR of 0.82 (95% CI 0.69–0.97, *P* = .022), corresponding to an absolute benefit of 6% to 7% in stages IB-IIIA, and 3% to 5% in IIIB (10). When the data from the European intergroup trial was added to this meta-analysis, the statistical significance was no longer present (HR 0.88, 95% CI 0.76–1.01, *P* = .07). However, this trial had 61% stage I patients and allowed any one of six adjuvant chemotherapy regimens. The only trial to compare neoadjuvant and adjuvant chemotherapy to date is the NATCH trial. This trial also had mostly stage I patients (75%) and used three cycles of carboplatin/paclitaxel. Patients with T1N0 to T3N1 disease were randomized to surgery alone, neoadjuvant, or adjuvant chemotherapy. Notably, 97% of the patients in the neoadjuvant arm received the planned chemotherapy versus 66.2% in the adjuvant arm, but there was no statistical difference in progression-free survival or OS. Although the strong adjuvant data may limit further studies, neoadjuvant chemotherapy with three cycles of a cisplatin-based doublet seems reasonable in stage IB-IIIA (N0–1), especially if there is a concern about ability to tolerate postoperative chemotherapy.

Treatment of Superior Sulcus Tumors

The approach to superior sulcus tumors, even in the earlier stages, has been slightly different, given the tumor

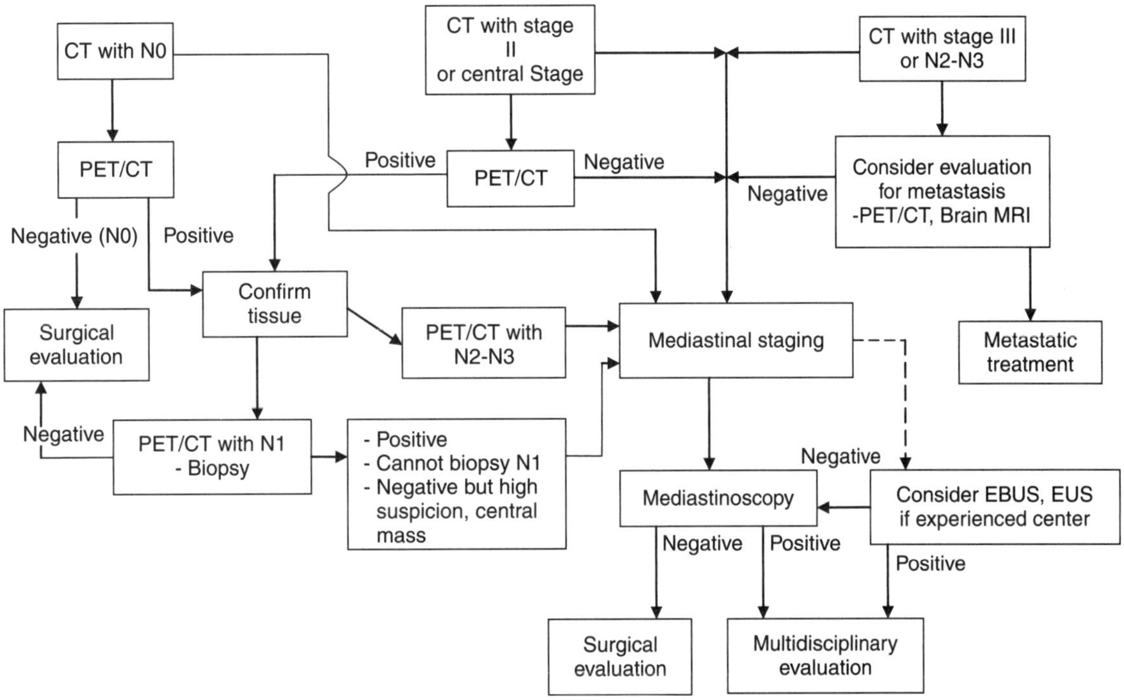

Figure 3.1B

Guidelines for locoregional lymph node staging in non-small cell lung cancer. PET/CT positive nodes must have tissue confirmation. Mediastinal staging with mediastinoscopy is still the gold standard for all but peripheral, PET/CT node negative tumors. Pos, positive; Neg, negative; EBUS, endobronchial ultrasound guided biopsy; EUS, esophageal ultrasound guided biopsy. Adapted from Ref. 9.

type and the risk to, or involvement of, adjacent structures. The classic presentation includes shoulder/arm pain or paresthesias, Horner's syndrome, and intrinsic arm muscle atrophy, caused by extrinsic tumor compression or direct brachial plexus involvement. Brachial plexus MRI imaging helps to determine resectability and extent of disease, as an MRI provides better resolution than a CT scan of the vascular and neurologic structures in this region. As these are relatively rare tumors (about 5% of all NSCLC), there is limited evidence-based data to guide treatment. The largest multi-institutional study, the Southwest Oncology Group (SWOG) Trial 9416, was a phase II trial to evaluate induction cisplatin/etoposide combined with radiation to 45 Gy, followed by surgery and two cycles of consolidation chemotherapy. With an 82-month median follow-up, the 5-year OS was 54% after an R0 resection, versus 44% for all patients. The median OS was not reached for those with a complete pathologic response at surgery (R0), but the median OS was 30 months for patients with minimal microscopic disease (R1) and 29 months for those with gross residual disease (R2). Institutional protocols differ, but cisplatin-based induction chemoradiation followed by surgery is the standard of care in the United States for resectable superior sulcus tumors. Microscopic residual disease clearly has a worse prognosis, but the protocols of additional chemotherapy and/or radiation also vary.

Treatment of Positive Margins

There are no data on the most effective treatment for positive surgical margins. In stage I and II disease, re-resection (with adjuvant chemotherapy in stage II) is preferred, since surgery is still the most definitive modality in early-stage disease. When re-resection is not possible, combination chemoradiation followed by chemotherapy is recommended, depending on patient performance status and ability to tolerate treatment postoperatively (7).

Regional (Stage III) NSCLC

S.S. is a 55-year-old woman with a history of mitral valve prolapse and anxiety, who presents with a persistent cough. A chest x-ray revealed a 3.5-cm right upper lobe mass. A subsequent chest CT showed a spiculated 3.5 × 3.3 cm^2 right upper lobe mass with right hilar lymphadenopathy and an enlarged 1.9-cm right paratracheal lymph node. A subsequent PET/CT demonstrated fludeoxyglucose (FDG) uptake in the lung mass and the paratracheal lymph node. A transbronchial core needle aspiration of both the mass and the 4R lymph node were both positive for poorly differentiated carcinoma, consistent with a lung primary. She has never smoked, but did have exposure working as a bartender for many years. She cares for her two young sons and teaches Pilates at the local gym. Her sister was diagnosed with breast cancer at the age of 33. Her brain MRI was negative and she had normal pulmonary function testing.

Evidence-Based Case Discussion

Stage III disease is heterogeneous, ranging from nonbulky, incidental N2 disease at resection to bulky, unresectable T4N3 disease. Definitive evidence regarding treatment, if available, does not necessarily apply to all patient populations. Data analysis is further complicated by varied imaging and diagnostic techniques, changes in staging, improvements in chemotherapy and radiation delivery, and small or underpowered studies. In general, primary tumor location, mediastinal lymph node involvement, patient performance status, and lung function are all considered in treatment planning. For most patients, the treatment goal is cure, but about 80% of patients recur, frequently locally or in the brain. Although there are limited retrospective data regarding routine screening for asymptomatic brain metastases, it is general practice that patients with stage III disease have either a head CT with IV contrast or an MRI.

Microscopic N2 Disease or Pathologic N2 Disease After Resection

Although not the case in S.S., if M.E. had had incidental N2 disease at surgical resection, radiation after completion of adjuvant chemotherapy is recommended, based on the previously mentioned Surveillance, Epidemiology and End Results (SEER) Medicare study, suggesting a benefit of PORT in patients with pN2 disease (8). There are also data from an unplanned subgroup analysis of patients on the Adjuvant Navelbine International Trialist Association (ANITA) trial. The data is only descriptive, as the allocation was not randomized. Patients with pN2 disease who received PORT after adjuvant chemotherapy had a median OS of 47 months versus 24 months for patients receiving only adjuvant chemotherapy. Corresponding 5-year OS were 47.4% and 34%, respectively. Adjuvant radiation typically follows chemotherapy, but the outcome is not clearly different if this sequencing is reversed (6).

Definitive Chemoradiotherapy

The standard of care in stage III disease is cisplatin-based chemotherapy with etoposide or vinblastine and concurrent radiation. This is the primary treatment for patients who are not operative candidates due to tumor size, location, or performance status. Multiple studies have indicated the benefit of concomitant chemoradiation over sequential chemotherapy and radiation or over radiation alone. A Cochrane meta-analysis of concurrent versus sequential chemotherapy and radiation had an HR of 0.74 (95% CI 0.62–0.89) and a 10% absolute survival benefit at 2 years (11). An NSCLC Collaborative Group meta-analysis found a significant but smaller absolute survival benefit of 5.7% at 3 years and 4.5% at 5 years (HR 0.84, 95% CI 0.74–0.95, *P* = .004) (12). Some of the difference in the latter analysis may be explained by the longer median follow-up (6 years) and the inclusion of three trials with single-agent cisplatin or carboplatin and two trials with split course radiation. All of the Cochrane analysis trials used cisplatin-based doublets and continuous radiation. Concomitant chemoradiation improved locoregional control, but distant progression was similar to sequential therapy. Chemoradiation also increased acute esophageal toxicity (grade 3–4) from 4% to 18% (*P* < .001), but acute pulmonary toxicity was similar. In poor performance status patients, weekly low-dose carboplatin/paclitaxel with concurrent thoracic radiation to 63 Gy, followed by two cycles of standard carboplatin/paclitaxel has been used, but not compared with full dose chemoradiotherapy in a randomized trial.

The optimal chemotherapy combination for chemoradiation is not clear and other agents, including pemetrexed, taxanes, and EGFR inhibitors, are also being examined. The radiation dose is typically 60 to 70 Gy. Newer 3-D and 4-D conformal techniques and respiratory gating have decreased the off-target delivery to the lungs, spinal cord, and esophagus. Various protocols have also used hyperfractionated radiation or intensity modulated radiotherapy (IMRT) to optimize radiation dosing. In IMRT, the radiation beam is modulated to increase the primary tumor radiation dose and decrease the normal tissue dose. Early results are promising. However, neither IMRT nor hyperfractionation should be used outside of a clinical protocol. For patients with very large radiation ports or significantly decreased performance status, sequential chemotherapy followed by radiation or radiation alone can still be used.

Both induction and consolidation chemotherapy have been used with chemoradiation in phase II studies, but have not been of proven benefit in randomized phase III studies. The CALGB 39801 study randomized patients to receive two induction cycles of carboplatin and paclitaxel followed by chemoradiation or to chemoradiation alone, but there was no survival benefit to induction. Initial SWOG phase II data was promising for docetaxel consolidation. However, a randomized phase III study showed increased toxicity in the consolidation docetaxel arm, without a difference in median OS. Therefore, neither induction nor consolidation chemotherapy is recommended with definitive chemoradiation outside of a clinical trial.

Multimodality Treatment

Because of the high incidence of locoregional failure (up to 83%) with chemoradiation, many have questioned if including surgery would provide any additional benefit. There has also been interest in trying to control micrometastatic disease and therefore distant recurrence with neoadjuvant chemotherapy. Most of the initial data for neoadjuvant chemotherapy relates to smaller trials, frequently with surgery alone as the comparison arm, which is inferior in stage III disease. Again, the analysis of these trials is complicated by mixed tumor burden, varied mediastinal disease assessment, and varied protocols. This topic was recently reviewed in depth (13), and several trials are still accruing data. The reader is encouraged to keep in mind that some patients designated as stage IIIB in these trials may now be classified as stage IIB (T4 same lobe nodule N0) or stage IIIA (T4 same lobe nodule N1-2, T4 ipsilateral lobe nodule N0-1).

Limited data suggest the emergence of two important classes of current stage IIIA patients that are often considered for multimodality therapy, T4N0-1 disease, and potentially resectable T3N2 disease. The interest in limited T4 disease began with SWOG 8805, a phase II study of two cycles of cisplatin/etoposide with 45 Gy of concurrent radiation, followed by surgery. Remarkably, 19 patients achieved complete pathologic response with a 50% 6-year survival. An exploratory multivariate analysis indicated that T4 non-N2 disease was the only independent predictor of long-term survival. SWOG 9019 was a phase II study evaluating only T4N0-3 patients, with the same induction regimen as 8805, but with completion to definitive radiation without interruption if there was no progressive disease. The median OS in this poor prognostic group was 15 months, but the prior improved response in the T4 N0-1 group was not seen (5-year OS 15%). Combined, these trials suggest that surgery after neoadjuvant chemoradiation may be beneficial in the T4 N0-1 group. Using neoadjuvant chemotherapy alone, the Spanish Lung Cancer Group Trial 9901 was a phase II study of three cycles of induction cisplatin, gemcitabine, and docetaxel, followed by surgery in 67 patients with T4N0-1 disease and 69 with T1-3N2 disease. The median OS was 15.9 months and not significantly different between T4 and N2 disease. The median OS was 48.5 months for all with a complete (R0) resection (33 stage IIIA and 29 stage IIIB), but was 60.6 months for the 29 T4N0-1 patients (53.2% 5-year survival rate). Interestingly, of the nine patients with complete pathologic response at surgery, eight had T4N0-1 disease, and the median OS was not reached after a median follow-up of 53.5 months (57% 5-year OS). Given these small numbers, it remains in question whether induction chemotherapy truly provides benefit for T4N0-1 disease, or if these tumors are less invasive by nature.

A recent summary of 15 cohort studies of patients that underwent primary surgery for T4 disease suggests that the 5-year OS in T4N0-N1 disease may be as high as 43% to 74% versus a 15% to 18% 5-year OS in T4N2 disease (14). Complete resection (5-year OS 38–46%) and T4 stage due to satellite nodules (5-year OS 48–57%) were also significant predictors of improved outcome. The improved prognosis of those with T4N0 ipsilateral tumor nodules who had an R0 resection (48% 5-year OS) was also seen in the data for the 7th edition of the American Joint Committee on Cancer (AJCC) staging criteria for NSCLC. However, the low prevalence makes a randomized trial determining the benefit of neoadjuvant or adjuvant chemotherapy in resectable T4N0-1 disease rather unlikely. Thus, complete surgical resection with or without additional chemotherapy and radiation could be considered in T4N0-1 disease (see Figure 3.2).

In patients, such as S.S., with potentially resectable T3N2 disease, multiple phase II and retrospective cohort studies suggest that nodal downstaging with neoadjuvant treatment is both predictive and prognostic. The European Organization for Research and Treatment of Cancer (EORTC) 08941 trial comparing sequential chemotherapy followed by radiation versus the same chemotherapy followed by surgery in surgically unresectable, stage IIIA N2 patients had 41.4% nodal downstaging to N0/1. This nodal downstaging group had a median OS of 22.7 months, compared to the OS of the radiation and surgery arms (17.5 and 16.4 months, respectively). Also, nodal downstaging, complete pathologic clearance, and no pneumonectomy were significant predictors of OS in the surgical arm. The phase III Intergroup 0139 trial hoped for more definitive data. Patients with biopsy-proven T1-3N2 disease received chemoradiation to 45 Gy with two cycles of cisplatin/etoposide. If there was no progression on CT scan, patients then proceeded to either completion radiation to 61 Gy or surgical resection, followed by two additional cycles of cisplatin and etoposide in both arms. The surgical group had a statistically improved PFS (12.8 months versus 10.5 months; HR 0.77, 95% CI 0.62–0.96, $P = .017$), but the OS was similar (23.6 months versus 22.2 months; HR 0.87, 95% CI 0.70–1.10, $P = .24$). The surgical group also had fewer local-only relapses, with

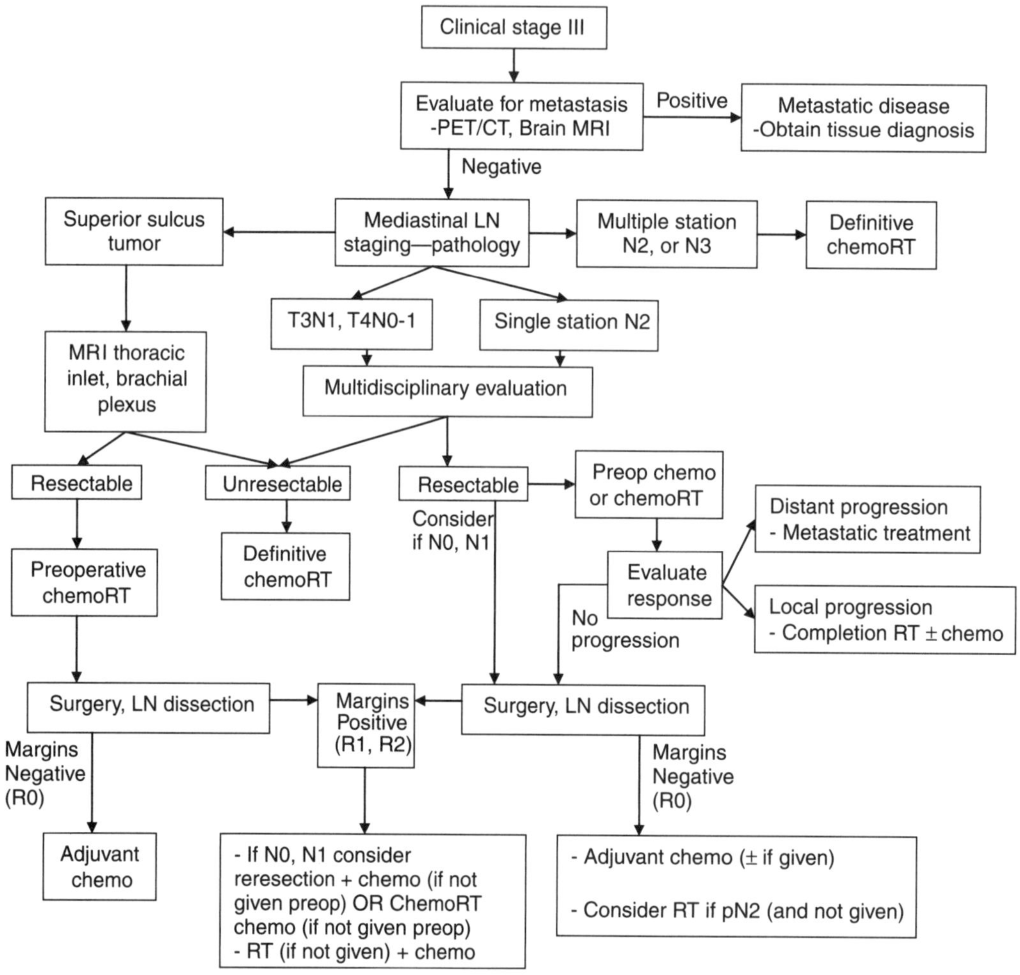

Figure 3.2

Pathway for diagnosis and clinical decision making in clinical stage III non-small cell lung cancer. Head CT with contrast is acceptable alternative to brain MRI. ChemoRT, chemoradiotherapy; RT, radiotherapy; pN2, pathologic N2; Preop, preoperative; R0, no residual tumor; R1, microscopic residual tumor; R2, macroscopic residual tumor. Adapted from National Comprehensive Cancer Network (7).

similar rates of distant metastases. Survival was complicated by a 26% perioperative mortality in pneumonectomy patients. Notably, the T0N0 and TanyN0 groups had a higher median and 5-year OS (39.8 months and 42%, and 34.4 months and 41%, respectively). However, the recurrence pattern of these groups is not described, and these groups might have responded well to any treatment. No comparison could be made to the nonsurgical arm, as it has been documented that in NSCLC CT scans do not accurately evaluate nodal response to chemotherapy and/or radiation. Surgical mediastinal staging has not been done in any nonsurgical arm to date, and it is unknown if PET/CT or staging by EUS could be an accurate alternative. Data from the 7th edition AJCC NSCLC staging had a similar OS in patients who had primary surgical resection in multistation N1 disease and in single-station N2 disease.

In comparison to the trial's mortality, retrospective reports of pneumonectomies after neoadjuvant treatment have shown a 90-day postoperative mortality rate as low as 3% at major tertiary care centers. Although a right-sided pneumonectomy can have increased early perioperative mortality related to bronchial stump covering, the long-term survival of right and left pneumonectomy patients is similar in experienced centers. Thus, induction chemotherapy or chemoradiation followed by surgery could be considered for selected patients with excellent performance status and nonbulky, stage IIIA N2 disease, especially those with single-station N2 disease and not requiring a right pneumonectomy. In summary, S.S. should have multidisciplinary evaluation to determine resectability and the type of surgery, followed by a risks and benefits discussion of standard definitive chemoradiation versus a trimodality treatment.

Prophylactic Cranial Irradiation

Although commonly used in small cell lung cancer, there is no indication for prophylactic cranial irradiation (PCI) in locally advanced NSCLC, as a survival benefit has not been shown. The Radiation Therapy Oncology Group (RTOG) 0214 trial randomizing 340 stage IIIA and IIIB patients to PCI or observation closed early due to slow accrual. There were no differences in OS or PFS, but the observation arm patients were 2.52 times more likely to develop CNS metastases than those in the PCI arm. Final recommendations regarding PCI may depend on whether significant differences in quality of life (QOL) measures are observed.

Metastatic NSCLC, Case 1

L.A. is a 55-year-old nonsmoking Asian woman from Hong Kong who was visiting her daughter in the United States. She reported an unrelenting cough productive of clear sputum associated with shortness of breath. A chest x-ray revealed a large right upper lobe lung mass and an elevated right hemidiaphragm. A subsequent chest CT revealed a 4.5 × 5 cm^2 right upper lobe mass, diffuse mediastinal lymphadenopathy, multiple subcentimeter lung nodules throughout, and a 3.5-cm mass in the right anterior lobe of the liver. A bronchoscopy with biopsy and a liver mass biopsy both demonstrated adenocarcinoma. She never smoked, but frequently inhaled cooking oil fumes in China. She is small, frail, and has dropped from 100 to 95 pounds in the past month.

Evidence-Based Case Discussion

EGFR Inhibitor

L.A.'s clinical characteristics, being female, Asian, a nonsmoker, and having adenocarcinoma, increase the likelihood that her tumor has an *EGFR* mutation. As previously mentioned, the incidence of this mutation in NSCLC is 30% to 40% in those of Asian descent and 10% to 15% in non-Asian populations. The IPASS trial was a phase III study of Asian, nonsmokers (80% women) with untreated, advanced NSCLC that were randomized to either first-line gefitinib or to carboplatin/paclitaxel (15). The study met its primary objective, illustrating noninferior PFS (HR 0.74, 95% CI 0.65–0.85, $P < .001$). An exploratory subgroup analysis revealed that gefitinib-treated patients with *EGFR*-mutated tumors had a significantly higher PFS (HR 0.48, 95% CI 0.36–0.64, $P < .001$), whereas gefitinib-treated patients with *EGFR* wild-type tumors had a significant decrease in PFS (HR 2.85, 95% CI 0.36–0.64, $P < .001$). Two subsequent randomized phase III trials included only patients with *EGFR*-mutated tumors. The North-East Japan (NEJ) 002 trial randomized patients to gefitinib or to carboplatin/paclitaxel. The gefitinib arm had a significantly better PFS, 10.8 months versus 5.4 months (HR 0.30, 95% CI 0.22–0.41, $P < .001$), and objective response rate (ORR) (73.7% versus 30.7%, $P < .001$). Ninety-five percent of the chemotherapy arm patients received second-line gefitinib, but only 58.5% had an objective response. The West Japan Trial Oncology Group (WJTOG) 3405 trial included a higher number of patients with postoperative relapses than NEJ002 trial (41% versus 9%). Patients were randomized to gefitinib or to cisplatin/docetaxel. The gefitinib arm had significantly better PFS, 9.2 months versus 6.3 months (HR 0.49, 95% CI 0.34–0.71, $P < .001$), and ORR (62.1% versus 32.2%, $P < .0001$). Although not a part of the preplanned analysis, a difference in PFS was not statistically significant between the two arms in the postoperative subgroup (13.7 months versus 8.1 months, $P = .069$). Both first-line treatment with gefitinib and postoperative disease were significant contributors to PFS in the multivariate model. The OS data from both trials are still immature, and neither trial showed survival difference between patients with an exon 19 deletion or the L858R substitution. In a pooled analysis of five phase II trials using first-line erlotinib or gefitinib in non-Asian populations, the ORR and time to progression in the *EGFR*-mutated patients was similar to that seen in the Japanese trials, 67% and 11.8 months, respectively (16). However, in this analysis, patients with exon 19 deletions had a better survival than those with the L858R mutation. Patients with wild-type *EGFR* did poorly, regardless of *K-ras* mutation status. Phase III trial data in non-Asian populations is pending, but the evidence is enough to consider first-line use of erlotinib in patients with a sensitizing *EGFR* mutation.

There is no clear evidence that concurrent erlotinib or gefitinib with first-line cytotoxic therapy provides benefit, nor is there sufficient evidence to suggest routine screening of all stage IV lung cancers for molecular markers. However, since L.A. had several indicators increasing her likelihood of having an *EGFR*-mutated tumor, and we would consider using erlotinib first line, it would be reasonable to check her tumor's mutation status (see Figure 3.3).

Standard Treatment +/– Bevacizumab or Cetuximab

Alternatively, if L.A. tests negative for the *EGFR* mutation, or if she was a non-Asian smoker, a platinum-based chemotherapy doublet would be indicated. Some debate the benefits of cisplatin over carboplatin in metastatic

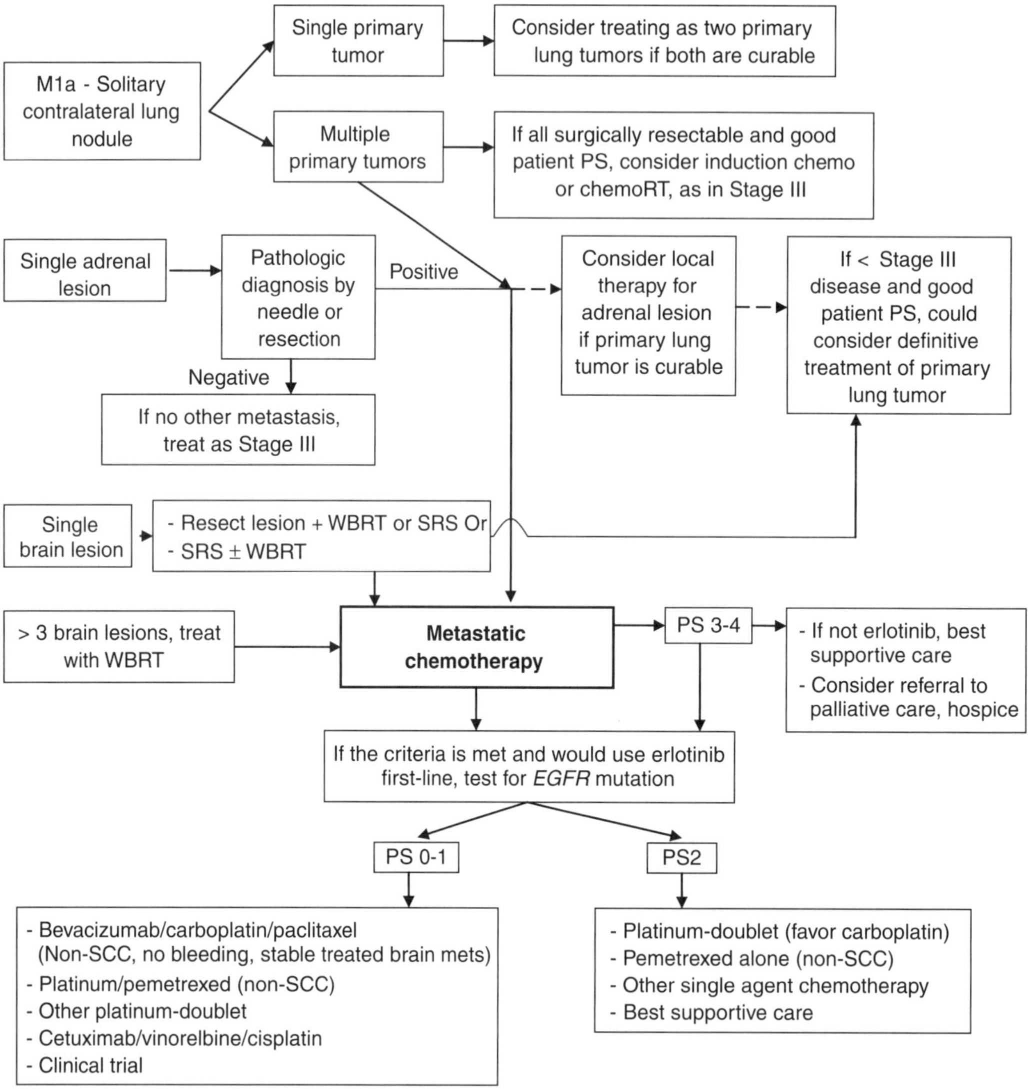

Figure 3.3

Pathway for clinical decision making in metastatic non-small cell lung cancer. Obtain brain MRI or head CT with contrast, if not already done. Consider PET/CT and/or CT abdomen pelvis if not already done. If bone pain, and no clear findings on CT or PET not available, consider bone scan. If treating with surgery, recommend mediastinal staging evaluation. PS, performance status; chemoRT, chemoradiotherapy; WBRT, whole brain radiotherapy; SRS, stereotactic radiosurgery, Non-SCC, non-squamous cell carcinoma. Adapted from National Comprehensive Cancer Network (7).

NSCLC. A meta-analysis of individual patient data from nine trials (2968 patients) showed that while the ORR was higher in patients treated with cisplatin, there was no significant OS difference between carboplatin and cisplatin regimens (HR 1.07, 95% CI 0.99–1.15, P = .10) (17). However, when the analysis was restricted to third-generation platinum-based regimens, the survival became significant (HR 1.11, 95% CI 1.01–1.21). Patients treated with cisplatin were more likely to have nausea, vomiting, and renal dysfunction. Patients treated with carboplatin were more likely to have thrombocytopenia. Given the importance of QOL in metastatic disease, the potential risk factors of cisplatin use should be taken into consideration, along with the small benefit. There is currently no evidence that one particular third-generation platinum-based doublet is better than another, and a three drug regimen (excluding targeted therapies) provides no additional benefit. If a patient cannot tolerate platinum-based chemotherapy, a nonplatinum-based doublet is recommended, but it is controversial whether this treatment is inferior. A meta-analysis of 37 phase I and II trials showed a significantly increased ORR with platinum-based treatment, with a 5% 1-year survival increase (P = .0003). However, when only third-generation agents were used, the survival difference was no longer apparent. In a separate meta-analysis of 11 phase III trials, all with newer agents, platinum-based treatment gave a 2.9% absolute reduction in the risk of death at 1 year (HR 0.88, 95% CI 0.78–0.99, P = .044), but with a higher risk of toxicity (18). Thus, a nonplatinum combination could be considered first line, if platinum agents are contraindicated.

Two targeted agents combined with standard chemotherapy doublets have improved response in metastatic disease. Bevacizumab and cetuximab are monoclonal antibodies targeted against the vascular endothelial growth factor receptor and EGFR, respectively. In a randomized phase III trial, Eastern Cooperative Oncology Group (ECOG) 4599 compared carboplatin and paclitaxel with or without bevacizumab in patients with newly diagnosed metastatic or recurrent NSCLC. Patients randomized to the bevacizumab arm continued bevacizumab alone after the initial six cycles, until disease progression or toxicity (19). The bevacizumab arm had significantly improved OS (12.3 months versus 10.3 months, HR 0.79, 95% CI 0.67–0.92, P = .003), PFS, and ORR, but higher toxicity rates, including clinically significant bleeding (4.4% versus 0.7%) and arterial thrombosis. AVAiL was a phase III trial comparing cisplatin/gemcitabine with or without bevacizumab, but even in the updated analysis, only response rate and PFS were statistically significant. Relative contraindications for bevacizumab use in lung cancer include recent significant bleeding, untreated or unstable brain metastases, major surgery in the past 28 days, squamous cell lung cancer, and any centrally located tumor with potential major vessel involvement. Patients who have had a treated and stable prior brain metastasis or those on stable long-term anticoagulation could be considered for treatment with bevacizumab after an informed discussion of the risks and benefits.

The FLEX trial was an open label phase III trial of cisplatin/vinorelbine with or without cetuximab in advanced lung cancer patients who had at least one tumor cell with EGFR expression by IHC. Up to six cycles of the initial regimen was followed by additional maintenance cetuximab in the cetuximab arm. The patients in this arm had a significantly improved OS (11.3 months versus 10.1 months; HR 0.87, 95% CI 0.762–0.996, P = .044). The BMS099 trial used carboplatin with paclitaxel or docetaxel, with or without cetuximab, but did not require *EGFR* status for enrollment, and saw no difference in DFS or OS. An optional correlative biomarker study with few samples showed no difference in response based on *EGFR* or *K-ras* mutations or on EGFR expression based on IHC or FISH. A meta-analysis combining the data from these two phase III trials and two phase II trials suggested an improvement in OS with a pooled HR of 0.87 (95% CI 0.79–0.96, P = .004) (20), but showed no benefit in PFS or 1-year survival. Given this data, cetuximab is not FDA approved for use in lung cancer.

Length of Treatment and Maintenance

To date, guidelines recommend that first-line chemotherapy be stopped after four cycles in patients who are not responding to treatment, or after a maximum of six cycles (7,21). A meta-analysis of 13 trials comparing a shorter versus a longer duration of chemotherapy found that longer chemotherapy durations improved both PFS (HR 0.75, 95% CI 0.69–0.81, P < .001) and OS (HR 0.92, 95% CI 0.86–0.99, P = .03) but also increased toxicity (21). However, the OS improvement was not significant when the data from one large trial (22) was excluded. Longer chemotherapy durations were also associated with more frequent adverse events and impaired QOL in two of the trials that collected QOL data. In a meta-analysis of a more uniform set of seven trials with third-generation platinum doublets, only PFS was improved (23).

Data from multiple maintenance treatment trials, either biologic/targeted or chemotherapy based, have been reviewed in several articles (24), and additional trials are ongoing. Continuation therapy, also called continuation maintenance, continues part of the initial regimen until disease progression or toxicity, such as in the trials with bevacizumab or cetuximab. However, these targeted trials were not designed to determine whether the benefit of the targeted agent is derived from the initial phase combined with chemotherapy, the maintenance phase alone, or both. To date, the strongest evidence is for early second-line therapy, also called "switch" maintenance, with either pemetrexed or erlotinib until disease progression.

In the JMEN trial, patients who had not progressed after four cycles of a non-pemetrexed containing platinum doublet were randomized 2:1 to pemetrexed or placebo (22). Both PFS (HR 0.5, 95% CI 0.42–0.61, $P < .0001$) and OS (HR 0.79, 95% CI 0.65–0.95, $P = .12$) were significantly improved in the pemetrexed arm. No difference in PFS or OS was seen in patients with SCC, about 30% of patients in each arm, but more benefit was seen in the non-squamous subgroup (PFS HR 0.44 and OS HR 0.70). In the SATURN trial, patients who had not progressed after four cycles of a platinum doublet were randomized 1:1 to erlotinib or placebo (25). Patients were stratified for EGFR IHC and not for *EGFR* mutations, but *EGFR* mutations were similar between the groups. Both PFS (HR 0.71, 95% CI 0.62–0.82, $P < .0001$) and OS (HR 0.81, 95% CI 0.70–0.95, $P = .0088$) were significantly improved in the erlotinib arm. The OS was also improved in the erlotinib arm patients with wild-type *EGFR* tumors (HR 0.77, 95% CI 0.61–0.97, $P = .0243$). The median OS for the erlotinib arm *EGFR*-mutation-positive patients had not been reached at the time of publication. In the placebo arm, 67% of *EGFR*-mutation-positive patients received erlotinib or gefitinib second line. However, neither trial delineates whether the benefit is from increased antineoplastic activity using three sequential treatment regimens or from receiving three different regimens at any time. An early second-line trial using docetaxel did not reach statistical significance for OS (26). In this trial, patients who had not progressed after four cycles of carboplatin and gemcitabine were randomized to receive immediate docetaxel (for a maximum of six cycles) or delayed docetaxel, given upon progression. PFS was statistically improved in the immediate docetaxel arm (5.7 months versus 2.7 months, $P = .001$), but not OS. In summary, switch-maintenance with pemetrexed or erlotinib may be reasonable in selected patients with nonprogressive disease after four cycles of platinum-based therapy (see Figure 3.3).

Metastatic NSCLC, Case 2

H.P. is a 60-year-old man with a smoking history of two packs a day, who presented to his physician with a month long history of persistent headaches, blurry vision, and cough after having been treated for community-acquired pneumonia. A head CT revealed a 2.5-cm right occipital lobe mass. Subsequent PET-CT showed a 4-cm left hilar lung mass with two FDG positive hilar lymph nodes and uptake in the occipital mass. A bronchoscopy and hilar lymph node biopsy were positive for SCC. Both EUS guided sampling of mediastinal lymph nodes and mediastinoscopy were negative for evidence of N2 involvement. He had since quit smoking and has had improvement of his headaches and vision with steroids. He is the primary care taker of his 85-year-old mother with dementia and has a good performance status.

Evidence-Based Case Discussion

Squamous Cell Carcinoma Versus Adenocarcinoma

The standard first-line treatment for metastatic SCC is a platinum-based doublet. The small molecule EGFR inhibitors (erlotinib and gefitinib) are not used because SCCs rarely carry *EGFR* mutations, and have not responded well to these drugs. Bevacizumab is not used due to the increased bleeding risk seen with this tumor type. Pemetrexed is also not indicated for use in SCC, based on data from two phase III trials (27). One was a front-line noninferiority trial in patients with Stage IIIB or IV NSCLC, randomized to either cisplatin/gemcitabine or cisplatin/pemetrexed. The other trial compared pemetrexed to docetaxel in the second-line setting. Non-squamous patients in both trials had a longer survival when treated with pemetrexed (HR 0.84, 95% CI 0.74–0.96, $P = 0.011$; HR 0.78, 95% CI 0.61–1.00, $P = .47$, respectively). It is hypothesized that this histologic difference in efficacy may be related to higher expression of thymidylate synthase (the primary target of pemetrexed) in SCC.

Treatment of Isolated Metastasis

In a patient with good PS and favorable prognostic factors (age younger than 65, controlled primary tumor in prior 3 months, and absence of extracranial metastasis) treatment of a solitary brain metastasis with either surgical resection followed by whole brain radiation (WBRT) or with WBRT and stereotactic radiosurgery (SRS) can improve OS and PFS (28), with a 5-year survival rate of 11% to 30%. SRS has been shown to be equivalent to surgery for single lesions <3 cm and without extensive edema or mass effect (29). Surgery should be considered with posterior fossa lesions, due to the risk of fourth ventricle compression and subsequent increased intracranial pressure. Limited data, mostly cases from series, suggest that SRS for up to three small brain lesions can still have a survival benefit over WBRT alone. Standard WBRT is given to 30 Gy in 10 fractions and can be used alone in cases where surgery or SRS are not indicated. However, there is limited data that WBRT provides any significant benefit to patients with poor performance status or advanced systemic disease. The effects of brain radiation on performance status, QOL, and neurologic function are now of concern in clinical trials. On completion of cranial treatment, systemic palliative chemotherapy or local radiation can be considered for the remaining extracranial disease, as tolerated.

However, in the case of H.P., a relatively young patient with good PS, aggressive treatment of both the lung primary and the solitary brain metastasis could be considered, based on retrospective analyses showing improved outcome in such patients (30). There are insufficient data to recommend concurrent chemotherapy and radiation with brain metastases. Therefore, the most aggressive treatment we could offer would be surgical resection followed by WBRT or SRS, and definitive treatment of his lung lesion with surgery and adjuvant chemotherapy. Less aggressive options should also be discussed, given the higher risks of side effects (see Figure 3.3).

Elderly or Poor Performance Status

If instead of being a healthy 60-year-old, the patient is a 76-year-old gentleman who is wheelchair bound from a recent stroke, the treatment options become much different. The median age of patients with newly diagnosed NSCLC is about 68; up to 40% of patients are older than 70. However, most trials are conducted in nonelderly patients with a good performance status. The American Society of Clinical Oncology (ASCO) recommends single-agent chemotherapy for patients with a performance status of 2 (31), based on several, mostly smaller trials, showing no difference in OS and increased toxicity using a doublet versus a single agent in these patients. Best supportive care and/or hospice should also be offered as options as part of a risk/benefit discussion. Age alone should not be used to guide treatment decisions, as older patients with good PS and minimal comorbidities derive the same benefit from treatment as younger patients do. However, older patients often have an increased risk of side effects. Patients with a PS 3 and an *EGFR* exon 19 or 21 mutation could be considered for treatment with erlotinib or gefitinib, based on the initial data in second-line use and on a small Japanese study in which 15 of 22 patients (68%) with a PS^{3}3 and an *EGFR* mutation improved to a PS ≤1, with a median OS of 18 months for the entire 29 patient group (32). However, other patients with a PS of 3 to 4 should be offered best supportive care, including palliative radiation for symptom control.

Recurrent NSCLC

Our first patient, M.E., had an uneventful left lower lobectomy and lymph node dissection. After an informed discussion, he opted not to have adjuvant chemotherapy. Two years later, he presented with chest pain and dyspnea. A chest CT showed multiple bilateral lung nodules, concerning for metastatic disease. A bronchoscopy and a fine-needle aspirate revealed AC, consistent with a lung primary. He had a good partial response to carboplatin and pemetrexed, but 6 months later had progression.

Evidence-Based Case Discussion

Few Areas, Long Time

If he presented with a single isolated recurrence, he could be considered for additional local therapy, including resection. Recurrences frequently occur in the first

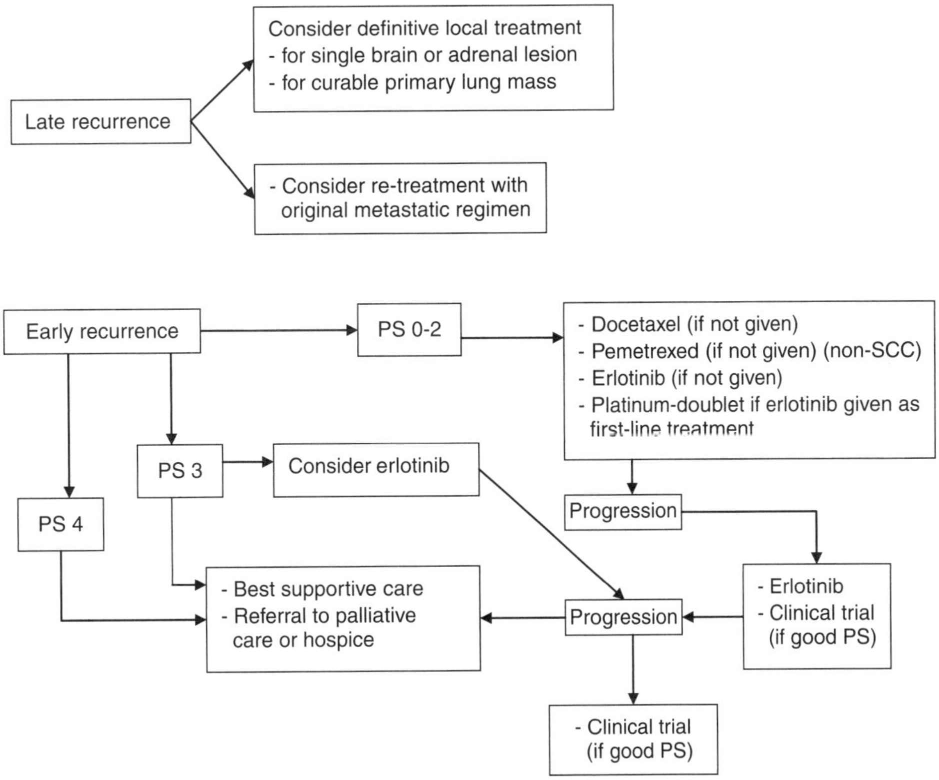

Figure 3.4

Pathway for clinical decision making in recurrent non-small cell lung cancer. PS, performance status; Non-SCC, non-squamous cell carcinoma. Adapted from National Comprehensive Cancer Network (7).

2 years, but patients with prior NSCLC have a 3% to 4% risk of developing a new primary every year. If the presentation is more consistent with a new primary lung cancer, he would also be a candidate for primary-stage appropriate treatment. If he presented with an isolated distant metastasis, such as to the brain, that could be treated with surgery or SRS with WBRT. However, there is no evidence for additional adjuvant chemotherapy for a treated isolated brain metastasis and no other disease.

Many Areas, Short Time

Docetaxel, erlotinib, gefitinib, and pemetrexed are second-line therapy options for patients who have progressed after first-line platinum-based treatment (31). The initial phase III erlotinib versus placebo trial in previously treated NSCLC patient provides evidence for erlotinib as both a second- and third-line treatment (33). Currently, there is no definitive evidence for third-line treatment with standard cytotoxic agents. If erlotinib was given first line, a platinum doublet could be considered in the second-line setting. However, there is no evidence to suggest benefit in switching from a cisplatin-based doublet to a carboplatin-based doublet, switching from erlotinib to gefitinib, or vice versa. Survival and response rates tend to decrease with each subsequent regimen, with increasing risk of toxicities. Best supportive care, including palliative care or hospice, would also be reasonable. Alternatively, additional clinical trials could be considered for patients that continue to have a good performance status (see Figure 3.4).

REFERENCES

1. William DT, Brambilla E, Noguchi M, et al. International Association for the Study of Lung Cancer/American Thoracic Society/European Respiratory Society International Multidisciplinary Classification of Lung Adenocarcinoma. *J Thorac Oncol.* 2011;6:244–285.
2. Larsen JE, Spinola M, Gazdar AF, and Minna JD. An overview of the molecular biology of lung cancer. In: Pass HI, Carbone DP, Johnson DH, et al., eds. *Principles and practice of lung cancer.* Philadelphia, PA: Lippincott Williams & Wilkins, 2010:60–61.
3. Gould MK, Fletcher J, Iannettoni, MD, et al. Evaluation of patients with pulmonary nodules: when is it lung cancer? *Chest.* 2007;132:108S–130S.
4. PORT meta-analysis trialists group. Postoperative radiotherapy for non-small cell lung cancer. *Cochrane Database Syst Rev.* 2005;(2):CD002142.
5. Pignon JP, Tribodet H, Scagliotti GV, et al. Lung adjuvant cisplatin evaluation: a pooled analysis by the LACE collaborative group. *J Clin Oncol.* 2008;26:3552–3559.
6. NSCLC Meta-analyses Collaborative Group. Adjuvant chemotherapy, with or without postoperative radiotherapy, in operable non-small-cell lung cancer: two meta-analyses of individual patient data. *Lancet.* 2010;375,1267–1277.
7. National Comprehensive Cancer Network. Practice guidelines in oncology – v.2.210. Non-small cell lung cancer. www.nccn.org, 2010, March 5.
8. Lally, BE, Zelterman D, Colasanto JM, et al. Postoperative radiotherapy for stage II or III non-small cell lung cancer using the surveillance, epidemiology, and end results database. *J Clin Oncol.* 2006;24:2998–3006.
9. Vansteenkiste J, Dooms C, De Leyn P. Early stage non-small-cell lung cancer: challenges in staging and adjuvant treatment: evidence-based staging. *Ann Oncol.* 2010; 21(Suppl 7):vii189–vii195.
10. Burdett SS, Stewart LA, Rydzewska L. Chemotherapy and surgery versus surgery alone in non-small cell lung cancer. *Cochrane Database Syst Rev.* 2007;(3):CD006157.
11. O'Rourke, NO, Figuls MR, Bernadó NF, Macbeth F. Concurrent chemoradiotherapy in non-small cell lung cancer. *Cochrane Database Syst Rev.* 2010;(6):CD002140.
12. Aupérin A, Péchoux CL, Rolland E, et al. Meta-analysis of concomitant versus sequential radiochemotherapy in locally advanced non-small-cell lung cancer. *J Clin Oncol.* 2010;28:2181–2190.
13. Lally BE, Pass HI, Albain KS. Preoperative chemotherapy/radiation therapy for early stage and locally advanced non-small cell lung carcinoma. In: Pass HI, Carbone DP, Johnson DH, et al., eds. *Principles and Practice of Lung Cancer.* Philadelphia, PA: Lippincott Williams & Wilkins, 2010:799–820.
14. Chambers A, Routledge T, Billè A, and Scarci M. Does surgery have a role in T4N0 and T4N1 lung cancer? *Interact CardioVasc Thorac Surg.* 2010;11:473–479.
15. Mok TS, Yi-Long Wu, Thongprasert S, et al. Gefitinib or carboplatin-paclitaxel in pulmonary adenocarcinoma. *N Engl J Med.* 2009;361:947–957.
16. Jackman DM, Miller VA, Cioffredi LA, et al. Impact of epidermal growth factor receptor and *KRAS* mutations on clinical outcomes in previously untreated non-small cell lung cancer patients: results of an online tumor registry of clinical trials. *Clin Cancer Res.* 2009;15(16):5267–5273.
17. Ardizzoni A, Boni L, Tiseo M, et al. Cisplatin versus carboplatin-based chemotherapy in first-line treatment of advanced non-small cell lung cancer: an individual patient data meta-analysis. *J Natl Cancer Inst.* 2007;99:847–857.
18. Pujol JL, Barlesi F, Duares JP. Should chemotherapy combinations for advanced non-small cell lung cancer be platinum-based? A meta-analysis of phase III randomized trials. *Lung Cancer.* 2006;51:335–345.
19. Sandler A, Gray R, Perry MC, et al. Paclitaxel-carboplatin alone or with bevacizumab for non-small-cell lung cancer. *N Engl J Med.* 2006;355:2542–2550.
20. Lin H, Jiang J, Liang X, et al. Chemotherapy with cetuximab or chemotherapy alone for untreated advanced non-small-cell lung cancer: a systematic review and meta-analysis. *Lung Cancer.* 2010;70:57–62.
21. Soon YY, Stockler MR, Askie LM, and Boyer MJ. Duration of chemotherapy for advanced non-small-cell lung cancer: a systematic review and meta-analysis of randomized trials. *J Clin Oncol.* 2009;27:3277–3283.
22. Ciuleanu T, Brodowicz T, Zielinski C, et al. Maintenance pemetrexed plus best supportive care versus placebo plus best supportive care for non-small-cell lung cancer: a randomized, double-blind, phase 3 study. *Lancet.* 2009;374:1432–1440.
23. Lima JP, dos Santos LV, Sasse EC, et al. Optimal duration of first-line chemotherapy for advanced non-small cell lung cancer: a systematic review with meta-analysis. *Eur J Cancer.* 2009;45:601–607.
24. Gridelli C, Rossi A, Maione P, et al. The role of maintenance treatment in advanced non-small cell lung cancer: reality or early second line? *Clin Lung Cancer.* 2010;11:374–382.
25. Capuzzo F, Ciuleanu T, Stelmakh L, et al. Erlotinib as maintenance treatment in advanced non-small-cell lung cancer: a multicentre, randomized placebo-controlled phase 3 study. *Lancet Oncol.* 2010;11:521–529.
26. Fidias P, Dakhil SR, Lyss AP, et al. Phase III study of immediate compared with delayed docetaxel after front-line therapy with

gemcitabine plus carboplatin in advanced non-small-cell lung cancer. *J Clin Oncol.* 2009;27(4):591–598.

27. Scagliotti G, Hanna N, Fossella F, et al. The differential efficacy of pemetrexed according to NSCLC histology: a review of two phase III studies. *Oncologist.* 2009;14:253–263.
28. Kalkanis SN, Kondziolka D, Gaspar LE, et al. The role of surgical resection in the management of newly diagnosed brain metastases: a systematic review and evidence-based clinical practice guideline. *J Neurooncol.*2010;96:33–43.
29. Linskey ME, Andrews DW, Asher AL, et al. The role of stereotactic radiosurgery in the management of patients with newly diagnosed brain metastases: a systematic review and evidence-based clinical practice guideline. *J Neurooncol.* 2010;96: 45–68.
30. Pfannschmidt J, Dienemann H. Surgical treatment of oligometastatic non-small cell lung cancer. *Lung Cancer.* 2010;69: 251–258.
31. Azzoli CG, Baker SB, Temin S, et al. American Society of Clinical Oncology clinical practice guideline update on chemotherapy for stage IV non-small cell lung cancer. *J Clin Oncol.* 2009;27:6251–6266.
32. Inoue A, Kobayashi K, Usui K, et al. First-line gefitinib for patients with advanced non-small-cell lung cancer harboring epidermal growth factor receptor mutations without indication for chemotherapy. *J Clin Oncol.* 2009;27:1394–1400.
33. Shepard FA, Pereira JR, Ciuleanu T, et al. Erlotinib in previously treated non-small-cell lung cancer. *N Engl J Med.* 2005;353: 123–132.

4

Small Cell Lung Cancer

IGOR I. RYBKIN AND GREGORY P. KALEMKERIAN

EPIDEMIOLOGY, RISK FACTORS, NATURAL HISTORY, AND PATHOLOGY

Small cell lung cancer (SCLC) is a distinct subtype of lung cancer that is characterized by neuroendocrine differentiation, early metastatic spread, and initial responsiveness to therapy. In 2010, it is estimated that there will be about 35,000 new cases of SCLC diagnosed in the United States. The incidence rate of SCLC peaked in the 1980s and has since been declining. The proportional incidence of SCLC as a fraction of all lung cancer cases has also decreased from 17–20% in the 1980s to 13–15% in 2002. Among patients with SCLC, the percentage of women has steadily increased from 28% in 1973 to 50% in 2002. These temporal trends in SCLC incidence directly reflect the prevalence of tobacco use among men and women over the past few decades.

The major cause of SCLC is a history of tobacco smoking, with over 95% of patients diagnosed being current or former smokers. The degree of risk is proportional to the overall exposure to tobacco smoke expressed as pack-years (packs smoked per day × years of smoking) and to the tar and nicotine content of the tobacco smoked. Other less common risk factors include exposure to second-hand smoke, radon, ionizing radiation, and bis(chloromethyl) ether (an industrial solvent).

SCLC typically presents as a large mass arising from a central airway with bulky hilar and mediastinal lymph node involvement. Most patients present with shortness of breath, cough, fatigue, and a variety of symptoms related to metastatic disease, such as weight loss, bone pain, and neurologic dysfunction. Bronchoscopic biopsy and brushings are usually diagnostic, though the bulk of the tumor is often submucosal, requiring a deeper biopsy or aspiration of the central mass or lymph nodes to obtain adequate diagnostic tissue.

SCLC is an aggressive disease with a high growth fraction and early metastatic potential. Historically, patients with SCLC who did not receive therapy had a very poor prognosis, with a median survival of 7 weeks for those with extensive stage (ES) and 14 weeks for those with limited stage (LS). The use of combination chemotherapy and radiation therapy has dramatically altered the course of SCLC due to the remarkable initial responsiveness of the disease. However, despite initial responses, most patients relapse and die with treatment-resistant disease. Between 1973 and 2002, the 2-year survival rate of patients with LS-SCLC improved from 15% to 22%, while the rate for those with ES-SCLC increased only slightly from 3.4% to 5.6%.

SCLC is a highly proliferative and invasive malignancy made up of small cells with a high nuclear-to-cytoplasmic ratio, frequent mitoses, nuclear molding, finely granular chromatin, and inconspicuous nucleoli. Usually, SCLC can be diagnosed by histology alone. However, in some cases, immunohistochemical studies can provide important supporting data. Like non-small cell lung cancer (NSCLC), SCLC usually expresses TTF1 and cytokeratin, but can be differentially characterized by the expression of neuroendocrine markers, such as synaptophysin, neural cell adhesion molecule (NCAM, CD56), chromogranin A, neuron-specific enolase (NSE), and Leu-7 (CD57). SCLC exhibits extensive cytogenetic abnormalities, including defects that cluster on chromosomes 1, 3 (particularly 3p), 5 and 17. In addition, many specific genetic abnormalities have been implicated in the pathogenesis of SCLC, including mutations of *p53*, *p16*, *RB1* and *ras*, and over-expression of *bcl-2*, *c-kit*, and *myc* family genes. Microarray expression analysis of lung cancers has revealed substantial differences in the expression profiles of SCLC and NSCLC. However, thus far, none of these cytogenetic or molecular markers has proven to be of additional diagnostic, prognostic, or therapeutic use in the clinical setting.

STAGING

Veterans' Administration Lung Study Group Staging for Small Cell Lung Cancer

Stage	Description
Limited	Tumor confined to one hemithorax, with or without regional lymph node involvement (including contralateral hilar and mediastinal and ipsilateral supraclavicular lymph nodes), and all disease can be safely contained within a tolerable radiation field
Extensive	Disease that has spread beyond limited stage, including contralateral supraclavicular lymph nodes, malignant pleural or pericardial effusion, and distant metastases

TNM Staging for Small Cell Lung Cancer

Stage	Description
IA	Primary tumor ≤3 cm (T1a, T1b) surrounded by lung or visceral pleura, without bronchoscopic invasion to the main bronchus, and no nodal or distant metastases (N0 M0)
IB	Primary tumor >3 cm, but ≤5 cm (T2a) and no nodal or distant metastases (N0 M0)
	Primary tumor ≤5 cm (T1a, T1b, T2a) that invades visceral pleura, involves the main bronchus (≥2 cm distal to the carina), or is associated with atelectasis or obstructive pneumonitis extending to the hilar region, but not involving the entire lung, and no nodal or distant metastases (N0 M0)
IIA	Primary tumor ≤5cm (T1a, T1b, T2a) and metastasis in ipsilateral peribronchial, hilar, and/or intrapulmonary lymph node(s) (N1), and no distant metastasis (M0)
	Primary tumor >5 cm, but ≤7 cm (T2b) and no nodal or distant metastases (N0 M0)
IIB	Primary tumor >5 cm, but ≤7 cm (T2b), and metastasis in ipsilateral peribronchial, hilar, and/or intrapulmonary lymph node(s) (N1), and no distant metastasis (M0)
	Primary tumor >7 cm (T3) *or* one directly invading the chest wall, diaphragm, phrenic nerve, mediastinal pleura, or parietal pericardium, or in the main bronchus <2 cm distal to the carina without involving the carina, or associated with atelectasis or obstructive pneumonitis of the entire lung (T3), *or* separate tumor nodule(s) in the same lobe as the primary tumor (T3), and no nodal or distant metastases (N0 M0)
IIIA	Primary tumor of any size that invades the mediastinum, heart, great vessels, trachea, recurrent laryngeal nerve, esophagus, vertebral body, or carina (T4), *or* separate tumor nodule(s) in a different lobe ipsilateral to that of the primary (T4), and no nodal or distant metastases (N0 M0)
	Primary tumor (T3, T4), and metastasis in ipsilateral peribronchial, hilar, and/or intrapulmonary lymph node(s) (N1), and no distant metastasis (M0)
	Primary tumor (T1–T3), and metastasis in the ipsilateral mediastinal and/or subcarinal lymph nodes(s) (N2), and no distant metastasis (M0)
IIIB	Primary tumor (T4), and metastasis in the ipsilateral mediastinal and/or subcarinal lymph nodes(s) (N2), and no distant metastasis (M0)
	Primary tumor of any size or invasion (T1–T4), and metastasis in the contralateral mediastinal, contralateral hilar, or ipsilateral or contralateral scalene or supraclavicular lymph node(s) (N3), and no distant metastasis (M0)
IV	Primary tumor of any size or invasion (T1–T4), with or without any lymph node metastasis (N0–N3) and separate tumor nodule(s) in a contralateral lobe *or* pleural nodules, *or* malignant pleural or pericardial effusion (M1a) or distant metastasis (M1b)

(*AJCC Cancer Staging Handbook*, 7th Edition)

CASE SUMMARIES

Limited-Stage SCLC: Combined Modality Therapy

M.R. is a 52-year-old woman who presents with progressive dyspnea on exertion over the past 4 weeks. She has also noted weight loss, fatigue, anterior chest pain, fever, and a nonproductive cough, though she continues to work full time. She is a current smoker with a 30-pack-year history. Her past medical history was otherwise unremarkable. Her physical examination revealed mild tachycardia and low grade fever with decreased breath sounds over the right lower lung field and no cervical or supraclavicular lymphadenopathy. Laboratory studies were remarkable for a slightly elevated white blood cell count, normal electrolytes, normal renal and hepatic function, and a serum LDH of 240 IU/L. Chest radiography showed right hilar fullness and a large right lower lobe density. A chest CT revealed a 4-cm right hilar mass with obstruction of the right lower lobe bronchus and partial atelectasis of the right lower lobe. There was bulky lymphadenopathy in the right paratracheal, precarinal, and subcarinal regions. A PET-CT showed intense FDG uptake in the right hilar mass and numerous mediastinal lymph nodes, but only mild uptake in the right lower lobe corresponding to the area of atelectasis. There was no abnormal FDG uptake elsewhere. An MRI of the brain revealed no suspicious lesions. Endobronchial biopsy of the right hilar mass and transbronchial aspiration of a subcarinal lymph node revealed SCLC.

Evidence-Based Case Discussion

The patient presented above is a middle-aged woman with a good performance status (ECOG PS 1) and no comorbid medical problems. After a complete staging evaluation, she is found to have LS-SCLC with a central primary tumor mass and mediastinal lymph node involvement that can all be safely treated with thoracic radiation. The right hilar mass is causing atelectasis in the right lower lobe and she has clinical evidence of mild postobstructive pneumonia for which initiation of oral, broad-spectrum antibiotics (e.g., amoxicillin-clavulanate) would be appropriate. Assistance with smoking cessation through aggressive counseling and pharmacologic means is also indicated to improve lung function, decrease the risks of treatment-related complications, and reduce the risk of second primary malignancy. She requires immediate referral to medical and radiation oncology in order to initiate treatment with curative intent in a timely manner.

Chemotherapy

The current standard-of-care for patients with LS-SCLC consists of 4 to 6 cycles of etoposide plus cisplatin (EP) along with early, concurrent thoracic radiotherapy. One small randomized trial has suggested that carboplatin can be safely substituted for cisplatin in patients with LS-SCLC with statistically similar outcomes. However, due to the paucity of comparative data, cisplatin should be used unless it is contraindicated (e.g., neuropathy, hearing loss, renal insufficiency). There is no data in the literature to justify the use of combinations other than platinum plus etoposide in patients with LS-SCLC. After completion of chemoradiotherapy, prophylactic cranial irradiation (PCI) should be strongly considered for those achieving a good response. It is important to remember that LS-SCLC is a curable disease and, as such, all patients should be offered optimal treatment as established by years of clinical research.

Thoracic Radiotherapy

Over the past three decades, most of the progress in the treatment of LS-SCLC has been due to advances in the use of radiotherapy. Two meta-analyses demonstrated that the addition of definitive thoracic radiation to chemotherapy significantly improved overall survival in patients with LS-SCLC by 5.4% at 2 to 3 years (P = .001) (1,2). Subsequent studies demonstrated that early thoracic radiotherapy (initiated within 9 weeks of starting chemotherapy or during the first 2 cycles of chemotherapy) improved local control and afforded a 5% overall survival benefit at 2 years when compared to late radiotherapy (P = .03) (3).

Despite the fact that a large, randomized trial reported a significant survival benefit with the use of hyperfractionated thoracic radiotherapy, this strategy remains controversial. Turrisi et al. randomized 417 patients with LS-SCLC to receive standard EP along with 45 Gy of early, concurrent thoracic radiotherapy given either once-daily over 5 weeks or twice-daily over 3 weeks (4). Patients receiving the twice-daily regimen had a significant improvement in overall survival compared to those receiving once-daily therapy (median, 23 vs. 19 months; 5-year, 26% vs. 16%; P = .04). Not surprisingly, twice-daily radiation also increased the risk of developing severe esophagitis (4). This study has been criticized for the relatively low total dose of radiation given to patients receiving once-daily therapy, resulting in a lack of biological equivalence between the radiation doses administered on the two arms. Conflicting results were reported from a trial of late, hyperfractionated radiotherapy in which 262 patients with LS-SCLC were randomized to receive standard EP along with either once-daily thoracic radiation to 50.4 Gy in 28 fractions or twice-daily radiation to 48 Gy in a split-course of 32 fractions (5). Radiation was started with the third cycle of chemotherapy in both arms. In this trial, there were no significant differences in progression-free (median, once-daily 19.5 months vs. twice-daily 18.8 months; P = .54) or overall survival (3-year, once-daily 34% vs. twice-daily 29%; P = .49). This trial has been criticized for the late initiation of radiation and the use of split-course therapy in the twice-daily arm. Therefore, the potential benefit of hyperfractionated radiation in LS-SCLC remains open to debate pending the results of on-going, well-designed, confirmatory trials. However, based on the available data, early, hyperfractionated, twice-daily radiation to 45 Gy should be strongly considered for patients in whom the potential toxicity of this approach is deemed acceptable by the treating physicians. Alternatively, in patients with poorer performance status or bulky disease that would require an excessively large treatment field, thoracic radiation may be administered once-daily to total dose of 60 to 70 Gy.

In patients with LS-SCLC, standard chemoradiotherapy yields an overall response rate of 80% to 95% and a complete response rate of 40% with median survival of 18 to 24 months and a 5-year survival rate of 20% (6). Owing to the high degree of responsiveness to therapy, even patients with impaired performance status should be considered for standard therapy with curative intent.

Prophylactic Cranial Irradiation

Over 50% of patients with SCLC will develop brain metastases during the course of their illness. A meta-analysis of randomized trials evaluating PCI versus no PCI reported a 25% absolute decrease in the incidence of brain metastases at 3 years (control, 58.6% vs. PCI, 33.3%; $P < .001$) and a 5.4% increase in 3-year overall survival (control, 15.3% vs. PCI, 20.7%; $P = .01$) (7). In this meta-analysis, 86% of patients had LS-SCLC. A retrospective analysis of patients with LS-SCLC from the SEER database also reported that PCI resulted in a significant increase in 2- and 5-year survival rates (8). On the basis of these data, PCI at 25 Gy in 10 fractions is recommended for patients with LS-SCLC who have good performance status, intact neurologic function, and complete or partial response to initial therapy.

Surgery

Less than 5% of all patients with SCLC present with clinical stage I (T1–2 N0 M0) disease. However, these patients comprise a special case in which surgical resection followed by adjuvant chemotherapy is a preferred treatment option. Prior to resection, all such patients should undergo surgical or endoscopic mediastinal staging to rule out occult nodal disease. If mediastinal staging shows no lymph node involvement, then patients should undergo lobectomy with further mediastinal lymph node dissection followed by adjuvant chemotherapy with cisplatin plus etoposide (9). Patients with pathologic stage I disease (T1–2 N0 M0) should receive adjuvant chemotherapy alone, while those with nodal metastases should undergo concurrent chemotherapy and postoperative mediastinal radiation. After complete resection and adjuvant therapy, PCI should also be considered.

Figure 4.1 shows the treatment algorithm for LS-SCLC.

Extensive-Stage SCLC: Systemic Palliative Therapy

D.F. is a 72-year-old man who presents with a 3-week history of worsening shortness of breath, abdominal fullness, weight loss, fatigue, right anterior chest pain, and swelling of his face and neck. He has also noted recent onset of difficulty standing up from a chair and walking upstairs. He has smoked one pack a day for 50 years. His past medical history was remarkable for chronic obstructive pulmonary disease, hypertension, and coronary artery disease. His physical examination revealed an elderly man who appears fatigued, but has an ECOG performance status of 1. There was moderate swelling of his face and neck and a palpable, hard, 3-cm

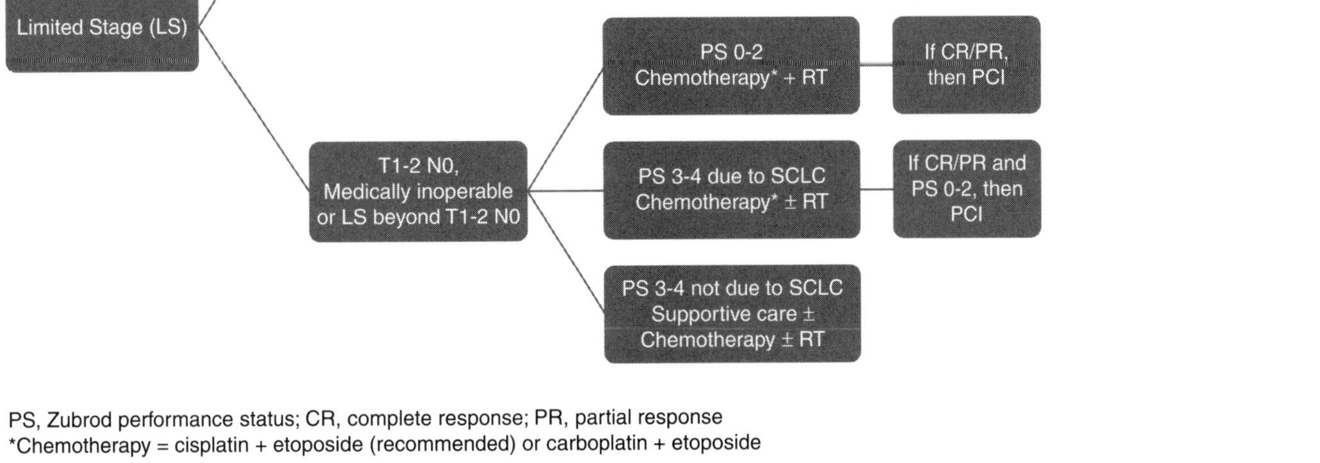

Figure 4.1

Treatment algorithm for LS-SCLC.

right supraclavicular lymph node. His breath sounds were diminished in all lung fields with coarse rhonchi in the right upper lung field. Abdominal exam revealed a firm, nodular, mildly tender liver edge 8 cm below the costal margin in the midline. Neurological examination revealed symmetrical proximal muscle weakness in upper and lower extremities. Laboratory studies were remarkable for normal electrolytes and blood counts, creatinine 1.3 mg/dL, LDH 450 IU/L, alkaline phosphatase 270 IU/L, AST 45 IU/L, ALT 56 IU/L, and total bilirubin 1.2 mg/dL. Paraneoplastic antibody panel revealed the presence of antibodies against voltage-gated calcium channels. Chest radiography revealed a widened mediastinum, a large right suprahilar mass, and emphysema. A CT of the chest and upper abdomen showed a 3.5-cm right supraclavicular lymph node, bilateral bulky mediastinal lymph nodes, a 7 × 5 cm right suprahilar mass with marked narrowing of the superior vena cava and the right upper lobe bronchus, multiple bilateral lung nodules ranging in size from 0.4 to 2.5 cm, postobstructive atelectasis in the right upper lobe, a 4.2-cm left adrenal mass, multiple liver nodules ranging in size from 1.2 to 5.7 cm, and numerous lytic bone lesions involving the vertebral bodies and ribs. An MRI of the brain was negative for metastatic lesions. A biopsy of a liver lesion showed metastatic SCLC.

Evidence-Based Case Discussion

The patient presented above is an elderly man with widely metastatic ES-SCLC causing superior vena cava syndrome and paraneoplastic Lambert-Eaton myasthenic syndrome. If left untreated, he would likely succumb to his disease in a few weeks. Although treatment with combination chemotherapy should afford him good palliation of symptoms, improved quality of life (QOL), and prolongation of survival, his prospects for long-term survival are limited. Owing to the high likelihood of achieving a brisk response and relief of symptoms with standard chemotherapy, palliative radiation is generally not indicated for the management of superior vena cava syndrome in patients with SCLC unless they have severe symptoms, such as confusion (due to cerebral edema) or stridor (due to laryngeal edema).

Chemotherapy

Many classes of chemotherapy agents have demonstrated relatively high response rates in patients with ES-SCLC, including platinums (cisplatin, carboplatin), epipodophyllotoxins (etoposide, tenoposide), camptothecin analogs (irinotecan, topotecan), alkylating agents (isofosfamide, cyclophosphamide), anthracyclines (doxorubicin, epirubicin), taxanes (paclitaxel, docetaxel), antimetabolites (methotrexate, gemcitabine), and vinca alkaloids (vincristine, vinblastine, vinorelbine). Alkylator-based combination chemotherapy regimens, such as cyclophosphamide, doxorubicin, and vincristine (CAV), were developed in the 1970s and resulted in significant improvements in response rate (60–80%) and overall survival (median 7–10 months) (10). During the 1980s, the combination of etoposide and cisplatin (EP) was found to yield response and survival rates similar to those of older alkylator-based regimens, with a relatively favorable toxicity profile (11). Randomized trials directly comparing CAV to EP failed to demonstrate the superiority of either regimen, and, recently, a phase III study comparing EP to cyclophosphamide, epirubicin, and vincristine (CEV) reported that overall survival was significantly better in patients assigned to the EP arm of the trial (10.2 vs. 7.8 months, P = .0004), with most of the difference noted in patients with LS-SCLC (12). Meta-analyses have also demonstrated a modest survival advantage for cisplatin-based therapy (13), and an analysis of randomized clinical trials performed over 20 years in patients with ES-SCLC revealed a slight survival improvement during the latter time interval when cisplatin-based trials predominated (14). EP has become the standard-of-care for both ES- and LS-SCLC since it results in less myelotoxicity and is easier to combine with thoracic irradiation in patients with LS-SCLC.

Phase II trials of several newer regimens have reported reasonable efficacy in patients with ES-SCLC. The combination of irinotecan plus cisplatin (IP) is one of the few regimens that has undergone phase III evaluation. The Japanese Clinical Oncology Group (JCOG) randomized 154 patients with previously untreated ES-SCLC to either EP or IP and reported that IP resulted in a significantly better response rate, progression-free survival, and overall survival (15). IP also induced significantly more severe diarrhea, while EP caused greater hematologic toxicity. Two randomized trials in Western patients have failed to confirm the superiority of IP over EP. A North American/Australian trial that compared a modified IP regimen to EP in 331 patients with previously untreated ES-SCLC reported similar efficacy in both arms in terms of response rate, progression-free survival, and overall survival (16). As in the JCOG trial, there was more myelosuppression and febrile neutropenia associated with EP and more diarrhea with IP. A SWOG trial in the United States randomized 651 patients with previously untreated ES-SCLC to receive IP or EP using the same regimens and schedules as reported by JCOG, and again found no significant difference in efficacy between the two arms (17). The combination of cisplatin plus oral topotecan, a topoisomerase 1 inhibitor related to irinotecan, was also compared to EP in 784 patients with previously untreated ES-SCLC with the finding that efficacy was similar in both arms (18). QOL analysis on this trial slightly favored EP (P = .049).

Although most of the randomized studies in ES-SCLC have utilized cisplatin-based combinations, there is evidence that carboplatin-based regimens yield similar response rates and survival. Studies directly comparing cisplatin plus etoposide to carboplatin plus etoposide have demonstrated equivalent efficacy in patients with ES-SCLC (19). Depending on the degree of response, a maximum of 4 to 6 cycles of initial chemotherapy should be administered. Elderly patients over 70 years of age have similar survival rates when compared with younger patients if they have a good performance status. Therefore, performance status and comorbidities, rather than age, should guide therapy. Overall, the combination of a platinum plus etoposide results in objective response rates of 60% to 70%, complete response rates of 10%, median survival of 8 to 10 months, and a 2-year survival of 5%. Despite these dismal long-term survival rates, platinum plus etoposide combinations remain the standard-of-care for patients with SCLC.

Encouraging data have been reported from phase II trials in patients with ES-SCLC with a variety of other doublet and triplet regimens incorporating newer chemotherapy agents, such as carboplatin plus paclitaxel and paclitaxel plus topotecan. However, it is highly unlikely that any of these empiric regimens will result in dramatic improvements in long-term survival. Numerous chemotherapy-based strategies, including dose-intensification, weekly administration, triplet therapy, high-dose consolidation, alternating or sequential non-cross-resistant regimens, and maintenance therapy, have failed to yield consistent or convincing improvements in survival, and several of these approaches have resulted in unacceptable toxicity.

Prophylactic Cranial Irradiation

The role of PCI in patients with ES-SCLC was evaluated by the EORTC in a trial in which 286 patients with ES-SCLC who had responded to initial chemotherapy were randomized to receive PCI or no PCI (20). In this trial, PCI significantly decreased the incidence of symptomatic brain metastases (14.6% vs. 40.4%; $P < .001$) and increased the 1-year survival rate (27.1% vs. 13.3%; $P = .003$). Although PCI did have a negative effect on quality-of-life (QOL) within the first 3 months of treatment, by 6 months there was no significant difference in global QOL scores between patients who did or did not receive PCI (21). Importantly, this trial excluded patients over 75 years of age, so the benefits of PCI in elderly patients remain unclear. PCI is now recommended for patients with ES-SCLC who have responded to initial therapy along the same guidelines as those noted above for patients with LS-SCLC.

Paraneoplastic Syndromes

The neuroendocrine nature of SCLC cells is responsible for the relatively common occurrence of neurologic and endocrine paraneoplastic syndromes in this disease. Hyponatremia, due to ectopic secretion of antidiuretic hormone (ADH) or atrial natiuretic peptide (ANP), is observed in up to 15% of patients with SCLC. Cushing's syndrome, due to ectopic ACTH secretion, occurs in 2% to 5% of patients (22). Both of these syndromes are reversible with successful treatment of the disease, though the metabolic derangements should be medically managed and controlled before initiating anticancer therapy. Neurologic paraneoplastic syndromes, typically caused by antibodies that crossreact between antigens on SCLC cells and neurons, occur less frequently, but are generally more debilitating. Most of these neurologic syndromes, such as subacute cerebellar degeneration and limbic encephalopathy, are irreversible since they are caused by antibodies that are cytotoxic to specific neurons. One notable exception is Lambert-Eaton myasthenic syndrome in which the proximal myopathy may improve as the disease is treated and the causative antibodies that interfere with presynaptic voltage-gated calcium channels are suppressed. Clinical recognition of paraneoplastic syndromes is important as it may allow for detection of SCLC at an earlier stage of disease.

Recurrent Disease

The majority of patients with SCLC will develop recurrent disease, which has been divided into two categories: refractory/resistant (primary progression or recurrence < 3 months after initial therapy) or relapsed/sensitive (recurrence > 3 months after initial therapy), with much lower responses to second-line therapy in patients with refractory/resistant disease. Trials have suggested that re-initiation of the initial chemotherapy regimen results in response rates of 50% to 60% in patients whose initial response duration was greater than 6 to 8 months (23). Therefore, re-induction with the initial chemotherapy regimen is recommended for patients relapsing after >6 months after the initial therapy, while a second-line agent, such as topotecan or paclitaxel, is more appropriate for those relapsing within 6 months.

The survival benefit of second-line chemotherapy was demonstrated in a randomized trial comparing oral topotecan to best supportive care in 141 patients with recurrent SCLC. Although the response rate to oral topotecan was only 7%, overall survival was significantly better in patients receiving chemotherapy (median, 26 vs. 14 weeks; 6-month, 49% vs. 26%; $P = .01$) (24). In phase II trials, combination chemotherapy regimens generally demonstrate higher response rates than single agents, but overall survival does not appear to be improved and the toxicity of combination regimens can be challenging. One randomized phase III trial directly compared single-agent topotecan to the combination of cyclophosphamide, doxorubicin, and vincristine (CAV) in 211 patients with SCLC who

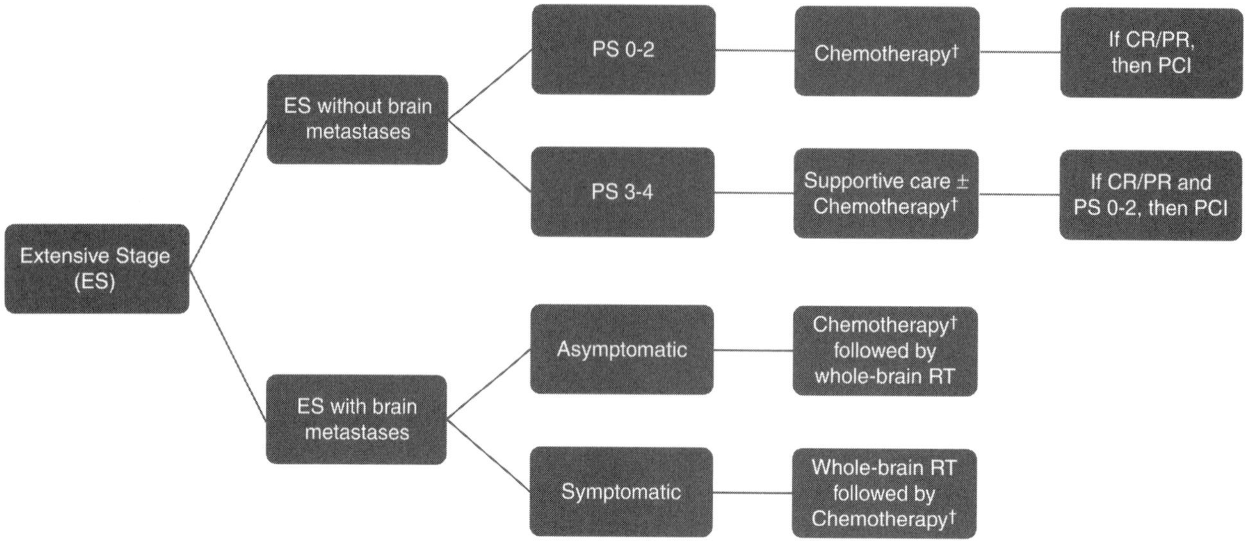

PS, Zubrod performance status; CR, complete response; PR, partial response
†Chemotherapy = platinum-based two-drug regimen (carboplatin + etoposide preferred)

Figure 4.2

Treatment algorithm for ES-SCLC.

had relapsed more than 60 days after initial therapy (25). This trial reported no significant difference in response rate (24% vs. 18%; *P* = .29), time to progression (13 vs. 12 weeks; *P* = .55), or overall survival (median, 25 vs. 25 weeks; *P* = .79) between patients treated with topotecan versus CAV, though toxicity was significantly greater with CAV (25). On the basis of these results, single-agent chemotherapy is considered the standard approach for patients with relapsed SCLC. Figure 4.2 is an algorithm for the treatment of patients with ES-SCLS.

Investigational Agents

Amrubicin is an investigational anthracycline that has promising activity in patients with SCLC. A phase II trial of single-agent amrubicin in 75 patients from the United States and Europe with refractory SCLC reported a response rate of 21%, disease control rate of 52%, median survival of 6 months, and 1-year survival of 16% (26). A small, randomized phase II trial from Japan comparing amrubicin to topotecan in 59 patients with recurrent SCLC reported a significantly better response rate (38% vs. 13%, *P* = .04) and disease control rate (79% vs. 46%, *P* = .02) in patients receiving amrubicin, but severe hematologic and nonhematologic toxicities were both more common in patients receiving amrubicin (27).

Over the past 30 years, we have gained extensive knowledge of the biology of SCLC, and preclinical studies have identified a plethora of molecular therapeutic targets. Many therapeutic agents aimed at these targets have been evaluated in phase II and III clinical trials in patients with SCLC, but thus far, none have demonstrated promising clinical activity. Among these failed approaches are anti-angiogenic agents (e.g., vandetinib, cediranib), metalloproteinase inhibitors (e.g., marimastat), growth factor inhibitors (e.g., dasatinib, imatinib), signal transduction pathway inhibitors (e.g., everolimus), retinoids (e.g., fenretinide), and pro-apoptotic agents (e.g., oblimersen). Despite these setbacks, an unprecedented number of novel, rational, molecular strategies are now being evaluated in preclinical and clinical trials in SCLC, including those targeting angiogenesis (e.g., bevacizumab), apoptotic pathways (e.g., small molecule Bcl-2 inhibitors), and cancer stem cells (e.g., Notch and hedgehog signaling). It is unlikely that empiric chemotherapy will lead to further significant improvements in patients with SCLC. Future advances will rely on on-going efforts to identify molecular targets that drive the survival, proliferation, and metastatic potential of cancer cells.

REFERENCES

1. Pignon JP, Arriagada R, Ihde DC, et al. A meta-analysis of thoracic radiotherapy for small-cell lung cancer. *N Engl J Med.* 1992;327:1618–1624.
2. Warde P, Payne D. Does thoracic irradiation improve survival and local control in limited-stage small-cell carcinoma of the lung? A meta-analysis. *J Clin Oncol.* 1992;10:890–895.
3. Fried DB, Morris DE, Poole C, et al. Systematic review evaluating the timing of thoracic radiation therapy in combined modality therapy for limited-stage small cell lung cancer. *J Clin Oncol.* 2004;22:4785–4793.

4. Turrisi AT, Kim K, Blum R, et al. Twice-daily compared with once-daily thoracic radiotherapy in limited small-cell lung cancer treated concurrently with cisplatin and etoposide. *N Engl J Med.* 1999;340:265–271.
5. Bonner JA, Sloan JA, Shanahan TG, et al. Phase III comparison of twice-daily split-course irradiation versus once-daily irradiation for patients with limited-stage small-cell lung carcinoma. *J Clin Oncol.* 1999;17:2681–2691.
6. Hann CL, Rudin CM. Management of small-cell lung cancer: incremental changes but hope for the future. *Oncology.* 2008; 22:1486–1492.
7. Auperin A, Arriagada R, Pignon JP, et al. Prophylactic cranial irradiation for patients with small-cell lung cancer in complete remission. Prophylactic Cranial Irradiation Overview Collaborative Group. *N Engl J Med.* 1999;341:476–484.
8. Patel S, Macdonald OK, Suntharalingam M. Evaluation of the use of prophylactic cranial irradiation in small cell lung cancer. *Cancer.* 2009;115:842–850
9. Tsuchiya R, Suzuki K, Ichinose Y, et al. Phase II trial of postoperative adjuvant cisplatin and etoposide in patients with completely resected stage I-IIIa small cell lung cancer: the Japan Clinical Oncology Lung Cancer Study Group Trial (JCOG9101). *J Thorac Cardiovasc Surg.* 2005;129:977–983.
10. Lowenbraun S, Bartolucci A, Smalley RV, et al. The superiority of combination chemotherapy over single agent chemotherapy in small cell lung carcinoma. *Cancer.* 1979;44:406–413.
11. Evans WK, Shepherd FA, Feld R, et al. VP-16 and cisplatin as first-line therapy for small-cell lung cancer. *J Clin Oncol.* 1985;3:1471–1477.
12. Sundstrøm S, Bremnes RM, Kaasa S, et al. Cisplatin and etoposide regimen is superior to cyclophosphamide, epirubicin, and vincristine regimen in small-cell lung cancer: results from a randomized phase III trial with 5 years' follow-up. *J Clin Oncol.* 2002;20:4665–4672.
13. Pujol JL, Carestia L, Duares JP. Is there a case for cisplatin in the treatment of small-cell lung cancer? A meta-analysis of randomized trials of a cisplatin-containing regimen versus a regimen without this alkylating agent. *Br J Cancer.* 2000;83: 8–15.
14. Chute JP, Chen T, Feigal, et al. Twenty years of phase III trials for patients with extensive-stage small-cell lung cancer: perceptible progress. *J Clin Oncol.* 1999;17:1794–1801.
15. Noda K, Nishiwaki Y, Kawahara M, et al. Irinotecan plus cisplatin compared with etoposide plus cisplatin for extensive small-cell lung cancer. *N Engl J Med.* 2002;346:85–91.
16. Hanna N, Bunn PA, Langer C, et al. Randomized phase III trial comparing irinotecan/cisplatin with etoposide/cisplatin in patients with previously untreated extensive-stage small-cell lung cancer. *J Clin Oncol.* 2006;24:2038–2043.
17. Lara PN, Natale R, Crowley J, et al. Phase III trial of irinotecan/cisplatin compared with etoposide/cisplatin in extensive-stage small-cell lung cancer: clinical and pharmacogenomic results from SWOG S0124. *J Clin Oncol.* 2009;27:2530–2535.
18. Eckardt JR, von Pawel J, Papai Z, et al. Open-label, multicenter, randomized, phase III study comparing oral topotecan/cislplatin versus etoposide/cisplatin as treatment for chemotherapy-naive patients with extensive-disease small-cell lung cancer. *J Clin Oncol.* 2006;24:2044–2051.
19. Okamoto H, Watanabe K, Kunikane H, et al. Randomised phase III trial of carboplatin plus etoposide vs split doses of cisplatin plus etoposide in elderly or poor-risk patients with extensive disease small-cell lung cancer: JCOG 9702. *Br J Cancer.* 2007;97:162–169.
20. Slotman B, Faivre-Finn C, Kramer G, et al. Prophylactic cranial irradiation in extensive small-cell lung cancer. *N Engl J Med.* 2007;357:664–672.
21. Slotman BJ, Mauer ME, Bottomley A, et al. Prophylactic cranial irradiation in extensive disease small-cell lung cancer: short-term health-related quality of life and patient reported symptoms: results of an international Phase III randomized controlled trial by the EORTC Radiation Oncology and Lung Cancer Groups. *J Clin Oncol.* 2009;27:78–84.
22. Marchioli CC, Graziano SL. Paraneoplastic syndromes associated with small cell lung cancer. *Chest Surg Clinics North Am.* 1997; 7:65–80.
23. Postmus PE, Berendsen HH, van Zandwijk N, et al. Retreatment with the induction regimen in small cell lung cancer relapsing after an initial response to short term chemotherapy. *Eur J Cancer Clin Oncol.* 1987;23:1409–1411.
24. O'Brien MER, Ciuleanu TE, Tsekov H, et al. Phase III trial comparing supportive care alone with supportive care with oral topotecan in patients with relapsed small-cell lung cancer. *J Clin Oncol.* 2006;24:5441–5447.
25. Von Pawel J, Schiller JH, Shepherd FA, et al. Topotecan versus cyclophosphamide, doxorubicin, and vincristine for the treatment of recurrent small-cell lung cancer. *J Clin Oncol.* 1999;17:658–667.
26. Ettinger DS, Jotte R, Lorigan P, et al. Phase II study of amrubicin as second-line therapy in patients with platinum-refractory small-cell lung cancer. *J Clin Oncol.* 2010;28:2598–2603.
27. Inoue A, Sugawara S, Yamazaki K, et al. Randomized phase II trial comparing amrubicin with topotecan in patients with previously treated small-cell lung cancer: North Japan Lung Cancer Study Group trial 0402. *J Clin Oncol.* 2008;26:5401–5406.

5

Breast Cancer

AIHUA EDWARD YEN, MICHELINA M. CAIRO, AND MOTHAFFAR F. RIMAWI

EPIDEMIOLOGY, RISK FACTORS, NATURAL HISTORY, AND PATHOLOGY

Breast cancer is the leading cause of cancer in women in the United States, representing 32% of all new cancer cases. It is the second most common cause of cancer death in the United States (15%) second only to lung cancer (25%) and is the most common cause of death from cancer in women aged 20 to 59 years. The lifetime risk of developing breast cancer is 12%, or 1 in 8, and more than 90% of women will have only localized disease at the time of diagnosis. Women with metastatic disease have a 20% chance of being alive for 5 years.

There are several known risk factors for breast cancer and some are modifiable thus allowing for preventative interventions. Age, family history, age at first full-term pregnancy, early menarche, late menopause, and breast density are not necessarily modifiable. However, postmenopausal obesity, use of menopausal hormones, alcohol consumption, and physical inactivity are associated with significantly increased breast cancer risk and intervention with lifestyle modifications may reduce that risk.

Besides female gender, age is the most important risk factor for developing breast cancer. The risk of developing breast cancer begins to climb at age 40 and accelerates after menopause. Therefore, breast cancer is considered to be largely a disease of postmenopausal age. Long-term exposure to hormones may contribute to the increased risk of developing breast cancer with increased age.

Women with a family history of breast cancer are at an increased risk of developing breast cancer. Having more than one first-degree relative with breast cancer confers higher risk and that risk increases the younger the relative was at the time of diagnosis. A history of ovarian cancer in first-degree relatives may be associated with certain breast cancer syndromes and increased breast cancer risk. Approximately 5% to 10% of breast cancer cases result from inherited mutations in the breast cancer susceptibility genes *BRCA1* or *BRCA2*. Women with *BRCA1* mutations are estimated to have an 87% risk for developing breast cancer by age 70. For *BRCA2* mutations, the corresponding risk is 49% to 87%. Breast cancer may also result from other less common syndromes such as Li Fraumeni or Cowden syndrome. Identified mutations only account for about 50% of heritable breast cancer.

Reproductive hormones are believed to influence breast cancer risk. Early menarche (<12 years) and older age at menopause (>55 years) increase the risk of breast cancer most likely by duration of exposure of breast tissue to reproductive hormones. For example, younger age at first full-term pregnancy (<30 years) and a greater number of pregnancies and longer duration of breastfeeding decreases the risk of breast cancer over the long term. Paradoxically, there is a transient increase in breast cancer risk following pregnancy. Recent use of hormones also appears to be a risk factor. Oral contraceptive use may slightly increase breast cancer risk, but it falls to normal risk after 10 years of nonuse.

Hormone replacement therapy with combined estrogen and progestin (but not with estrogen only) has been shown to increase breast cancer with risk increasing with longer use. The risk appears to decrease within 5 years of discontinuation of hormone use.

Though the incidence of breast cancer is higher in white women, black women are more likely to die of the disease. While the 5-year survival for white women is 90%, it is 77% for black women. Younger age at diagnosis, more advanced stage at diagnosis, and higher probability of triple negative cancer may in part explain this discrepancy.

Other factors that increase the risk of breast cancer include breast density. Women with dense breasts by BIRADS criteria have a four to six fold increase in breast cancer risk. Increased bone mineral density in postmenopausal women increases risk of breast cancer, which may be mediated by hormonal effects.

Atypical proliferative lesions including atypical ductal hyperplasia (ADH) and atypical lobular hyperplasia

(ALH) are associated with 4 to 5 times the risk of breast cancer. Radiation exposure is also a breast cancer risk factor, with the highest risk involving women treated with high-dose radiation for cancer in childhood such as mantle radiation for Hodgkin's Lymphoma.

Early-stage breast cancer has a high probability of cure. Women with localized breast cancer that has not spread to locoregional lymph nodes have a 98% 5-year relative overall survival (OS) (compared with women who do not have cancer). Tumor size is one of the best-validated clinical factors. Studies have shown that tumors less than 1 cm in size have good prognosis in patients without lymph node involvement. Once the tumor spreads to regional lymph nodes, survival falls to 83%. The number of positive axillary lymph nodes is the most powerful prognostic indicator and is a poor prognostic sign. The risk increases with the number of lymph nodes involved. However, even metastatic breast cancer may be treatable and has a 23.4% 5-year survival.

Although rare pathologic subtypes can be seen, most breast cancers are adenocarcinomas that are subdivided into noninvasive (carcinoma in situ) and invasive. Among invasive adenocarcinomas, there are two dominant subtypes, invasive lobular carcinoma (ILC) and invasive ductal carcinoma (IDC), which carry a similar prognosis stage for stage.

Ductal carcinomas account for about 90% of all breast cancers. The majority of invasive ductal carcinomas are no special type (NST). Tubular and mucinous carcinomas are special subtypes of ductal carcinomas and account for 5% to 8%. They are almost universally ER-positive and they have an excellent prognosis.

Medullary carcinomas represent another special type of breast cancer and include 3% to 5% of ductal carcinomas. They tend to be negative for estrogen receptor (ER), the progesterone receptor (PR), and the human epidermal growth factor-2 (HER2) (triple negative) and are found more commonly in patients with *BRCA1* gene mutations. Poorly differentiated histology and higher nuclear grade have a worse prognosis.

Certain biomarkers have emerged as important factors affecting the natural history and treatment of breast cancer. The three most validated biomarkers in breast cancer are the ER, the progesterone receptor PR, and HER2. They are valuable prognostic markers and also predict for response to therapy. The majority of breast cancers (70% or more) are positive for the hormone receptors (ER and/or PR), and 25% are HER2-amplified or over-expressing (HER2-positive). Although ER-positive and/or PR-positive breast cancer has a better prognosis, it is also responsive to hormonal therapy. HER2 over-expressing breast cancer has a worse prognosis as it correlates to a more aggressive tumor subtype but is also a valuable target for HER2 targeted therapy.

In the last decade, molecular expression profiling has led to the identification of molecular subtypes of breast cancer, namely, luminal A and B, basal type, HER2-positive, and normal-like. The molecular portraits revealed in the patterns of gene expression do have characteristics in common with clinical phenotypes; ER-positive breast cancer correlates to luminal A and B molecular subtypes, HER2 over-expressing breast cancer correlates to the HER2-positive subtype, and triple negative breast cancer correlates to the basal-type subtype. Although not yet used in clinical practice, these molecular subtypes shed light on the heterogeneity of breast cancer and are the subjects of ongoing research to characterize clinical and biological behavior and develop new therapeutics.

Gene profiling assays have become important prognostic and predictive tests in the appropriate setting. As described later in the chapter, two gene-expression tests are available to assist in the management of breast cancer: Oncotype DX and MammaPrint. Both gene assays are used routinely in clinical practice to determine risk of recurrence and aid the decision on adjuvant chemotherapy in appropriate patients.

STAGING

The AJCC staging system for breast cancer is shown below.

Breast Cancer Clinical Staging

Stage	Definition
0	Ductal carcinoma in situ
IA	Tumor less than 2 cm in greatest dimension (T1); no regional lymph node metastases
IB	No evidence of primary tumor (T0) or a T1 tumor either with microscopic invasion of 1–3 ipsilateral axillary lymph nodes (N1 mic)
IIA	No evidence of primary tumor (T0) or a T1 tumor either with metastases in 1–3 ipsilateral, mobile axillary lymph nodes (N1), OR a tumor of >2 cm but <5 cm (T2) with no axillary lymph nodes (N0)
IIB	Tumor <5 cm (T2) with invasion in 1–3 ipsilateral, mobile axillary lymph nodes (T1) OR a tumor >5 cm (T3) with no axillary lymph node metastases (N0)
IIIA	Tumor of any size (T0, T1, T2, or T3) with invasion into ipsilateral fixed or matted axillary lymph nodes, clinically apparent internal mammary lymph nodes, or pathological involvement of 4–9 axillary lymph nodes (N2), OR a tumor >5 cm (T3) with metastases in 1–9 ipsilateral, mobile, or fixed axillary lymph nodes (N1, N2)
IIIB	Tumor of any size with direct extension to the chest wall or the skin (T4) with or without metastases to ipsilateral, axillary lymph nodes (N0 to N2)
IIIC	Tumor of any size with metastases to ipsilateral infraclavicular and axillary, ipsilateral internal mammary and axillary, or ipsilateral supraclavicular lymph nodes; or pathological involvement of >10 axillary lymph nodes (N3)
IV	Tumor of any size, presence or absence of lymph node metastases, with distant metastatic disease (M1)

CASE SUMMARIES

Ductal Carcinoma In Situ

L.P. is a healthy 48-year-old woman who was found to have an abnormal screening mammogram, with a cluster of pleomorphic calcifications in the left breast. Her physical exam showed no palpable masses, dimpling, nipple discharge, or lymphadenopathy. A stereotactic core biopsy showed ductal carcinoma in situ (DCIS), ER-positive and PR-positive. Her mother died of metastatic breast cancer, and she was referred to a multidisciplinary breast care clinic seeking treatment recommendations.

Evidence-Based Case Discussion

L.P. has DCIS. Annually in the United States there are more than 50,000 cases of DCIS. By definition, it is noninvasive, and the basement membrane of the ductal unit is preserved. However, recurrences may present even after 15 years, and half of those recurrences become invasive cancer. DCIS represents a heterogeneous group, and various treatment options exist. Surgery is the primary treatment modality for this localized breast cancer and may be offered as mastectomy or breast conservation surgery (also known as segmental mastectomy, partial mastectomy, or lumpectomy).

Regarding the choice of surgery, lumpectomy followed by radiation therapy is equivalent to mastectomy as shown by the NSABP B-06 trial. Comparing breast conserving surgery plus postoperative radiotherapy with breast conserving surgery alone showed an increased risk of local recurrence if radiotherapy is omitted (39% chance of ipsilateral breast tumor vs. 14.3%; $P < .001$) (1). Cosmetically acceptable breast preservation was achieved in a subset of patients who underwent lumpectomy and axillary lymph node dissection plus radiation therapy. After 20 years of follow-up there continue to be no significant differences in overall survival (OS) and disease-free survival (DFS) between the group of patients who underwent total mastectomy and the group treated with lumpectomy and breast radiation.

Adjuvant radiotherapy is beneficial for DCIS, but not all experts agree on its use across all cases of DCIS. Large prospective trials such as NSABP B-17 and EORTC 10853 showed that radiation following breast conservation therapy significantly reduced local recurrences, but did not translate to an OS benefit. These findings are limited by trial design. In both trials, only DCIS with smaller sizes were included in the studies, and margin widths were not quantified. Also, postsurgical mammograms were not routinely performed, making confirmation of successful resection impossible.

Data from retrospective and small prospective studies have consistently showed that tumor size, pathologic grade, histologic type, presence of necrosis, patient age, and margin width are associated with recurrence. Four risk factors, including pathologic classification, margin size, tumor size, and age, were incorporated into the Van Nuys Prospective Index (VNPI) for use as a risk-adapted clinical tool for adjuvant management. A scoring number is assigned to each risk factor, and the sum is then classified as low—4 to 6; intermediate—7 to 9; or high risk—10 to 12. Risk-dependent management decisions may include breast conservation therapy and observation alone, breast conservation therapy and radiotherapy, or mastectomy. Unfortunately, subsequent prospective trials using the VNPI have produced conflicting results, and there has not yet been a large prospective, randomized trial validating the VNPI. It should be used only with caution and in selected patients.

The role of adjuvant hormonal therapy is also being investigated. The NSABP B-24 trial, a prospective, randomized study, evaluated adjuvant tamoxifen after lumpectomy and radiation in women with extensive DCIS, or those with close margins (2). At 7 years, the tamoxifen-treated group had a 10.3% recurrence rate in breast cancer events compared with 16.9% in the placebo arm. Also in the tamoxifen arm, invasive breast cancer events were reduced by 48% and contralateral breast cancer events were reduced from 3.2% to 1.8%. The UK CCCR DCIS trial failed to achieve the same significant results with adjuvant tamoxifen after lumpectomy and surgery. Tamoxifen only reduced the risk from 15% to 13%. However, their study group excluded patients with older age and positive margins. Neither group initially evaluated ER status, but a post hoc analysis of NSABP B-24 did report that in those women with ER-positive DCIS, tamoxifen significantly reduced incidence of breast cancer by 59% versus 20% in those who were ER-negative (2). Ongoing trials are evaluating the use of adjuvant aromatase inhibitors versus tamoxifen in postmenopausal women with DCIS after breast conservation therapy and radiation.

For L.P., the recommendations should include breast conservation therapy and adjuvant radiation. The VNPI may be applied cautiously as a guideline. Tamoxifen should be offered to further decrease the low chances of contralateral breast cancer and ipsilateral recurrence. Figure 5.1 provides a treatment algorithm for patients with DCIS.

Early-Stage ER-Positive Breast Cancer

J.S. is a 51-year-old perimenopausal woman who underwent a routine screening mammogram that showed a 1.3 cm × 1.4 cm spiculated mass in the left breast. On physical examination, her axillary lymph nodes were not palpably enlarged. An ultrasound-guided core needle biopsy revealed IDC, ER-positive, PR-positive, HER2-negative by immunohistochemistry.

After multidisciplinary clinical evaluation, J.S. opted for breast conservation therapy and underwent left breast

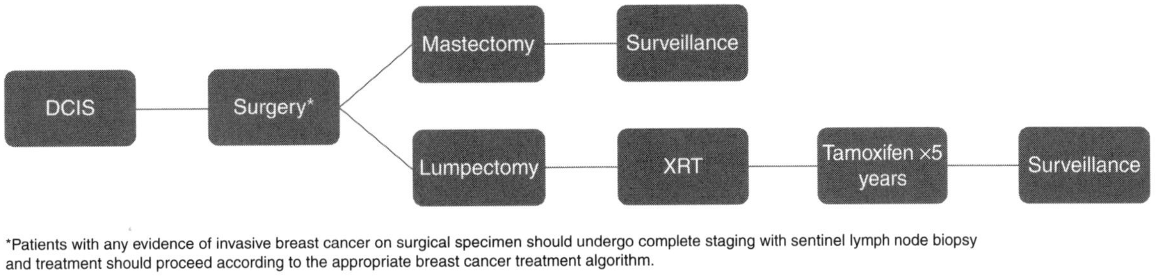

Figure 5.1

Treatment algorithm for DCIS.

lumpectomy with sentinel lymph node biopsy. The surgical pathology revealed IDC, 1.9 cm in greatest diameter, histological grade 2, Ki67 31%, ER-positive (90% staining, 3+ intensity), PR-positive (50% staining, 2+ intensity), and HER2-negative (2+ IHC, FISH ratio 1.3). Surgical margins were free of tumor. Three sentinel lymph nodes were removed and were not involved with cancer.

Evidence-Based Case Discussion

J.S. has a T1 N0 (stage I) left breast IDC. Regarding the choice of surgery, lumpectomy followed by radiation therapy is equivalent to mastectomy as shown by the NSABP B-06 trial discussed earlier (1). Sentinel lymph node biopsy provides adequate axillary lymph node staging when negative. A more recent study, the ACOSOG Z0011, suggests that there is no survival advantage to axillary lymph node dissection compared to sentinel lymph node biopsy even when 1 to 2 nodes are positive (3). It is noteworthy that this study was done in patients with clinically negative axillary nodes, with tumors less than 5 cm in size, who underwent lumpectomy and received no neoadjuvant targeted therapy or chemotherapy. In this select group of patients that includes J.S., it is therefore possible to rely on sentinel lymph node biopsy and spare them the potential morbidity of axillary lymph node dissection. Studies are ongoing to determine whether micrometastases detected by hematoxylin and eosin (H&E) stain or IHC on sentinel lymph node biopsy influence survival. The data from ACOSOG Z0010 and NSABP B-32 are thus far concordant with Z0011 (3,4).

The question then arises as to whether or not J.S. would benefit from systemic adjuvant therapy, and there are several factors to be considered. Adjuvant systemic therapy for hormone receptor positive, HER2-negative breast tumors can include endocrine therapy alone or chemotherapy followed by endocrine therapy. When considering chemotherapy, there are factors relating to the disease and factors relating to the patient's general health. Competing comorbidities need to be weighed against the potential benefits of therapy. First we consider the patient factors. J.S. is an otherwise healthy woman who has no contraindications to adjuvant therapy.

We then consider the features of her tumor. This patient has multiple favorable indicators including a small tumor that is node-negative. Her tumor is ER-positive and PR-positive, which predicts better outcome and response to hormone therapy. Estrogen receptor content is reported as positive or negative based on the Allred score (see Table 5.1). The tumor cells are stained with the hormone receptor antibody and both the percentage of positively staining tumor cells and the average intensity of the staining are independently graded. The resulting estrogen receptor proportion score and intensity score are added together resulting in the Allred score. The Allred score has been prospectively validated to correlate to endocrine therapy responsiveness. In prospectively validated clinical trials, patients with Allred scores of 3 to 8 derive additional benefit from endocrine therapy. Allred scores of 0 to 2 are reported as negative because patients with these scores did not derive additional benefit from adjuvant endocrine therapy. J.S. has an Allred score of 8 given the 90% ER staining and strong intensity, so she would be expected to have a favorable response to endocrine therapy. In some patients, the progesterone content may not correlate to the estrogen content. Retrospective analysis of endocrine therapy treatment outcomes in women whose estrogen receptor was positive but whose progesterone receptor was negative revealed that these patients had worse outcomes than those patients whose progesterone receptor was positive.

In addition, J.S's tumor is negative for HER2 overexpression. Measurement of HER2 expression by IHC has also been standardized. ASCO-CAP recommendations suggest that HER2 staining of 0 to 1+ is negative. 3+ staining is positive and these patients benefit from targeted HER2 therapy. 2+ staining is equivocal and requires additional testing with fluorescence in situ hybridization (FISH) gene amplification. FISH score is reported as a ratio of HER2 expression compared to a standard marker CEP-17. A ratio less than 1.8 is negative, 1.8 to 2.2 is intermediate, and greater than 2.2 is positive. Less commonly, the results can be reported in terms of HER2 gene copy number. A HER2 gene copy number less than 4 is negative, 4 to 6 is intermediate, and greater than 6 is positive. J.S.'s

Table 5.1 Allred Score

Allred Score for ER Status

Proportion Score	Percentage of Positive Staining Cells	Intensity Score	Average Intensity of Positively Stained Cells
0	None	0	None
1	<1	1	Weak
2	1–10	2	Intermediate
3	10–33	3	Strong
4	33–66		
5	66–100		

Interpretation of Allred Score

Sum of Proportion and Intensity Score	Interpretation
0, 2	Negative
3–8	Positive

Derived from JM Harvey et al. (5).

ratio of HER2 to CEP-17 expression is 1.3 so she does not qualify for HER2 targeted therapy. J.S.'s tumor also has two less favorable pathologic features. The tumor grade, a measure of aggressiveness derived from the degree of cellular atypia, is intermediate. In addition, the proliferation index, Ki67, is high suggesting rapid growth. Considering J.S.'s tumor is ER-positive and HER2-negative, which portends a good prognosis, but intermediate grade with a high Ki67, which suggests poor prognosis, we conclude that this is an intermediate-risk case based on the clinical and pathologic features.

As illustrated by this case, it can be difficult to determine from clinical and pathologic features which patients are at highest risk of recurrence and would benefit most from adjuvant treatment and which patients could be spared the toxicity and risks associated with chemotherapy. On the basis of the intermediate clinical and pathologic features, the option of administering systemic chemotherapy prior to hormonal therapy will be discussed with J.S.

In the circumstance in which the clinical and pathologic features do not help to make a clear treatment decision, molecular tests have become available to provide additional information about the risk of recurrence. These include the 21-gene signature, Oncotype DX, and the 70-gene signature, MammaPrint. MammaPrint uses fresh frozen tissue from node-negative, ER-positive or ER-negative patients <61 years of age with tumor size <5 cm. This assay reports 10-year survival rates as either high risk or low risk. Oncotype DX analyzes expression of 21 genes in formalin-fixed paraffin-embedded tissue from node-negative, ER-positive patients. This assay reports a recurrence score that determines the 10-year risk of distant recurrence and categorizes it as low, medium, or high risk. Oncotype DX was retrospectively validated on the NSABP B14 trial in which tamoxifen was compared to tamoxifen plus CMF. Patients were both pre- and postmenopausal. The gene-expression array was performed on the stored tumor blocks and the scores correlated to the clinical outcome. Patients with high scores benefit from adjuvant chemotherapy while those with low scores may be treated with adjuvant endocrine therapy alone. In the intermediate group there is no conclusive evidence on which to make a treatment decision, but the Tailor Rx trial was designed to address this question. ER-positive, node-negative patients who underwent Oncotype DX testing were eligible to participate in the trial. If their recurrence score was low or high they were treated with endocrine therapy or chemotherapy, respectively. In the case of intermediate recurrence scores, patients were randomized to chemotherapy or endocrine therapy. Tailor Rx recently completed accrual and it is hoped the results will help objectively determine whether intermediate risk patients would benefit from chemotherapy.

Large randomized studies have shown that the adjuvant use of tamoxifen—a selective ER modulator—for 5 years decreases the risk of recurrence of breast cancer by 45% to 50% and the risk of death by 31%, and the benefit persists for years after therapy is discontinued (6). Treatment beyond 5 years offers no additional benefit and there is potential for an increase in the risk of toxicities such as endometrial cancer and thromboembolism. Tamoxifen is effective in both premenopausal and postmenopausal women, though a greater benefit was seen in postmenopausal patients.

Several trials have assessed the utility of aromatase inhibitors in postmenopausal women with ER-positive or PR-positive breast cancer (Table 5.2). These agents

Table 5.2 Clinical Trials of Adjuvant Endocrine Therapy in Postmenopausal Women with Hormone Receptor-Positive Tumors: A Comparison of Therapy Involving the Use of Aromatase Inhibitors as Compared to Tamoxifen Alone

Trial Design	Median Follow-Up (Months)	Aromatase Inhibitor	Disease-Free Survival		Overall Survival	
			Hazard Ratio	*P*-value	Hazard Ratio	*P*-value
Sequential						
ABCSG 8	72	Anastrozole	0.85	0.067	0.78	0.032
ARNO 95	30	Anastrozole	0.66	0.049	0.53	0.045
IES	55.7	Exemestane	0.76	<.001	0.85	0.08
ITA	64	Anastrozole	0.57	0.005	0.56	0.1
TEAM*	61	Exemestane	0.97	0.604	1	0.999
BIG 1-98*	71	Letrozole	0.96	NR	0.9	NR
Upfront						
ATAC	100	Anastrozole	0.9	0.025	1	0.99
BIG 1-98	76	Letrozole	0.88	0.030	0.81	0.08
ABCSG 12	47.8	Anastrozole	1.1	0.590	1.8	0.7
Extended						
ABCSG 6a	62	Anastrozole	0.62	0.031	0.89	0.57
MA-17	30	Letrozole	0.68	<.001	0.98	0.853
NSABP B-33	30	Exemestane	0.68	0.070	NR	NR

*In TEAM and BIG 1–98, hazard ratio is reported for sequential therapy compared to AI alone, rather than to tamoxifen alone.

Extended refers to treatment with aromatase inhibitor after 5 years of tamoxifen therapy; *sequential* refers to treatment with aromatase inhibitor before or after 2–3 years of tamoxifen therapy; *upfront* refers to initial treatment with aromatase inhibitor. NR is not reported.

Adapted from ASCO Clinical Practice Guidelines (7).

have a different mechanism of action and a distinct side-effect profile compared to the selective ER modulators. Aromatase inhibitors are less likely than tamoxifen to increase the risk for thrombotic events or endometrial cancer; however, they are more likely to be associated with arthralgias and osteoporosis. In the largest clinical trials, arthralgias was reported in 11% to 36% of patients taking aromatase inhibitors compared with 5% to 30% of patients on tamoxifen. Bone mineral density is also more likely to be affected by aromatase inhibitors with a 2- to 3-fold decrease in bone mineral density, a 1.5-fold risk of osteoporosis, and a 1.5-fold risk of fracture when compared with tamoxifen. Tamoxifen use is associated with an increased risk of venous thrombotic events (3.9% vs. 1.7% in BIG 1–98) compared to aromatase inhibitors, but no increased incidence of cerebrovascular events. In addition, the risk of endometrial cancer was increased in patients taking tamoxifen compared to aromatase inhibitors (0.8% vs. 0.2% in the ATAC trial). There were no reported deaths from endometrial cancer in either group.

In several clinical studies including the ATAC, BIG 1–98, and EIS trials, there is a small but significant (2–5%) absolute advantage in DFS over tamoxifen alone when aromatase inhibitors were used in postmenopausal patients either upfront for 5 years or after 2 to 3 years of initial tamoxifen (8–10). Several studies included in Table 5.2 sought to determine the optimal sequence of adjuvant endocrine therapy.

On the basis of these data, the choice of hormone therapy in a postmenopausal woman should include an aromatase inhibitor, either upfront or after initial therapy with tamoxifen. As described later in the evidence-based discussion of metastatic breast cancer, aromatase inhibitors alone are not effective in premenopausal or perimenopausal women. Studies are underway comparing ovarian suppression therapy plus aromatase inhibitors to tamoxifen in premenopausal women. At this time, this strategy is reserved for patients with relative contraindications to tamoxifen therapy such as previous venous thromboembolic events.

In summary, in the case of J.S., a perimenopausal woman with a 1.9-cm, node- negative, ER-positive, PR-positive, HER2-negative IDC, who underwent breast conservation therapy, the decision to administer systemic chemotherapy can be made based on clinical and pathologic features alone. Alternatively, additional testing with a gene signature may be pursued. Should the result show high-risk disease, the patient would benefit from adjuvant systemic chemotherapy. If it shows low-risk disease, chemotherapy can be forgone as it offers little or no benefit to the patient. Evidence of benefit in patients with an intermediate risk is inconclusive and participation on a clinical

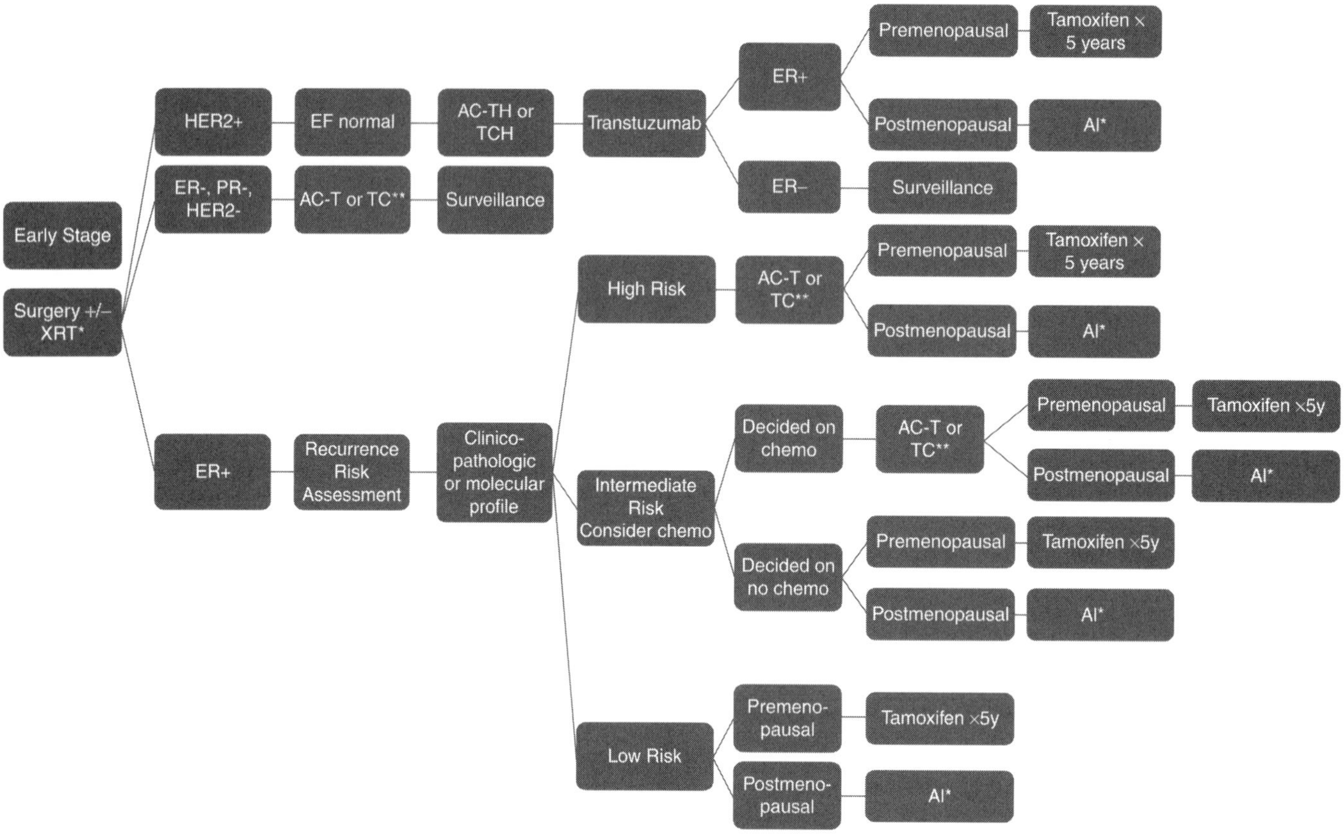

#Radiotherapy (XRT) is given to appropiately selected patients after the completion of adjuvant chemotherapy. It may be given concurrently with adjuvant HER2 targeted therapy or endocrine therapy.

+In the case of HER2+ tumors, trastuzumab (H) is added in combination with a taxane most commonly after AC.

**Adjuvant chemotherapy for breast cancer involves a combination of A (doxorubicin), C (cyclophosphamide), and T (taxane, either docetaxel or paclitaxel). In clinical trials they have been administered: sequentially AC-T, or concurrently TAC, or without anthracyclines (TC). TCH refers to docetaxel, carboplatin, and trastuzumab.

*AI = Aromatase inhibitor may be given for 5 years or for 2–3 years followed by tamoxifen to complete 5 years of adjuvant endocrine therapy. If tamoxifen was started when a patient was premenopausal it may be switched to AI when she is verifiably postmenopausal.

Figure 5.2

Treatment algorithm for early stage breast cancer.

trial may be appropriate where available. Otherwise, the decision needs to be based on the available clinicopathologic features and incorporating the patient's preferences.

Since J.S. is not verifiably postmenopausal, adjuvant hormonal therapy with tamoxifen is most appropriate. If the patient has spontaneous amenorrhea for 12 months (24 months for chemotherapy induced amenorrhea, preferably with a hormone profile consistent with postmenopausal status in either case), her therapy can be switched to an aromatase inhibitor after 2 to 3 years of tamoxifen for a total treatment time of 5 years. Figure 5.2 includes a suggested treatment algorithm for ER-positive, early-stage breast cancer.

Early-Stage ER-Positive Breast Cancer, Stages I or II

T.J. is a 48-year-old woman who underwent a yearly screening mammogram and was found to have an abnormal 1.3 × 1.0 cm mass in the right breast. No palpable axillary masses were found on examination, and ultrasound-guided core needle biopsy showed IDC, ER weakly positive, PR-negative, and HER2-negative (1+ by IHC). She had lumpectomy and sentinel lymph node biopsy, and the pathologic review of the surgical specimen showed IDC, 1.1 cm in greatest diameter, intermediate ER staining in 10% of the specimen, PR-negative, HER2-negative, grade 3, Ki67 of 46%, with two sentinel lymph nodes negative for malignancy. All margins were free of malignant involvement.

Evidence-Based Case Discussion

T.J. has right breast IDC, pathologic stage I (T1 N0). Although the staging is identical to the previous case, it is important to note that T.J. is younger and that the pathologic characteristics suggest a more aggressive tumor biology. Several features in this case speak toward a greater benefit from adjuvant chemotherapy than hormonal therapy: the patient's young age, the weak hormone receptor status, the high pathologic grade, and high proliferation rate. Oncotype DX testing may be performed to confirm her high risk, but it is reasonable to recommend adjuvant chemotherapy based on the characteristics described above. Since patients with high-risk, lymph-node-negative or lymph-node-positive disease generally benefit from adjuvant chemotherapy, the following discussion will apply to both subsets of patients.

Adjuvant chemotherapy may prolong survival and decrease the risk of relapse in early breast cancer. A large meta-analysis by the Early Breast Cancer Trialists' Collaborative Group (EBCTCG) pooled the results of 194 randomized trials for adjuvant chemotherapy and hormonal therapy initiated before or in 1995 (6). Overall, adjuvant chemotherapy reduced recurrences and improved mortality after 15 years of follow-up, particularly in patients younger than 50 years old compared with those 50 to 69 years old (12.3% vs. 4.5% recurrence rate reduction and 10% vs. 3% death rate reduction respectively). The use of an anthracycline-containing, polychemotherapy regimen showed significantly superior efficacy (0.89 recurrence rate ratio and 0.84 breast cancer death rate ratio) over those regimens without it (e.g., CMF—cyclophosphamide, methotrexate, fluorouracil). The benefit of chemotherapy appeared to be greater in ER-negative disease compared with that in ER-positive disease, with relative risk reductions in those 50 to 69 years old of 33% versus 14%. These cumulative results provided the rationale for anthracycline-containing regimens to be a standard of care for adjuvant treatment of breast cancer.

The use of taxanes in adjuvant chemotherapy has been explored in many trials (Table 5.3). Adding paclitaxel sequentially after an anthracycline-containing chemotherapy combination was shown in two phase III trials (NSABP B-28 and CALGB 9344) to improve disease-free survival. The E1199 trial evaluated two different taxanes, paclitaxel, and docetaxel, each in two different schedules. After treatment with four cycles of standard doxorubicin (Adriamycin) and cyclophosphamide (AC) chemotherapy, patients were randomized in a two-by-two factorial design to receive either paclitaxel or docetaxel administered on either a weekly or every 3-week regimen for 3 months. Approximately 10% of the study group had no nodes involved, and two-thirds had less than four lymph nodes involved. A small but significant benefit in 5-year OS was shown when paclitaxel was administered weekly as compared to every 3 weeks (89.7% vs. 86.5%; $P = .01$). Five-year DFS was also greatest in the same arm (81.5% vs. 76.9%; $P = .006$). Docetaxel given every 3 weeks was equivalent to weekly paclitaxel. Peripheral neuropathy was more frequently associated with weekly paclitaxel.

The role of dose density and different sequential scheduling including taxanes were compared in the CALGB 9741 trial. One hypothesis evaluated by this study was whether a dose-dense schedule (2-week cycle with filgrastim) or conventional length schedule (3-week cycle) was more efficacious. Total doses of chemotherapy agents were equivalent. The 4-year DFS (82% vs. 75%) and 3-year OS (92% vs. 90%) were improved in the dose-dense schedules, without a prohibitive increase in toxicity, due to primary filgrastim prophylaxis. A subgroup analysis showed most of the benefit to be derived by patients with ER-negative tumors.

The BCIRG 001 and the GEICAM 9805 trials demonstrated the feasibility and efficacy of combining a taxane with an anthracycline in the adjuvant therapy of node-positive and node-negative breast cancers, respectively (Table 5.3). In BCIRG 001, six cycles of TAC (docetaxel,

Table 5.3 Prospective, Randomized Controlled Trials for Adjuvant Chemotherapy for HER2-Negative Breast Cancer

Reference	Trial Name	*N*	Comparative Arms	DFS (%)*	OS (%)*
Mamounas et al., JCO 2005	NSABP B-28	3060	AC vs.	72	NS
			AC – paclitaxel	76	
Henderson et al., JCO 2003	CALGB 9344	3121	AC vs.	65	77
	(Intergroup 148)		AC – paclitaxel	70	80
Sparano et al., NEJM 2008	ECOG 1199	4950	AC – paclitaxel Q week vs.	81.5	89.7
			– docetaxel Q 3 weeks vs.	81.2	86.2
			– paclitaxel Q 3 weeks	76.9	86.5
Citron et al., JCO 2003	CALGB 9741	2005	Dose-dense schedule vs.	82	92
			Conventional schedule	75	90
Martin et al., NEJM 2005	BCIRG 001	1491	TAC vs.	62	76
			FAC	55	69
Martin et al., NEJM 2010	GEICAM 9805	1060	TAC vs.	87.8	NS
			FAC	81.8	
Jones et al., JCO 2009	US oncology 9735	1016	TC vs.	81	87
			AC	75	82
Joensuu et al., Lancet 2009	FinXX	1500	DX-CEX vs. D-FEC	NS	NS

*Unless indicated by NS, the DFS and OS differences in the comparison groups were statistically significant.

doxorubicin, and cyclophosphamide) showed superior efficacy over FAC (5-FU, doxorubicin, and cyclophosphamide) in node-positive patients at 10 years, with an improved DFS (62% vs. 55%; *P* = .004). TAC was associated with a significantly higher incidence of grade 3 and 4 neutropenia as compared to FAC, since primary prophylaxis with G-CSF was not allowed. Patients in the TAC arm also demonstrated an improved OS at 10 years (76% vs. 69%; *P* = .002). Similar findings were observed in the GEICAM 9805 trial at first interim analysis, which randomized node-negative patients to TAC versus FAC (87.8% vs. 81.8%; HR 0.68, 95% CI 0.49–0.93, *P* = .01) but this did not translate into a benefit in OS (HR 0.76, 95% CI 0.45–1.26). Concurrent chemotherapy is being directly compared with sequential, dose-dense chemotherapy in NSABP B-38, which has completed accrual but has not yet been reported.

The role of anthracyclines-based chemotherapy as a stand-alone regimen was challenged in the U.S. Oncology Research Trial 9735 (Table 5.3). After 7 years' follow-up, this study, which included node-positive and node-negative patients, confirmed that four cycles of docetaxel and cyclophosphamide (TC) was superior to four cycles of doxorubicin (Adriamycin) and cyclophosphamide (AC) not only in DFS (81% vs. 75%; *P* = .033) but also in OS (87% vs. 82%; *P* = .032). Approximately half of the cases were node-negative, and most cases had less than four nodes involved. A superior DFS and OS were seen in both older and younger patients. Although febrile neutropenia occurred twice as frequently in the TC group, three deaths in the AC group were attributed to cardiomyopathy and congestive heart failure, myelodysplasia, and myelofibrosis. This trial provided a rationale for TC as an attractive non-anthracycline-containing alternative standard of care regimen.

Agents other than taxanes and anthracyclines have been tested in the adjuvant setting. Recently, capecitabine in combination with docetaxel, epirubicin, and cyclophosphamide was evaluated in the FinXX trial. This study randomized 1500 women with node-positive or high-risk, node-negative breast cancer either to three cycles of capecitabine and docetaxel followed by three cycles of cyclophosphamide, epirubicin, and capecitabine, or to three cycles of docetaxel followed by three cycles of cyclophosphamide, epirubicin, and fluorouracil. Most patients had ER-positive and HER2-negative tumors less than 5 cm, histologic grade 2 or 3, and less than four positive axillary lymph nodes. At the 5-year analysis, there was no difference in the recurrence-free or overall survival. However, an unplanned subgroup analysis showed a benefit in the capecitabine-containing arm in patients with triple negative breast cancer, although this requires prospective validation and characterization.

For T.J., with her higher-risk, node-negative, stage I IDC, the rationale of adjuvant therapy should be explained, and treatment recommendations should begin with adjuvant combination chemotherapy, with a regimen containing taxane and anthracycline. After she completes subsequent radiotherapy, further treatment with hormonal therapy should be recommended. Figure 5.2 features a treatment algorithm for patients with high-risk node-negative cancer (which is also applicable to patients with node-positive disease).

Early-Stage Triple Negative Breast Cancer

P.L. is a 39-year-old African-American woman who presented to her physician with a left breast mass. Her mother and older sister had breast cancer, and she is worried about having it as well. A mammogram and ultrasound showed a 3.8 × 2.6 × 3.6 cm left breast mass. A core biopsy of the mass revealed an ER-negative, PR-negative, and HER2-negative IDC. A diagnostic MRI showed the mass to be 3.5 × 3.2 × 3.0 cm with no other lesions in either breast. A staging bone scan and CT scans were performed to assess for regional or distant metastatic disease and were negative.

Evidence-Based Case Discussion

P.L. has clinically stage IIA (cT2 N0 M0) triple negative breast cancer (TNBC). TNBC is a molecularly heterogeneous category of aggressive breast cancer, comprising approximately 15% to 20% of breast cancers. Unlike other types of breast cancer, it lacks the advantage of having hormone receptor targets for treatment, and the backbone of medical treatment for this group is cytotoxic chemotherapy. Despite superior sensitivity and response to chemotherapy, TNBCs exhibit higher recurrence rates and patients have worse survival, especially after recurrence.

The clinicopathologic features and behavior of TNBC are distinct from other breast cancers. Epidemiologic associations include younger age, Hispanic or African-American background, obesity, and lower socioeconomic levels. Tumors tend to be larger at presentation and are known to arise in between yearly screening mammograms (interim cancers). Unlike other breast cancer types, tumor size and node status do not predict the prognosis of TNBC behavior very well. Histopathologic characteristics and receptor status dominate the prognostic picture, as shown in repeated studies.

Metastatic disease occurs more frequently in the central nervous system (CNS), lungs, and viscera, and less often in bone. With the occurrence of metastases, patients with TNBC do more poorly than those with other subtypes, with a one-year median OS rate. Taxanes, antimetabolites, anthracyclines, and alkylating agents are among the active agents in TNBC. Trials with single-agent and combination chemotherapy regimens in the neoadjuvant setting have shown pathologic complete response rates ranging from 20% to 66%. However, despite the responsiveness of TNBC to initial chemotherapy, recurrence and survival rates are worse, an observation that has been named the "triple negative paradox." This was best demonstrated in a study of Liedtke et al. that examined 1118 patients, including 255 who had TNBC. The TNBC group demonstrated a trend toward a higher incidence of pathologic complete response (pCR) after neoadjuvant chemotherapy (22% vs. 11%; $P = .34$) compared to non-TNBC group, but the 3-year DFS (63% vs. 76%) and OS (74% vs. 89%, HR = 2.53, 95% CI 1.77–3.57; $P < .0001$) were significantly worse (11). However, patients with TNBC who achieved pCR with neoadjuvant chemotherapy had similar OS as non-TNBC cohorts (94% v 95%; $P = .24$). Research is ongoing toward finding more efficient treatment for chemotherapy-resistant TNBC.

The recent advent of molecular profiling has provided some exciting and promising insight into newer treatment strategies for TNBCs. Genomic expression profiling of TNBC, BRCA hereditary breast cancer, and basal-like breast cancer revealed overlapping signatures among these groups, implying common features in their pathophysiology. *BRCA1* and *2* encode proteins that are crucial for DNA repair, in which germline mutations cause hereditary cancer syndromes. These cancers have been found to be particularly sensitive to chemotherapy agents that corrupt DNA repair, such as PARP inhibitors, alkylating agents, and platinum salts, both in cell culture and in xenograft models. This strategy of exploiting the inherently faulty DNA repair mechanism by using therapies that cause further impediments is now an attractive avenue for experimental therapeutics. Data from a phase II trial evaluating response rates in metastatic TNBC to a combination regimen of carboplatin and gemcitabine with or without BSI-201, a PARP inhibitor, showed a nearly 5-month improvement in median OS in the chemotherapy plus targeted therapy arm, 12.3 versus 7.7 months (HR=0.5, 95% CI 0.30–0.82; $P = .005$) (12). With the goal of confirming these promising results, a randomized phase III trial was recently completed, but based on a press release from the sponsor, the study failed to demonstrate an improvement in DFS and OS. However, a planned subgroup analysis showed that there was significant benefit in patients receiving the PARP inhibitor regimen as second- or third-line therapy (NCT00938652 ClinicalTrials.gov).

For P.L., recommendations for her clinical T2 N0 triple negative, IDC breast cancer should begin with a surgical evaluation and staging. Surgical pathology will yield the final tumor size and lymph node status, but given the clinical tumor size alone, she is likely to be treated with adjuvant combination chemotherapy with an anthracycline-containing regimen followed by a taxane. Figure 5.2 includes a treatment algorithm for patients like P.L. who have triple negative, early-stage breast cancer.

Given her strong family history of breast cancer and her diagnosis at a young age, genetic evaluation for *BRCA1* and *2* mutations is warranted. If P.L. is found to be a carrier of a mutation, genetic testing should be offered to her first-degree relatives. In patients with *BRCA1* and *2* mutations, there is a lifetime risk of up to 87% breast cancer and up to 45% ovarian cancer. Several risk reduction strategies exist but the most effective is prophylactic surgery with bilateral mastectomy and bilateral oophorectomy. Mutation carriers (affected and unaffected) should be counseled extensively on these surgeries and their timing by a multidisciplinary team, and issues such as fertility, reconstructive surgeries, and psychological impact need to be taken into consideration.

Locally Advanced Breast Cancer

S.R. is a 58-year-old postmenopausal woman who was referred to the oncologist by her primary care physician because of a 5 × 7 cm right breast mass along with matted right axillary lymphadenopathy (3.5 × 4 cm) both of which have been increasing in size since the patient first noticed them 9 months ago. There were no palpable cervical, supraclavicular, or contralateral axillary lymph nodes. The skin overlying the tumor was erythematous and the surrounding tissue was indurated. The total area involved by erythema and induration comprised one third of the breast, and the tumor contours were clearly palpable just below the surface of the skin. A mammogram showed a 5.1 × 4.3 cm right breast mass without other suspicious lesions in either breast. An ultrasound confirmed the mammographic findings as well as the 4-cm right axillary lymphadenopathy. A core needle biopsy of the breast mass revealed IDC, grade 3, with Ki67 of 74%. Tumor markers were ER-positive, PR-positive, and HER2-positive. The patient was concerned that the tumor was going to extrude through the skin in the near future and was anxious about starting therapy as soon as possible to remove the tumor.

Evidence-Based Case Discussion

S.R. has presented with stage III, locally advanced breast cancer (LABC). Further basic staging studies are indicated to rule out metastatic disease at presentation. A complete physical examination looking for other regional lymph nodes as well as signs of metastatic disease, such as bone tenderness or enlarged organs, is always indicated but particularly important in this case. Laboratory studies including blood counts and chemistries, including liver enzymes, as well as a chest x-ray and a bone scan should be ordered. A CT scan of the chest and abdomen to assess for systemic metastases in the lungs and liver should be performed as well.

In the case of S.R., these studies showed no evidence of metastatic disease. Although HER2-positive disease has a tendency to metastasize to the brain, routine imaging with MRI or CT scan is not indicated unless the patient presents with symptoms of CNS metastases.

Certain features of S.R.'s physical examination could raise concern for inflammatory breast cancer (IBC). IBC is a clinically aggressive subtype of breast cancer found in 2% of breast cancer patients marked by rapid onset, diffuse erythema and edema over two third of the breast, peau d'orange, tenderness, warmth, enlargement of the breast, and diffuseness or even absence of identifiable tumor on palpation. On microscopic examination of a skin biopsy, tumor infiltration of the dermal lymphatics may also be observed but IBC is ultimately a clinical diagnosis. The aggressive clinical features of IBC correlate to a poor prognosis with 5-year survival of only 20% to 50%. Because the induration and erythema involve less than 50% of S.R.'s breast she does not meet the clinical criteria for IBC. In addition, the fact that she noted a mass 9 months ago and that the tumor outlines are clearly visible just below the skin suggest a locally advanced breast cancer with secondary inflammatory features rather than an IBC.

Although the patient's first inclination may be to proceed directly to surgery, she may be best served by starting with neoadjuvant therapy. Clinical trials have shown an advantage for systemic therapy, including chemotherapy and targeted anti-HER2 therapy at the beginning of treatment, rather than after surgery. Several combination regimens have been shown to produce significant tumor shrinkage (>50% by WHO criteria) in >70% of patients; however, complete clinical response and pCR are less frequent. Tumor progression is very uncommon (1–2%) so that operable patients rarely become inoperable. In up to 63% of patients who have undergone neoadjuvant chemotherapy, it may be possible to consider breast conservation therapy, depending on the tumor to breast ratio. In an EORTC 10902 study, neoadjuvant therapy with a combination of 5-FU, epirubicin, and cyclophosphamide (FEC) reduced the size of locally advanced breast tumors such that 23% of patients were downstaged at surgery and 16% of previously unresectable tumors became resectable (13). Similar results were observed in the NSABP B-18 trial in which neoadjuvant chemotherapy with anthracyclines increased the possibility of breast conserving therapy. Patients who achieved a pCR had significantly better DFS and OS than those who did not.

It was the goal of the NSABP B-27 trial to determine the optimal neoadjuvant chemotherapy regimen. The addition of neoadjuvant docetaxel to doxorubicin and cyclophosphamide (AC) in women with surgically resectable tumors doubled the pCR rate from 13% to 26% ($P > .00001$) (14). In both NSABP trials, patients who achieved a pCR had significantly better DFS and OS than those who did not (14).

In HER2-positive tumors, the results may be even more dramatic with pCR rates up to 40% as observed in the GeparQuattro trial. When the pCR rates of IBCs and LABCs treated with neoadjuvant chemotherapy were compared with that of (smaller) operable breast cancers, there was no difference between the groups suggesting that tumor size does not predict the probability of pathologic complete response (15). Very large tumors should not be excluded from neoadjuvant therapy because it is the chemosensitivity of the tumor rather than the size that determines the response to therapy.

Neoadjuvant treatment can include cytotoxic chemotherapy, hormonal therapy, and targeted biological agents. Although potentially as effective, hormonal therapy is not as commonly used as neoadjuvant chemotherapy. Hormonally sensitive tumors are usually lower grade and slower growing, and therefore their rate of shrinkage in response to treatment is usually slower. Carefully selected patients may receive neoadjuvant hormonal therapy if their tumor type is likely to respond (high ER content, low grade, postmenopausal age) or if their comorbidities prohibit the use of the more toxic chemotherapy.

The rationale for administering adjuvant HER2 targeted therapy is based on its dramatic survival benefit over that of chemotherapy alone. The NSABP B-31 trial compared doxorubicin and cyclophosphamide followed by paclitaxel with the same regimen plus 52 weeks of trastuzumab. At 3 years, the trastuzumab group had an absolute difference in DFS of 12% over the control group and trastuzumab therapy was associated with a 33% reduction in the risk of death ($P = .015$) (16). Another trial, the BCIRG 006 used a non-anthracyline containing regimen (docetaxel, carboplatin, and trastuzumab) and compared it to AC followed by docetaxel with or without trastuzumab. This trial also showed the trastuzumab containing arms to have a superior outcome (17). These findings changed the standard of care to include 12 months of treatment with trastuzumab to adjuvant chemotherapy of patients with HER2-positive breast cancer.

One concern with this strategy was a 3% increase in heart failure symptoms in patients on anthracycline-containing regimens who then received trastuzumab. However, subsequent safety analyses both on and off trial have found no significant increase in clinically significant heart failure. Cardiac monitoring at baseline and periodically during therapy is advised as a means of identifying early cardiac toxicity prior to clinical manifestations.

Resistance to trastuzumab is an important clinical problem and has led to the development of additional HER2 targeted agents, such as the small molecule dual EGFR and HER2 inhibitor, lapatinib. In a randomized clinical trial in women with locally advanced or metastatic HER2-positive breast cancer who had progressed on a trastuzumab-containing regimen, lapatinib in conjunction with capecitabine improved time to progression from 4.4 months to 8.4 months as compared to capecitabine alone (hazard ratio 0.49; $P < .001$) (18). Currently, only trastuzumab is indicated in the adjuvant setting and lapatinib is reserved for recurrent, trastuzumab-refractory tumors. Ongoing trials described above are testing the role of lapatinib in early-stage and curable breast cancer.

Mounting clinical and preclinical evidence suggests combination targeted anti-HER2 therapy may be a superior therapeutic strategy to single-agent targeted therapy. Recently, three neoadjuvant clinical trials were reported that assessed the relative efficacy of anti-HER2 agents (including trastuzumab, pertuzumab, and lapatinib) used singly or in combination with each other and with cytotoxic chemotherapy.

On the GeparQuinto study, patients received neoadjuvant chemotherapy with epirubicin and cyclophosphamide followed by docetaxel combined with trastuzumab or lapatinib. The primary endpoint, pCR was significantly higher in the trastuzumab arm as compared to the lapatinib arm (31.3% versus 21.7%; $P < .05$) (19).

In the phase II Neosphere trial, patients were treated with neoadjuvant pertuzumab, trastuzumab, or their combination, with or without docetaxel. The combination targeted therapy arm of trastuzumab + pertuzumab + docetaxel had a 45% pCR rate, which was significantly higher than that seen in the docetaxel + trastuzumab arm (29%; $P = .014$), which was in turn significantly higher than observed in the trastuzumab + pertuzumab arm (16.8%; $P = .019$) (20). In this phase II study, the combination of trastuzumab and pertuzumab did not cause an increased risk of serious adverse events.

The NeoALLTO trial was a phase III neoadjuvant study of lapatinib, trastuzumab, or their combination along with paclitaxel. The pCR rate in the combination lapatinib + trastuzumab + paclitaxel arm was significantly higher than the trastuzumab + paclitaxel arm (51.3% versus 29.5%; $P = .001$) (21). The rate of grade 3 diarrhea was higher in lapatinib-containing arms compared to trastuzumab.

In these trials, combination targeted therapy plus chemotherapy outperformed single-agent anti-HER2 therapy with chemotherapy. If the improved pCR reported in these trials translates to improved DFS and OS, then combination targeted therapy may play an important role in HER2-directed therapy.

S.R. underwent neoadjuvant therapy with docetaxel and trastuzumab for four cycles with an excellent clinical response in which her breast and axillary masses were no longer palpable with a resolution of the skin changes and breast contraction. She was able to undergo lumpectomy and axillary lymph node dissection, and the pathology assessment revealed a pathologic complete response with no residual carcinoma in the breast or lymph nodes.

S.R. was advised to undergo adjuvant chemotherapy consisting of doxorubicin (Adriamycin) and cyclophosphamide (AC). Cardiac studies to monitor for anthracycline cardiotoxicity remained normal throughout treatment. After completion of AC chemotherapy, trastuzumab was restarted for nine additional months (for a total treatment time of 12 months). Since her tumor was ER- and PR-positive, subsequent hormonal therapy with upfront aromatase inhibitors or sequential therapy with tamoxifen followed by an aromatase inhibitor are appropriate strategies for this postmenopausal woman.

Radiation therapy to the breast and axilla (to decrease the chance of local recurrence) were recommended after completion of adjuvant chemotherapy (and may be administered concurrently with trastuzumab). Radiation therapy is indicated to decrease the risk of local recurrence in women after breast conserving therapy as we discussed earlier. It is also indicated in women with tumors larger than 5 cm (T3), involvement of skin or chest wall (T4), and involvement of four or more lymph nodes (N2-N3).

Surveillance during the 5 years of hormonal therapy includes yearly mammography. There is no evidence supporting surveillance with whole-body imaging at this time. Figure 5.3 represents a treatment algorithm for locally advanced breast cancer.

Metastatic Breast Cancer

G.T. is a 62-year-old woman with a prior history of a T2 N0 M0 IDC of the left breast (ER-positive, PR-positive, HER2-negative) that was diagnosed 7 years ago and treated with partial mastectomy and radiation followed by adjuvant hormonal therapy with a nonsteroidal aromatase inhibitor for 5 years. She came to her oncologist complaining of shortness of breath for 3 months. She had previously been physically active until she experienced left leg pain for 3 weeks, and a swollen painful right underarm, both interfering with her ability to work. Her physical examination revealed a left breast with a healed lumpectomy scar without suspicious lesions. However, right axillary lymphadenopathy and point tenderness at the lumbar spine (L5) were detected.

CT scans confirmed the axillary masses and also demonstrated presence of three subcentimeter nodules in the upper lobe of the right lung, but showed no evidence of metastasis in the liver. A bone scan revealed technetium uptake in the lumbar vertebrae, ribs, and pelvis. An MRI showed a compression fracture of the involved vertebrae, with greater than 50% loss of height, and also T2 flair signal along the spinal cord.

Evidence-Based Case Discussion

G.T. has now developed a metastatic (State IV) recurrence of her breast cancer to bone, lymph nodes, and possibly lungs. Metastatic breast cancer (MBC) is an incurable group of cancers, with widely ranging survival times. With the advent of effective screening for early-stage breast cancer, most cases of MBC are recurrences of earlier breast

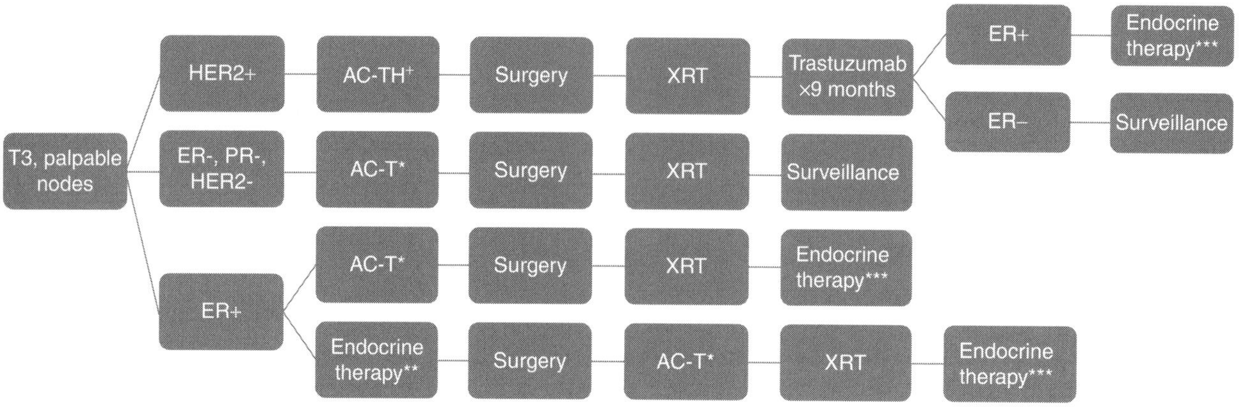

*Neoadjuvant chemotherapy for breast cancer involves a combination of A (doxorubucin), C (cyclophosphamide), and T (taxane, either docetaxel or paclitaxel). The optimal sequence has not yet been determined. In clinical trials they have been administered: sequentially AC-T, concurrently TAC, or before and after surgery AC-surgery-T, or T-surgery-AC.

**The optimal neoadjuvant endocrine therapy regimen has not yet been defined. With low pathologic complete response rates, neoadjuvant endocrine therapy is uncommon and reserved for a specific subset of patients.

***For details of adjuvant endocrine therapy treatment by menopausal status please see the endocrine therapy section of the early stage breast cancer treatment algorithm

+In the case of HER2+ tumors, trastuzumab (H) is added in combination with a taxane most commonly after AC.

Figure 5.3

Treatment algorithm for locally advanced breast cancer.

cancers treated with curative intent. Of the women with invasive breast cancer, 20% to 30% will develop metastases, most frequently in the first 5 to 10 years after diagnosis. Once metastases arise, the median OS is approximately 2 years but this varies by tumor subtype.

The goals of treatment are to prolong life, to optimize quality of life, to control symptoms, and to control the disease burden. Treatment modalities include chemotherapy, hormonal therapy, radiation, and palliative surgery. Breast cancer recurrence may occur locally or distantly. Involvement of almost every known organ by metastatic lesions has been described in the literature. Disease progression represents a growing population of resistant cells from the original tumor, and the pattern of progression is influenced by the histology of the cancer. For example, IDC recurs more commonly in lung ($P < .05$), pleura ($P < .05$) and brain ($P < .05$), when compared with ILC, which more commonly spreads to the bone marrow ($P < .01$) and peritoneum ($P < .01$) (22). Bone involvement as the initial presentation of distant metastases occurred in significantly more women with ILC, than with IDC (50% vs. 34%, $P < .01$).

Histology also influences prognosis. In a 2009 study, patients with IDC had poorer 5-year (80%) and 10-year (61%) survival compared with patients with ILC (87% and 68%) and mixed (84% and 69%) cancers ($P = .029$) (23). CNS metastases are more frequently associated with HER2 over-expressing breast cancer.

Hormonal therapy is the preferred initial treatment for metastatic, hormone- responsive breast cancer without visceral metastases and associated organ dysfunction. Advantages for hormonal therapy include a milder side-effect profile, ease of administration, and a proven survival benefit. Ovarian suppression or ablation, antiestrogens, estrogen receptor modulators, progestins, and aromatase inhibitors are among the hormonal treatment strategies used.

Twenty to thirty-five percent of patients may have a clinical response to initial hormonal therapy, with an additional 30% to 35% experiencing stable disease. Clinical response may take 2 to 3 months to achieve maximum benefit, and the mean response duration may extend to 1 or 2 years or longer. If there is a response to first-line treatment, the likelihood of response to second-line treatment is 50%. If both ER and PR are positive, the response rate may be up to 70% to 80%, the response rate may be slightly less if only one receptor is positive. Other positive predictive factors include postmenopausal status, longer DFS, no liver involvement, slower tumor growth, and older age. The menopausal status influences the initial choice of hormonal treatment.

For premenopausal women, surgical ovarian ablation, now more than a century old, remains in use although it is now largely replaced by medical therapy. Tamoxifen, a selective estrogen receptor modulator (SERM), was approved by the FDA in 1977. It is the most popular first-line hormonal therapy in metastatic, premenopausal females, showing an approximate 50% clinical benefit (combined objective response and stable disease) for an average duration of 12 months. When compared to oophorectomy in a phase III trial, there was an insignificant trend favoring tamoxifen. However, tamoxifen failure does not preclude response to oophorectomy. A tumor flare is possible with initiation of tamoxifen and predicts an excellent response. The flare symptoms, if they occur, generally resolve spontaneously after a few weeks but may be attenuated by steroids.

Chemical ablation with GnRH analogs has also been compared to oophorectomy in premenopausal women. Compared to oophorectomy, monthly, low-dose goserelin showed similar failure-free survival and OS in patients with hormone receptor positive, metastatic disease. Tamoxifen added to hormonal ablation demonstrated superiority over ablation alone. In a meta-analysis of four trials, this combination suggested better response rates, median response duration, progression-free survival (PFS), and OS (24). After progression, aromatase inhibitors (with ovarian ablation), progestins, and high-dose estrogen can still be utilized.

Unlike premenopausal women, the principal source of estrogen in postmenopausal women is from peripheral tissue conversion of adrenal hormones by the aromatase enzyme, rather than from ovarian production. Aromatase inhibitors (AI) are currently into their third and fourth generation and are being used in postmenopausal women as treatment for MBC and in the adjuvant setting. In earlier studies, the AI anastrozole was found have equivalent efficacy as Tamoxifen, but in a multicenter, phase III study of 900 metastatic postmenopausal women, another AI, letrozole, demonstrated superior median time to progression (9.4 vs. 6 months; $P < .0001$) and overall objective response (32% vs. 21%; $P = .0002$), with a median OS trend favoring the AI as compared to tamoxifen (25). Headaches, arthralgias, musculoskeletal pain, fatigue, weight gain, and hot flashes are common side effects of AIs, but are generally well tolerated. After progression with AI, fulvestrant and exemestane have shown clinical benefit. Aromatase inhibitors should not be used as single-agent therapy in premenopausal women.

Chemotherapy in metastatic breast cancer can be used to treat hormone therapy-refractory disease, or to treat patients de novo with significant visceral metastases. Choosing a single-agent sequential or combination strategy is an area of some controversy in MBC. Compared to sequential single-agent therapy, MBC is more likely to respond to combination regimens with an improved PFS, but with more toxicity. Overall survival among patients receiving combination versus single-agent regimens was evaluated in a large meta-analysis of 189 randomized controlled trials spanning from 1975 to 1997. Overall survival between the two strategies favored combination regimens by 18%, translating to an absolute survival benefit of 9% at 1 year, 5% at 2 years, and 3% at 5 years (26). For most patients, the goals are to achieve disease stabilization, palliate symptoms, and maintain a favorable quality of life.

The choice of agents in the treatment of MBC is based on extensive clinical trial experience. Anthracyclines, such as doxorubicin and epirubicin, are among the most active agents. When used in first-line combination regimens, response rates range from 50% to 80% with an associated response duration of 8 to 15 months. Myelosuppression is the dose-limiting factor, and prophylactic G-CSF support is commonly used. Dose-related cardiotoxicity is well described and can result in permanent cardiac dysfunction, which has been associated with poor prognosis. The incidence of clinically apparent congestive heart failure with cumulative doses of 320 mg/m^2 is less than 1%, and up to 10% after 550 mg/m^2. Pretreatment and serial cardiac function monitoring is recommended throughout anthracycline administration.

Taxanes are also active in metastatic breast cancer, initially finding their role in anthracycline-resistant cancers, with response rates of 20% to 30%. As first-line treatment, paclitaxel response rates are 32% to 62% with response durations of approximately 6 months in phase III trials. Docetaxel is another active taxane. When compared to doxorubicin salvage therapy in a phase III randomized multicenter trial of women whose MBC progressed after previous alkylating therapy, docetaxel demonstrated a significantly higher overall response rate (47.8% vs. 33.3%; $P = .008$) with a median time to treatment failure (22 vs. 18 weeks; $P = .01$) (27). Early data from the TAX 311 trial also showed a significantly improved median OS of 15.4 versus 12.7 months ($P = .03$) favoring docetaxel over paclitaxel. Important toxicities to consider when using taxanes include edema, hypersensitivity, and neuropathy. Early success with nab-paclitaxel, a second-generation taxane that eliminates cremaphor from its preparation, led to its FDA approval in 2005 for use in relapsed MBC.

Conflicting results from several large prospective trials comparing anthracyclines to taxanes led to a meta-analysis published in 2007 by Piccart-Gebhart (28). Compiled results from eight randomized prospective trials comparing anthracycline plus taxane versus anthracycline plus cyclophosphamide combinations, and three single-agent trials comparing a taxane versus an anthracycline were included. In the single-agent trials, the response rates were similar in the taxane and in the anthracycline arms (38% and 33%; $P = .08$), but the hazard ratios for PFS favored anthracyclines over taxanes (1.19, 95% CI 1.04–1.36; $P < .011$) with no difference in OS (1.01, 95% CI 0.88–1.16; $P < .90$). In combination trials, the response rate was 57% (10% complete) in taxane-based combinations as compared to 46% (6% complete) in control arms ($P < .001$). The hazard ratio for PFS in the taxane-based combinations compared with control arms was 0.92 (95% CI 0.85–0.99; $P < .031$) and 0.95 (95% CI 0.88 –1.03; $P < .24$) for survival. These results suggest that as single agents, taxanes are inferior to anthracyclines in PFS but not in response or OS. However, when taxanes are added to anthracyclines, the response rates and PFS are significantly improved as compared to non-taxane combinations, but with no advantage in OS.

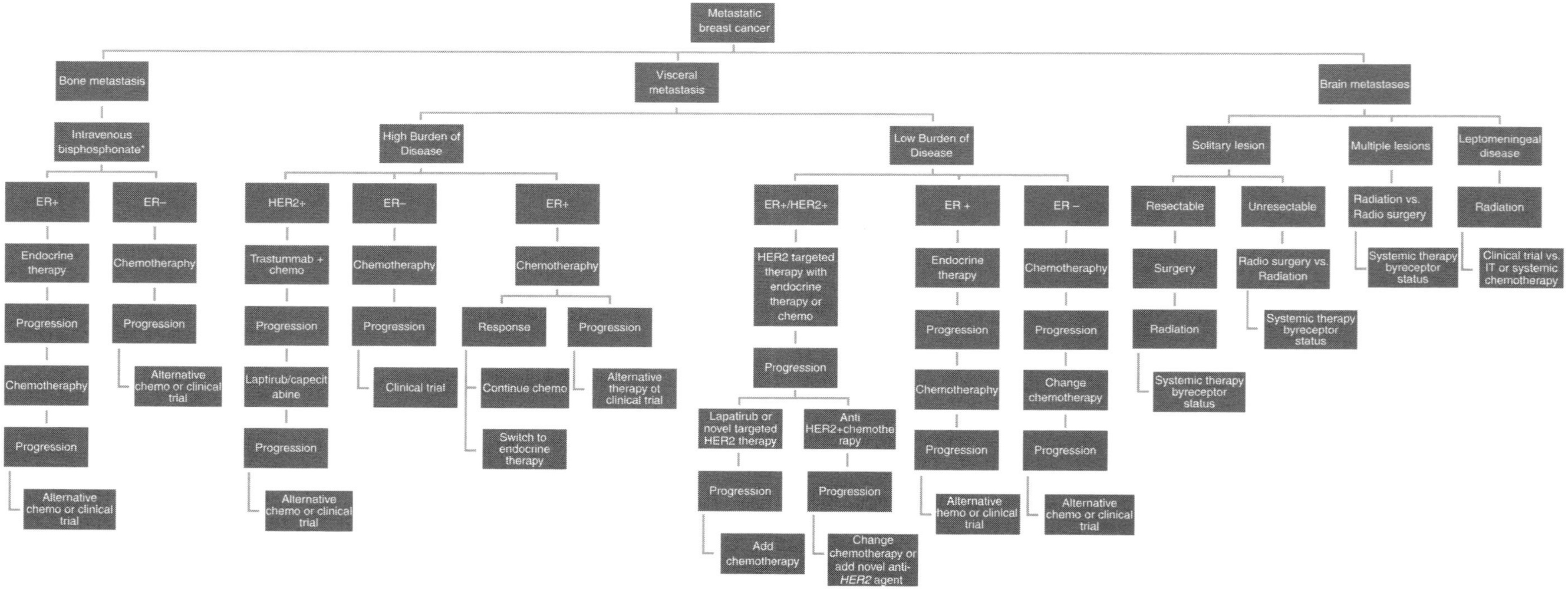

Figure 5.4

Treatment algorithm for metastatic breast cancer.

Capecitabine is an oral prodrug of 5-FU that has activity and utility as a salvage treatment after anthracycline and taxane therapy. In a phase III trial, the addition of capecitabine to docetaxel extended survival from 11.5 to 14.5 months ($P < .01$) with improvements in both response and time to disease progression as well (29). After failing anthracyclines, taxanes, and capecitabine, third-line treatment with gemcitabine and vinorelbine may still have effect.

In addition to these active drugs, new agents, which selectively inhibit the molecular pathways active in malignancy, have shown utility in MBC. In addition to trastuzumab, which targets the HER2 receptor pathway, anti-angiogenesis agents such as bevacizumab have also been tested in combination with conventional chemotherapy. In the E2100 trial, the addition of bevacizumab to paclitaxel significantly doubled the response rate from 14.2% to 28.2% ($P < .0001$), also resulting in a doubling of median PFS from 5.9 to 11.8 months (HR 0.67; $P < .001$) (30). Unfortunately, there was no benefit in the OS rate in this and confirmatory studies that led to the withdrawal of bevacizumab as an FDA-approved agent in MBC.

For patients with bone metastases, intravenous bisphosphonates can improve quality of life and pain control, reduce incidence of fractures, and treat hypercalcemia of malignancy. Accordingly, the ASCO consensus statement supports the administration of pamidronate or zoledronate every 3 to 5 weeks for metastatic bone lesions. When compared with pamidronate, zoledronate significantly improved skeletal related events (SRE, including incidence of pathologic fracture, cord compression, or need for radiation or surgical treatment) by an additional 20% ($P = .025$) and by an additional 30% in patients receiving hormonal therapy ($P = .009$) (31). Side effects include osteonecrosis of the jaw, renal insufficiency, and ocular inflammation.

Though the patient in this case has not yet developed brain metastases, the CNS is a known site of metastasis for breast cancer. The management of CNS metastases in breast cancer are similar to those in other tumors. Selected solitary metastases may be removed surgically followed by whole brain or stereotactic radiotherapy. Treatment of multiple metastases and leptomeningeal disease are outlined in Figure 5.4. Participation on a clinical trial should be considered since the optimal management of brain metastases is still being defined.

In summary, G.T. has hormone receptor positive, metastatic breast cancer to the lymph nodes, bone, and lung, with a long disease-free interval. Surgical stabilization of her spine should be considered. Once addressed and treated, her breast cancer can be treated with a palliative intent. The burden of disease in the lungs is small and not eliciting symptoms, and therefore a reasonable initial approach may be to administer hormonal therapy with close monitoring. Exemestane, a steroidal AI, is a reasonable option given evidence of its efficacy after progression on a nonsteroidal AI.

Once refractory to hormone therapy (she may benefit from the use of sequential hormonal agents), her chemotherapy management may include use of an anthracycline, taxane, and perhaps capecitabine, as determined by her performance status, cardiac function, and comorbidities. Bisphosphonates should be included in her plan of care. Figure 5.4 provides a treatment algorithm for patients with metastatic breast cancer.

REFERENCES

1. Fisher B, Anderson S, Bryant J, et al. Twenty-year follow-up of a randomized trial comparing total mastectomy, lumpectomy, and lumpectomy plus irradiation for the treatment of invasive breast cancer. *N Engl J Med.* 2002;347(16):1233–1241.
2. Fisher B, Dignam J, Wolmark N, et al. Tamoxifen in treatment of intraductal breast cancer: National Surgical Adjuvant Breast and Bowel Project B-24 randomised controlled trial. *Lancet.* 1999;353(9169):1993–2000.
3. Giuliano AE, Hunt K, Ballman E, et al. Dissection vs no axillary dissection in women with invasive breast cancer and sentinel node metastasis: a randomized clinical trial. *JAMA.* 2011;305: 519–575.
4. Weaver DL, Ashikaga T, Krag DN, et al. Effect of occult metastases on survival in node-negative breast cancer. *N Engl J Med.* 2011;364(5):412–421.
5. Harvey JM, Clark GM, Osborne CK, Allred DC. Estrogen receptor status by immunohistochemistry is superior to the ligand-binding assay for predicting response to adjuvant endocrine therapy in breast cancer. *J Clin Oncol.* 1999;17(5): 1474–1481.
6. Early Breast Cancer Trialists Collaborative Group (EBCTCG). Effects of chemotherapy and hormonal therapy for early breast cancer on recurrence and 15-year survival: an overview of the randomised trials. *Lancet.* 2005;365 (9472):1687–1717.
7. ASCO Clinical Practice Guidelines: Updates on adjuvant endocrine therapy for women with hormone receptor positive breast cancer. July 12, 2010.
8. Howell A, Cuzick J, Baum M, et al. Results of the ATAC (Arimidex, Tamoxifen, Alone or in Combination) trial after completion of 5 years' adjuvant treatment for breast cancer. *Lancet.* 2005;365(9453):60–62.
9. BIG 1-98 Collaborative Group. Letrozole therapy alone or in sequence with tamoxifen in women with breast cancer. *N Engl J Med.* 2009;361(8): 766–776.
10. Coombes RC, Hall E, Gibson LJ, et al. A randomized trial of exemestane after two to three years of tamoxifen therapy in postmenopausal women with primary breast cancer. *N Engl J Med.* 2004;350(11):1081–1092.
11. Liedtke C, Mazouni C, Hess KR, et al. Response to Neoadjuvant Therapy and Long-Term Survival in Patients with Triple-Negative Breast Cancer. *J Clin Oncol.* 2008;26(8):1275–1281.
12. O'Shaughnessy J, Osborne C, Pippen JE, et al. Iniparib plus chemotherapy in metastatic triple-negative breast cancer. *N Engl J Med.* 2011;364(3): 205–214.
13. van der Hage JA, van de Velde CJ, Julien JP, et al. Preoperative Chemotherapy in Primary Operable Breast Cancer: Results from the European Organization for Research and Treatment of Cancer Trial 10902. *J Clin Oncol.* 2001;19(22):4224–4237.

14. Rastogi P, Anderson SJ, Bear HD, et al. Preoperative chemotherapy: updates of National Surgical Adjuvant Breast and Bowel Project Protocols B-18 and B-27. *J Clin Oncol*. 2008;26:778–785.
15. Costa SD, Loibl S, Kaufmann M, et al. Neoadjuvant chemotherapy shows similar response in patients with inflammatory or locally advanced breast cancer when compared with operable breast cancer: a secondary analysis of the GeparTrio trial data. *J Clin Oncol*. 2010;28(1):83–91.
16. Romond EH, Perez EA, Bryant J, et al. Trastuzumab plus adjuvant chemotherapy for operable HER2-positive breast cancer. *N Engl J Med*. 2005;353(16):1673–1684.
17. Slamon D, Eiermann W, Robert N, et al. Phase III randomized trial comparing doxorubicin and cyclophosphamide followed by docetaxel (ACT) with doxorubicin and cyclophosphamide followed by docetaxel and trastuzumab (ACTH) with docetaxel, carboplatin and trastuzumab (TCH) in Her2neu positive early breast cancer patients: BCIRG 006 study. *Cancer Res*. 2009;69(24 Supplement):62.
18. Geyer CE, Forster J, Lindquist D, et al. Lapatinib plus capecitabine for HER2-positive advanced breast cancer. *N Engl J Med*. 2006;355(26):2733–2743.
19. Untch M, Loibl S, Bischoff J, et al. Lapatinib vs trastuzumab in combination with neoadjuvant anthracycline-taxane-based chemotherapy: primary efficacy endpoint analysis of the GEPARQUINTO study (GBG 44). *SABCS*. 2010;Abstract S3–1.
20. Gianni L, Pienkowski T, Im Y-H, et al. Neoadjuvant pertuzumab (P) and trastuzumab (H): antitumor and safety analysis of a randomized phase II study (NeoSphere) *SABCS*. 2010;Abstract S3–2.
21. Baselga J, Bradbury I, Eidtmann H, et al. First results of the NeoALTTO trial (BIG 01–06 / EGF 106903): a phase III, randomized, open label, neoadjuvant study of lapatinib, trastuzumab, and their combination plus paclitaxel in women with HER2-positive primary breast cancer. *SABCS*. 2010; Abstract 291.
22. Jain S, Fisher C, Smith P, et al. Patterns of metastatic breast cancer in relation to histological type. *Eur J Cancer*. 1993;29A(15): 2155–2157.
23. Bharat A, Gao F, Margenthaler JA. Tumor characteristics and patient outcomes are similar between invasive lobular and mixed invasive ductal/lobular breast cancers but differ from pure invasive ductal breast cancers. *Am J Surg*. 2009;198(4):516–519.
24. Klijn JG, Blamey RW, Boccardo F, et al. Combined Hormone Agents Trialists' Group and the European Organization for Research and Treatment of Cancer. Combined tamoxifen and luteinizing hormone-releasing hormone (LHRH) agonist versus LHRH agonist alone in premenopausal advanced breast cancer: a meta-analysis of four randomized trials. *J Clin Oncol*. 2001;19(2):343–353.
25. Mouridsen H, Gershanovich M, Sun Y, et al. Phase III study of letrozole versus tamoxifen as first-line therapy of advanced breast cancer in postmenopausal women: analysis of survival and update of efficacy from the International Letrozole Breast Cancer Group. *J Clin Oncol*. 2003;21:2101–2109.
26. Fossati R, Confalonieri C, Torri V, et al. Cytotoxic and hormonal treatment for metastatic breast cancer: a systematic review of published randomized trials involving 31,510 women. *J Clin Oncol*. 1998;16:3439–3460.
27. Chan S, Friedrichs K, Noel D, et al. Prospective randomised trial of docetaxel versus doxorubicin in patients with metastatic breast cancer: The 303 Study Group. *J Clin Oncol*. 1999;17: 2341–2354.
28. Piccart-Gebhart MJ, Burzykowski T, Buyse M, et al. Taxanes alone or in combination with anthracyclines as first-line therapy of patients with metastatic breast cancer. *J Clin Oncol*. 2008;26:1980–1986.
29. O'Shaughnessy J, Miles D, Vukelja S, et al. Superior survival with capecitabine plus docetaxel combination therapy in anthracycline-pretreated patients with advanced breast cancer: Phase III trial results. *J Clin Oncol*. 2002;20:2812–2823.
30. Miller KD, Wang M, Gralow J, et al. E2100: a randomized phase III trial of paclitaxel plus bevacizumab as first-line therapy for locally recurrent or metastatic breast cancer. Proceedings of the 41st Annual Meeting of the American Society of Clinical Oncology. Orlando, FL. 2005; Educational Session.
31. Rosen LS, Gordon D, Kaminski M, et al. Long-term efficacy and safety of zoledronic acid compared with pamidronate disodium in the treatment of skeletal complications in patients with advanced multiple myeloma or breast carcinoma. *Cancer*. 2003; 98:1735–1744.

6

Esophageal Cancer

DAVID SHEPARD AND SUSAN URBA

EPIDEMIOLOGY, RISK FACTORS, NATURAL HISTORY, AND PATHOLOGY

Despite advances in staging and treatment, esophageal cancer continues to be associated with a high mortality rate. Among all forms of cancer, it ranks eighth in incidence throughout the world, and the American Cancer Society estimates that in 2010 there will be 16,640 new diagnoses of esophageal cancer and 14,500 deaths in the United States. In parallel with the increased prevalence of obesity and reflux disease, the incidence of esophageal cancer has been increasing in the United States. There has been a marked increase in diagnoses of esophageal adenocarcinoma in young white males, a population whose incidence rate rose 463% since the late 1970s (1).

Esophageal cancers are seen far more frequently in men than in women with a median age at diagnosis of 69 years. There are predominantly two types of esophageal cancer: adenocarcinoma and squamous cell carcinoma. Adenocarcinoma is now the most common histologic subtype of esophageal cancer in the United States and Western world, accounting for approximately 75% to 80% of patients. Squamous cell carcinoma of the esophagus has decreased in incidence, but still remains the most common histologic subtype seen in African Americans.

Strong risk factors for squamous cell cancer are alcohol and tobacco. Other relatively rare predisposing conditions are long-standing achalasia, tylosis, esophageal webs, and human papilloma virus. For adenocarcinoma of the esophagus, gastroesophageal reflux and intestinal metaplasia of the lower esophagus (Barrett's esophagus) are well-recognized risk factors, with approximately 0.5% of patients with Barrett's esophagus progressing to adenocarcinoma annually. Obesity may be an indirect risk factor, by increasing the incidence of reflux disease. *Helicobacter pylori* is a type of bacterium that is found in the stomach in about two thirds of the world's population. Although it is a risk factor for gastric cancer and MALT lymphoma, it is not a risk factor for esophageal cancer. As a matter of fact, *H. pylori* infected persons may actually have a decreased incidence of esophageal cancer.

Most commonly, patients will present with dysphagia and weight loss. Patients who are deconditioned at presentation with >10% of body weight loss have a worse overall prognosis. Swallowing difficulties are worst with meats and breads, and often a patient is eating primarily soft foods and liquids when he seeks medical attention. Pain may also occur with swallowing. Anemia secondary to GI blood loss, or frank GI bleeding, may be the first signs of esophageal cancer. Patients who have cough associated with swallowing may have a tracheoesophageal fistula and should undergo bronchoscopy as part of the evaluation. Unfortunately, because the esophagus has a rich lymphatic network, the cancer has an early tendency to metastasize, and approximately two-thirds of patients have metastatic disease at the time of diagnosis.

STAGING

The AJCC staging system for esophagus and esophagogastric junction cancer are shown below.

Squamous Cell Carcinoma of the Esophagus

Stage	Description
IA	Well-differentiated (G1) tumor invades the lamina propria, muscularis mucosa, or submucosa (T1), no lymph nodes (N0), no metastases (M0)
IB	Moderate to poorly differentiated (G2–G3) tumor invades the lamina propria, muscularis mucosa, or submucosa (T1), no lymph nodes (N0), no metastases (M0) OR Well-differentiated (G1) tumor invades the muscularis propria or adventitia (T2–T3) of lower esophagus, no lymph nodes (N0), no metastases (M0)
IIA	Well-differentiated (G1) tumor invades the muscularis propria or adventitia (T2–T3) of upper or middle esophagus, no lymph nodes (N0), no metastases (M0) OR Moderate to poorly differentiated (G2–G3) tumor invades muscularis propria or adventitia (T2–T3) of lower esophagus, no lymph nodes (N0), no metastases (M0)
IIB	Moderate to poorly differentiated (G2–G3) tumor invades muscularis propria or adventitia (T2–T3) of upper or middle esophagus, no lymph nodes (N0), no metastases (M0) OR Any grade (G1–G4) tumor invades the lamina propria, muscularis mucosa, submucosa, or mucularis propria (T1–T2), 1–2 regional lymph nodes involved (N1), no metastases (M0)
IIIA	Any grade (G1–G4) tumor invades the lamina propria, muscularis mucosa, submucosa, or muscularis propria (T1–T2), 3–6 regional lymph nodes involved (N2), no metastases (M0) OR Any grade (G1–G4) tumor invades adventitia (T3), 1–2 regional lymph nodes involved (N1), no metastases (M0) OR Any grade (G1–G4) resectable tumor invades pleura, pericardium, or diaphragm (T4a), no lymph nodes (N0), no metastases (M0)
IIIB	Any grade (G1–G4) tumor invades adventitia (T3), 3–6 regional lymph nodes involved (N2), no metastases (M0)
IIIC	Any grade (G1–G4) resectable tumor involves pleura, pericardium, or diaphragm (T4a), 1–6 regional lymph nodes involved (N1–N2), no metastases (M0) OR Any grade (G1–G4) unresectable tumor invades other adjacent structures, such as aorta, vertebral body, trachea (T4b), any lymph node involvement (N0-N3), no metastases (M0) OR Any grade (G1–G4) tumor with invasion to any depth (T1–T4b), 7 or more regional lymph nodes involved (N3), no metastases (M0)
IV	Any grade (G1–G4) tumor with invasion to any depth (T1–T4b), any regional lymph node involvement (N0–N3), distant metastasis (M1)

Adenocarcinoma of the Distal Esophagus and Esophagogastric Junction

Stage	Description
IA	Well to moderately differentiated (G1–G2) tumor invades the lamina propria, muscularis mucosa, or submucosa (T1), no lymph nodes (N0), no metastases (M0)
IB	Poorly differentiated (G3) tumor invades the lamina propria, muscularis mucosa, or submucosa (T1), no lymph nodes (N0), no metastases (M0) OR Well to moderately differentiated (G1–G2) tumor invades the muscularis propria (T2), no lymph nodes (N0), no metastases (M0)
IIA	Poorly differentiated (G3) tumor invades the muscularis propria (T2), no lymph nodes (N0), no metastases (M0)
IIB	Any grade (G1–G4) tumor invades the adventitia (T3), no lymph nodes (N0), no metastases (M0) OR Any grade (G1–G4) tumor invades the lamina propria, muscularis mucosa, submucosa, or muscularis propria (T1–T2), 1–2 regional lymph nodes involved (N1), no metastases (M0)
IIIA	Any grade (G1–G4) tumor invades the lamina propria, muscularis mucosa, submucosa, or muscularis propria (T1–T2), 3–6 regional lymph nodes involved (N2), no metastases (M0) OR Any grade (G1–G4) tumor invades adventitia (T3), 1–2 regional lymph nodes involved (N1), no metastases (M0) OR Any grade (G1–G4) resectable tumor invades pleura, pericardium, or diaphragm (T4a), no lymph nodes (N0), no metastases (M0)

IIIB	Any grade (G1–G4) tumor invades adventitia (T3), 3–6 regional lymph nodes involved (N2), no metastases (M0)
IIIC	Any grade (G1–G4) resectable tumor involves pleura, pericardium, or diaphragm (T4a), 1–6 regional lymph nodes involved (N1–N2), no metastases (M0) OR Any grade (G1–G4) unresectable tumor invades other adjacent structures, such as aorta, vertebral body, trachea (T4b), any lymph node involvement (N0–N3), no metastases (M0) OR Any grade (G1–G4) tumor with invasion to any depth (T1–T4b), 7 or more regional lymph nodes involved (N3), no metastases (M0)
IV	Any grade (G1–G4) tumor with invasion to any depth (T1–T4b), any regional lymph node involvement (N0-N3), distant metastasis (M1)

CASE SUMMARIES

Locally Advanced Resectable Esophageal Cancer

J.D. is a 53-year-old man with a past medical history significant for tobacco use, obesity, and gastroesophageal reflux disease (GERD). His reflux had become progressively worse over the past 2 years, but for the most part he responded to his over-the-counter proton pump inhibitor. He began to have difficulty swallowing and presented to his primary care physician complaining of solid food getting stuck in his throat. He denied any trouble with liquids. He stated that his appetite had decreased and he believed that this was secondary to nervousness regarding pain with swallowing. He had not been to see a doctor recently but believed his weight was stable. He reported that he was very active, working as a carpenter without any limitations. His physical examination was negative with no palpable masses or adenopathy in the neck or abdomen. He was surprised that his weight had dropped approximately 5 pounds from what he considered his usual weight, without him realizing it. His laboratory studies were unremarkable with a hemogram and a comprehensive metabolic panel within normal limits.

He was referred to a gastroenterologist for further evaluation and an upper endoscopy revealed a partially obstructing mass in the distal portion of the thoracic esophagus. The lesion was biopsied and the pathology review revealed a grade 2 adenocarcinoma. On receiving the diagnosis, his primary care physician ordered a CT of the chest, abdomen, and pelvis to rule out metastatic disease. The only abnormalities identified were the known esophageal mass that measured 2.8 cm and a suspiciously enlarged paraesophageal lymph node. A PET scan was performed that did not identify any other worrisome lesions. An endoscopic ultrasound showed that the tumor invaded the muscularis propria and demonstrated an enlarged hypoechoic node measuring approximately 1.8 cm. On the basis of this staging evaluation, J.D. was judged to have T2 N1 M0, stage IIB disease. The gastroenterologist referred J.D. to an oncologist for treatment discussion.

Evidence-Based Case Discussion

To assess the appropriate treatment options, this patient must be seen by three major disciplines: surgery, radiation oncology, and medical oncology. This is done most expeditiously in a Tumor Board setting, if one exists. Ideally, the surgeon would see J.D. first to make sure that he is a surgical candidate, both from the standpoint of extent of disease, and medical comorbidities. The surgeon met J.D. and determined that he had locally advanced esophageal cancer that appeared amenable to resection, and he had no medical conditions that would preclude him going through surgery. Therefore, the next step would be referral to the medical oncologist and radiation oncologist for evaluation.

J.D.'s risk factors include GERD and obesity. His tumor, having penetrated the submucosa into the muscularis, significantly increased the chance for spread to the lymphatics as well as distant metastases. Survival with surgical treatment alone in this setting is poor, 20% to 30% at 2 years (2). Recent evidence supports the use of multimodality therapy. However, there are several possible standards of care for management of stage II and III disease. They include preoperative chemoradiation, preoperative chemotherapy, and surgery followed by chemoradiation. The decision regarding which is the best treatment for this patient depends on his performance status, his personal wishes, and the level of expertise of participating specialists.

Preoperative Chemoradiation

Preoperative chemoradiation followed by surgery is the most common treatment approach in the United States for patients with resectable locally advanced esophageal cancer. For the rare patients who present with very early disease, it is not necessary to give trimodality therapy. For instance, patients with T1a disease (tumor limited to the mucosa) may be treated with endoscopic mucosal resection or esophagectomy, and those with T1b (tumor invades the submucosa) may be treated with esophagectomy. However, most patients present with locally advanced disease, T2 or higher tumors, and often with lymph nodes that are involved with cancer. It is for this group that combination therapy is a major consideration. Several randomized trials have shown to benefit from this approach (Table 6.1). Historically, cisplatin plus 5-fluorouracil (5-FU) has been the chemotherapy regimen most frequently given in the neoadjuvant setting with concurrent radiation. More recently, other chemotherapy agents have been used, including carboplatin, paclitaxel, irinotecan, oxaliplatin, and capecitabine.

One of the first trials showing a survival benefit was an Irish trial reported in 1996 by Walsh and colleagues, in which 113 patients with adenocarcinoma were randomized to either surgery alone or concurrent cisplatin, 5-FU, and radiation therapy (40 Gy) followed by surgery (3). A statistically significant survival benefit was shown favoring the combined modality arm: 32 versus 6% of patients alive at 3 years. While this survival benefit was promising, the data were interpreted with some caution because of the unexpectedly low survival rate for the patients treated with surgery alone on the standard arm.

At the University of Michigan, an aggressive neoadjuvant regimen was evaluated, in which 100 patients with esophageal cancer were randomized to either preoperative chemoradiation consisting of cisplatin, 5-FU, and vinblastine versus surgery alone (4). Median survival was similar between the two groups, and although the 3-year survival was 30% with multimodality therapy compared with 16% in the surgery only arm, this did not meet statistical significance. Interestingly, the survival rate for patients treated with trimodality therapy was similar for this trial and the Irish trial described earlier—30% and 32%. However, the survival in the surgical arm was different in each of the studies—16% in the Michigan trial and 6% in the Irish trial.

More recently, the CALGB designed a large randomized trial conducted by the Intergroup to compare surgery alone to preoperative cisplatin, 5-FU, and radiation (5). Unfortunately, the trial had to close early after only 56 of the projected 500 patients were enrolled, due to poor accrual. Surprisingly, even with such small numbers, the median survival was superior for the group treated with multimodality therapy, 4.5 versus 1.8 years, ($P = .02$).

A pressing question is whether surgery really has to be added to a patient's regimen after chemoradiation. A group from Germany enrolled 172 patients with squamous cell carcinoma of the esophagus in a trial that directed them to receive induction chemotherapy followed by chemoradiation followed by surgery, or the same induction chemotherapy followed by chemoradiation without surgery (6). The induction chemotherapy was three cycles of cisplatin, 5-FU, leucovorin, and etoposide, and the chemotherapy given concurrently with radiation was cisplatin and etoposide. Three-year survival was similar between the two arms—31% with surgery versus 24% with chemoradiation only. Local progression-free survival at 2 years was better in the surgery group—64.3% versus 40.7%, $P = .003$. However, this trial only included patients with squamous cell carcinoma, and it is not clear if these results can be extrapolated to patients with the more commonly seen adenocarcinoma of the distal esophagus or GE junction (GEJ). Also, only 66% of the patients randomized to surgery actually underwent resection of their tumor. While surgery is still typically added to most patients' treatment plan if possible, there are circumstances where a surgeon skilled in performing an esophagectomy may not be available, and definitive chemoradiation is therefore administered to these patients.

One of the most recently reported trials is by the CROSS study group from the Netherlands, which

Table 6.1 Select Randomized Preoperative Chemoradiation Trials for Potentially Resectable Esophageal Cancer

Author (ref #)	No. of Patients	Histology	Regimen	Survival
Walsh (3)	113	AC – 100%	Cisplatin/5FU/40 Gy XRT + Surgery Surgery alone	3 yr: 32% 6% ($P = .01$)
Urba (4)	100	AC – 75% SCC – 25%	Cisplatin/5FU/vinblastine/45 Gy XRT +Surg Surgery alone	3 yr: 30% 16% ($P = .15$)
Tepper (5)	56	AC – 75% SCC – 25%	Cisplatin/5-FU/50.4 Gy XRT + Surgery Surgery alone	5 yr: 39% 16% ($P = .002$)
Stahl (6)	172	SCC – 100%	Induct: Cisplatin/ 5FU/ Leucovorin/ Etoposide Concurrent: Cisplatin/Etoposide/40 Gy XRT + Surgery Same Chemotherapy + 65 Gy XRT, No Surgery	3 yr: 31% 25% ($P = .02$, equivalence)
Gaast (CROSS) (7)	363	AC – 74% SCC – 23%	Carboplatin/paclitaxel/41.4 Gy XRT + Surgery Surgery alone	3 yr: 59% 48% ($P = .011$)

XRT, radiation therapy; AC, adenocarcinoma; SCC, squamous cell carcinoma.

convincingly demonstrated the benefit of preoperative combined modality therapy (7). Three hundred sixty three patients with resectable T2–3 N0–1 M0 esophageal cancers were randomized to receive either surgical resection alone or preoperative paclitaxel and carboplatin given concurrently with 41.4 Gy of radiation over 23 fractions, followed by surgery 6 weeks later. The median age of the patients who enrolled for the study was 60 years, and the median WHO performance status was 0. Three fourths of the patients had adenocarcinoma, reflecting the national average. Chemotherapy consisted of paclitaxel 50 mg/m^2 and carboplatin area under the curve (AUC) = 2 mg/ml.min, which was administered weekly on days 1, 8, 15, 22, and 29 of radiation. The treatment was extremely tolerable, and resection was performed in a high percentage of patients: 90% of patients in the combined modality arm, and 86% of patients in the surgery alone arm. Complete (R0) resections were possible in 92.3% of patients in the trimodality arm compared to 67% of the patients in the surgery alone arm ($P < .002$). This was an important factor in the results, because unless patients have an R0 resection (microscopic negative margins) the chance of disease recurrence is high. The three-year overall survival favored the multimodality arm: 59% versus 48% alive at 3 years. The median survival was 49 months versus 26 months ($P = .011$, HR 0.67).

The Australasian G.I. Trials Group published a meta-analysis of 10 trials and 1209 patients that assessed preoperative chemoradiotherapy versus surgery alone (8). The results showed a 2-year absolute survival benefit of 13% for chemoradiation (HR 0.81, $P = .002$). At present, preoperative chemoradiation followed by surgery is the most common approach used by physicians in the United States. Chemotherapy doublets that are used most commonly contain a platinum agent or a fluoropyrimidine, coupled with a taxane, irinotecan, or oxaliplatin.

The National Comprehensive Center Network guidelines for Esophageal and Esophagogastric Junction Cancers affirm preoperative chemoradiation as a standard treatment approach to localized esophageal cancer. The guidelines list a sample of 18 possible chemotherapy combinations that have been utilized and reported in this setting. This underscores the fact that the final choice of the chemotherapy agents can be determined by the oncologist, taking into consideration factors related to the patient's medical condition and the physician's own interpretation of reported data.

Preoperative Chemotherapy

Another possible approach to the treatment of esophageal cancer is preoperative chemotherapy. Since the most common site of disease recurrence after surgery is distant disease, theoretically it would be very important to deliver chemotherapy to a patient as soon as possible after diagnosis to minimize the chance of micrometastatic disease. Three large randomized trials tested this concept (Table 6.2). Two showed survival benefit for preoperative chemotherapy before esophagectomy, and one did not.

The Medical Research Council in the United Kingdom showed evidence for the superiority of giving two cycles of preoperative epirubicin, cisplatin, and fluorouracil versus surgery alone for 802 patients (9). Median survival was 16.8 months in the combined modality arm and 13.3 months in the surgery alone arm. The results of this trial were updated in 2007, and the difference in overall survival at 5 years persisted—23% for the dual modality arm versus 17% for the surgery alone arm.

In addition, the MAGIC trial provided more evidence for the benefit of three cycles of preoperative chemotherapy with a triplet regimen consisting of epirubicin, cisplatin, and infused fluorouracil, with an additional three cycles of the same triplet post-op (10). The study randomized 503 patients with resectable adenocarcinoma of the lower esophagus, gastroesophageal junction, or stomach to perioperative therapy and surgery versus surgery alone. All patients had an Eastern Cooperative Oncology Group (ECOG) performance status of 0 or 1. Although gastric cancers were the predominant tumor type (74%), the remaining 26% of patients in the trial had cancer of the esophagus or GEJ. Chemotherapy was well tolerated and rates of postoperative complications were similar between the two groups. With a median follow-up of 4 years, the perioperative chemotherapy group had a 5-year overall survival of 36% versus 23% for those treated with surgery ($P = .009$). This difference was observed despite the fact that only 42% of the patients in the perioperative

Table 6.2 Select Randomized Preoperative Chemotherapy Trials for Resectable Esophageal Cancer

Author (ref#)	No. of Patients	Histology	Regimen	Survival
Medical Research Council (9)	802	AC – 66% SCC – 31%	Cisplatin/5FU + surgery Surgery alone	2 yr: 43% 34% ($P = .004$)
Cunningham (MAGIC) (10)	503 (75% gastric, 25% esophageal)	AC – 100%	Epirubicin/cisplatin/ 5FU + surgery Surgery alone	5 yr: 36% 23% ($P = .008$)
Kelsen (11)	440	AC – 54% SCC – 46%	Cisplatin/5FU + surgery Surgery alone	3 yr: 23% 26% ($P = .74$)

treatment group completed all protocol treatment, and 34% of patients who completed the preoperative chemotherapy and surgery did not go on to receive any postoperative treatment.

In contrast, the results and conclusions were different in an American Intergroup trial in which Kelsen and colleagues randomized 440 patients with esophageal cancer to either surgery alone or three cycles of cisplatin and 5-FU given preoperatively, followed by two additional cycles in the postoperative setting (11). There was no significant survival difference between the two arms: 2-year survival was 35% for patients treated with preoperative chemotherapy and 37% for those treated with surgery alone. This trial also demonstrated that for patients with localized esophageal cancer, whether or not preoperative chemotherapy is given, an R0 resection plays a crucial role in long-term survival. Even a microscopically positive margin is a poor prognostic factor. This negative trial possibly contributed to the bias of American physicians against preoperative chemotherapy and in favor of preoperative chemoradiation.

In 2007, two meta-analyses reported some benefit for preoperative chemotherapy compared to surgery alone. The Australasian G.I. Trials Group, with a sample of eight trials and 1724 patients reported a 2-year absolute survival benefit of 7% favoring preoperative systemic therapy (8). The Meta-Analysis of Chemotherapy in Esophagus Cancer Collaborative Group with a sample size of nine trials containing 2012 patients reported a 5-year absolute survival increase of 4% in preoperative chemotherapy arms (12). Accordingly, the National Comprehensive Cancer Network (NCCN) guidelines currently include perioperative chemotherapy as an acceptable treatment option for adenocarcinoma of the distal esophagus and GEJ. The suggested chemotherapy regimen is epirubicin, cisplatin, and 5-FU, and possible modifications include substituting oxaliplatin for cisplatin, or substituting capecitabine for 5-FU.

Postoperative Chemoradiation

Another approach to the treatment of locally advanced esophageal cancer is to perform surgery first, and then to follow up with chemoradiation in some patients. Reasons for starting with surgery may include patient preference, a borderline medical condition of the patient that causes concern about the ability to deliver trimodality therapy, a very elderly patient who may not tolerate long periods of aggressive treatment, or the occasional rare instance when an esophageal perforation occurs during a diagnostic endoscopy and necessitates immediate surgery.

Patients with stage II/III esophageal cancer should be considered for postoperative chemoradiation if no neoadjuvant therapy was administered. An Intergroup trial that included 556 patients with surgically resected adenocarcinoma of the stomach or GEJ demonstrated a 9-month median survival advantage favoring postoperative chemoradiation compared with surgery alone (13). Patients were randomized to either surgery alone or postoperative chemoradiation. The adjuvant therapy was 5-FU 425 mg/m^2 daily for 5 days, followed by 45 Gy of radiation over 5 weeks with two more cycles of chemotherapy delivered concurrently, and then two more 5-day cycles of 5-FU. T3 tumors predominated in both groups, with similar representation of patients having more than four positive lymph nodes. With a median follow-up of 5 years, the median duration of survival was 36 months in the chemoradiation group and 27 months in the control arm. At 3 years, 50% of patients in the chemoradiation arm were alive versus 41% in the surgery alone arm ($P = .005$).

The NCCN guidelines recognize postoperative chemoradiation as a standard of care for patients with adenocarcinoma of the stomach or GEJ, particularly for those patients who either have T3 tumors, are node positive, or had an R1 (microscopic positive margins) or R2 (macroscopic positive margins) resection. Because the trial that generated this recommendation used 5-FU and leucovorin, those agents are the ones listed in the guidelines as the major recommendation. However, it is acceptable to substitute capecitabine for 5-FU, or to use the regimen of paclitaxel and 5-FU.

Summary

With three reasonable therapeutic options (see Figure 6.1), how does a physician choose the appropriate treatment? The selection and dosing of anticancer treatment is complex, and must take into account patient variability, comorbidities, and nutritional status. If a patient has a very good performance status and wants aggressive treatment, then preoperative chemoradiation is a very reasonable choice. This practice is particularly common in the United States, and is supported by a substantial survival difference compared to surgery in meta-analyses. Occasionally, there might be some concern about a compromised patient being able to tolerate full chemoradiation and its accompanying toxicities, or a patient may have had prior radiation for another cancer in the past, which would make current administration of radiation difficult or impossible. This type of patients could be treated with perioperative chemotherapy to give some additional benefit over surgery alone. This approach is supported by meta-analyses comparing perioperative chemotherapy to surgery, although the survival benefit noted was slightly lower than that observed in the meta-analyses done for preoperative chemoradiation. And lastly, some patients may get surgery first for a variety of reasons. In that case, if the surgery was well tolerated and the patient's disease was T3 tumor, lymph node positive, or positive surgical margins, evaluation should be done to determine if postoperative

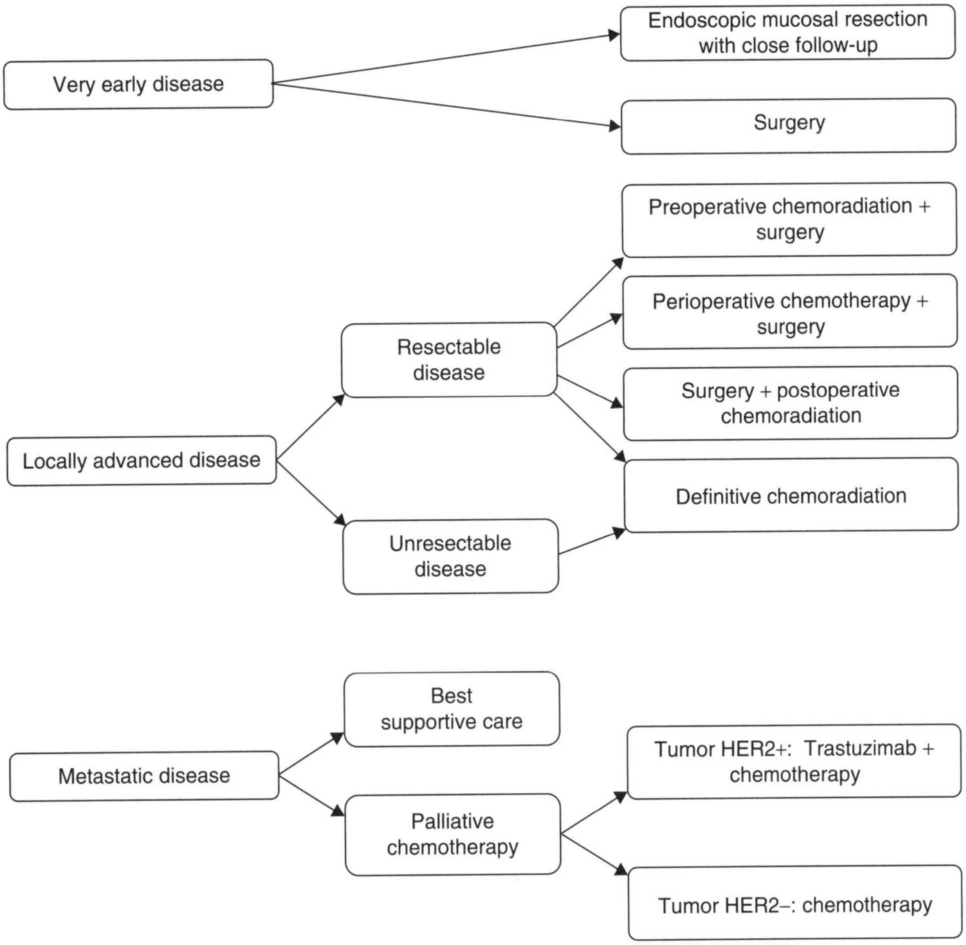

Figure 6.1

Algorithm for the treatment of esophageal cancer.

chemoradiation would be appropriate for that patient to improve the patient's overall and disease-free survival. In the case of J.D., his relatively young age, good performance status, and desire for aggressive treatment would lead to treatment with preoperative chemoradiation. The chemotherapy agents would most likely include a doublet of a platinum, or a fluoropyrimidine, or a taxane.

Locally Advanced Unresectable Esophageal Cancer

M.W. is a 68-year-old man who has been a heavy smoker for most of his life. He was also an alcoholic who has been sober for the past 2 years. He developed throat and neck pain and was seen by an otolaryngologist who did not find any abnormality during an office examination. He was then referred on for an upper endoscopy, and a fungating tumor was noted less than 25 cm from the incisors. The biopsy was positive for squamous cell carcinoma. His CT scan of the neck, chest, and abdomen showed no visceral metastases but did suggest that the tumor was growing posteriorly to involve a cervical vertebral body. His tumor stage was therefore IIIC (T4b N0 M0). He was evaluated by a thoracic surgeon who deemed his tumor to be unresectable. He was referred to Medical Oncology and Radiation Oncology for possible concurrent chemoradiation.

Evidence-Based Case Discussion

This patient's tumor is surgically unresectable for 2 reasons. First, the lesion appears to invade the vertebral body, making it technically difficult or impossible to achieve clear margins. Second, even if there was no bony involvement, the tumor is very high in the upper esophagus and would require a pharyngolaryngoesophagectomy, which would be too morbid with too little chance of cure. Therefore, definitive chemoradiation is the best choice for this patient. Evidence shows that patients who will not receive surgery should be treated with chemoradiation rather than radiation alone, if they can tolerate the side effects of combined modality treatment.

The Intergroup conducted a trial that was reported by Herskovic et al. (14). This was a phase III prospective, randomized trial that enrolled 121 patients and randomized them to either radiation alone or a combination of radiation with concurrent cisplatin and 5-FU. The dose of radiation as a single modality was 64 Gy. The treatment in the combination therapy arm consisted of 50 Gy of radiation given concurrently with cisplatin 75 mg/m^2 and 5-FU 1000 mg/m^2/day over 4 days for four cycles. The majority of patients in both arms had squamous cell cancers: 84% in the chemoradiation arm and 92% in the radiation alone/control arm. Most patients were between the ages of 60 and 69 and the

Karnofsky performance status (KPS) was greater than 80 in 92% to 95% of all patients. The combined treatment was more toxic overall with severe side effects in 44% and life threatening in 20% of patients receiving chemoradiation compared with 25% and 3%, respectively, in the radiation alone arm. The median survival was 12.5 months for patients in the combined modality arm, compared with 8.9 months for patients treated with single-agent radiation. Five-year survival rates for chemoradiotherapy versus radiotherapy were 26% and 0%. The authors concluded that concurrent therapy with cisplatin, 5-FU, and radiation is superior to radiation therapy alone, but at the cost of increased side effects (Table 6.3).

A subsequent Intergroup trial took the concept of definitive concurrent chemoradiation with cisplatin and 5-FU a step further, by testing whether it was more effective to give a higher dose of radiation with concurrent chemotherapy—64.8 Gy versus the standard 50.4 Gy (15). Two hundred and eighteen patients were randomized, of which 85% had squamous cell carcinoma and 15% had adenocarcinoma. There was no significant difference in survival between the arms: median survival was 13 months for the high-dose radiation and 18.1 months for the standard radiation; 2-year survival was 31% versus 40% (Table 6.3). Therefore, cisplatin and 5-FU in combination with 50.4 Gy of radiation was considered the standard of care.

The NCCN guidelines note that numerous regimens and dosing schedules of chemotherapy have been used in combination with radiation as definitive therapy for patients with esophageal cancer. Some of the agents listed in various combinations include cisplatin and 5-FU/capecitabine, oxaliplatin and a fluoropyrimidine, a taxane and cisplatin, paclitaxel and carboplatin, irinotecan and cisplatin, a taxane with a fluoropyrimidine, or even triplet therapy. Very recent trials are also exploring the addition of targeted agents to chemoradiation.

Summary

Nonsurgical therapy is best for bulky, inoperable disease, for patients who are not surgical candidates due to significant comorbidities, or for patients whose tumors are so proximal that the surgery required would be very extensive and extremely morbid with minimal chance of cure. For these patients who have a good performance status and desire aggressive treatment, concurrent chemoradiation is indicated (Figure 6.1). However, although survival is better with chemoradiation, the physician must remember that it is also significantly more toxic, and so radiation alone may be the best option for very frail patients. Our patient, M.W., is relatively young and relatively healthy. After a frank discussion about the substantial possibility of severe hematologic and gastrointestinal side effects, concurrent chemoradiation would be initiated. These patients have to be monitored closely for nutrition, fluid intake, and pain.

Metastatic Esophageal Cancer

L.J. is a 66-year-old male veteran. He had been married for 36 years and his wife had prompted him to go to his primary care physician because he had been losing weight. His past medical history was significant for diabetes and he attributed his recent 62 pound weight loss over the past 7 months to his recent limitation of sweets from his diet. His wife reported to the physician that he looked relatively pale. His energy was decreasing, which he attributed to old age. On review of symptoms he reported epigastric pain and difficulty swallowing solid foods. He could ingest food, but had to take several drinks of water to accomplish this. He described the pain as dull and fairly constant, but low in intensity. He denied any change in his bowel habits.

On examination, L.J. had conjunctival pallor, and his sclera were anicteric. Palpation of his neck revealed a Virchow's node. His lung examinatiolar rales. His cardiac examination was unremarkable. He was tender in the epigastrum and there was a vaguely palpable mass. He did not have abdominal distention and no lower extremity edema.

A hemogram revealed a hemoglobin of 10.1 mg/dL and a comprehensive metabolic panel demonstrated a mild elevation of his transaminases. A CT scan of the chest, abdomen, and pelvis was ordered in addition to a GI referral for endoscopy. At the time of endoscopy, L.J. was found to have a circumferential narrowing at the GEJ with a friable and ulcerated mass. Biopsies of the mass were taken and revealed a moderately well-differentiated adenocarcinoma. The CT scan demonstrated a 6 × 7 cm mass at the GEJ, multiple low attenuation lesions in the liver ranging in size from 5 mm to 2.3 cm, diffuse adenopathy

Table 6.3 Select Randomized Definitive Chemoradiation Trials for Unresectable Esophageal Cancer

Author (ref)	No. of Patients	Histology	Regimen	Survival
Herskovic (14)	121	AC – 13%	Cisplatin/5FU + 50 Gy XRT	2 yr: 38%
		SCC – 87%	64 Gy XRT	10% (p=.001)
Minsky (15)	218	AC – 14%	Cisplatin/5FU + 50.4 Gy XRT	2 yr: 40%
		SCC – 86%	Cisplatin/5FU + 64.5 Gy XRT	31% (NSD)

consistent with metastatic disease involving celiac, lesser curvature, posterior mediastinal, and a left supraclavicular node. There were scattered lung nodules bilaterally all less than 5 to 8 mm in diameter. One of the liver nodules was biopsied and unfortunately was also positive for adenocarcinoma. The biopsy was tested for HER2/neu with immunohistochemistry and the results were 3+ positive.

Evidence-Based Case Discussion

Determination of treatment for a patient with metastatic esophageal cancer starts with a discussion between the physician and patient regarding goals of care. In order to make a reasonable decision for the best quality of life, the patient must understand that this stage of disease is incurable, and that chemotherapy is palliative in nature. If the patient has no symptoms to palliate, the best decision might be to elect no treatment. However, this patient has abdominal pain and dysphagia, so he has symptoms to palliate. It may be possible to relieve his dysphagia with placement of a stent, but because he has a reasonable performance status, palliative chemotherapy is also an option (Figure 6.1).

Chemotherapy

The choices for chemotherapy typically include a combination of two to three drugs, and the most commonly used active agents are the platinums (cisplatin, carboplatin, oxaliplatin), the fluoropyrimidines (5-FU and capecitabine), the taxanes (paclitaxel and docetaxel), irinotecan, and epirubicin (see Table 6.4). In 2008 the "REAL-2" trial conducted in the United Kingdom compared four triplet chemotherapy regimens: all regimens contained epirubicin, combined with either cisplatin and 5-fluorouracil (ECF), cisplatin and capecitabine (ECX), oxaliplatin and 5-fluorouracil (EOF), or oxaliplatin and capecitabine (EOX) (16). In the study, 1002 patients were enrolled and the endpoint was noninferiority in overall survival for triplet therapies comparing the newer agents, oxaliplatin and capecitabine, as opposed to the older agents, cisplatin and infusional 5-FU. Patients enrolled in the study had either metastatic or locally advanced cancers of the esophagus, GEJ, or stomach. At a minimum, 87% of patients in each arm had an ECOG performance status of 0 or 1. Eighty-six percent to 90% of patients had adenocarcinomas. The median number of cycles of therapy in each group was six. Regarding the primary endpoint, both capecitabine and oxaliplatin performed well with hazard ratios for death of 0.86 and 0.92 compared to infusional 5-FU and cisplatin, respectively. The overall response rate in the EOX arm was 47.9% versus 40.7%, 46.4%, and 42.4% for the ECF, ECX, and EOF arms respectively. Progression-free survival was 7 months in the EOX arm versus 6.2 to 6.7 months in the three comparator arms. The EOX arm was associated with a 11.2-month median survival compared with 9.9, 9.9, and 9.3 months in the ECF, ECX, and EOF arms respectively. Cisplatin containing regimens were associated with greater frequencies of hair loss and grade 3 or 4 leukopenia, whereas oxaliplatin containing regimens were associated with a greater incidence of grade 3 or 4 peripheral neuropathy. The primary endpoint was achieved and capecitabine and oxaliplatin were proven noninferior to 5-FU and cisplatin, respectively. Since this trial, EOX has become a frequently used regimen for metastatic disease.

The NCCN guidelines list numerous possible chemotherapy combinations, involving cisplatin, carboplatin, oxaliplatin, 5-FU, capecitabine, paclitaxel, docetaxel, irinotecan, and epirubicin. The regimen is typically chosen by weighing its potential side effects and the patient's characteristics and medical history.

Targeted Therapy

Recent studies have shown that approximately 20% of adenocarcinomas of the esophagus express the receptor for HER2. This suggested the possibility of therapeutic

Table 6.4 Select Randomized Chemotherapy Trials for Metastatic Esophageal Cancer

Author (ref#)	No. of Patients	Regimen	Response Rate (%)	Median Survival (months)	Survival
Cunningham (REAL-2) (16)	1002	Epirubicin/cisplatin/5FU (ECF)	40.7	9.9	1 yr: 37.7%
		Epirubicin/cisplatin/ capecitabine (ECX)	46.4	9.9	40.8%
			42.4	9.3	40.4%
		Epirubicin/oxaliplatin/5FU (EOF)	47.9	11.2	46.8%
		Epirubicin/oxaliplatin/ capecitabine (EOX)			
Bang 2010 (ToGA) (17)	584 HER2+ patients	Cisplatin/5-FU or capecitabine	35	11.1	
		Cisplatin/5FU or capecitabine + Trastuzumab	47	13.8 (P = .0046)	
Kang (AVAGAST) (18)	774	Cisplatin/capecitabine	37	10.1	
		Cisplatin/capecitabine + bevacizumab	46	12.1 (P = .1002)	

utility for trastuzumab, which is a monoclonal antibody that binds to the HER2 receptor. Therefore, a phase 3 randomized, open labeled controlled study, called the ToGA trial, was conducted (17). In the ToGA study, 3665 patients were screened, and 810 had tumors that were HER2 positive, for an overall positivity rate of 22%, which included 20% of gastric cancers and 34% of GEJ cancers. HER2 receptor positivity was determined by immunohistochemistry (3+), or FISH (HER2:CEP17 ratio≥2). Five hundred eighty four patients were included in the primary analysis and were randomized to either the control arm (cisplatin 80mg/m^2 on day 1 and either capecitabine 1000 mg/m^2 orally twice per day for 14 days of a 21-day cycle or fluorouracil 800 mg/m^2 by continuous infusion on days 1 to 5 of each cycle) or the experimental arm (the same chemotherapy plus trastuzumab 8 mg/kg on day 1 of the first cycle, followed by 6 mg/kg every 3 weeks). Approximately 90% of patients in each treatment arm had good ECOG performance status, and 80% to 83% of patients had gastric cancer. Median overall survival was 13.8 months for those assigned to the trastuzumab plus chemotherapy arm, and 11.1 months for those assigned to chemotherapy alone (HR 0.74). The rates of grade 3 or 4 toxicities including cardiac toxicities did not differ greatly between the treatment arms. The authors concluded that trastuzumab plus chemotherapy is a new standard option for patients with advanced HER2 positive GEJ and gastric cancers.

Bevacizumab is a monoclonal antibody that binds to the vascular endothelial growth factor receptor (VEGF-R). The AVAGAST trial was a randomized, double-blind, placebo controlled trial that recently compared outcomes of 774 patients treated with capecitabine and cisplatin plus bevacizumab, versus the same chemotherapy alone (18). The study unfortunately did not meet its primary objective of demonstrating a significant increase in overall survival. Within the intent to treat population, the median overall survival was 10.1 months with chemotherapy and placebo, as compared to 12.1 months in the chemotherapy plus bevacizumab arm (HR 0.87, P = .1002). However, progression-free survival significantly favored the bevacizumab-containing arm: 29.5 months in the placebo arm compared with 38.0 months in the treatment arm (P = .0121). Bevacizumab was well tolerated overall.

Although it is disappointing that the bevacizumab did not contribute to an improvement in overall survival, we await the results of several ongoing trials using this agent. The MAGIC-B trial is continuing in the United Kingdom, in which patients with resectable cancer are randomized to receive preop and postop chemotherapy consisting of epirubicin, cisplatin, and capecitabine, plus or minus bevacizumab. The Dana Farber Cancer Institute is treating patients with metastatic esophageal cancer in a randomized trial, giving cisplatin, irinotecan, and bevacizumab in both arms, plus or minus docetaxel. However, until these results are available, and because of the negative outcome of the AVAGAST trial, bevacizumab should not be used routinely outside of a clinical trial for patients with esophageal cancer.

Summary

L.J.'s tumor was 3+ positive for HER2 receptor, he had a reasonable performance status, and he wished to pursue at least one regimen of palliative chemotherapy to try to relieve his discomfort and dysphagia. Therefore, we can elect to offer to treat him with cisplatin, 5-FU or capecitabine, and trastuzumab. We first need to address that he has an adequate means of maintaining nutrition, possibly a feeding tube or stent if he cannot swallow enough on his own, before initiating the chemotherapy.

REFERENCES

1. Hongo M, Nagasaki Y, Shoji T. Epidemiology of esophageal cancer: Orient to Occident. Effects of chronology, geography and ethnicity. *J Gastroenterol Hepatol.* 2009;24(5):729–735.
2. Girling DJ, Bancewicz J, Clark PI, et al. Surgical resection with or without preoperative chemotherapy in oesophageal cancer: a randomized controlled trial. *Lancet.* 2002;359(9319):1727–1733.
3. Walsh TN, Noonan N, Hollywood D, et al. A comparison of multimodal therapy and surgery for esophageal adenocarcinoma. *N Engl J Med.* 1996;335(7):462–467.
4. Urba S, Orringer M, Turrisi A, et al. Randomized trial of preoperative chemoradiation vs surgery alone in patients with locoregional esophageal cancer. *J Clin Oncol.* 2001;19(2):305–313.
5. Tepper J, Krasna M, Niedzwiecki D, et al. Phase III trial of trimodality therapy with cisplatin, fluorouracil, radiotherapy, and surgery compared with surgery alone for esophageal cancer: CALGB 9781. *J Clin Oncol.* 2008;26(7):1086–1092.
6. Stahl M, Stuschke M, Lehmann N, et al. Chemoradiation with and without surgery in patients with locally advanced squamous cell carcinoma of the esophagus. *J Clin Oncol.* 2005;23(10):2310–2317.
7. Gaast AV, van Hagen P, Hulshof M, et al. Effect of preoperative concurrent chemoradiotherapy on survival of patients with resectable esophageal or esophagogastric junction cancer: results from a multicenter randomized phase III study. *J Clin Oncol.* 2010;28(15s):abstract #4004.
8. Gebski V, Burmeister B, Smithers BM, et al. for the Australasian Gastro-Intestinal Trials Group. Survival benefits from neoadjuvant chemoradiotherapy or chemotherapy in oesophageal carcinoma: a meta-analysis. *Lancet Oncol.* 2007;8:226–234
9. Medical Research Council Oesophageal Cancer Working Party. Surgical resection with or without preoperative chemotherapy in oesophageal cancer: a randomized controlled trial. *Lancet.* 2002;359(9319):1727–1733.
10. Cunningham D, Allum WH, Stenning SP, et al. Perioperative chemotherapy versus surgery alone in resectable gastroesophageal cancer. *N Engl J Med.* 2006;355(1):11–20.
11. Kelsen DP, Ginsberg R, Pajak TF, et al. Chemotherapy followed by surgery compared with surgery alone for localized esophageal cancer. *N Engl J Med.* 1998;339(27):1979–1984.
12. Thirion PG, Michiels S, Le Maitre A, Tierney J, on behalf of the Meta-Analysis of Chemotherapy in Esophagus Cancer Collaborative Group. Individual patient data-based meta-analysis assessing pre-operative chemotherapy in resectable oesophageal carcinoma. *J Clin Oncol.* 2007;25(18S):abstract #4512.

13. Macdonald JS, Smalley SR, Benedetti J, et al. Chemoradiotherapy after surgery compared with surgery alone for adenocarcinoma of the stomach or gastroesophageal junction. *N Engl J Med.* 2001;345(10):725–730.
14. Herskovic A, Martz K, al-Sarraf M, et al. Combined chemotherapy and radiotherapy compared with radiotherapy alone in patients with cancer of the esophagus. *N Engl J Med.* 1992;326(24): 1593–1598.
15. Minsky BD, Pajak TF, Ginsberg RJ et al. INT 0123 (Radiation Therapy Oncology Group 94-05) Phase III trial of combined modality therapy for esophageal cancer: high-dose versus standard-dose radiation therapy. *J Clin Oncol.* 2002;20(5): 1167–1174.
16. Cunningham D, Starling N, Rao S, et al. Capecitabine and oxaliplatin for advanced esophagogastric cancer. *N Engl J Med.* 2008;358(1):36–46.
17. Bang YJ, Van Custem E, Feyereislova A, et al. Trastuzumab in combination with chemotherapy versus chemotherapy alone for treatment of HER2-positive advanced gastric or gastro-oesophageal junction cancer (ToGA): a phase 3, open-label, randomised controlled trial. *Lancet.* 2010;376 (9742): 687–697.
18. Kang AY, Ohtsu E, Van Cutsem E, et al. AVAGAST: A randomized, double-blind, placebo-controlled, phase III study of first-line capecitabine and cisplatin plus bevacizumab or placebo in patients with advanced gastric cancer (AGC). *J Clin Oncol.* 2010;28:abstract #4007.

7

Gastric Cancer

EDUARDO VILAR AND MARK M. ZALUPSKI

EPIDEMIOLOGY, NATURAL HISTORY, RISK FACTORS, AND PATHOLOGY

In 2010, in the United States, around 21,130 new cases of gastric cancer were diagnosed, and around 10,620 deaths occurred due to this neoplasm. The incidence of gastric cancer shows wide geographic variation, with high rates of this disease in Japan, Korea, China, and certain countries in Latin America and Eastern Europe. In contrast, low incidence rates are observed in Northern Africa, South and Southeast Asia, and North America. This regional variation is probably related to differences in epidemiological factors, but it may also be attributable to molecular differences in the biology of the disease. In addition, the incidence of gastric cancer has steadily decreased in the United States and Western European countries during the last three decades. This observation is likely related to changes in dietary habits, improvement in food preparation and storage, and treatment of *Helicobacter pylori* infection.

On the basis of the NCI SEER Cancer Statistic Review, the median age of diagnosis of gastric cancer in the time period 2003 to 2007 was 70, with 27% of the patients diagnosed between the ages of 75 and 84, and 12% more than 85 years of age. Twenty three percent of the patients presented with localized disease, 32% with locally advanced, and 34% with distant metastasis. Survival correlated with stage, with 5-year survival rates of 62%, 27% and 3% for localized, regional, and distant disease, respectively. The majority of the patients are diagnosed with advanced disease, and therefore are considered for systemic treatment based on their performance status and comorbidities. Selection of systemic treatment options should take into account the toxicity profile of the agent(s) used and the resultant tolerance in patients who are generally elderly.

Analytical epidemiology studies have identified several risk factors involved in the pathogenesis of this disease, reflecting the multifactorial nature of gastric cancer. The strength of the association of each factor varies depending on the subtype of gastric cancer analyzed. Traditional risk factors for gastric carcinoma have been linked to the intestinal subtype. These include high salt diet, presence of nitrates in cured foods, tobacco exposure, and *H. pylori* infection. The *H. pylori* infection leads to the development of chronic gastritis and progression through atrophy, intestinal metaplasia, dysplasia, and malignancy. Protective factors such as a diet rich in fruits and vegetables, refrigeration of food, and exposure to vitamin C and carotenoids have been related to decreased risk. It is noteworthy that the decrease in the incidence of gastric cancer observed during the last few decades is clearly attributable to interventions leading to the modifications of these risk factors, thus impacting on the burden of intestinal gastric cancer. Genetic predisposition has also been recognized as important to the development of intestinal subtype, such as deficiency of mismatch repair proteins and a diagnosis of Lynch Syndrome.

Conversely, relationships between diffuse gastric cancer and specific environmental factors have not been clearly identified, although *H. pylori* may also account for an increase in the risk of the diffuse subtype. Genetic factors, however, have been strongly associated with the development of early onset, diffuse gastric carcinoma. The presence of germline truncating mutations in *CDH1*, which encodes for the protein E-Cadherin, leads to the autosomal dominant cancer genetic syndrome known as hereditary diffuse gastric cancer (HDGC), which is also associated with the development of lobular breast cancer. The diagnosis of HDGC confers, by age 80, an estimated cumulative risk of gastric carcinoma of 67% for men (95%

confidence interval [95% CI], 39–99) and 83% for women (95% CI, 58–99). In addition, in women the cumulative risk of breast cancer is approximately 39% (95% CI, 12–84). Strikingly, immunohistochemistry (IHC) evidence for the loss of E-Cadherin is also observed in approximately 50% of sporadic gastric cancer, although these cases are typically associated with the presence of missense mutations of *CDH1*.

Finally, risk factors for the development of gastroesophageal junction (GEJ) tumors include alcohol, tobacco, past medical history of gastroesophageal reflux, and obesity. The incidence of GEJ tumors among young white individuals has increased in the past decade in Western countries secondary to the relative increase in the rates of obesity and reflux disease.

Gastric cancer spreads by local invasion, lymphatic extension, distant hematogenous metastasis, and peritoneal dissemination. Initially, the malignancy invades locally into, along, and through the gastric wall, further advancing into neighboring organs and anatomic structures. Intestinal type gastric carcinomas are commonly limited to a restricted area of the stomach. In contrast, diffuse carcinomas tend to widely invade the entire stomach, inducing a linitis plastica and often extending into the duodenum. Lymph node involvement usually correlates with size and depth of the primary tumor and follows an orderly fashion when spreading into regional lymph node stations. This behavior influences the surgical principles underlying the extent of lymphadenectomy in those patients who are candidates for surgical resection. Venous invasion leads to the development of distant metastasis that are most commonly located in the liver, lungs, and bone. Finally, local invasion of the serosal surface precedes the development of peritoneal metastases. Not uncommonly, bilateral ovarian metastases are observed in premenopausal women diagnosed with gastric carcinoma, the so-called Krukenberg's tumor.

Generally, intestinal gastric cancer will develop distant metastasis via hematogenous dissemination. Diffuse tumors often present with extensive lymph node and peritoneal involvement. Tumors of the GEJ resemble the behavior of esophageal tumors. Not infrequently, the esophagus is involved through submucosal progression. In addition, lymph node metastases may be located in the lower mediastinum (upward progression) or in the esophagogastric angles and other para-aortic structures (downward progression).

Gastric cancer is not a single disease. Its classification can be established based on the anatomic location of the primary tumor and/or the histologic pattern displayed. On the basis of the anatomic location in the stomach, gastric carcinoma is subdivided into cardiac (involving the GEJ) and noncardiac tumors (the majority located in the corpus or the antral area). When differentiated by histological pattern, gastric cancer is divided into intestinal or diffuse subtypes (1). At the present time, both classifications are used simultaneously because the epidemiological factors, precursor lesions, and phenotypic and clinical features correlate specifically with each subtype (Table 7.1). Therefore, a three-category classification is widely used: GEJ/cardiac, intestinal noncardia, and diffuse subtype.

The Lauren classification distinguishes between intestinal and diffuse gastric cancer. Intestinal gastric cancer forms rudimentary glands and displays different degrees of differentiation, from well through moderately and

Table 7.1 Summary of the Characteristics of Gastric Cancer Based on Tumor Subtypes

	Cardiac GE Junction	Noncardiac Intestinal	Noncardiac Diffuse
Epidemiology	Incidence increasing in Western countries	Incidence decreasing worldwide	Incidence stable
Biology	Possible link with HER2 biology	HNPCC-related	*CDH1* mutations Loss of E-Cadherin
Clinical features	GERD Obesity	*H. pylori* infection Tobacco/Alcohol Salt intake Poor fruit/vegetable diet	No clear relation to classical risk factors
Pathology		Stepwise progression model: – Chronic gastritis – Intestinal metaplasia – Dysplasia	No stepwise progression No precursor lesion Signet ring cells Interstitial mucin
HER2 status	32% +ve GEJ	32% +ve Intestinal	6% +ve Diffuse

GERD, gastroesophageal reflux disease; GEJ, gastroesophageal junction; HNPCC, hereditary nonpolyposis colorectal cancer; GC, gastric cancer; +ve, positive.

poorly differentiated tumors. This subtype usually arises from a background of intestinal metaplasia. It follows a stepwise progression model that begins with chronic gastritis triggered by factors such as *H. pylori* infection and is promoted by a diet that is poor in fruits and vegetables and rich in nitrates. Chronic gastritis induces atrophy of the gastric epithelium followed by replacement of the atrophic cells by cells resembling the intestine, a condition called intestinal metaplasia. This metaplasia may transition into increasing grades of dysplasia, eventually extending through the basement membrane and becoming an invasive carcinoma. In the other histologic subtype, that is, diffuse gastric cancer, tumors contain cells that fail to form any recognizable structures, resembling glands with the classical appearance of signet ring cells. Sometimes small amounts of interstitial mucin are observed. Diffuse gastric cancer does not have any well-defined precursor lesion, although it may arise in a background of chronic gastritis. It is not uncommon to find evidence of *H. pylori* infection as well.

More recently, a molecular subtype of gastric cancer has been identified based on overexpression of the oncoprotein HER2. The HER2 protein is a 185-kDa *trans*-membrane tyrosine kinase receptor that is a member of the family of the epidermal growth factor receptors (EGFR). HER2 is encoded by a gene located at chromosome 17q21. It has been shown to be overexpressed and/or amplified in 13% to 22% of gastric cancers (2). Overexpression may be determined using IHC with a monoclonal antibody (Herceptest) and amplification using fluorescent in situ hybridization (FISH), following the same procedures as in breast cancer. The ToGA trial analyzed a total of 1527 gastric cancers for HER2 overexpression using both IHC and FISH, with an observed frequency of 22%. These analyses showed a higher correlation between HER2 overexpression and the intestinal subtype (versus the diffuse and mixed subtypes) and the GEJ location (versus the noncardiac origin). The role of HER2 as a prognostic factor in gastric cancer is debated. The majority of studies, however, have shown a negative prognostic effect for those tumors overexpressing HER2. Importantly, therapeutic implications for HER2-positive tumors will be discussed in further detail in the metastatic disease section of this chapter.

STAGING

Gastric cancer is staged by using TNM classification, which is based on the extent of tumor and involvement of local and distant structures. The American Joint Committee on Cancer (AJCC) staging of gastric tumors is shown below.

Carcinoma of the Stomach Staging Classification

Stage	Definition
0	Carcinoma in situ: intraepithelial tumor without invasion of the lamina propria
IA	Tumor invades lamina propria, muscularis mucosae, or submucosa without lymph node involvement or metastasis
IB	Tumor invades muscularis propia without lymph node involvement or metastasis, *or* tumor invades lamina propria, muscularis mucosae, or submucosa with metastasis in 1–2 regional lymph nodes
IIA	Tumor penetrates subserosal connective tissue without invasion of visceral peritoneum or adjacent structures without lymph node involvement or metastasis; *or* tumor invades muscularis propia with metastasis in 1–2 regional lymph nodes; *or* tumor invades lamina propria, muscularis mucosae, or submucosa with metastasis in 3–6 regional lymph nodes
IIB	Tumor invades serosa (visceral peritoneum) without lymph node involvement or metastasis *or* tumor penetrates subserosal connective tissue without invasion of visceral peritoneum or adjacent structures with metastasis in 1–2 regional lymph nodes *or* tumor invades muscularis propia with metastasis in 3–6 regional lymph nodes *or* tumor invades lamina propria, muscularis mucosae, or submucosa with metastasis in 7 or more regional lymph nodes
IIIA	Tumor invades serosa (visceral peritoneum) with metastasis in 1–2 regional lymph nodes *or* tumor penetrates subserosal connective tissue without invasion of visceral peritoneum or adjacent structures with metastasis in 3–6 regional lymph nodes *or* tumor invades muscularis propia with metastasis in 7 or more regional lymph nodes
IIIB	Tumor invades adjacent structures with metastasis in 0–2 regional lymph nodes *or* tumor invades serosa (visceral peritoneum) with metastasis in 3–6 regional lymph nodes *or* tumor penetrates subserosal connective tissue without invasion of visceral peritoneum or adjacent structures with metastasis in 7 or more regional lymph nodes
IIIC	Tumor invades adjacent structures with metastasis in 3 or more regional lymph nodes *or* tumor invades serosa (visceral peritoneum) with metastasis in 7 or more regional lymph nodes
IV	Distant metastasis

Source: American Joint Committee on Cancer (AJCC), 7th edition.

CASE SUMMARIES

Resectable Gastric Cancer

S.C. is a 66-year-old man with a past medical history relevant for myocardial infarction secondary to coronary artery disease, hyperlipidemia, peripheral vascular disease with intermittent claudication, and sleep apnea. He has a 20-pack-year history of tobacco exposure and no history of alcohol use. S.C. presented with epigastric pain over a 3-month period and subsequently had one episode of gastrointestinal bleeding that required admission to a local hospital. During that admission a complete workup was performed, including an EGD that revealed the presence of an ulcerated and friable mass in the gastric fundus as well as mild gastritis in the antrum. Biopsies demonstrated invasive adenocarcinoma. A CT scan of chest, abdomen, and pelvis showed thickening of the fundus and cardia of the stomach with adjacent pathologically enlarged lymph nodes. There was no evidence of distant metastatic disease. A combined positron emission tomography and CT scanning (PET-CT) confirmed the presence of increased uptake in the posterior aspect of the fundus and in regional lymph nodes. Endoscopic ultrasound (EUS) examination revealed tumor in the gastric wall involving the muscularis propria, with enlarged lymph nodes in the vicinity (uT2 N1 Mx). S.C. was evaluated by surgery and considered to be a candidate for total gastrectomy with Roux-en-Y esophagojejunostomy and placement of jejunostomy feeding tube. At this point S.C. was referred to the medical oncology clinic for evaluation.

Evidence-Based Case Discussion

The staging workup for gastric cancer should include history and physical examination, blood count and differential, liver, and renal function tests, upper endoscopy (EGD), computed tomography (CT) of the abdomen and pelvis, and either x-ray or CT scan of the thorax. The role of EGD is crucial in the diagnosis of gastric cancer since it enables the visualization of the tumor as well as the evaluation of its localization and extent. Moreover, EGD allows biopsy and diagnosis of the tumor and simultaneously determines the presence of *H. pylori* infection or Barrett's esophagus. EUS is helpful in determining the depth of tumor invasion and the proximal and distal extent of the tumor, although it is less useful for this purpose in those tumors located in the antrum. In women, pelvic CT or ultrasound (US) may help to rule out the presence of ovarian metastasis. PET-CT has been shown to be superior for preoperative staging when compared to CT scan or PET alone. PET-CT is especially useful to evaluate the presence of distant metastasis and to help accurately determine the nodal staging. The use of laparoscopy, with or without cytology of peritoneal washings, is debated. Some institutions perform it routinely as an initial maneuver in all patients who are medically fit and candidates for surgical resection. Especially in those patients to be treated with neoadjuvant therapy with the intention of downstaging, laparoscopy may be performed prior to therapy in order to exclude the presence of metastatic disease. The staging classification of gastric cancer is based on the data collected with these procedures and is depicted above. However, in clinical settings, a more often used classification, based on the potential for resection and evidence for extent of disease, divides patients into three categories: resectable, locally advanced unresectable, and metastatic gastric cancer (Figure 7.1).

An attempt at curative resection is often the initial treatment for gastric cancer. However, complete resection is sometimes not possible. In Western countries, fewer than half the patients are candidates for curative resection at the time of their initial presentation. The major surgical issues include the extent of the luminal resection and the lymph node dissection. Regarding the extent of luminal resection, tumors located distally can be addressed either by a total gastrectomy or a distal subtotal gastrectomy. Several prospective studies have shown no difference in terms of survival between these two approaches. However, the quality of life is superior after a subtotal gastrectomy. For those tumors located more proximally, factors such as an association with Barrett's esophagus, the exact location (i.e., within the GE junction versus subcardial region) and the grade of differentiation of the tumor (well/moderately versus poorly differentiated) need to be considered. Proximal subtotal gastrectomy can be a valid approach for either well or moderately differentiated tumors that arise within the GE junction, but not for those associated with Barrett's esophagus or tumors located in the subcardial region. Poorly differentiated tumors, those associated with Barrett's esophagus, and those extending into any portion of the esophagus require total gastrectomy with some extent of esophagectomy and a Roux-en-Y reconstruction.

An area of controversy in the surgical treatment of gastric cancer is the extent of the lymph node dissection. Lymph node dissection is classified into different categories designated D0–3 as the extent of lymphadenectomy increases. D1 dissection includes perigastric lymph nodes located in the lesser and greater curvatures and is a minimum standard surgical treatment. A classical D2 dissection includes nodes located along the hepatic, left gastric, celiac, and splenic arteries including the splenic hilum, thus requiring a splenectomy for proximal tumors. D3 involves dissection and removal of the portahepatic and periaortic nodes, areas sometimes considered metastatic locations. D2 dissection requires a high degree of expertise and should be performed only in those centers with sufficient experience. Studies have analyzed the effect of D1 versus D2 dissection on survival. Generally, it is believed that D2 dissections offer a survival advantage over D1 dissections.

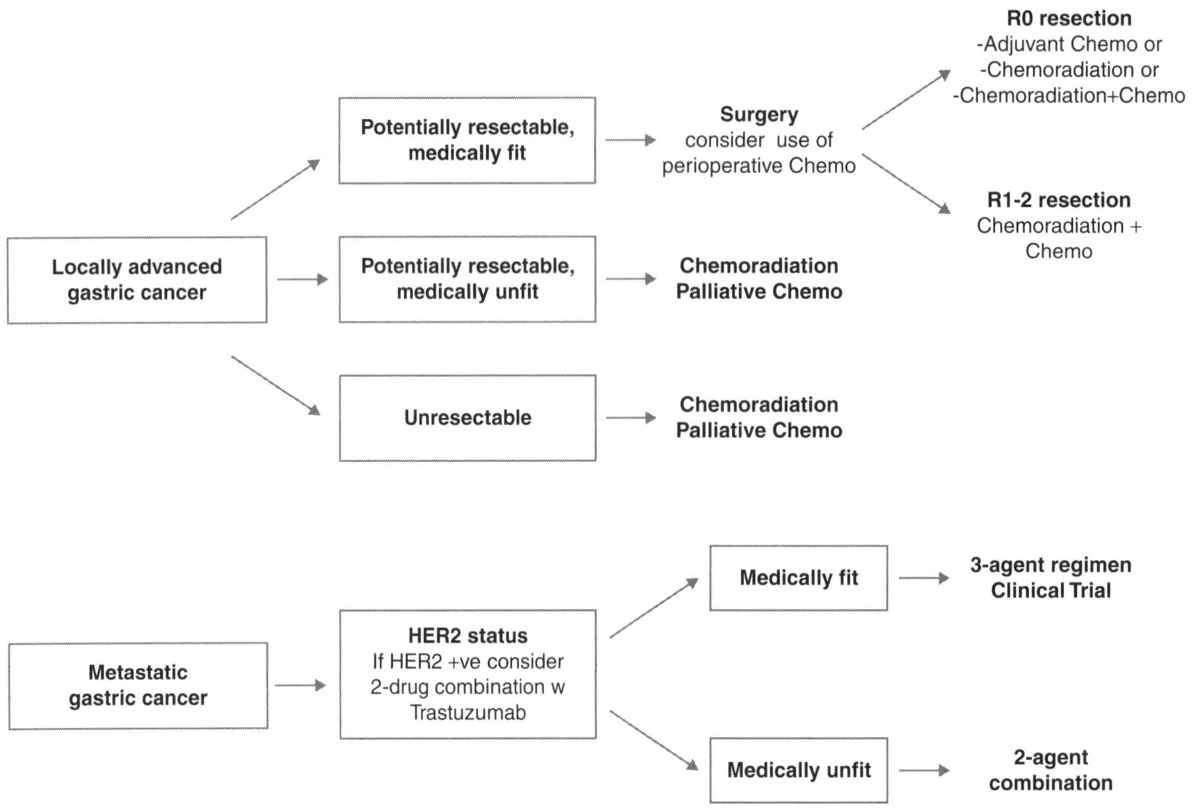

Figure 7.1

Algorithm for the treatment of gastric cancer.

In Asian countries, the standard of care includes the classical D2 dissection, whereas in Western countries the standard is a modified D2 dissection, excluding splenectomy or pancreatectomy and achieving the goal of removing at least 15 lymph nodes.

In addition to resection, therapeutic strategies that have been studied for resectable gastric cancer include the use of perioperative chemotherapy, postoperative adjuvant chemotherapy, and postoperative adjuvant chemoradiation. To date, however, these different approaches have not been directly compared with one another.

The rationale for the use of perioperative chemotherapy (pre- and postoperative treatment) includes downstaging of the tumor to improve the rate of complete resection; earliest possible treatment of micrometastasis when the cell growth fraction is high; treatment of tumors when the cell heterogeneity is low and tissue oxygenation is high; and avoidance of disruption in the delivery of adjuvant therapy following surgery due to postoperative complications that may delay or prevent its use. The UK Medical Research Council (MRC) Adjuvant Gastric Infusional Chemotherapy (MAGIC) trial was a phase III randomized controlled study including 503 patients (3). This study demonstrated a significant survival benefit with six cycles of perioperative chemotherapy using a regimen that included epirubicin, cisplatin, and 5-fluorouracil (ECF) as compared to surgery alone. Survival rates at 5 years were improved from 23% with surgery alone to 36% with surgery and chemotherapy ($P = .009$). The use of perioperative chemotherapy did not affect the rate of surgical resection (91.6% in the chemotherapy arm versus 94.6% in the surgery arm). However, a significant downstaging effect was observed in the perioperative arm with regard to tumor stage (T1-2 disease 52% in the chemotherapy arm versus 37% in the surgery-only arm, P-value = .002) and nodal disease described by an increase in the fraction of patients with N0-1 disease (84% in the chemotherapy arm versus 70% in the surgical arm, $P = .01$). Regarding the extent of lymphadenectomy in this trial, approximately 40% of patients underwent some type of D2 dissection, 21% had D1 dissections, 20% had surgical resection of the primary without lymph node dissection, and the rest had a non-resectional surgery. These data reflect the quality of the surgery performed in those patients enrolled in the MAGIC trial, and should be taken into account when comparing trials testing other modalities of adjuvant treatment such as the ACTS-GC trial or the Intergroup 0116.

The Adjuvant Chemotherapy Trial of S-1 for Gastric Cancer (ACTS-GC) study was a Japanese trial in which postoperative patients with D2 nodal dissection were randomized to receive S-1 (a combination of the oral fluoropyrimidine tegafur with the dihydropyrimidine dehydrogenase inhibitors 5-chloro-2,4-dihydroxypyridine and potassium oxonate) or observation (4). The investigators reported a significant improvement in 3-year survival from 70% with surgery alone to 80% with the addition of S-1 (HR, 0.68; 95% CI 0.52–0.87; *P* = .002). However, questions remain as to the benefit of adjuvant chemotherapy with S-1 in non-Japanese populations, since clinical trials performed in Western populations in the advanced disease setting with this agent have shown less benefit. A recent meta-analysis in resected gastric cancer compared adjuvant chemotherapy to observation and demonstrated an overall survival benefit with chemotherapy (5). This study retrieved single-patient data from 17 randomized clinical trials that completed accrual before 2004, thus not including the positive results from the ACTS-GC trial. Adjuvant chemotherapy was associated with a statistically significant benefit in terms of overall survival (HR, 0.82; 95% confidence interval, 0.76–0.90; *P* = 0.001) and disease-free survival (HR, 0.82; 95% CI, 0.75–0.90; *P* = 0.001). The mortality hazard was reduced by 18%, with an absolute improvement in survival of 6% observed at 5 years, maintaining this improvement through 10 years. Therefore, although the value of S-1 in Western populations is debated, the use of adjuvant chemotherapy with other agents is a reasonable option.

Finally, a study conducted in North America (Intergroup 0116) compared surgery alone to surgery followed by combined modality adjuvant treatment (6). A total of 556 patients were randomized. Adjuvant therapy consisted of one cycle of 5-FU/leucovorin, followed by chemotherapy concurrent with radiation to the gastric bed and regional lymph nodes, followed by two additional cycles of chemotherapy. Five-year survival in the surgery-alone group was 41% compared with 50% in the adjuvant treatment group (HR, 1.31; 95% CI 1.09–1.59; *P* = .005). The majority of the patients included in this trial underwent D0 dissections, whereas 36% had D1 and only 10% had D2 dissections, raising the question of a possible compensatory effect of the chemoradiotherapy in a suboptimally resected population.

Characterization of failure patterns in patients following surgical treatment of gastric cancer suggests that two thirds of patients will relapse with locoregional disease and one third with distant metastatic disease. Therefore, there is rationale for adjuvant strategies to combine multimodality approaches, including the use of chemotherapy and radiation. There are several ongoing phase III clinical trials exploring multimodality therapies. The CRITICS study is investigating the value of postoperative radiation therapy as compared to chemotherapy alone. The trial has a targeted recruitment of 788 patients with stage IB-IVA gastric cancer. The plan is randomization to perioperative chemotherapy with three cycles of epirubicin, cisplatin, and capecitabine (ECX) before and after surgery, versus three cycles of neoadjuvant ECX followed by adjuvant radiation with concurrent cisplatin and capecitabine. The CALGB-80101 trial has enrolled 826 patients with the same staging and will test the value of combination chemotherapy as compared to 5-FU/LV only. All patients receive chemoradiation with concurrent 5-FU/LV, with randomization to adjuvant chemotherapy with 5-FU/LV or to combination chemotherapy with ECF. These two trials are a reflection of a multimodality paradigm for localized and locally advanced gastric cancer combining surgery, chemotherapy, and radiotherapy to reduce the rate of locoregional and distant relapses and subsequently improve survival in this patient population.

Locally Advanced Unresectable and Metastatic Gastric Cancer

D.K. is a 35-year-old man with no significant past medical history who presented with chest pain. He was initially evaluated at the emergency department and underwent a complete cardiologic workup, which was negative. Subsequently, under the diagnostic suspicion of dyspepsia, he was initiated on treatment with a proton pump inhibitor without clinical response. During the course of the following 2 weeks he began to complain of abdominal pain in a band-like region across the upper abdomen, along with bloating and burping. He also noted the presence of fevers and night sweats at that time. His primary care physician ordered an abdominal US that revealed the presence of multiple liver lesions. A CT scan of the chest, abdomen, and pelvis confirmed the presence of more than 30 low-attenuation liver lesions, an enhancing mass rising from the lesser curvature of the stomach, and multiple enlarged lymph nodes along the gastrohepatic ligament. An US-guided biopsy of one of the liver lesions was positive for undifferentiated carcinoma. An endoscopy was subsequently performed and visualized a large, fungating, ulcerated mass arising in the cardia that extended into the gastric body in the lesser curvature of the stomach. Biopsies were positive for anaplastic carcinoma. Immunohistochemical staining for HER2/neu on the stomach lesion was negative. Laboratory studies demonstrated, mildly decreased hemoglobin of 10.6 g/dL, a normal creatinine value of 0.7 mg/dL, and abnormal liver function tests relevant for AST of 42 IU/L, ALT of 79 IU/L, ALK of 194 IU/L but with a total bilirubin within the normal range. D.K. was referred to medical oncology with the diagnosis of stage IV gastric cancer. At the initial visit, the performance status of the patient was ECOG 1 and his pain was well controlled with a regimen of long-acting slow release morphine. Following discussion with the patient and family, it was decided to initiate chemotherapy with a regimen combining intravenous epirubicin and oxaliplatin and oral capecitabine.

Evidence-Based Case Discussion

The standard treatment for patients diagnosed with locally advanced unresectable or metastatic gastric cancer is systemic chemotherapy. This is based on several meta-analyses performed to assess the value of chemotherapy on quality of life and overall survival, the two main therapeutic endpoints in this patient population. The most recent update of these series of meta-analyses from the Cochrane Collaboration published in 2010 shows a significant benefit in survival for chemotherapy versus best supportive care (BSC) (11 versus 4.3 months; HR 0.37; 95% CI 0.24–0.55). Moreover, the average quality-adjusted survival was longer in the group of patients randomized to chemotherapy compared with the BSC group. Of note, between 10% and 24% of patients who were treated with chemotherapy were alive after 2 years. Therefore, future phase III studies looking at therapeutic interventions in advanced gastric cancer require a chemotherapy arm (7).

Numerous drugs have been demonstrated to have single-agent activity in gastric cancer, including 5-FU and fluoropyrimidine analogs (S-1 and capecitabine); topoisomerase inhibitors (irinotecan, etoposide); taxanes (paclitaxel, docetaxel); platinum analogs (cisplatin, oxaliplatin, carboplatin); anthracyclines (doxorubicin, epirubicin); and antibiotics (mitomycin-C). Although the majority of these agents show only modest benefit, with response rates in the range of 20% to 30%, single-agent studies have pointed toward the more active drugs to be considered for combinations in further studies. Additional clinical trials in the advanced setting have addressed two important questions: (1) Is combination chemotherapy superior to single-agent therapy? and (2) Which drugs should be incorporated into combination chemotherapy regimens?

Several meta-analyses have provided the answer to the first question. Across the literature it has been consistently demonstrated that combination chemotherapy is superior to single-agent treatment in terms of overall survival (HR 0.82; 95% CI 0.74–0.90), progression-free survival, and response rate, the latter two measures often correlating with improvement or maintenance of quality-of-life measures. Various combinations have shown significant activity with relatively tolerable toxicity. Cisplatin and 5-FU often serve as a comparator or backbone of the majority of regimens studied. Other agents or classes of drugs combined or added include the anthracyclines, taxanes, and topoisomerase inhibitors. The most studied three-drug regimens include ECF (epirubicin, cisplatin, and 5-FU) and DCF (docetaxel, cisplatin, and 5-FU). Although ECF has never been compared to standard cisplatin and 5-FU (CF) in a phase III clinical trial, ECF has become an accepted standard regimen. A total of 274 patients were randomized in a phase III clinical trial to receive either ECF or FAMTX (5-FU, doxorubicin, and methotrexate) as first-line treatment in advanced disease. Median survival was significantly improved for ECF (8.7 versus 6.1 months: $P < .01$) as was tumor response (45% versus 21%; $P < .0002$) (8). Conversely, the DCF regimen was compared with CF in a phase III clinical trial (the V325 trial) showing a statistically significant prolongation time to progression (5.6 versus 3.7 months; $P < .001$) and survival (9.2 versus 8.6 months; $P = 0.02$). The toxicity of the DCF combination is concerning, however, with 82% of the patients developing grade 3/4 neutropenia and 29% febrile neutropenia (9). This effect was attenuated when patients treated with DCF received G-CSF as secondary prophylaxis. Regarding the use of fluoropyrimidine analogs, two Japanese studies have shown noninferiority of the combination of cisplatin plus S-1 compared to cisplatin plus infusional 5-FU (10). Finally, an irinotecan based regimen combining 5-FU and folinic acid has been compared in a phase III trial to the CF regimen, but did not show superiority in terms of time to progression or survival.

The REAL-2 study evaluated the equivalency of oxaliplatin to cisplatin, and capecitabine to infusional 5-FU. This study of 1002 patients had a 2 × 2 factorial design where patients were assigned to ECF, EOF (substituting oxaliplatin for cisplatin), ECX (substituting capecitabine for 5-FU), and EOX (substituting both oxaliplatin and capecitabine), and was sample sized for noninferiority assumptions. The results demonstrated that oxaliplatin was equivalent to cisplatin, as was capecitabine to infusional 5-FU. Another randomized phase III clinical trial (ML17032) addressed the question of the equivalence of capecitabine and infusional 5-FU added to cisplatin with a similar noninferiority design. In this study patients were randomized to receive CF or cisplatin plus capecitabine (CX), and the response rate was statistically superior for those patients receiving CX compared to CF (41 versus 29%, $P = .03$). However, no differences were seen for the primary end points of this trial, progression-free survival (5.6 versus 5.0 months) and overall survival (10.5 versus 9.3 months). A meta-analysis combining 1318 patients treated with an oral fluoropyrimidine versus infusional 5-FU in the context of the REAL-2 and ML17032 studies observed that overall survival was superior for those receiving capecitabine (11). In summary, we have learned that combination therapy is the preferred option for the treatment of metastatic gastric cancer, and that several platinum and fluoropyrimidine analogs have effects equivalent to other formulations in their class, allowing for more alternatives in the administration of chemotherapy.

The ability to use three-drug combinations to treat advanced gastric cancer is dependent on the suitability of the patient for chemotherapy, and only those patients with high performance status should be considered for such regimens. Although two-drug regimens have shown lower response rates as compared to three-drug combinations, many are quite active as described in phase II/III clinical trials in the first-line setting (Table 7.2).

Table 7.2 Activity of Two-Drug Combination Regimens in Gastric Cancer Based on Data Extracted from Phase II and III Clinical Trials

Treatment	N	RR (%)
5-FU/leucovorin/oxaliplatin	112	34
5-FU/leucovorin/cisplatin	110	27
5-FU/leucovorin/irinotecan	172	32
5-FU/doxorubicin	49	27
Docetaxel/cisplatin	158	26
Docetaxel/oxaliplatin	71	38
Docetaxel/capecitabine	44	39
Cisplatin/5-FU	165	26
Cisplatin/capecitabine	160	41
Cisplatin/S-1	153	54
Cisplatin/paclitaxel	41	51

RR, response rate.

Table 7.3 Targeted Therapies for Gastric Cancer

Drug	Pathway	Status
Trastuzumab	HER2	Approved by the FDA
Lapatinib	EGFR, HER2	Phase III
Erlotinib	EGFR	Phase II
Gefitinib	EGFR	Phase II
Cetuximab	EGFR	Phase III
Panitumumab	EGFR	Phase III
Bevacizumab	VEGF	Phase III
Sunitinib	VEGFR, PDGFR, KIT, FLT3, RET	Phase II
Sorafenib	VEGFR2/3, PDGFR, KIT, RAF	Phase II
Everolimus	mTOR	Phase III

Therefore, two-drug regimens may also be considered in those patients not suitable for polychemotherapy based on lower performance status, comorbid conditions, advanced age, or previous intolerance to chemotherapy.

Newer targeted agents have also been evaluated in advanced gastric cancer, with varying degrees of success (Table 7.3). Following the discovery of the overexpression of HER2 in gastric cancer, a logical therapeutic consequence was the application of agents known to target this pathway. The ToGA trial was a phase III multicenter study conducted in 130 institutions worldwide evaluating the cisplatin/fluoropyrimidine doublet, with or without trastuzumab in advanced, untreated HER2 positive gastric cancer (12). A total of 584 patients were enrolled. Those receiving trastuzumab had improved survival as compared to those not receiving targeted therapy (13.8 vs. 11.1 months; HR 0.74, 95% CI 0.60–0.91; $P = .0046$) (1). This trial has led to the approval of trastuzumab use in metastatic gastric cancer. Tyrosine kinase inhibitors targeting HER2, including lapatinib, are currently undergoing evaluation in combination with chemotherapy in the first-line setting.

Therapeutic strategies targeting the EGFR pathway have been tested, with uncertain benefit. EGFR tyrosine kinase inhibitors, including erlotinib and gefitinib, have not shown single-agent activity. On the other hand, the addition of a monoclonal antibody targeting EGFR to active chemotherapy regimens (such as FOLFIRI or FOLFOX) has shown some benefit, but the incremental value of the antibody is difficult to discern in phase II trials. Therapeutic interventions targeting angiogenesis are also ongoing. A phase II trial combining bevacizumab with modified DCF in untreated advanced gastric cancer patients reported a response rate of 65%, a time to progression of 8.3 months, and a median overall survival of 12.3 months. A pivotal phase III trial randomizing patients to cisplatin and capecitabine with or without bevacizumab failed to show a survival benefit from bevacizumab, as initially presented at ASCO 2010. Interestingly, there were continental differences noted, with efficacy suggested in North American populations. Finally, multitargeted tyrosine kinase inhibitors, such as sunitinib and sorafenib, that exert antiangiogenic effects have also been studied. Phase II trials of sunitinib as a single agent in the second-line setting and sorafenib combined with cisplatin and docetaxel as first-line therapy reported encouraging response rates and further evaluation was warranted.

Following progression on first-line treatment, there is no standard second-line therapy for advanced gastric cancer. One randomized phase II clinical trial compared single-agent irinotecan to BSC and observed a significant survival advantage for the treated group. Other groups have conducted single-arm phase II trials with two-drug regimens such as irinotecan/capecitabine, irinotecan/docetaxel, docetaxel/capecitabine, FOLFIRI, and FOLFOX. Strikingly, most studies show very similar median progression-free (~4 months) and overall survival times (~9 months). This observation stresses that it is not the particular agent or combination but the adequate patient selection and good performance status that are essential in decision making for treatment in the second-line setting.

In conclusion, although the incidence of gastric cancer is declining in Western countries, the mortality associated with this disease continues to be high. Surgery is the only curative treatment for this malignancy. Multimodality approaches that include the use of chemotherapy and radiation therapy are needed in those with resectable disease, in order to reduce relapse rates. In the advanced setting, combination chemotherapy is the best option to improve quality of life and extend survival. Treatment selection should be based on the performance status of the patient and goals of therapy. Finally, improvement in our knowledge of the molecular biology of gastric cancer has recently led to the approval of a new treatment for this disease, trastuzumab, while other targets for therapy, including EGFR and angiogenesis, are under intense investigation and development.

REFERENCES

1. Shah MA, Kelsen DP. Gastric cancer: a primer on the epidemiology and biology of the disease and an overview of the medical management of advanced disease. *J Natl Compr Canc Netw.* Apr;8(4):437–447.
2. Gravalos C, Jimeno A. HER2 in gastric cancer: a new prognostic factor and a novel therapeutic target. *Ann Oncol.* 2008;19(9):1523–1529.
3. Cunningham D, Allum WH, Stenning SP, et al. Perioperative chemotherapy versus surgery alone for resectable gastroesophageal cancer. *N Engl J Med.* 2006;355(1):11–20.
4. Sakuramoto S, Sasako M, Yamaguchi T, et al. Adjuvant chemotherapy for gastric cancer with S-1, an oral fluoropyrimidine. *N Engl J Med.* 2007;357(18):1810–1820.
5. Paoletti X, Oba K, Burzykowski T, et al. Benefit of adjuvant chemotherapy for resectable gastric cancer: a meta-analysis. *JAMA.*;303(17):1729–1737.
6. Macdonald JS, Smalley SR, Benedetti J, et al. Chemoradiotherapy after surgery compared with surgery alone for adenocarcinoma of the stomach or gastroesophageal junction. *N Engl J Med.* 2001;345(10):725–730.
7. Wagner AD, Unverzagt S, Grothe W, et al. Chemotherapy for advanced gastric cancer. *Cochrane Database Syst Rev.* 2010;3: CD004064.
8. Webb A, Cunningham D, Scarffe JH, et al. Randomized trial comparing epirubicin, cisplatin, and fluorouracil versus fluorouracil, doxorubicin, and methotrexate in advanced esophagogastric cancer. *J Clin Oncol.* 1997;15(1):261–267.
9. Van Cutsem E, Moiseyenko VM, Tjulandin S, et al. Phase III study of docetaxel and cisplatin plus fluorouracil compared with cisplatin and fluorouracil as first-line therapy for advanced gastric cancer: a report of the V325 Study Group. *J Clin Oncol.* 2006;24(31):4991–4997.
10. Van Cutsem E, Van de Velde C, Roth A, et al. Expert opinion on management of gastric and gastro-oesophageal junction adenocarcinoma on behalf of the European Organisation for Research and Treatment of Cancer (EORTC)-gastrointestinal cancer group. *Eur J Cancer.* 2008;44(2):182–194.
11. Okines AF, Norman AR, McCloud P, et al. Meta-analysis of the REAL-2 and ML17032 trials: evaluating capecitabine-based combination chemotherapy and infused 5-fluorouracil-based combination chemotherapy for the treatment of advanced oesophago-gastric cancer. *Ann Oncol.* 2009;20(9): 1529–1534.
12. Bang YT, Van Cutsem E, Feyereislova A, et al. Trastuzumab in combination with chemotherapy alone for treatment of HER-2 positive advanced gastric cancer or gastro-esophageal junction cancer (ToGA): A phase 3, open-label, randomised controlled trial. *Lancet.* 2010; 9742(376):687–97.

8

Pancreatic Cancer

AHMED A. EID AND DONGXIN LIU

EPIDEMIOLOGY, RISK FACTORS, NATURAL HISTORY, AND PATHOLOGY

Pancreatic cancer is the second most common gastrointestinal malignancy with 9 cases per 100,000 population in the United States, but it is the fourth cause of cancer death following lung, breast/prostate, and colorectal cancers. There were 42,470 new cases diagnosed in 2009 and 35,240 estimated deaths from pancreatic cancer (1). The incidence of pancreatic cancer increases steadily with age starting from age 50 and peaks around age 70. The disease is extremely unusual in patients younger than age 30 and rarely occurs before age 50. There are racial and geographic differences in the incidence of pancreatic cancer: the incidence is higher in African Americans than in Caucasians, and is also higher in developed countries than underdeveloped countries.

The most important risk factor for pancreatic cancer is age. People in the eighth decade of life experience a risk approximately 40 times that of those in the fourth decade. Cigarette smoking is another important risk factor for pancreatic cancer with a relative risk of at least 1.5. The risk increases with the number of cigarettes consumed and returns to baseline 15 years after smoking cessation. Diet also appears to be a risk factor: diets rich in fat and meat seem to be associated with the development of pancreatic cancer, whereas fruits and vegetables seem to have a protective effect. This could explain the geographic difference in pancreatic cancer incidence. Other possible risk factors for pancreatic cancer may include coffee and alcohol consumption, use of aspirin and NSAIDs, obesity, and *Helicobacter pylori* infection. However, these relationships are not consistent across studies and are therefore unreliable. Several medical conditions, such as diabetes and chronic pancreatitis, have been shown to be associated with increased risk of pancreatic cancer. Approximately 5% to 10% of patients have a genetic predisposition for pancreatic cancer. Hereditary pancreatitis, multiple endocrine neoplasia (MEN), hereditary nonpolyposis colon cancer (HNPCC), Gardner syndrome, von Hippel-Lindau syndrome (VHL) and *BRCA1*/*BRCA2* gene mutations have been found to increase the risk of pancreatic cancer.

Pancreatic cancer is a highly lethal disease with less than a 5% 5-year survival rate in all stages. Its incidence rate is ranked tenth, but it is the fourth leading cause of cancer death in the United States. The poor prognosis of pancreatic cancer is due, in part, to a delay in diagnosis and low resection rate. Approximately 80% of patients would have developed local and/or distant metastasis at time of diagnosis, which makes the tumor unresectable. Chemotherapy and radiation therapy offer only modest survival benefit for those patients. Even for those patients who undergo surgical resection, the 5-year survival is only 25% to 30% for node-negative disease and 10% for node-positive disease due to the fact that most of them will develop recurrence within 2 years.

The pancreas consists of exocrine and endocrine components, and pancreatic cancers can arise from either portion. More than 90% of pancreatic cancers are adenocarcinomas derived from ductal cells of the exocrine portion, of which two thirds occur in the head of the pancreas, and one third occurs in other parts of the pancreas such as the body or tail. A variety of other malignant tumors arising from the ductal epithelia of pancreas include acinar cell carcinoma, cystadenocarcinoma, giant cell carcinoma, and so on. Tumors such as adenosquamous carcinomas and carcinosarcomas can also occur. Pancreaticoblastoma arises from multipotential cells that can differentiate into mesenchymal, endocrine, or acinar cells, and it occurs primarily in children. Other uncommon pancreatic tumors including small cell carcinoma, schwannoma, leiomyosarcoma, liposarcoma, and malignant fibrous histocytoma can also arise in the pancreas.

Pancreatic endocrine tumors (PETs) are rare. They arise from the islet cells of the pancreas. Functional endocrine tumors are named after the hormone or the peptide they secrete. Insulinomas are the most common, followed by gastrinomas, glucagonomas, VIPomas, and somatostatinomas in terms of frequency. Nonfunctional pancreatic endocrine tumors (NF-PETs) are not associated with an excess production of any hormone or peptide. PETs are relatively slow growing with better survival compared with ductal adenocarcinoma of the exocrine pancreas.

STAGING

Pancreatic cancer is staged by using TNM classification, which is based on the extent of tumor and involvement of local and distant structures. The 7th edition of the American Joint Committee on Cancer (AJCC) staging of endocrine and exocrine pancreatic tumors is shown below.

AJCC 7th Edition Staging System for Pancreatic Cancer

Stage	Definition
0	Carcinoma in situ (Tis) without regional lymph nodes (N0) or distant metastasis (M0) (Tis N0 M0)
IA	Tumor limited to the pancreas (≤2 cm) (T1) without regional lymph nodes (N0) or distant metastasis (M0) (T1 N0 M0)
IB	Tumor limited to the pancreas (>2 cm) (T2) without regional lymph nodes (N0) or distant metastasis (M0) (T2 N0 M0)
IIA	Tumor extends beyond the pancreas but without involvement of the celiac axis or the superior mesenteric artery (T3) and also without regional lymph nodes (N0) or distant metastasis (M0) (T3 N0 M0)
IIB	Tumor with T1–3 with regional lymph nodes metastasis (N1) but without distant metastasis (M0) (T1–3 N1 M0)
III	Tumor involves the celiac axis or the superior mesenteric artery (unresectable primary tumor) (T4) with or without regional lymph nodes metastasis (Tany) but without distant metastasis (T4 Nany M0)
IV	Tumor with distant metastasis (M1) (Tany Nany M1)

CASE SUMMARIES

Resectable Pancreatic Adenocarcinoma

G.S. is a 61-year-old woman with a 70-pack-year history of smoking who presented with constant dull abdominal pain for the last few months. Two weeks prior to presentation, she started to notice dark tea-colored urine, clay-colored white stools and yellowing of her eyes and skin. She also complained of progressive fatigue, loss of appetite, and unintentional weight loss of 30 lbs during the last several months. She denied fever/chills, emesis, shortness of breath, chest pain, or urinary symptoms. She denied alcohol consumption as well. Her past medical/surgical history was only significant for hypertension. Her physical examination was remarkable for icteric sclerae, jaundice, and periumbilical tenderness on deep palpation without rebound or guarding. Blood tests showed markedly elevated total and direct bilirubin (10.9/mg/dL and 9.7 mg/dL, respectively) with a modest elevation of her alkaline phosphatase and transaminases. Complete cell count (CBC), basic metabolic panel (BMP), amylase and lipase were within normal limits. A CT scan of the abdomen and pelvis revealed an ill-defined heterogeneous mass in the pancreatic head measuring approximately 2.5 × 2.6 × 2.7 cm with marked dilatation of the common bile duct as it narrowed to complete/near complete occlusion at the level of the pancreatic head. Intrahepatic biliary ductal dilation was also observed. No hepatic lesions or abdominal lymphadenopathy was seen. The serum CA19-9 was elevated to 221.57 U/mL (reference range 0–37 U/mL).

Since pancreatic adenocarcinoma was highly suspected, endoscopic ultrasonography (EUS) and EUS-guided fine needle aspiration (FNA) biopsy were performed and revealed a T3 N0 M0 pancreatic adenocarcinoma (stage IIA). On the basis of a discussion in a multidisciplinary tumor board, G.S. was judged to be a good candidate for surgical resection. She underwent a complete (R0) resection and started adjuvant chemotherapy with gemcitabine 6 weeks after the surgery.

Evidence-Based Case Discussion

G.S. represents a patient with early-stage pancreatic adenocarcinoma (stage IIA). With a risk factor of heavy cigarette smoking, she presented with abdominal pain and obstructive jaundice as well as other nonspecific symptoms that included fatigue, anorexia, and weight loss. Her diagnosis was suggested by history and physical examination findings, suspicious abnormalities seen on CT imaging, and a markedly elevated CA19-9 level. The clinical suspicion of pancreatic cancer was confirmed by EUS-guided FNA. The treatment for this patient was surgery followed by adjuvant therapy.

The diagnosis of pancreatic cancer is often made on the basis of history, imaging studies, and laboratory tests (Figure 8.1). There are no good screening tests for pancreatic cancer, and therefore, the early clinical diagnosis of pancreatic cancer is hampered by the nonspecificity and subtle onset of symptoms. Pain is the most common presenting symptom, typically mid-epigastric in location with radiation to the back. When the cancer

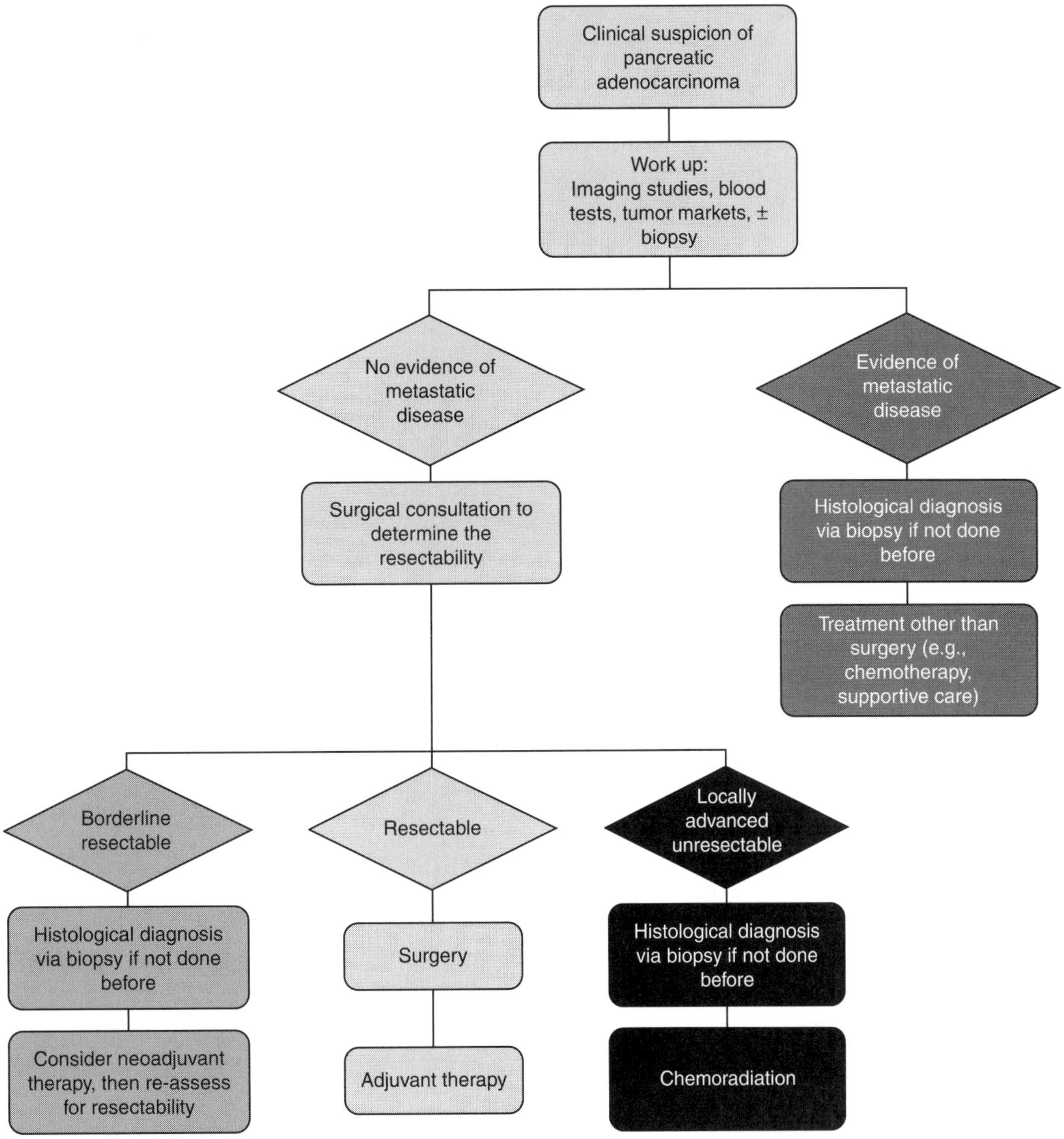

Figure 8.1

Algorithm of diagnosis and treatment for resectable pancreatic adenocarcinoma.

is located in the head of the pancreas, obstructive jaundice is the most characteristic sign. Patients usually notice jaundice, pruritis, the darkening of urine, and lightening of the color of stools. Significant weight loss is another characteristic feature of pancreatic cancer. Other common presenting symptoms include fatigue, anorexia, nausea, vomiting, early satiety, constipation, and glucose intolerance. Migratory thrombophlebitis and venous thromboses (Trousseau's sign) occur with high frequency in patients with pancreatic cancer and could be the first manifestation. Depression is found to be more common in patients with pancreatic cancer. Physical examination may reveal jaundice, temporal wasting, hepatomegaly, or ascites without any characteristic physical findings.

Routine laboratory findings in pancreatic cancer are usually nonspecific such as elevated bilirubin, elevated alkaline phosphatase and transaminases levels, elevated amylase and/or lipase, coagulopathy, thrombocytosis, and a low serum albumin level due to malnutrition. Several tumor markers such as CA19-9 or carcinoembryonic antigen (CEA) may be elevated in pancreatic cancer, but they all lack sensitivity and specificity. CA19-9 seems to have the greatest sensitivity (70%) and specificity (87%) for the diagnosis of pancreatic cancer. CA19-9 is also useful in monitoring recurrent or advanced disease. CEA has been used as a tumor marker in gastrointestinal malignancies, but only 40% of patients with pancreatic adenocarcinoma have elevated CEA levels. In general, CEA is neither sensitive nor specific for pancreatic cancer.

A number of imaging modalities are available to assist in the diagnosis and staging of pancreatic cancer. These include computing tomography (CT) scanning, magnetic resonance imaging (MRI), endoscopic retrograde cholangiopancreatography (ERCP), transcutaneous ultrasonography (TUS), endoscopic ultrasonography (EUS), and positron emission tomography (PET) scanning. The abdominal CT scan is the mainstay modality for the diagnosis of pancreatic cancer as well as assessing resectability. Dual or triple phase thin-cut spiral CT (pancreatic protocol) has approximately 70% sensitivity for tumors less than 1.5 cm and almost 100% for tumors larger than 1.5 cm. It also has 90% accuracy in the determination of resectability of pancreatic cancer. EUS is excellent for tumor staging and can detect the presence of portal vein invasion, hepatic lesions, and lymph node involvement. Concurrent EUS-guided FNA allows the simultaneous cytologic confirmation of pancreatic adenocarcinoma. The role of MRI in pancreatic cancer has been less well studied than CT scanning, but is not superior to spiral CT scanning. PET scanning by itself does not appear to offer additional benefits to a high-quality CT scan, but PET scanning with simultaneous CT imaging may be more sensitive than conventional imaging. Pathologic diagnosis can be achieved with EUS-guided or CT-guided biopsy, brush cytology and forceps biopsy via ERCP, peritoneal cytology, or laparoscopy. If patients have obvious liver metastatic disease based on the initial imaging findings, they should undergo biopsy of liver lesions for diagnosis.

Preoperative staging laparoscopy is indicated if there is high likelihood of unresectability not confirmed by imaging tests. For example, when liver or other suspicious lesions seen on imaging studies are not confirmed by initial tissue biopsy, laparoscopy allows for direct visualization of the liver and peritoneal surfaces with biopsy of any suspicious area. However, if metastatic disease is confirmed, surgical resection of the primary tumor is not indicated.

Despite the advances in cancer therapy, the treatment of pancreatic cancer still remains challenging. To date, the radical surgical resection of pancreatic ductal adenocarcinoma is the only treatment with survival benefit. Unfortunately, only 10% to 20% of patients present with resectable disease at the time of diagnosis. The management of patients with pancreatic carcinoma depends on the stage of the disease at diagnosis. Patients with pancreatic adenocarcinoma can be classified into four groups: resectable, borderline resectable, locally advanced unresectable, and disseminated (Figure 8.1). In general, stage 0-IIA tumors are usually considered resectable. Some of the stage IIB tumors are also resectable if involved lymph nodes are contained within the resection area. Stage III and IV tumors are unresectable. For patients with resectable disease, surgical resection followed by adjuvant therapy is the standard of care.

Curative resection options include pancreaticoduodenectomy (Whipple procedure), total pancreatectomy or distal pancreatectomy depending on the anatomic location of the tumor. Each procedure is associated with its own set of perioperative complications and risks. If a tumor is located in the head of the pancreas, patients will most likely benefit from a Whipple procedure, which consists of removal of the distal half of the stomach (antrectomy), the gall bladder and its cystic duct (cholecystectomy), the common bile duct (choledochectomy), the head of the pancreas, duodenum, proximal jejunum, and regional lymph nodes with surgical drainage of the distal pancreatic duct and biliary system, usually accomplished through anastomosis to the jejunum. Pancreaticoduodenectomy is considered, by any standard, a major surgical procedure with a significant mortality rate. Many studies have shown that hospitals with high-volume pancreaticoduodenectomy will have better overall results than low-volume hospitals. Even at high-volume hospitals, morbidity has been found to vary by a factor of almost four depending on the experience of the surgeon in performing the procedure. Distal pancreatectomy is done for tumors located in the body and tail of the pancreas. Total pancreatectomy is the least commonly done procedure with the highest associated mortality. However, it still remains a viable option in the surgical treatment of pancreatic cancer.

Even with surgery, patients often have poor long-term survival due to early relapse. At least 80% of patients who undergo surgery will develop local or distant relapse within 2 years of surgery. In an attempt to reduce the incidence of relapse and death, postoperative adjuvant treatment in the form of systemic chemotherapy alone or concurrent chemotherapy and radiotherapy is commonly administered. Adjuvant therapy should only be considered for patients who have adequately recovered from surgery, and treatment should ideally be initiated within 4 to 8 weeks after surgery.

There is as yet no consensus regarding the standard of adjuvant therapy after resection of pancreatic cancer. The potential benefit of adjuvant therapy with either chemotherapy alone or chemoradiation has been studied, whereas very few clinical trials have addressed the benefit of adjuvant radiation alone. The approach is different in the United States and Europe. Chemotherapy alone is the current standard adjuvant therapy in Europe based on the results of the ESPAC-1 trial (European Study Group for Pancreatic Cancer) and the CONKO-001 trial.

ESPAC-1 was a multicenter trial that randomized patients with pancreatic adenocarcinoma undergoing "curative" resection to either concurrent chemoradiotherapy alone (radiation plus fluorouracil), or chemotherapy alone (fluorouracil), or concurrent chemoradiotherapy followed by chemotherapy or observation. Patients who received chemotherapy had a statistically significant survival benefit over patients who did not receive chemotherapy (median survival 20.1 months vs. 15.5 months, 2-year survival rate 40% vs. 30%, 5-year survival rate 21% vs. 8%, *P* = .009), while patient in the chemoradiotherapy arm showed worse median survival compared with patients who did not receive chemoradiotherapy (median survival 15.9 months vs. 17.9 months, 2-year survival rate 29% vs. 41%, 5-year survival rate 10% vs. 20%). This study concluded that adjuvant chemotherapy has a significant survival benefit in patients with resected pancreatic cancer, whereas adjuvant chemoradiotherapy has a deleterious effect on survival (2). However, the design and interpretation of this study were complicated, and were subject to criticism.

A subsequent European trial CONKO-001 was conducted to evaluate the role of adjuvant chemotherapy with gemcitabine for pancreatic cancer. Three hundred sixty-nine patients with early-stage pancreatic cancer were randomly assigned to adjuvant gemcitabine for 6 months versus observation after completing surgical resection. There was a statistically significant improvement in disease-free survival (DFS) (13 months vs. 7 months) with adjuvant gemcitabine. However, the improvement in overall survival was very modest (2-month improvement with gemcitabine, 22.8 months vs. 20.2 months, *P* = .005). The difference in overall survival became apparent only after 2 years. Five-year survival was 21% for gemcitabine group and 9% with observation (3,4).

Chemoradiation has become the standard adjuvant treatment in the United States. In 1985, the Gastrointestinal Tumor Study Group (GITSG) conducted a small postresection trial in which 22 patients were randomized to observation and 21 to chemoradiation (5- fluorouracil [5-FU]) treatment followed by 2 years of 5-FU as maintenance. The median survival was significantly longer in the patients who received adjuvant treatment compared with those who did not receive it (20 months vs. 11 months) and the 2-year survival rate was 43% versus 18%, respectively (5). On the basis of these results, 5-FU-based chemoradiation became the standard of care for nearly two decades.

The Radiation Therapy Oncology Group (RTOG) conducted a phase III study to determine if the addition of gemcitabine to adjuvant fluorouracil chemoradiation improved survival for patients with resected pancreatic adenocarcinoma. Chemotherapy with either fluorouracil or gemcitabine was administered for 3 weeks prior to standard chemoradiation therapy, and for 12 weeks after. Chemoradiation with a continuous infusion of fluorouracil was the same for all patients. Patients with pancreatic head tumors had a median survival of 20.5 months and a 3-year survival of 31% in the gemcitabine group versus a median survival of 16.9 months and a 3-year survival of 22% in the fluorouracil group (*P* = .09). After adjustment for nodal status, tumor size and surgical margin status on multivariant analysis, the treatment effect was in favor of improved survival for the gemcitabine group (*P* = .05). However, there was significant increased grade 4 hematologic toxicity in the gemcitabine group than the fluorouracil group (14% vs. 1%, *P* < .001) without a difference in the incidence of febrile neutropenia or infection. These results suggested that the addition of gemcitabine to adjuvant fluorouracil-based chemoradiation was associated with a survival benefit for patients with resected pancreatic cancer, although this improvement was not statistically significant (6).

ESPAC-3 is a multicenter open-label phase III trial that randomized 1088 patients with pancreatic ductal adenocarcinoma who had undergone surgical resection to either bolus fluorouracil plus folinic acid or gemcitabine for 6 months. The median survival was 23 months for patients treated with fluorouracil plus folinic acid and 23.6 months for those treated with gemcitabine (*P* = .39). There were no significant differences in either progression-free survival or global quality-of-life scores between the treatment groups. There were more treatment-related serious adverse events in the group of patients who received fluorouracil plus folinic acid (14 %) compared with the group of patients who received gemcitabine (14% vs 7.5%, *P* < .001). The study concluded that gemcitabine did not result in improved overall survival in patients with completely resected pancreatic cancer compared with fluorouracil plus folinic acid. (7)

The use of chemotherapy and/or radiation therapy in the neoadjuvant setting is controversial. Several clinical trials conducted at MD Anderson Cancer Center have shown improved median survival as long as 25 months using neoadjuvant chemotherapy and/or radiation therapy. However, at present, no form of neoadjuvant therapy in pancreatic carcinoma should be considered as a standard of care, and this remains an experimental area.

Metastatic (Unresectable) Pancreatic Cancer

P.Y. is a 67-year-old male who came to his primary care physician (PCP) with a complaint of left arm swelling for 3 days. Notably, he had been diagnosed with right lower extremity deep vein thrombosis (DVT) and pulmonary embolism (PE) 2 months previously, and he was anticoagulated with warfarin. His INR was monitored by his PCP regularly and the level was very stable in the therapeutic range (2.7 on the day of presentation). His other past medical history was limited to treatment for hypertension. He had a 40-pack-year history of smoking and quit after he was diagnosed with PE and DVT. He did not have a family history of cancer.

Further review of systems revealed that for the last 3 months, P.Y. had experienced vague abdominal discomfort with decreased appetite and > 10 lbs of unintentional weight loss. His physical exam was remarkable for left arm and right leg swelling and mild abdominal tenderness in the periumbilical area. A venous doppler ultrasound of the left upper extremity revealed an acute thrombus in the left axillary vein. His anticoagulation was switched from warfarin to enoxaparin.

Trousseau's syndrome was suspected and additional imaging tests were ordered. An abdominal CT scan showed a 3-cm mass in the pancreatic head with evidence of multiple hepatic lesions ranging in size from 1 cm to 2 cm. Laboratory analysis revealed a markedly elevated CA19-9 and CEA level. Other routine laboratory tests were within normal limits except for a slightly elevated total bilirubin, transaminases, and alkaline phosphatase. A core biopsy of the liver lesion revealed moderately differentiated adenocarcinoma consistent with metastasis from pancreatic carcinoma.

Because of the presence of hepatic metastasis (stage IV), his disease was unresectable and he was referred to the medical oncology clinic, where the decision was made to initiate palliative chemotherapy.

Evidence-Based Case Discussion

P.Y. represents a patient with unresectable stage IV pancreatic adenocarcinoma. More than 50% of patients with pancreatic adenocarcinoma have metastatic disease at the time of diagnosis because of relatively nonspecific symptoms, the lack of an effective screening modality, and the aggressive biology of this cancer. This patient presented with Trousseau syndrome, which prompted the workup for malignancy. Thromboembolic disease including DVT, PE, thrombophlebitis migrans is one of the common complications of pancreatic cancer with an incidence of 17% to 57%, which is one of the highest among all forms of cancer. There is some evidence that prophylactic anticoagulation reduces the incidence of thromboembolic events and is associated with improved response to chemotherapy and improved overall survival. The choice of treatment for this patient was chemotherapy.

Despite some progress in the understanding of the molecular biology and pathogenesis of pancreatic cancer, minimal progress has been made in the treatment of patients with advanced disease. The goal of currently available systemic chemotherapy is palliative with the aims of improving quality of life and extending survival, at least to a modest extent. However, given the limited sensitivity of pancreatic adenocarcinoma to chemotherapy and radiation therapy, the survival benefit of chemotherapy is minimal. The median survival for patients with untreated metastatic disease is about 2 to 3 months, and 6 months for patients who are treated.

Symptom relief is a very important aspect of management for patients with advanced or metastatic pancreatic cancer. In patients with obstructive jaundice or gastric outlet obstruction, surgical bypass or endoscopic stent placement should be considered. Advanced pancreatic cancer can be extremely painful since the tumor commonly invades neural and perineural tissues. Therefore, the pain associated with advanced pancreatic cancer is a major debilitating symptom and needs to be treated aggressively with a combination of long-acting narcotics for baseline pain control and short-acting narcotics for breakthrough pain. In cases of refractory pain, celiac plexus neurolysis is recommended. Nutritional support is required for all patients with pancreatic cancer. Pancreatic enzyme supplements can help ameliorate malabsorption and provide good relief for patients with bloating, diarrhea, or gas after meals. Megestrol acetate, dronabinol, or steroids can help stimulate appetite in some patients. Nutritional supplements are also highly recommended.

Before offering chemotherapy it is important to determine if the patient is a suitable candidate for chemotherapy (Figure 8.2). Considerations should include performance

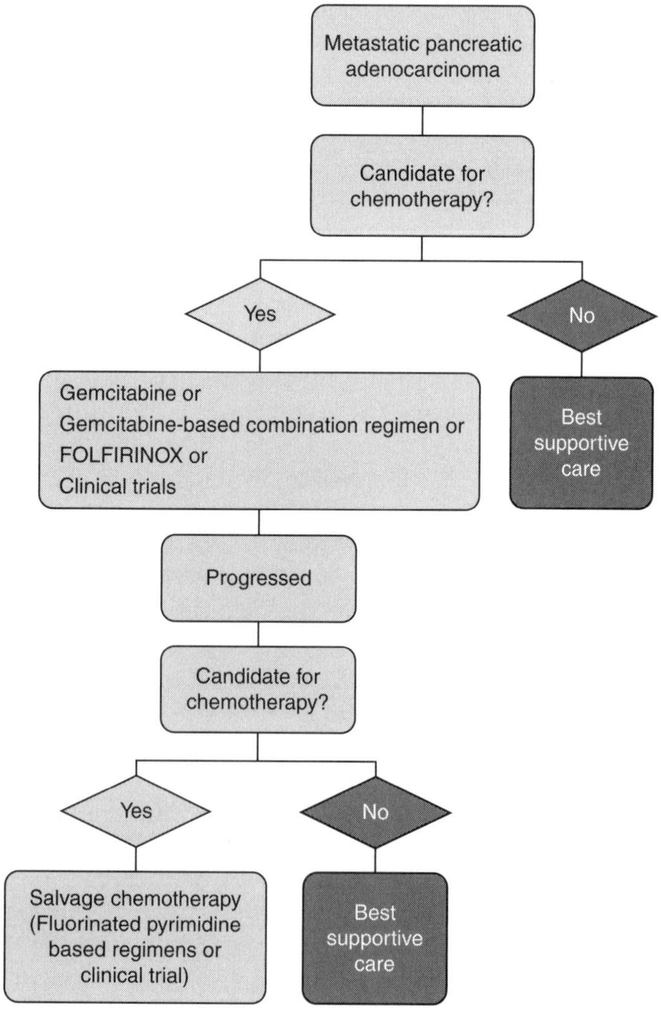

Figure 8.2

Algorithm of diagnosis and treatment for metastatic pancreatic adenocarcinoma.

status; adequate hematological, renal, and hepatic function; nutritional status; and the potential toxicity of the proposed therapy. Patients who are debilitated with poor performance status are generally not candidates for chemotherapy since the possibility of deriving benefit from chemotherapy is extremely low. For these patients, best supportive care should be the treatment option. However, for patients with good performance status who desire therapy, chemotherapy may be offered in addition to supportive management, or, whenever possible, they should be encouraged to participate in clinical trial. Major phase III clinical trials of front-line chemotherapy for advanced pancreatic cancer including metastatic pancreatic cancer are summarized in the following sections, and outlined in Table 8.1.

Monotherapy With Gemcitabine

Historically, 5-FU-based chemotherapy was the principal treatment regimen for patients with advanced pancreatic cancer. Although there were studies suggesting survival benefit with 5-FU over the best supportive care alone, the survival gain was quite modest. 5-FU-based combination therapy (such as with doxorubicin or leucovorin) did not offer any advantage over 5-FU alone.

Gemcitabine is a pyrimidine antimetabolite inhibiting DNA synthesis of cells. The pivotal trial published by Burris et al. in 1997 established single-agent gemcitabine as the current standard of care for first-line treatment of metastatic pancreatic adenocarcinoma. Of the patients receiving gemcitabine, 23.8% experienced a partial response as compared to 4.8% of patients receiving 5-FU bolus therapy ($P = .0022$). Gemcitabine also conferred a modest survival advantage over 5-FU treatment with median survival of 5.65 months versus 4.41 months ($P = .0025$) and 1-year survival rate of 18% versus 2%. (8).

Pharmacokinetic data suggested that a longer infusion time of gemcitabine may be more effective than shorter infusion times. This prompted a phase II study in which patients with advanced pancreatic cancer were randomized to receive gemcitabine either at a fixed or constant dose rate. Whereas the results of this trial demonstrated an improved median and overall survival for patients who received fixed dose gemcitabine, this observation was not confirmed in the subsequent phase III E6201 trial (9). Currently, fixed dose rate administration is considered as a category 2B recommendation by the NCCN guidelines.

Combination Therapy With Cytotoxic Agents

A meta-analysis of randomized trials showed that patients with minimal disease-related symptoms and good performance status may benefit from combination chemotherapy with gemcitabine and either a platinum agent or a fluoropyrimidine (10,11) (Figure 8.2). For now, the acceptable combination regimens (doublets) recommended by the NCCN include gemcitabine/oxaliplatin, gemcitabine/cisplatin, and gemcitabine/ fluoropyrimidine. The clinical trials that evaluated these doublets are reviewed below.

The combination of gemcitabine and oxaliplatin was studied in a randomized clinical trial in which 326 patients were randomized to receive GemOX (gemcitabine [fixed dose rate] plus oxaliplatin) versus gemcitabine alone (constant dose rate). The GemOX arm produced a significantly superior response rate (27% vs. 17%, $P = .04$), progression-free survival (5.8 months vs. 3.7 months, $P = .04$), and clinical benefit (38.2% v 26.9%, $P = 0.03$). Although there was a trend toward better median survival for the GemOX arm (9 months vs. 7 months), it was not statistically significant ($P = .13$). The GemOx arm was associated with a higher incidence of toxicity such as thrombocytopenia, vomiting, and neuropathy (12). One flaw of this trial was the nonuniform administration of gemcitabine between the study arms. In response to this concern, another phase III trial (ECOG 6201) compared fixed dose rate gemcitabine with or without oxaliplatin to constant dose rate gemcitabine. There was no statistically significant difference in overall survival among the three study arms (6.0 months vs. 5.9 months vs. 4.9 months, respectively) (9).

To assess the potential benefit of a combination of gemcitabine with fluoropyrimidine, a randomized phase II study enrolled 319 patients to receive either gemcitabine/capecitabine (GemCap) or gemcitabine alone (Gem). Post hoc subset analysis of patients with good Karnofsky performance status (KPS; score of 90 to 100) showed a significant prolongation of median OS time in the GemCap arm compared with the Gem arm (10.1 vs. 7.4 months, $P = .014$) (13). A phase III European trial of similar design randomized 533 patients with advanced pancreatic cancer to a combination of gemcitabine/capecitabine versus gemcitabine alone. The combination significantly improved objective response rate (19.1% vs. 12.4%; $P = .034$) and progression-free survival (5.3 months vs. 3.8 months; $P = .004$) and was associated with a trend toward improved OS (7.1 months vs. 6.2 months, $P = .08$) compared with gemcitabine alone (14).

To determine the effectiveness of gemcitabine plus cisplatin as the first-line chemotherapy for advanced pancreatic cancer, a phase III study was conducted in which 195 patients were randomly assigned to receive either gemcitabine with cisplatin (GemCis arm) or gemcitabine alone (Gem arm). The GemCis arm was associated with a prolonged median progression-free survival (5.3 months vs. 3.1 months, $P = 0.053$) and a trend toward an improved median overall survival (7.5 months vs. 6.0 months), although the advantage did not reach statistical significance ($P = .15$) (15). Whereas these results supported the efficacy and safety with gemcitabine plus cisplatin, a larger (400 enrollees) phase III trial of similar design (the GIP-1

Table 8.1 Summary of Major Phase III Clinical Trials of Front-Line Chemotherapy for Advanced Pancreatic Adenocarcinoma

Chemotherapy Regimen	*n*	Response Rate (%)	PFS (Months)	Median OS (Months)	Reference
Cytotoxic agents					
Gem vs. 5-FU	126	23.8 vs. 4.8[†] (*P* = .0022)	n/a	5.65 vs. 4.41 (*P* = .0025)	Burris et al., *JCO* 1997
Gem/5-FU vs. gem	327	6.9 vs. 5.6*	3.4 vs. 2.2 (*P* = .022)	6.7 vs. 5.4 (NS)	Berlin et al., *JCO* 2002 (ECOG2297 trial)
IG vs. gem	145	15 vs. 10 (NS)	2.8 vs. 2.9 (NS)	6.4 vs. 6.5 (NS)	Stathopoulos et al., *Br J Cancer* 2006
IRINOGEM vs. gem	360	16.1 vs. 4.4 (*P*<.001)	3.5 vs. 3.0 (NS)	6.3 vs. 6.6 (NS)	Rocha Lima et al., *JCO* 2004
Gem/ pemetrexed vs. gem	565	14.8 vs. 7.1 (*P* = .004)	3.9 vs. 3.3 (NS)	6.2 vs. 6.3 (NS)	Oettle et al., *Annal Onc* 2005
GemOX vs. gem	326	27 vs. 17 (*P* = .04) 38.2 vs. 26.9[†] (*P* = .03)	5.8 vs. 3.7 (*P* = .04)	9 vs. 7 (NS)	Louvet et al., *JCO* 2005 (GERCOR/ GISCAD study)
GemOX vs. gem FDR vs. gem	832	9 vs. 10 vs. 6 (NS)	2.7 vs. 3.5 vs. 2.7 (NS)	5.7 vs. 6.2 vs. 4.9 (NS)	Poplin et al., *JCO* 2009 (ECOG6201 trial)
GemCap vs. gem	319	32 vs. 30*	4.3 vs. 3.9 (NS)	8.4 vs. 7.2 (NS) 10.1 vs. 7.4 (*P* = .014) for KPS 90–100	Herrmann et al., *JCO* 2007
GemCap vs. gem	533	19.1 vs. 12.4 (*P* = .034)	5.3 vs. 3.8 (*P* = .004)	7.1 vs. 6.2 (*P* = .08)	Cunninghams et al., *JCO* 2009
GemCis vs. gem	195	10.2 vs. 8.2*	5.3 vs. 3.1 (*P* = .053)	7.5 vs. 6.0 (NS)	Heinemann et al., *JCO* 2006
GemCis vs. gem	400	10.1 vs. 12.9 (NS)	3.9 vs. 3.8 (NS)	8.3 vs. 7.2 (NS)	Colucci et al., *JCO* 2010 (GIP study)
FOLFIRINOX vs. gem	342	31.6 vs. 9.0 (*P*< .001)	6.4 vs. 3.3 (*P* < .0001)	11.1 vs. 6.8 (*P* < .0001)	Conroy et al., *JCO* 2010 (PRODIGE 4/ ACCORD 11 trial)
Combination with targeted agents					
Gem/ erlotinib vs. gem	569	8.6 vs. 8.0*	3.75 vs. 3.55 (*P* = .004)	6.4 vs. 5.9 (*P* = .025)	Moore et al., *JCO* 2007
Gem/ cetuximab vs. gem	766	*n/a*	3.5 vs. 3.0 (*P* = .058)	5.8 vs. 5.9 (NS)	Philip et al., *JCO* 2007 (SWOG S0202)
Gem/ bevacizumab vs. gem	602	13 vs. 10*	3.8 vs. 2.9 (*P* = .07)	5.8 vs. 6.1 (NS)	Kindler et al., *JCO* 2010 (CALGB 80303)
Gem/ erlotinib/ bevacizumab vs. gem	607	13.5 vs. 8.6 (*P* = .057)	4.6 vs. 3.6 (*P* = .0002)	7.1 vs. 6.0 (NS)	Van Cutsem et al., *JCO* 2009

PFS, progression-free survival; OS, overall survival; KPS, Karnofsky performance status; Gem, gemcitabine; IG, irinotecan/gemcitabine; IRINOGEM, irinotecan/gemcitabine; GemOx, gemcitabine/oxaliplatin; GemCap, gemcitabine/capecitabine; GemCis, gemcitabine/cisplatin; FLOLFIRINOX, oxaliplatin/irinotecan/fluorouracil/leucovorin; NS, not significant.
**P*-value not reported.
[†]Clinical response, all others refer to tumor response.

study) demonstrated no benefit in either overall survival or progression-free survival favoring the GemCis arm (16).

Three- and four-drug combinations have also been studied, but the data are limited so far. It is worth mentioning the interim results of a randomized phase III trial comparing the FOLFIRINOX regimen (oxaliplatin and irinotecan plus fluorouracil and leucovorin) to gemcitabine, which demonstrated an improved response rate (31.6% vs. 9.4%), median progression-free survival (6.4 vs. 3.3 months), and median overall survival (11.1 vs. 6.8 months, $P < .0001$) for the four-drug combination. Despite a significantly higher rate of grade 3–4 toxicity, the final results of this trial (17) could establish FOLFIRINOX as a new standard front-line therapy for patients with good performance status.

Combination Therapy With Targeted Agents

The potential benefit of combining cytotoxic chemotherapy with agents that target angiogenesis and growth factor pathways has been tested in several clinical trials. Whereas most have failed to show improved survival relative to gemcitabine alone, the combination of erlotinib (an EGFR tyrosine kinase inhibitor [TKI]) with gemcitabine demonstrated promising results. A phase III study conducted by National Cancer Institute of Canada randomized 569 patients to receive either gemcitabine with erlotinib or gemcitabine alone and showed a small but statically significant survival benefit favoring the combination arm (6.4 months vs. 5.9 months, $P = .025$, HR 0.81 with 95% confidence interval 0.67–0.97). The 1-year survival rate was 24% and 17% respectively (18). On the basis of the results of this trial, the combination of gemcitabine and erlotinib is considered an acceptable first-line treatment option for metastatic pancreatic cancer.

In contrast, phase III trials of similar design comparing combinations of cetuximab (anti-EGFR antibody) or bevacizumab (anti-VEGF antibody) plus gemcitabine versus gemcitabine alone failed to demonstrate statistically significant improvements in overall survival (19,20).

Trials in which other targeted agents administered in combination with gemcitabine including sorafenib (multitargeted TKI), sunitinib (multitargeted TKI), aflibercept (multitargeted TKI), axitinib (VEGF trap), lapatinib (EGFR and HER2 TKI), and trastuzumab (anti-HER2 monoclonal antibody) were similarly negative, failing to demonstrate a survival benefit for the combination.

Salvage Therapy

Although gemcitabine monotherapy or selected gemcitabine combinations have emerged as acceptable standards of care in the first-line setting, there is no standard second-line chemotherapy for patients who progress or relapse after first-line therapy. Those patients with excellent performance status and organ reserve may be candidates for clinical trial or, in the absence of clinical trial availability, may be offered single-agent or combination therapy using potentially active drugs not employed in first-line therapy (e.g., FOLFOX, CapOx, 5-FU/leucovorin, or single-agent capecitabine) (Figure 8.2).

Metastatic Pancreatic Neuroendocrine (Islet) Carcinoma

R.G. is a 56-year-old man who presented to his PCP complaining of constant and worsening mid-epigastric pain of several months' duration having previously experienced mid-epigastric abdominal pain with nausea and bloating for 2 years. Over the previous 12 months, he lost 20 lbs unintentionally. An over-the-counter proton pump inhibitor (PPI), initially improved his symptoms but failed to provide long-term relief. His review of systems was negative except for the gastrointestinal complaints as described above. He denied fatigue, vomiting, diarrhea, flushing, shortness of breath, or chest pain. His physical examination was remarkable only for the mild tenderness at the mid-epigastric area.

A CT of abdomen and pelvis revealed a 3-cm hypodense mass in the area of the pancreatic head and multiple diffuse liver lesions. Serum measurements of CA19–9, CEA, and AFP were within normal limits as were other laboratory tests including CBC, metabolic panel, and coagulation profile. However, a serum chromogranin A level was found to be markedly elevated. A CT-guided biopsy of the liver mass was performed, and showed a well-differentiated neuroendocrine carcinoma. Immunohistochemical stains were positive for cytokeratin as well as neuroendocrine markers chromogranin A and synaptophysin.

Having unresectable stage IV disease, R.G. then underwent hepatic artery chemoembolization for his hepatic metastases, and tolerated the procedure well without major complications. After the procedure, he was subsequently treated with octreotide.

Evidence-Based Case Discussion

[Please see following Chapter 9, Neuroendocrine Tumors, for a fuller discussion of pancreatic neuroendocrine tumors, PNETs.]

This patient presented with a metastatic nonfunctional pancreatic neuroendocrine tumor (NF-PNET) with nonspecific symptoms of abdominal pain of several years' duration, weight loss, and so on. More than 50% of patients with PNET have metastatic disease at presentation, and nearly all of these have evidence of liver metastases. The diagnosis for this case was made by imaging study (CT scanning), laboratory tests (elevated chromogranin A level) and definitive pathology via biopsy (Figure 8.3). Since the patient was symptomatic and had significant tumor burden in the liver, he required treatment intervention. He was not a surgical candidate due to the bilobar

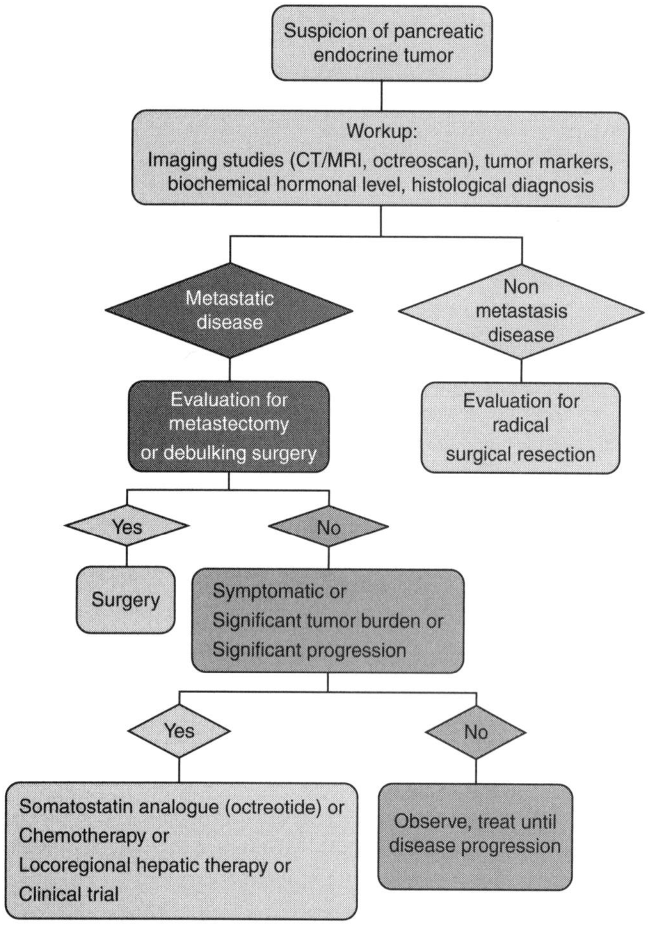

Figure 8.3

Algorithm of diagnosis and treatment for pancreatic endocrine tumor.

distribution of his liver metastases. Since he had hepatic dominant disease, he underwent nonsurgical intervention with hepatic artery embolization in order to reduce the tumor burden in the liver. Octereotide LAR was also administered for subsequent disease control.

Pancreatic neuroendocrine tumors arise from the exocrine component of the pancreas and constitute less than 5% of pancreatic neoplasms. The prognosis and overall survival of patients with these tumors are much better than for patients with pancreatic adenocarcinomas. The majority of PNETs are sporadic, but may be associated with genetic syndromes such as MEN-1, von Hippel-Lindau (VHL) disease, neurofibromatosis, and tuberous sclerosis.

PNETs are divided into two groups clinically: functional and nonfunctional PNETs. Functional PNETs (F-PNETs) secrete biologically active peptides causing endocrine tumor syndromes. The relatively common tumor syndromes are insulinoma with secretion of insulin, gastrinoma (Zollinger-Ellison syndrome) with secretion of gastrin, glucagonoma with secretion of glucagon, VIPoma with secretion of VIP, and somatostatinoma with secretion of somatostatin. NF-PETs are not associated with a specific hormonal syndrome either because no peptide or hormone is secreted or the substance secreted does not cause specific symptoms. NF-PNETs are more frequent than F-PNETs, and also have worse survival rates than F-PNETs.

In 2000, the WHO introduced a histological classification system for gastroenteropancreatic neuroendocrine tumors (GEP-PNETs) including PNETs, in which tumor location, extension, proliferative capacity, and angio-/perineural invasion are assessed. This grading system discriminates well-differentiated endocrine tumors with benign features from well-differentiated and poorly differentiated endocrine carcinomas. Well-differentiated endocrine carcinomas demonstrate slow growth, low proliferative index, and late spread with metastasis. In contrast, poorly differentiated endocrine carcinomas have high Ki-67 proliferation and mitotic rate and rapid progression with lymph node and other distant metastases (to liver, bone, lung, etc.).

The diagnostic assessment for PNET should include localization of the primary tumor, nodal status, metastatic disease, presence of functional syndrome, histological classification of the tumor and the familial genetic background (Figure 8.3). Imaging studies are essential for the management of patients with PNETs. Conventional imaging techniques such as CT, MRI, and US are still the most commonly used modalities. For identifying patients with liver metastases, high-resolution spiral CT and MRI are much more sensitive than US. EUS/FNA is useful for tissue diagnosis to distinguish PNETs from adenocarcinoma and also to localize tumors not imaged with conventional studies. EUS is more effective at localizing intrapancreatic PNETs, and can identify tumors in approximately 90% of cases, particularly when the tumor is small and frequently missed by conventional studies. Functional imaging studies play an important role in the diagnosis of PNETs. Most PNETs express high levels of somatostatin receptors that have high affinity for the somatostatin analogues such as octreotide. Radiolabeled octreotide scanning (octreoscan) has been proved sensitive and specific for localizing both primary PNETs and metastases. Standard fluorodeoxyglucose (FDG)-PET scanning is not useful because of the low metabolic activity of most PNETs.

In addition to the specific hormone released by a functional PNET, other tumor markers have been used for initial diagnosis and treatment response, most notably the serum chromogranin A that is elevated in 88% to 100% of PNETs.

Surgery is the only treatment modality with the potential to cure patients with PNETs. Even for PNETs with liver or lung metastases, they should be evaluated for metastectomy or radical resection whenever possible (Figure 8.3). When curative surgery is not feasible, tumor debulking may also render medical therapy more effective by decreasing the secretion of bioactive substances. Most of the PNETs present at advanced stage, therefore nonsurgical treatments play a crucial role in controlling symptoms, improving quality of life, and prolonging survival. Nonsurgical treatment approaches include biotherapies with somatostatin analogues and interferon, systemic chemotherapy, and targeted therapy. For patients with hepatic dominant diseases, nonsurgical regional hepatic therapy such as hepatic artery embolization, radiofrequency ablation, cryoablation, and radioembolization can be considered as treatment options. Liver transplantation should be considered in only highly selected patients.

Depending on the secreted hormone, symptom management for F-PNETs may significantly improve quality of life. PPI and H2-receptor antagonists are useful in the symptomatic management of gastrinomas. Diazoxide, an insulin-release inhibitor, and glucagon are useful for treatment of insulinoma in conjunction with frequent high-carbohydrate meals. Patients with glucagonoma syndrome are treated symptomatically with insulin.

Somatostatin analogues are the mainstay of treatment for palliating symptoms by decreasing the secretion of peptides and inhibiting tumor growth. Even in patients presenting with metastatic PNET, excellent survival can still be achieved by using a multimodality approach.

Biotherapy With Somatostatin Analogues and Interferon

Somatostatin is an endogenous inhibitor of various hormones secreted from the endocrine system including insulin, glucagon, and gastrin. However, it has limited clinical use due to its short half-life (<3 min). Somatostatin analogues such as octreotide, lanreotide, and pasireotide have been developed and used as the first-line medical therapy for well-differentiated NETs including PNETs. Octreotide was the first available somatostatin analogue, and was introduced into clinical practice in 1983 for treatment of neuroendocrine tumors. The development of a long-acting release (LAR) formulation, which is administered monthly, eliminates the need for daily injection. The result of a double-blind, placebo-controlled randomized phase III study (PROMID) treating well-differentiated metastatic midgut NETs with either octreotide LAR or placebo demonstrated that octreotide LAR significantly improved time to tumor progression compared with placebo in patients with functionally active and inactive metastatic midgut NETs (14.3 vs. 6.0 months, *P* = .000072, HR= 0.34) (21). After 6 months of treatment, stable disease was observed in 66.7% of patients in the octreotide LAR group and 37.2% of patients in the placebo group. Moreover, the survival benefit of octreotide was independent of tumor functionality, chromogranin A level, performance status, or age. Because of the low number of observed deaths, survival analysis was not confirmatory. The response to octreotide may depend on the cell type. For example, insulinomas are marginally responsive to octreotide, while gastrinomas and VIPomas often respond.

Interferon therapy is generally recommended as a second-line approach in treatment of PNETs. IFN-α can inhibit tumor growth by inhibiting proliferation and hormone synthesis as well as by stimulating T cells and NK cell function. As a single agent, IFN-α can produce ~40% biochemical response and ~10% of objective tumor response (22), but with a less favorable toxicity profile than the somatostatin analogues.

Cytotoxic Chemotherapy

If biotherapy with either somatostatin analogues or interferon fails to control well-differentiated PNETs, chemotherapy could be considered. Streptozocin is a broad spectrum antibiotic isolated from *Streptomyces achromogenes* and was the first agent shown to have significant benefit as monotherapy for PNETs (23). A phase II study conducted in 1973 demonstrated a biochemical and a measurable disease (tumor size) response of 64% and 50%, respectively, for patients with metastatic islet cell carcinoma treated with streptozocin (24). Combinations of streptozocin with 5-FU and/or doxorubicin showed improved overall survival and response rates in the earlier studies, but subsequent trials failed to confirm the success. At present, streptozocin is the only drug approved by FDA for treatment of NETs including PNETs. For poorly differentiated PNETs, chemotherapy with cisplatin and etoposide is recommended. Temozolomide-based regimens such as temozolomide with thalidomide or capecitabine have also been tested in small phase II clinical trials.

Targeted Therapy

The expression of several signaling pathways has been shown to be enhanced in PNETs including VEGF, PDGF, IGF-1, and so on. Accordingly, agents that inhibit the activity of various tyrosine kinases and mTOR have been assessed for activity against PNETs. In a recent phase III trial, 171 patients with advanced, well-differentiated PNETs (all with documented disease progression) were randomized to treatment with either sunitinib, a multi-targeted TKI, or to placebo. The objective response rate and median progression-free survival was 9.3% and 11.4 months, respectively, in the sunitinib group vs. 0% and 5.5 months, respectively, in the placebo group (hazard ratio for progression of death, 0.42; 95% confidence interval [CI], 0.26 to 0.66; P< 0.001) (25). In a phase II trial, treatment with sorafenib (another TKI) produced an objective partial response in 11% of patients with PNETs, and a minor response in 14% (26). Another target of therapy is mTOR, a threonine kinase that regulates downstream signaling pathways. In a phase III study, 410 patients with advanced, low-grade of intermediate-grade, progressive PNETs, were randomized to treatment with either everolimus (an mTOR inhibitor) or placebo. Similar to the results of the sunitinib phase III trial, treatment with everolimus was associated with an improved progression-free survival of 11.0 months as compared to 4.6 months in the placebo group (hazard ratio for disease progression or death from any cause for everolimus, 0.35; 95% CI of 0.27 to 0.45; P<0.001) (27).

REFERENCES

1. Jemal A, Siegel R, Ward E, Hao Y, Xu J, Thun MJ. Cancer statistics, 2009. *CA Cancer J Clin.* 2009;59(4):225–249.
2. Neoptolemos JP, Stocken DD, Friess H, et al. European Study Group for Pancreatic Cancer. A randomized trial of chemoradiotherapy and chemotherapy after resection of pancreatic cancer. *N Engl J Med.* 2004;350(12):1200–1210.
3. Oettle H, Post S, Neuhaus P, et al. Adjuvant chemotherapy with gemcitabine vs observation in patients undergoing curative-intent resection of pancreatic cancer: a randomized controlled trial. *JAMA.* 2007;297(3):267–277.
4. Trappe R, Riess H, Anagnostopoulos I, et al. Efficiency of antiviral therapy plus IVIG in a case of primary EBV infection associated PTLD refractory to rituximab, chemotherapy, and antiviral therapy alone. *Ann Hematol.* 2009;88(2):167–172.
5. Kalser MH, Ellenberg SS. Pancreatic cancer. Adjuvant combined radiation and chemotherapy following curative resection. *Arch Surg.* 1985;120(8):899–903.
6. Regine WF, Winter KA, Abrams RA, et al. Fluorouracil vs gemcitabine chemotherapy before and after fluorouracil-based chemoradiation following resection of pancreatic adenocarcinoma: a randomized controlled trial. *JAMA.* 2008;299(9):1019–1026.
7. Neoptolemos JP, Stocken DD, Bassi C, et al. European Study Group for Pancreatic Cancer. Adjuvant chemotherapy with fluorouracil plus folinic acid vs gemcitabine following pancreatic cancer resection: a randomized controlled trial. *JAMA.* 2010;304(10):1073–1081.
8. Burris HA III, Moore MJ, Andersen J, et al. Improvements in survival and clinical benefit with gemcitabine as first-line therapy for patients with advanced pancreas cancer: a randomized trial. *J Clin Oncol.* 1997;15(6):2403–2413.
9. Poplin E, Feng Y, Berlin J, et al. Phase III, randomized study of gemcitabine and oxaliplatin versus gemcitabine (fixed-dose rate infusion) compared with gemcitabine (30-minute infusion) in patients with pancreatic carcinoma E6201: a trial of the Eastern Cooperative Oncology Group. *J Clin Oncol.* 2009;27(23):3778–3785.
10. Heinemann V, Boeck S, Hinke A, Labianca R, Louvet C. Meta-analysis of randomized trials: evaluation of benefit from gemcitabine-based combination chemotherapy applied in advanced pancreatic cancer. *BMC Cancer.* 2008;8:82.
11. Heinemann V, Labianca R, Hinke A, Louvet C. Increased survival using platinum analog combined with gemcitabine as compared to single-agent gemcitabine in advanced pancreatic cancer: pooled analysis of two randomized trials, the GERCOR/GISCAD intergroup study and a German multicenter study. *Ann Oncol.* 2007;18(10):1652–1659.
12. Louvet C, Labianca R, Hammel P, et al.; GERCOR; GISCAD. Gemcitabine in combination with oxaliplatin compared with gemcitabine alone in locally advanced or metastatic pancreatic cancer: results of a GERCOR and GISCAD phase III trial. *J Clin Oncol.* 2005;23(15):3509–3516.
13. Herrmann R, Bodoky G, Ruhstaller T, et al.; Swiss Group for Clinical Cancer Research; Central European Cooperative Oncology Group. Gemcitabine plus capecitabine compared with gemcitabine alone in advanced pancreatic cancer: a randomized, multicenter, phase III trial of the Swiss Group for Clinical Cancer Research and the Central European Cooperative Oncology Group. *J Clin Oncol.* 2007;25(16):2212–2217.
14. Cunningham D, Chau I, Stocken DD, et al. Phase III randomized comparison of gemcitabine versus gemcitabine plus capecitabine in patients with advanced pancreatic cancer. *J Clin Oncol.* 2009;27(33):5513–5518.
15. Heinemann V, Quietzsch D, Gieseler F, et al. Randomized phase III trial of gemcitabine plus cisplatin compared with gemcitabine alone in advanced pancreatic cancer. *J Clin Oncol.* 2006;24(24):3946–3952.
16. Colucci G, Labianca R, Di Costanzo F, et al.; Gruppo Oncologico Italia Meridionale (GOIM); Gruppo Italiano per lo Studio dei Carcinomi dell'Apparato Digerente (GISCAD); Gruppo Oncologico Italiano di Ricerca Clinica (GOIRC). Randomized phase III trial of gemcitabine plus cisplatin compared with single-agent gemcitabine as first-line treatment of patients with advanced pancreatic cancer: the GIP-1 study. *J Clin Oncol.* 2010;28(10):1645–1651.
17. Conroy T, Desseigne F, Ychou M, et al. III FOLFIRINOX versus gemcitabine for metastatic pancreatic cancer. *N Engl J Med.* 2011;364:1817–1825.
18. Moore MJ, Goldstein D, Hamm J, et al.; National Cancer Institute of Canada Clinical Trials Group. Erlotinib plus gemcitabine compared with gemcitabine alone in patients with advanced pancreatic cancer: a phase III trial of the National Cancer Institute of Canada Clinical Trials Group. *J Clin Oncol.* 2007;25(15):1960–1966.
19. Philip PA, Benedetti J, Fenoglio-Preiser C, et al. Phase III study of gemcitabine plus cetuximab versus gemcitabine in patients with locally advanced or metastatic pancreatic adenocarcinoma: SWOG S0205 study. *J Clin Oncol.* 2007;25(18S):LBA 4509 (abstract)
20. Kindler HL, Niedzwiecki D, Hollis D, et al. Gemcitabine plus bevacizumab compared with gemcitabine plus placebo in patients with advanced pancreatic cancer: phase III trial of the Cancer and Leukemia Group B (CALGB 80303). *J Clin Oncol.* 2010;28(22):3617–3622.
21. Rinke A, Müller HH, Schade-Brittinger C, et al.; PROMID Study Group. Placebo-controlled, double-blind, prospective, randomized study on the effect of octreotide LAR in the control of tumor growth in patients with metastatic neuroendocrine midgut tumors: a report from the PROMID Study Group. *J Clin Oncol.* 2009;27(28):4656–4663.
22. Dirix LY, Vermeulen PB, Fierens H, De Schepper B, Corthouts B, Van Oosterom AT. Long-term results of continuous treatment with recombinant interferon-alpha in patients with metastatic carcinoid tumors–an antiangiogenic effect? *Anticancer Drugs.* 1996;7(2):175–181.
23. Murray-Lyon IM, Eddleston AL, Williams R, et al. Treatment of multiple-hormone-producing malignant islet-cell tumour with streptozotocin. *Lancet.* 1968;2(7574):895–898.
24. Broder LE, Carter SK. Pancreatic islet cell carcinoma. II. Results of therapy with streptozotocin in 52 patients. *Ann Intern Med.* 1973;79(1):108–118.
25. Raymond E, Dahan L, Raoul J-L, et al. Sunitinib malate for the treatment of pancreatic neuroendocrine tumors. *N Engl J Med.* 2011;364:501–513.
26. Hobday TJ, Rubin J, Holen K, et al. MC044h, a phase II trial of sorafenib in patients (pts) with metastatic neuroendocrine tumors (NET): a Phase II Consortium (P2C) study. *J Clin Oncol.* 2007;25(18S):4504 (abstract)
27. Yao JC, Shah M, Tetshide I, et al. Everolimus for advanced pancreatic neuroendocrine tumors. *N Engl J Med.* 2011;364:514–523.

9

Neuroendocrine Tumors

MARIELA BLUM AND GARRETT R. LYNCH

EPIDEMIOLOGY, RISK FACTORS, NATURAL HISTORY, AND PATHOLOGY—GENERAL

In comparison to other cancers, neuroendocrine tumors (NETs) are fairly rare. The Surveillance, Epidemiology, and End Results (SEER) registry demonstrated an annual age-adjusted incidence of 5.25 new cases per 100,000 people in 2004. The risk of developing NETs is higher in African American individuals (high overall NET incidence of 6.50) compared to Caucasians. NETs comprise a diverse group of neoplasms that share morphologic and cellular features, biologic behavior, and functional abilities. NETs originate in tissues derived from neuroectoderm and endoderm. These tumors can develop from various endocrine glands, such as the pituitary, the parathyroid, or the neuroendocrine portions of the adrenal glands, as well as in endocrine islets within the thyroid or pancreas. They can also develop from endocrine cells found dispersed among the exocrine cells of the digestive and respiratory tracts. NETs can occur in virtually all tissues and organs but are more frequently located in the digestive tract. Most NETs have endocrine function and secrete peptides and neuroamines that cause clinical syndromes; however, many are clinically silent or nonfunctional until late presentation when mass effects result. Diagnosis of NETs is complex and often requires sophisticated laboratory and scanning techniques (1).

Unlike many other cancers, a unified classification system for NETs does not exist. These tumors share certain features, including their microscopic appearance and immunohistochemistry characteristics, as well as their biology and functions. Given their diversity, a variety of different nomenclature systems have been developed based on organ or embryonic site of origin for use in grading and staging of NETs (2).

However, these classification schemas became outdated since it has been observed that patient prognosis is highly dependent on the biological behavior of the tumor and its histological differentiation, rather than its site of origin.

In current clinical practice, NETs are typically divided into well-differentiated and poorly differentiated, with differentiation being linked to tumor grade. Low-grade NETs are considered indolent, whereas high-grade tumors behave very aggressively. Intermediate-grade tumors tend to be less predictable but often follow a moderately aggressive course (2). Well-differentiated NETs are either low or intermediate grade, whereas poorly differentiated NETs are always considered high grade.

Functionality also should be considered when referring to NETs. Functionality is defined based on the presence of excess hormone secretion that causes different clinical symptoms. This is particularly important in pancreatic tumors, where such tumors are designated according to their primary hormone production and related clinical syndrome (e.g., insulinomas, gastrinomas, VIPomas, glucagonomas and nonfunctioning islet cell tumors). The current recommended practice is to describe NETs according to their location of primary origin (e.g., pancreas, duodenum, small intestine, etc.), their grade, differentiation, and reference to the resultant hormone secretion or symptoms.

The pathologic diagnosis of NETs is based on morphological and immunohistochemical features including positive IHC staining for neuroendocrine markers, which include chromogranin, synaptophysin, and neuron-specific enolase (NSE).

WELL-DIFFERENTIATED NEUROENDOCRINE TUMORS

Epidemiology, Risk Factors, Natural History, and Pathology

Oberndofer first coined the term carcinoid (or "Karzinoid") in 1907 to describe all NETs. He chose the term "carcinoid" for these tumors because they grew so slowly that he considered them to be "cancer-like" rather than truly cancerous. In 1929, he reported that some such tumors in the pancreas were not as indolent as previously thought. He used the term neuroendocrine tumors to distinguish these from what most authorities call carcinoids. Today the term carcinoid has been retained and is used synonymously with the term well-differentiated NET, as well as for the low-grade carcinoma associated with the classic carcinoid syndrome.

Carcinoid tumors are the most commonly occurring endocrine tumors of the gut, with the small bowel being the most common site, followed by the appendix. Carcinoids, however, occur in the bronchus, pancreas, rectum, ovary, lung, and thymus. Approximately 2500 new cases of carcinoid tumor are diagnosed annually in the United States. These tumors grow slowly and are often clinically silent for many years before metastasizing. The most common sites for metastases in order of frequency are regional lymph nodes, liver, lung, and bone. Carcinoid tumors can secrete various hormones, including adrenocorticotropic hormone, antidiuretic hormone, gastrin, pancreatic polypeptide, somatostatin, serotonin, histamine, and tachykinins. Carcinoid syndrome occurs in less than 10% of patients with carcinoid tumors. The carcinoid syndrome describes symptoms related to the secretion of serotonin, histamine, or tachykinins into the systemic circulation resulting in classic symptoms of episodic cutaneous flushing, abdominal cramps, and diarrhea. For gut-derived carcinoid tumors, carcinoid syndrome most commonly occurs in the setting of hepatic metastases that provides access to the systemic circulation.

The major clinical manifestation of carcinoid syndrome include the following:

- Cutaneous flushing (90%)
- Gastrointestinal hypermotility with diarrhea (70%)
- Abdominal pain (40%)
- Heart disease (right-sided) (37%)
- Severe sweating (15%)
- Bronchial constriction/wheezing (17%)
- Myopathy (7%)
- Pellagra, dermatitis (5%)

Two of these clinical manifestations deserve further comment. Carcinoid heart disease is reported in approximately 50% of all patients with malignant carcinoid syndrome and is severe in approximately 25% of cases. Carcinoid heart disease occurs primarily on the right side of the heart but may involve the left side to a lesser degree. It is caused by serotonin-induced fibrosis of the tricuspid and pulmonary valves, and by fibrous deposits in the endocardium. These deposits are thought to be responsible for the thickening of the endocardium of the cardiac chambers and papillary muscles. Thickening and deformation of the valve cusps and chordae tendineae can be seen and may result in heart failure, valvular dysfunction, or combined functional lesions. The tricuspid valve is most commonly affected.

Another condition that can develop with carcinoid tumors is pellagra. Pellagra is niacin deficiency (vitamin B3) characterized by diarrhea, dermatitis, dementia, and death. It can develop through several mechanisms, but it develops primarily via the action of functioning tumor cells in diverting tryptophan toward serotonin production and thereby away from the niacin production pathway. Anorexia and diarrhea, frequently present in the carcinoid syndrome, reduce the availability of exogenous niacin by decreasing the amount ingested and absorbed. The decreased availability of endogenous and exogenous niacin eventually results in the depressed tissue niacin levels responsible for the development of pellagra.

The occurrence and severity of the carcinoid syndrome are directly related to elevation of serotonin or its metabolites and tumor size. The patient often has a long history of vague abdominal symptoms, a series of visits to his or her primary care practitioner, and referral to a gastroenterologist. Many individuals with carcinoid tumors are initially misdiagnosed with irritable bowel syndrome.

The diagnosis includes a strong clinical suspicion in patients who present with flushing, diarrhea, wheezing, myopathy, or right-sided heart disease. Appropriate biochemical confirmation and imaging studies are often needed to assess disease burden and evaluate primary location.

In clinical practice, the following constitute the best markers for diagnosis and follow-up of carcinoid tumors: chromogranin A, 24-hour urine 5-hydroxyindoleacetic-acid (5-HIAA), gastrin, serotonin, pancreastatin, and NSE.

Commonly used standard imaging techniques include computed tomography (CT) (triple phase studies are required when CT is used in the evaluation of liver metastases), magnetic resonance imaging (MRI), and octreotide scans. The majority of carcinoid tumors possess high-affinity receptors for somatostatin, and an octreotide scan (radiolabeled somatostatin receptor scintigraphy [SRS]) can be used in diagnosis.

Staging

As recently as a few years ago, no formal TNM-based staging systems existed for NETs for any anatomical site. Recently, TNM staging systems that include NETs of all anatomical sites have been proposed (3). The American Joint Committee on Cancer (AJCC) has recently published TNM staging systems for NETs of the stomach, small bowel, large bowel, and appendix (4). To exemplify the AJCC staging system, the following table outlines the system for NETs of the colon or rectum.

AJCC Staging for NETs of the Colon or Rectum

Stage	Description
I	Primary tumor <2 cm in greatest dimension (T1) with invasion of lamina propria or submucosa with no regional lymph node (N0) or distant metastases (M0)
IIA	Tumor invades muscularis propria or >2 cm with invasion of lamina propria or submucosa (T2) with no regional lymph node (N0) or distant metastases (M0)
IIB	Tumor invades through the muscularis propria into the subserosa or into nonperitonealized pericolic or perirectal tissues (T3) with no regional lymph node (N0) or distant metastases (M0)
IIIA	Tumor directly invades peritoneum or other adjacent organs (T4) without lymph node (N0) or distant metastases (M0)
IIIB	Any T with regional lymph node metastases (N1); no distant metastases (M0)
IV	Any T, any N, with distant metastases (M1)

Case Summary

Well-Differentiated Neuroendocrine Tumors

A.C. is a 58-year-old man with history of gastroesophageal reflux disease (GERD) who had been well until 2 years ago when he developed loose stools. He was treated initially for reflux and his symptoms were attributed to a long-term history of proton pump inhibitors use. Two months prior to evaluation he became increasingly fatigued. He noticed a metallic taste in his mouth, flushing in his face, sweats, and worsening diarrhea (small volume stools up to 20 times a day). He also experienced a 33-pound weight loss over a 2-month period. The patient presented to his primary care physician, who admitted him to the hospital with dehydration and malnutrition.

He underwent esophagogastroduodenoscopy (EGD) and colonoscopy, which revealed only teleangiectasias. He underwent further evaluation with CT of the chest, abdomen, and pelvis, which revealed numerous poorly defined enhancing lesions throughout the liver, with the largest lesion measuring 12 by 15 cm. Oncology was consulted, and at that time, he denied any dizziness, lightheadedness, fevers, or chills. He reported some dysphagia without odynophagia. He denied any nausea, vomiting, or abdominal pain but had lost 38 pounds in a 4-week period.

His past medical history was positive for GERD, hypertension, hypercholesterolemia, and colonic polyps, and his family history was significant for leukemia. Previous surgical procedures included a cholecystectomy and incisional hernia repair. His Eastern Cooperative Oncology Group performance status was 1. He rarely drank alcoholic beverages and denied any illicit drug use. He had smoked cigarettes for 20 years but stopped 10 years ago. His medications included atenolol, ranitidine, amlodipine, and a multivitamin. He has had prior allergic reactions to penicillin and iodine.

On physical examination, he appeared ill. His weight was 193 pounds, and he was afebrile. His blood pressure was 102/71 mm Hg and his pulse was 70 beats per minute. He had no lymphadenopathy. The lung and cardiac examinations were normal. His abdomen was soft with normal bowel sounds and no tenderness or hepatosplenomegaly. Skin and neurologic examinations were normal.

Laboratory test results for hemoglobin and comprehensive metabolic panel were normal, but serum chromogranin A was elevated at 4900 ng/mL (normal value < 225 ng/mL) as well as urine 5-HIAA at 361 mg/24h (normal value < 6 mg/24h). Other selective tumor marker results included normal serum levels of neurospecific enolase, insulin growth factor I, and gastrin. An octreotide scan was performed, which showed octreotide uptake in the liver, as well as the terminal ileum.

Cytologic examination of a specimen obtained via a CT-guided fine-needle aspiration biopsy of one of the liver lesions showed metastatic low-grade NET.

Evidence-Based Case Discussion

Diarrhea is a common symptom, with multiple causes making determination of its etiology sometimes difficult. Common causes of chronic diarrhea include irritable bowel syndrome, inflammatory bowel disease, malabsorption syndromes, chronic infections, and neoplasm. Irritable bowel syndrome, in particular, should be treated as a diagnosis of exclusion; and patients should initially undergo assessment for "alarm symptoms," such as weight loss, nocturnal diarrhea, rectal bleeding, or anemia. Upper gastrointestinal endoscopy with small bowel biopsy and colonoscopy are indicated and will assist in the diagnosis of the above conditions. Our patient's characteristic symptoms of flushing and diarrhea raised the concern for an NET, and biomarker data accompanied by imaging and pathology confirmed the presence of a metastatic low-grade NET with a likely primary in the terminal ileum.

Depending on the results obtained from imaging studies, carcinoid tumors are classified as being locoregional or metastatic disease.

Therapy for Localized Disease

For localized disease, surgical resection should be performed (5).

Appendix: For appendiceal tumor of 2 cm or less, simple appendectomy is recommended, and no further follow-up is required. If the tumor is more than 2 cm in diameter, right hemicolectomy with lymph node resection should be performed.

Small bowel: For tumors 2 cm or less, segmental resection with operative search for other sites is recommended. If the tumor is more than 2 cm or multifocal, hemicolectomy is advised. If primary is not discovered, mesenteric resection to minimize bowel obstruction should be considered.

Colon: For colonic tumors, hemicolectomy with appropriate lymph node resection is recommended

Rectal: For lesions 2 cm or less, transanal or endoscopic resection and regular follow-up is recommended. For tumors more than 2 cm, abdominoperineal resection or lower anterior resection should be considered.

Figure 9.1 shows an algorithm of the management of localized disease.

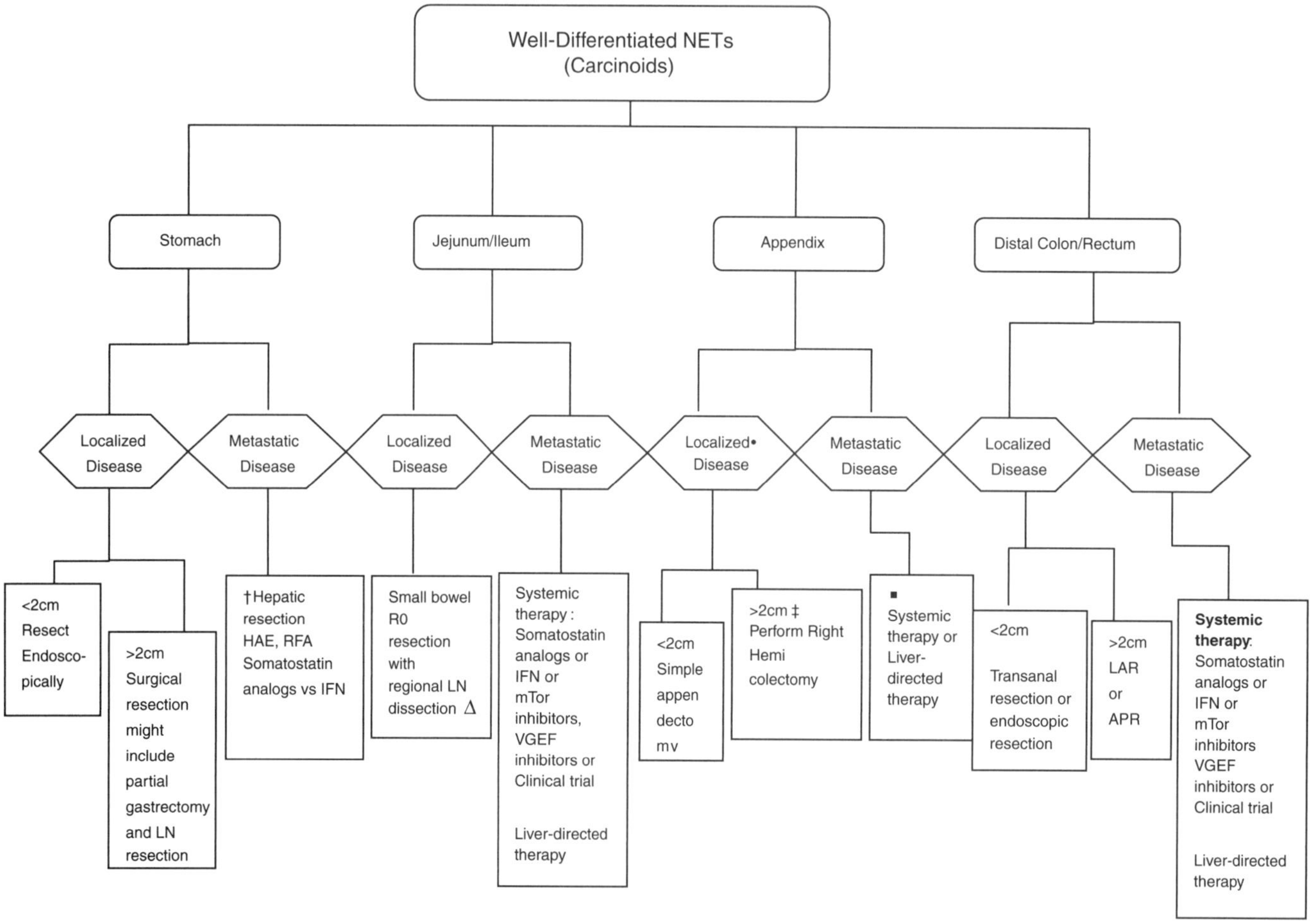

†A small percentage of patients with a limited number of hepatic metastasis localized predominantly to one lobe may be successfully treated with hepatic resection.other options include hepatic arterial embolization (HAE), radiofrecuency ablation (RFA), or cryoablation.

Δ Making a concerted effort to preserved bowel length and the ileocecal valve

‡Formal right hemicolectomy in patients with tumor invasion at the base of the appendix, with tumor greater than 2 cm, in those with tumor where size cannot be determined, with incompletely resected tumors, with evidence of lmphovascular invasion, with invasion into the mesoappendix, with intermediate to high grade tumors, and in with mixed histology (globet cell carcinoid, adenocarcinoid).

▪ Please see systemic therapy for jejunum/ileum

•NETs of the cecum are more aggressive than appendiceal carcinoid. Surgical excision with attention to resection of mesenteric lymph nodes

Figure 9.1

Therapeutic algorithm for well-differentiated NETS.

Therapy for Metastatic Disease

For metastatic disease or unresectable carcinoid tumors in symptomatic patients, somatostatin analogs are indicated for symptom control (5). In the United States, octreotide is the only somatostatin analog approved for the management of carcinoid syndrome. Octreotide comes in two forms: immediate release and sustained release. When there is need for immediate symptom management, a subcutaneous rescue injection of short-acting octreotide (100–500 μg every 8–12 hours) should be administered. For long-term treatment, octreotide-LAR with a starting dose of 20 mg I.M. every 4 weeks should be used. The results from the PROMID study showed that octreotide-LAR significantly lengthened the time to tumor progression compared with a placebo: 14.3 months for octreotide-LAR versus 6 months for the placebo group in patients with functionally active and inactive metastatic midgut low-grade NETs. After 6 months of treatment, stable disease was observed in 66.7% of the patients in the Octreotide LAR group and 37.2% of the patients in the placebo group (6).

Whether symptomatic or not, resection of liver metastases should be considered if feasible. In cases where liver metastases are unresectable, local ablative radiofrequency therapy, cryotherapy, or microwave therapy should be considered. Hepatic regional therapy (arterial embolization, chemoembolization, or radioembolization) or cytoreductive surgery are also available options. If none of these options can be offered, systemic therapy with cytotoxic agents such as interferon, temozolamide, dacarbazine, 5-fluorouracil, and capecitabine can be used in patients with progressive metastases. Figure 9.1 provides an algorithm of the management of metastatic disease.

A number of investigational therapies have shown preliminary evidence of activity in patients with advanced carcinoid tumors. These include inhibitors of the vascular endothelial growth factor receptor (VEGFR) pathway (bevacizumab, sunitinib, and sorafenib), as well as inhibitors of mammalian target of rapamycin (mTOR inhibitors).

Surveillance

Patients with carcinoid tumors should be reevaluated 3 to 12 months after resection, and annually thereafter by performing a complete patient history and physical examination as well as CT or MRI imaging studies. Serum chromogranin A and urinary 5-HIAA in 24-hour samples may be used as tumor markers.

For A.C., treatment with octreotide-LAR was initiated, and within 2 months, the patient's overall condition improved. He gained approximately 10 lbs and his diarrhea resolved. After 6 months, the patient was back to his baseline weight and was completely asymptomatic. Previously elevated levels of serum chromogranin A and urinary 5-HIAA both declined to near normal. Even though excellent control of the patient's symptoms was achieved with the use of octreotide, surgical resection of the hepatic metastases, which has been shown to prolong survival, should be considered.

PANCREATIC NEUROENDOCRINE TUMORS (INTERMEDIATE GRADE)

Epidemiology, Risk Factors, Natural History, and Pathology

The adult endocrine pancreas contains "micro-organs" called islets of Langerhans. The average human islet consists of approximately 3000 cells producing insulin (β-cells, 54%), glucagon (α-cells 34%), somatostatin (δ-cells, 10%), vasoactive intestinal polypeptide (VIP) (δ2 cells), pancreatic polypeptide (PP cells), and substance P/serotonin (enterochromaffin cells). Pancreatic neuroendocrine tumors (PNETs), or Islet cell tumors, are assumed to originate in these islets of Langerhans. In theory, each pancreatic endocrine cell type could give rise to a PNET (7).

PNETs are rare neoplasms. Although the peak incidence is between ages 40 and 60 years, a significant number of patients diagnosed with islet cell tumors are under the age of 35. PNETs are classified as functional or nonfunctional. Of the patients with PNETs, 15% to 30% have nonfunctioning tumors whereas 70% to 80% of patients manifest with clinically evident hormonal symptoms. Clinical presentations of PNETs are summarized in Table 9.1.

The pathogenesis of PNETs is poorly understood. The majority of PNETs are sporadic, but PNETs may also be associated with genetic syndromes such as multiple

Table 9.1 Clinical Syndromes Associated With PNET

Tumor (Secreted Product)	Clinical Presentation
Gastrinoma (gastrin)	Zollinger-Ellison syndrome (ZES)
Insulinoma (insulin)	Whipple's triad
Glucagonoma (glucagon)	Glucagonoma syndrome
Vasoactive intestinal peptidoma	Verner Morrison syndrome
Well-differentiated NF-PNETs	Mass effect (jaundice, hemorrhage)
Poorly differentiated	Mass effect/ syndromes reported

Source: Ehehalt F, Saeger HD, Schmidt CM, Grutzmann R. Neuroendocrine tumors of the pancreas. *Oncologist.* 2009;14(5):456–467.

Table 9.2 Hereditary Syndromes Associated with PNET

Genetic Syndrome	Gene Abnormality	Associated NET Type
MEN 1	Menin 11q13	Gastrinoma, Insulinoma, Thymic
MEN 2	RET	Medulary thyroid carcinoma (CMT) and pheochromocytoma
Neurofibromatosis type I	Hamartin 17q11	Duodenal somatostatinoma
VHL disease	pVHL 3q25	NFNET
Tuberous sclerosis	Tuberin	Rarely NFNET, insulinoma, and gastrinoma
Familial carotid paraganglioma	11q	

Source: Ehehalt F, Saeger HD, Schmidt CM, Grutzmann R. Neuroendocrine tumors of the pancreas. *Oncologist.* 2009;14(5):456–467.

endocrine neoplasia (MEN-1), von Hippel-Lindau (VHL) disease, neurofibromatosis 1 (NF-1), and tuberous sclerosis (TSC) (Table 9.2).

In 2000, the WHO introduced a histological classification system for PNETs. This system was intended to allow benign tumors to be distinguished from malignant tumors. For the WHO classification system, tumor localization, extension, proliferative capacity, and vascular and perineural invasion are assessed (7) (Table 9.3).

Staging

Because PNETs do not arise in the luminal gut, separate TNM staging systems are used for PNETs (4).

AJCC Staging of Pancreatic NET

Stage	Description
IA	Tumor limited to the pancreas, <2 cm in greatest dimension (T1) without regional lymph node (N0) or distant metastases (M0)
IB	Tumor limited to the pancreas, >2 cm in greatest dimension (T2) without regional lymph node (N0) or distant metastases (M0)
IIA	Tumor extends beyond the pancreas, but without involvement of celiac axis or the superior mesenteric artery (T3) without regional lymph node (N0) or distant metastases (M0)
IIB	T1, T2, or T3 tumor with regional lymph node metastases (N1); no distant metastases (M0)
III	Tumor involves the celiac axis or the superior mesenteric artery (T4; unresectable) without regional lymph node (N0) or distant metastases (M0)
IV	Any T, any N, with distant metastases (M1)

Table 9.3 WHO Classification of PNETs

1. Well-differentiated endocrine tumor (WDET)
   1.1. Benign behavior. Confined to the pancreas, <2 cm in diameter, <2 mitosis per 10 high-power fields <2 % Ki67 positive cells, no angioinvasion or perineural invasion
   1.2. Uncertain behavior. Confined to the pancreas and one or more of the following features: >2 cm in diameter, >2 mitosis per 10 HPF, >2% Ki67 positive cells, angioinvasion, perineural invasion
2. Well-differentiated endocrine carcinoma (WDEC)
   2.1. Low-grade malignant
   2.2. Gross local invasion and/or metastases
3. Poorly differentiated endocrine carcinoma (PDEC)
   3.1. High-grade malignant
   3.2. >10 mitoses per HPF

Source: Ehehalt F, Saeger HD, Schmidt CM, Grutzmann R. Neuroendocrine tumors of the pancreas. *Oncologist.* 2009;14(5):456–467.

Case Summary

Pancreatic Neuroendocrine Tumors

R.B. is a 33-year-old woman who was referred to the outpatient cancer center for further evaluation and therapy of a PNET. The patient had been well until 2 weeks prior to this visit when she developed jaundice and dark urine. She had been having intermittent abdominal pain, nausea, and postprandial diarrhea for 2 months. She presented to the emergency room of an outside hospital where she was found to have elevated liver enzymes. Her total bilirubin was 8.4 mg/dL, direct bilirubin 4.0 mg/dL, alkaline phosphatase 99 IU/L, AST 539 IU/L, ALT 539 IU/L. An ultrasound of the abdomen was performed that showed liver masses with bile duct dilatation. Computerized tomography of the abdomen confirmed multiple liver masses, bile duct dilatation, and a pancreatic mass with retroperitoneal lymphadenopathy.

Two days later, she underwent endoscopic retrograde cholangiopancreatography (ERCP) with fine-needle aspiration of the pancreatic mass, as well as stent placement in the common bile duct. The ERCP visualized a pancreatic mass involving the head of the pancreas that appeared highly vascular. There was vascular involvement of the splenic and portal vessels. Cytology from the aspirate revealed an NET based on immunohistochemistry that was positive for synaptophysin, S-100, and chromogranin. Ki67 was positive in 50% of the cells and there were 6 mitoses per 10 high-power fields. Six days later, a colonoscopy was performed, which was normal. A diagnostic laparoscopy with liver biopsy was performed 2 days later. The cytology report from the liver biopsy confirmed a neuroendocrine carcinoma. The patient presented to the Cancer Center for further recommendation.

On examination, the patient appeared well. Her vital signs were normal. Her abdomen was soft with no tenderness, hepatomegaly, splenomegaly, or palpable masses. The remainder of the examination was normal. Basic laboratory test results, including a complete blood count, electrolytes, glucose, total protein, globulin, albumin, and calcium, as well as tests of coagulation and renal and hepatic function, were normal. Other specific markers were as follows: chromogranin A and neurospecific enolase were elevated at 970 ng/m (normal less than 225 ng/mL) and 58 ng/mL (normal less than 15 ng/mL), respectively. Serum vasoactive intestinal polypeptide, gastrin, and urinary 5-HIAA were within the normal range.

Evidence-Based Case Discussion

R.B. presented with a pancreatic mass and liver metastases. The biopsy was consistent with an NET with 6 mitoses per 10 high-power fields, a feature consistent with an intermediate-grade NET. Her tumor was nonfunctional, but had she presented with symptoms characteristic of a functional PNET, the diagnostic evaluation described in the next section would have been performed.

Diagnostic Evaluation of Functional Pancreatic Neuroendocrine Tumors

The classic description of an *insulinoma* is the Whipple's triad, which includes symptoms of hypoglycemia, a measured low blood glucose concentration, and resolution after the ingestion of glucose. Ninety percent of these tumors are benign. The major symptoms caused by insulinomas are those of hypoglycemia, which include the adrenergic symptoms of nervousness, sweating, palpitations, and diaphoresis.

The gold standard test for diagnoses is a positive 72-hour fasting blood glucose and insulin levels. This test excludes all differential diagnoses of hypoglycemia. Patients with insulinoma have elevated levels of C-peptide. An insulin level greater than 3 μU/mL (and often found to be greater than 6 μU/mL) when blood glucose is less than 45 mg/dL and an insulin to glucose ratio is 0.3 or less is diagnostic, reflecting the inappropriate secretion of insulin at the time of hypoglycemia.

Preoperative localization of tumors over 0.5 cm can be achieved with abdominal ultrasound, endoscopic ultrasound, CT, or MRI. Somatostatin receptor scintigraphy (SRS) is positive in 60% of all benign insulinomas. Percutaneous selective arterial calcium stimulation and portal venous sampling are used when other localization studies fail to identify the tumor.

Most of insulinomas are benign, but malignancy might be found in tumors larger than 2 cm. It is important to document any possible site of metastases by CT scan or MRI since this may change the treatment strategy.

Gastrinomas are NETs that produce gastrin. The chronic effects from hypergastrinemia result in a marked gastric acid hypersecretion that ultimately causes severe peptic ulcer disease. They are often accompanied by refractory diarrhea and GERD (Zollinger-Ellison syndrome). Fifty to sixty percent of gastrinomas are malignant.

Diagnosis of a gastrinoma requires measuring fasting gastrin levels (basal level, stimulated level, and gastric acidity). Gastrin levels (basal and stimulated) should be measured after the patient is off proton pump inhibitor therapy for at least 1 week. If the fasting serum gastrin level (FSG) is elevated less than tenfold and the gastric pH is less than 2, then a basal acid output (BAO) measurement should be performed. In patients with Zollinger-Ellison syndrome, serum parathormone, fasting calcium, and prolactin levels should be assessed to rule out MEN-1 (7).

Tumor localization involves upper gastrointestinal endoscopy, CT scan, SRS, or PET Octreotide. If these tests fail to localize the gastrinoma, endoscopic ultrasonography and selective angiography with secretin stimulation and hepatic venous sampling should be considered.

Surgical exploration for gastrinoma should include investigation of the pancreas with intraoperative ultrasonography, duodenal transillumination, and duodenotomy. Laparoscopic approaches are typically not feasible.

Glucagonomas are generally large tumors associated with liver metastases. They are characterized by glucose intolerance, weight loss, and a pathognomonic rash called migratory necrolytic erythema. This rash has a characteristic annular pattern of erythema with central crusting and bullae. The diagnosis of glucagonoma requires the demonstration of increased plasma glucagon levels (usually 500 to 1000 pg/mL, whereas normal is less than 50 pg/mL) in the presence of symptoms (3).

VIPomas (Verner-Morrison syndrome) are PNETs that secrete vasoactive intestinal peptide (VIP) that leads to large-volume diarrhea, hypokalemia, and achlorhydria.

Their diagnosis requires the demonstration of an elevated VIP plasma level.

Somatostatinoma are PNETs that can occur in the duodenum or pancreas. Most cases reported in the literature are PNETs containing somatostatin by immunohistochemistry, without a specific somatostatinoma syndrome, which is a classic clinical pentad of diabetes mellitus, cholelithiasis, weight loss, steatorrhea and diarrhea, and hypochlorhydria and achlorhydria.

The diagnosis is made by the presence of a PNET with the appropriated elevated somatostatin hormone assay result (3). For functioning and nonfunctioning tumors, global neuroendocrine parameters such as chromogranin A and neurospecific enolase should be assessed. SRS, octreotide scan, or other radionucleotide PET should be performed to evaluate octreotide receptor status and localization. Additional imaging modalities include contrast-enhanced ultrasound (CEUS), CT scan, and MRI (7).

Treatment for Localized Disease

Surgical resection is the optimal treatment for localized PNETs. For gastrinomas, gastrin hypersecretion may be treated with histamine H2 receptor antagonists or with proton pump inhibitors. For insulinomas, stabilization of glucose levels with diet or diazoxide (200 to 600 mg/d) is advised. Treatment of electrolyte imbalance with IV fluids and octreotide (if octreotide scan results are positive) may be useful in patients with VIPoma or glucagonoma.

Laparoscopic enucleation is the preferred procedure for insulinomas less than 2 cm, whereas central or distal partial pancreatectomy may be required in certain cases (7). If laparoscopic enucleation is not possible due to the size of tumor or invasion, then pancreaticoduodenectomy or distal pancreatectomy with lymphadenectomy and removal of resectable liver metastases is recommended.

In nonresectable cases, palliative tumor debulking may be justified to achieve hypoglycemic control and may prolong survival. Other procedures such as radiofrequency ablation (RFA), cryotherapy, or transarterial chemoembolization (TACE) for liver metastases can also be considered.

The treatment approach for gastrinomas usually depends on the results of preoperative localization studies. In patients with occult gastrinoma (i.e., no primary tumor or metastases seen on imaging), observation is recommended. Alternatively, if the tumors are identified at surgery, duodenectomy with removal of periduodenal lymph nodes can be performed. Gastrinomas in the head of the pancreas, but not adjacent to the pancreatic duct, should be resected via duodenectomy. Gastrinomas that are deeper or invasive in proximity to the main pancreatic duct should be managed by pancreaticoduodenectomy with periduodenal node dissection. Because most tumors are located in the "gastrinoma triangle" (pancreatic head, duodenum, and surrounding lymph nodes), a distal pancreatectomy allows for removal of the extremely rare distally located gastrinomas. Because primary lymph node gastrinomas have been reported, lymphadenectomy should always be performed, even in the absence of a pancreatic or duodenal primary (8).

Most glucagonomas are malignant, calcified, and located in the tail of the pancreas with regional node involvement. The recommended treatment includes either excision of the tumor with peripancreatic nodal dissection or distal pancreatectomy with resection of lymph nodes and splenectomy.

As with nonfunctioning tumors, depending on the size, location, and invasiveness of the tumor, recommended options for VIPomas are excision, distal pancreatectomy, resection of peripancreatic lymph nodes and spleen. Pancreaticoduodenectomy with dissection of peripancreatic nodes are recommended for tumors in the head of the pancreas.

Long-acting somatostatin analogs (e.g., octreotide, lanreotide) are generally successful in the initial management of patients with glucagonomas, VIPomas and in some patients with somatostatinomas (3).

See Figure 8.3 in Chapter 8 for algorithm for the management of PNETs.

Management of Locoregional Unresectable Disease and or Metastatic Pancreatic Neuroendocrine Tumors

PNETs demonstrate a highly variable growth pattern, with most insulinomas being benign (>85%), whereas greater than 50% of the other symptomatic PNETs and the nonfunctioning PNETs demonstrate liver metastases (9). Surgical excision of both the primary tumor and liver metastases should be considered when possible.

For symptomatic or significant disease progression, patients with a positive octreotide scan or elevated biomarkers can be treated with short-acting octreotide of 150 to 250 mcg subcutaneously three times a day. If a symptomatic response occurs, then an initial monthly dose of 20 to 30 mg LAR octreotide I.M. is recommended. Systemic chemotherapy should also be considered in rapidly progressive disease (see Figure 8.3 in Chapter 8, Pancreatic Cancer). A number of chemotherapy agents alone or in combination, such as doxorubicin, streptozocin, 5-fluourouracil, temozolamide, and dacarbazine, have established antitumor effects in PNETs. A retrospective analysis of 84 patients with either locally advanced or metastatic disease who received streptozocin, 5-fluorouracil, and doxorubicin showed that this regimen was associated with an overall response rate of 39% and median survival duration of 37 months (10). In patients with poorly differentiated PNETs, chemotherapy is recommended with the combination of cisplatin and etoposide or its analogs (3).

Recently, a number of newer chemotherapeutic agents with some efficacy in malignant PNETs have been described. Temozolamide-based regimens represent an alternative to streptozocin-based therapy in patients with advanced PNETs. Temozolamide has been commonly administered as a single agent or in combination with capecitabine (3). The results of two recently completed phase III trials have demonstrated the utility of inhibitors of multiple tyrosine kinases associated with receptors for platelet-derived growth factor (PDGFR), stem cell factor (c-kit), and vascular endothelial growth factor (VEGFR), and inhibitors of the mammalian target of rapamycin (mTOR). A randomized double-blinded trial of sunitinib (an oral multitargeted tyrosine kinase inhibitor) versus placebo as salvage therapy in advanced, well-differentiated PNET after documented progression (86 patients in the sunitinib group and 85 patients in the placebo group) showed a median progression-free survival of 11.4 months in the sunitinib arm versus 5.5 months for the patients who received placebo. The objective response rate was 9.3% in the sunitinib arm and 0% in the placebo arm (11). Equally promising phase III results have also been reported with the mTOR inhibitor everolimus. Four hundred ten patients with advanced-, low-, or intermediate-grade PNET with recent radiographic progression were randomized to receive oral everolimus (207 patients) or placebo (203 patients) both in conjunction with best supportive care. The median progression-free survival in the everolimus group was 11.0 months as compared with 4.6 months in the control group (the hazard ratio for disease progression or death from any cause with everolimus was 0.35, 95% confidence interval [CI] = 0.27–0.45, $P < 0.001$). At 18 months' follow-up, the proportion of patients who were alive and free of progression was 34% (CI = 26–43) in the everolimus group versus 9% (CI = 4–16) in the placebo group (12).

For patients with incurable liver metastases and dominant metastases, treatment options include hepatic regional therapies such as arterial embolization, radioembolization, chemoembolization, and local ablative therapy (RFA, cryotherapy, microwave), which may provide cytoreductive therapy of the liver metastases (9).

In the case of R.B., as described above, she was initiated on chemotherapy with adriamycin, streptozocin, and 5-fluourouracil, which resulted in a sustained progression-free interval.

ADRENOCORTICAL CARCINOMA

Epidemiology, Risk Factors, Natural History, and Pathology

Adrenocortical carcinomas (ACC) are rare malignancies (incidence of 1 to 2 per million population) with a heterogeneous presentation and a variable but generally poor prognosis (13). There is a bimodal age distribution with an initial peak in childhood and a second higher peak in the fourth or fifth decade of life. Women are more affected than men; the female to male ratio is approximately 1.5 to 1.

The majority of cases are sporadic; nevertheless, cases of adrenal carcinoma have been seen in association with several hereditary syndromes including the Li-Fraumeni syndrome, Beckwith-Wiedmann syndrome, and multiple endocrine neoplasia. The molecular pathogenesis of ACC is still poorly understood. However, inactivating mutations at the 17p13 locus, including the *p53* tumor suppressor gene, and alterations of the 11p15 locus, leading to IGF-II overexpression are frequently observed (13).

Approximately 60% of patients present with signs and symptoms of adrenal steroid hormone excess, usually in the form of rapidly progressing Cushing's syndrome, with or without virilization. Signs and symptoms of Cushing's syndrome are caused by hypercortisolism and include weight gain with centripetal obesity, a rounded face (moon face), increased fat deposition around the neck (buffalo hump), relatively proximal muscle wasting, psychiatric disturbances, hyperglycemia, and hypokalemia. Androgen secreting ACCs in women may induce hirsutism, deepening of the voice, male pattern baldness, and oligomenorrhea. In men, estrogen secreting tumors may induce gynecomastia and testicular atrophy. Aldosterone producing ACCs present with hypertension and marked hypokalemia. Nonfunctioning or hormone-inactive ACCs, usually present with abdominal discomfort associated with nausea, vomiting, abdominal fullness, or back pain caused by the mass effect of a large tumor.

Staging

AJCC Staging of Adrenocortical Carcinoma

Stage	Description
I	Tumor <5 cm in greatest dimension without invasion (T1) without regional lymph node (N0) or distant metastases (M0)
II	Tumor >5 cm in greatest dimension without invasion (T2) without regional lymph node (N0) or distant metastases (M0)
III	T1 or T2 tumor with regional lymph node metastases (N1) OR tumor extends beyond adrenal invading fat (T3) without regional lymph node (N0); no distant metastases (M0)
IV	T3 or T4 tumor with regional lymph node metastases (N1) without distant metastases (M0) OR any T, any N, with distant metastases (M1)

Case Summary

Metastatic Adrenocortical Carcinoma

G.H. is a 32-year-old woman who was referred to the Cancer Center because of an adrenal mass. She had been in her usual state of health until 2 months prior to her evaluation when she began to experience back pain and generalized swelling. Her back pain was most noticeable in her cervical and lumbar areas. She reported increased irritability, facial hair, and easy bruising. She also became more anxious over the previous 3 months and noticed an elevation in her blood pressure. The patient presented to her primary care physician who believed her symptoms were related to polycystic ovarian syndrome. She underwent a dexamethasone suppression test, which revealed an elevated cortisol level. The urinary free cortisol was also found to be elevated. Subsequently, an ultrasound of the abdomen revealed a 5.3 by 1.5 cm mass in the superior margin of the right kidney, which was suspected to be of adrenal origin. This was followed by an MRI, which confirmed the mass to be located in the adrenal gland. One week prior to her Cancer Center referral, she was admitted to the hospital with hypokalemia and hypertension. Her potassium was replaced and blood pressure medications were adjusted. On the basis of her evaluation to date, she was diagnosed with Cushing's syndrome secondary to an adrenocortical mass concerning for malignancy.

At her Cancer Center visit, G.H. reported anxiety and episodes of flushing. She had gained approximately 12 pounds in the last month. She had difficulty sleeping for the last 2 months and she had recently noticed a numbness and tingling sensation in her upper extremities. Her medications were metoprolol, potassium chloride, alprazolam, and zolpidem. She did not drink alcohol, smoke, or use illicit drugs. Her father had prostate cancer, and one grandmother had a history of cervical carcinoma.

On physical examination, the patient was overweight with a moon face with increased facial hair. Her blood pressure was elevated at 157/99 mm Hg with a normal pulse. Her BMI was 32. There was an unusual distribution of her body fat, particularly noticeable at the top of her back. Her lungs were clear to auscultation and her heart was regular without murmurs. The abdomen was soft, with no tenderness, hepatomegaly, splenomegaly, or palpable masses. The remainder of the examination was normal. Her cortisol level was elevated to 50.4 µg/dL (reference range 4.3–22 µg/dL) but her ACTH, free metanephrines, aldosterone, and renin levels were within the normal range. Dehydroepiandrosterone and testosterone levels were also elevated at 626 mcg/dL (31–228 mcg/dL) and 314 ng/dL (14–76 ng/dL), respectively. Other laboratory-test results were normal, including complete blood cell count, electrolytes, glucose, total protein, globulin, albumin, and calcium. Renal and hepatic functions were also normal.

Review of CT scans of the abdomen and pelvis confirmed the presence of a large heterogeneous mass with central calcification arising from the superior portion of the right adrenal gland, and also showed multiple scattered ring-enhanced lesions in the liver and numerous pulmonary nodules in lung bases consistent with metastases. A small lytic lesion was identified in the costochondral junction suggestive of bone metastasis in her eighth rib. An MRI of the cervical, thoracic, and lumbosacral spine was requested due to the patient's symptoms of numbness and tingling in the upper extremities. It revealed a severe compression fracture of C6 with retropulsion, and an epidural tumor causing mild C6 cord compression. Epidural metastases from C5 to C7, as well as S4 and S5 epidural disease was noted in addition to multiple other bone metastases. G.H. underwent a fine-needle aspiration of the right adrenal mass. Pathological examination showed adrenal carcinoma.

Evidence-Based Case Discussion

G.H. is a patient with adrenocortical carcinoma with metastases to liver, lung, and bone.

Diagnosis and Evaluation

In the evaluation of adrenal masses, screening should be performed to exclude a pheochromocytoma. Pheochromocytomas are NETs derived from adrenal chromaffin cells, which produce, store, metabolize, and secrete catecholamines or their metabolites. About 10% of these tumors are malignant, and 90% arise in the adrenal medulla, while extra-adrenal pheochromocytomas usually occur within the para-aortic sympatic chain. Pheochromocytomas may occur sporadically or as a part of a hereditary syndrome (such as MEN 2A, MEN 2B, neurofibromatosis type I, von Hipper-Lindau, and Osler-Weber-Rendu syndrome). The main signs and symptoms of catecholamine excess include hypertension, palpitations, headache, sweating, and pallor. According to the degree of catecholamine excess, patients can present with myocardial infarction, arrhythmia, stroke or other signs of ischemic events resulting in serious morbidity and mortality. Because imaging often cannot reliably differentiate between ACC and pheochromocytoma, screening should include a 24-hour urinary estimation of catecholamines (epinephrine, norepinephrine, and dopamine) and its metabolites, including metanephrines and normetanephrines. In addition, plasma metanephrines and catecholamines can be assayed in order to establish the diagnosis in most patients. For functional adrenocortical carcinomas, a thorough hormonal work-up is needed to identify the type of hormone hypersecretion occurring, as well as for monitoring trends after surgical treatment and identifying subsequent tumor recurrence (see Table 9.4) (13).

Evaluation with CT or MRI is recommended for initial tumor localization, and more recently, 18F-fluorodeoxyglucose positron emission tomography (FDG-PET) has been used to distinguish benign and malignant lesions. According to the National Institute of Health consensus conference, tumors larger than 6 cm are highly suspicious for malignancy. On unenhanced CTs, the Hounsfield Unit (HU) number is typically higher in carcinomas than in adenomas and a threshold value of 10 HU has been proposed as a means of distinguishing benign from malignant adrenal tumors (14). Adrenal lesions with an attenuation value of more than 10 HU in unenhanced CTs, or an enhancement washout of less than 50% and a delayed attenuation of more than 35 HU (on 10–15 minute delayed enhanced CT) are suspicious for malignancy. Because the lung and liver are the most common sites of metastatic spread, thoracic and abdominal scans are integral to the staging work-up of ACCs.

Because histologic analysis of an adrenal mass may be unreliable, fine or core tissue needle aspiration biopsies (percutaneous) are generally not recommended except in possible metastatic deposits. Laparoscopic excision of the tumors is the preferred method of removal of benign adrenal tumors. When tumors are thought to be malignant, an open or laparoscopic-assisted operation should be done since these malignant tumors are prone to rupture. If pheochromocytoma is suspected, patients should receive a preoperative blocking agent in order to counteract the significant release of catecholamines on target tissues due to anesthesia and surgical manipulation of the tumor. Nuclear atypia, atypical and frequent mitoses (more than 5 per 50 high-power fields), vascular and capsular invasion, and necrosis are suggestive of malignancy. Several studies have demonstrated the value of Ki67 staining in differentiating benign from malignant lesions. In addition, Ki67 expression may be of prognostic relevance, as high expression (greater than 10%) has been associated with poor survival (13).

Table 9.4 Hormonal Work-Up and Imaging in Patients With Suspected or Proven ACC*

Glucocorticoid excess (minimum 3 of 4 test)	Dexamethasone suppression test (1mg, 23:00h)
	Excretion of free urinary cortisol (24-h urine)
	Basal cortisol (serum)
	Basal ACTH (plasma)
Sexual steroids and steroid precursors	DHEA-S (serum)
	17-OH-progesterone (serum)
	Androstendione (serum)
	Testosterone (serum)
	17 B-estradiol (serum, only in men and postmenopausal women)
Mineralcorticoid excess	Potassium (serum)
	Aldosterone to renin ratio (only in patients with arterial hypertension and/or hypokalemia)
Exclusion of a pheochromocytoma (1 of 2 tests)	Catecholamine excretion (24- h urine)
	Meta-and normetanephrines (plasma)
Imaging	CT or MRI of abdomen and thorax
	Bone scintigraphy (when suspecting skeletal metastases)
	FDG-PET (optional)

*As per recommendations of the ACC working group of the European Network of the Study of Adrenal Tumors (ENSAT), May 2005.
From Allolio and Fassnacht (13).

Therapy for Localized and Advanced ACC

Adrenal carcinomas are rare; therefore, clinical series are small, and only limited prospective evaluation of treatment strategies exists.

In stages I through III, complete tumor removal by a specialized surgeon offers the best chance of cure. Surgical resection is often extensive with en bloc resection of the invaded organs and lymph nodes. At present there is a consensus that open adrenalectomy remains the operation of choice for ACC with invasion to adjacent organs, enlarged regional lymph nodes, and tumors larger than 10 to 12 cm in size (13).

Owing to its rarity, there are no published randomized prospective trials for adjuvant therapy. The majority of retrospective trials of adjuvant therapy have included the use of mitotane, an oral adrenocorticolytic agent. Mitotane exerts a specific cytotoxic effect on adrenocortical cells, producing focal degeneration of the fascicular, and particularly the reticular zone, whereas changes in the zona glomerulosa are minimal. The main side effects of mitotane are weakness, fatigue, dizziness, loss of appetite, nausea, vomiting, and diarrhea. The largest study thus far retrospectively analyzed 177 patients who underwent tumor resection and subsequent treatment in Italy and Germany. In the Italian cohort, 47 of the 102 patients received adjuvant mitotane at doses ranging from 1 to 5 g daily, whereas none of the 75 German patients received adjuvant mitotane. Recurrence-free survival was significantly prolonged in the mitotane group as compared with the two control groups (median recurrence-free survival was 42 months as compared with 10 months in control group 1 and 25 months in control group 2). Hazard ratios for recurrence were 2.91 (95% confidence interval [CI], 1.77–4.78; $P < .001$) and 1.97 (95% CI, 1.21–3.20; $P = .005$), suggesting that adjuvant mitotane may be an effective postoperative strategy (15). Due to the adrenolytic effects of mitotane, replacement doses of corticosteroids (hydrocortisone or prednisone) should be prescribed in order to prevent adrenal insufficiency.

For patients with high-grade adrenal carcinoma suspected of having residual disease due to invasion and incomplete resection, the National Comprehensive Cancer Network (NCCN) recommends adjuvant mitotane or radiation therapy to the adrenal tumor bed. Follow-up with imaging and biomarkers every 3 to 6 months in functional tumors is also recommended. Figure 9.2 demonstrates an algorithm for the management of patients with localized ACC.

G.H. presented with stage IV adrenocortical carcinoma with metastases to the liver, lungs, and bones. In advanced stages, such as this case, the treatment is often palliative (see Figure 9.2 for treatment algorithm).

Treatment strategies include treatment of endocrine excess syndromes in functional adrenal carcinomas, the use of mitotane or several multiagent chemotherapy regimens and/or radiation for low-grade tumors, or palliative chemotherapy or radiation for high-grade tumors. The role of tumor debulking in the presence of metastatic disease is debatable. Incomplete resection of the primary tumor or metastatic disease not amenable to surgery is associated with a particularly poor prognosis (13). In most studies, the overall survival is less than 12 months.

Several studies have evaluated the combination of mitotane with cytotoxic agents, including cisplatin and etoposide. In a large prospective phase II trial, the combination of cisplatin, etoposide, and doxorubicin with mitotane 4 g daily yielded an overall response rate of 49% (by WHO criteria). Median time to tumor progression and overall survival of the entire cohort were 9.1 and 28.5 months, respectively (18.2 and 47.7 months, respectively, in the patient subset attaining a disease response) (16). Another study reported an objective response rate of 36% with the combination of mitotane plus streptozocin. The overall 2-year and 5-year survival rates were 70% and 32.5%, respectively (17). An international phase III trial called the First International Randomized Trial in Locally Advanced and Metastatic Adrenocortical Carcinoma Treatment (FIRM-ACT) trial is currently underway comparing etoposide, doxorubicin, cisplatin, and mitotane against streptozocin and mitotane. Currently the first-line chemotherapy treatment for advanced metastatic adrenocortical carcinoma includes the combination of cisplatin, adriamycin, etoposide, and mitotane, while second-line therapy is mitotane plus streptozocin.

For most bone and brain metastases, radiation therapy is the treatment of choice. In the case of G.H., palliative radiation was initiated for the epidural metastases from C6 to C7 in order to relieve the mild cord compression. Mitotane was given concurrently. Subsequently, she received a chemotherapy combination of cisplatin, adriamycin, etoposide, and mitotane with few reported side effects.

POORLY DIFFERENTIATED (HIGH-GRADE) EXTRAPULMONARY NEUROENDOCRINE CARCINOMAS

Epidemiology, Risk Factors, Natural History, and Pathology

The terms poorly differentiated and high-grade neuroendocrine carcinoma (PD NECA) are used interchangeably. The classic small cell carcinoma occurs in the lung, but extrapulmonary poorly differentiated

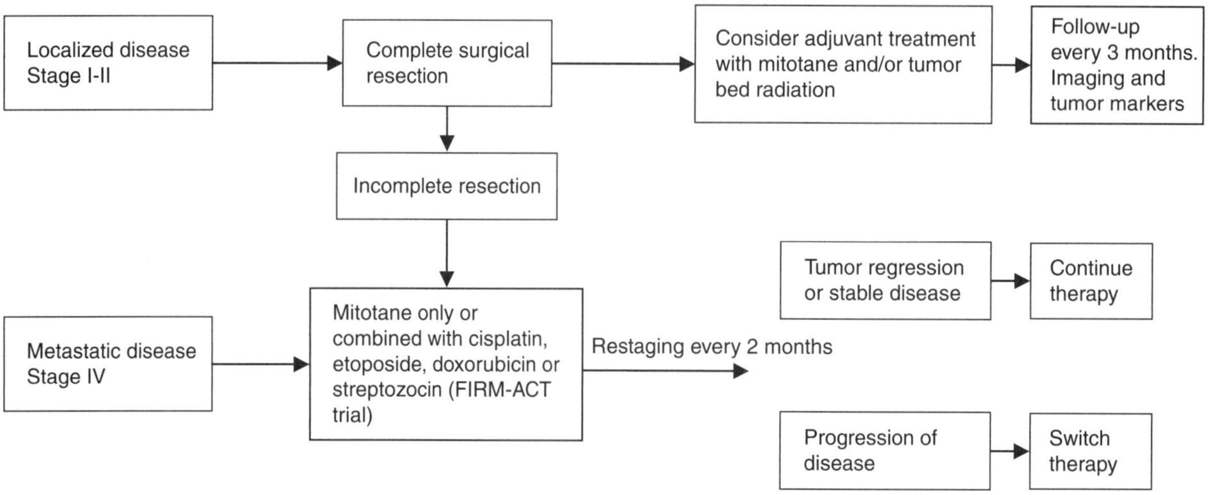

Figure 9.2

Management algorithm for adrenal cortical carcinoma.

neuroendocrine carcinomas can originate in the skin, larynx, gastrointestinal tract, bladder, cervix, and prostate. NECAs are characterized by a high mitotic rate (greater than 10–20 mitoses per 10 high-power fields) and extensive necrosis (18).

Extrapulmonary poorly differentiated NECAs are exceedingly rare and they confer a poor prognosis with median survival durations in patients with localized, regional, and distant disease of 34, 14, and 5 months respectively.

Case Summary

High-Grade/Poorly Differentiated Neuroendocrine Tumor

M.M. is a 32-year-old man who was seen in consultation by oncology during inpatient hospitalization because of a high-grade NET. The patient had been well until approximately 3 weeks before this evaluation when he developed abdominal pain, heartburn, cramping, nausea, vomiting, and constipation. The pain was most noticeable after eating. He had been vomiting for 2 weeks and reported a weight loss of 30 pounds over the same time period. He presented to the emergency room with the above symptoms and the gastroenterology service was consulted. CT scans of the abdomen, obtained on the day of admission, showed a large mass in the gastrohepatic area that abutted the stomach and the esophagus, as well as multiple large liver lesions. An upper gastrointestinal endoscopy showed a large, lobular mass in the body of the stomach. Biopsies were taken and the pathology was consistent with a poorly differentiated neuroendocrine carcinoma with 20 mitosis per 10 high-power fields.

He did not have any medical and surgical history in the past. He had lost approximately 40 pounds of body weight during the previous month, which he attributed to emesis. He exercised regularly, drank alcohol, and smoked socially but denied any illicit drug use. There was no history of cancer in the family.

On physical examination, the patient appeared well and his vital signs were normal. His BMI was 25. The abdomen was soft, with tenderness in the epigastric area. There was no distention, hepatomegaly, splenomegaly, lymphadenopathy, or palpable masses. The remainder of the examination was also normal. Other laboratory test results, including the hematocrit, complete blood cell count, glucose, total protein, globulin, albumin, and calcium, as well as tests of coagulation, renal, and hepatic function were normal. Immunohistochemistry examination of the pathology specimen was positive for synaptophysin, chromogranin, CK7, CAM 5.2, CK 5/6. Morphologic and immunophenotypic features were consistent with a high-grade NET.

Evidence-Based Case Discussion

Management of Limited Disease

Similar to small cell lung carcinoma, poorly differentiated neuroendocrine carcinomas tend to metastasize even in patients with apparently localized tumors. Surgery alone is rarely curative. Given their aggressive behavior, surgical resection followed by adjuvant chemotherapy (4 or 6 cycles of cisplatin or carboplatin and etoposide), with or without radiation, is recommended. Based on the treatment for limited stage small cell lung cancer, a course of definitive chemotherapy with 4 to 6 cycles of cisplatin or carboplatin and etoposide with radiation can be considered in patients with localized extrapulmonary involvement, particularly when surgical resection is difficult. Concurrent chemotherapy with radiation is more efficacious as reported in clinical trials for limited stage small cell lung cancer, but at the expense of increased toxicity (18).

Data on extrapulmonary PD NECAs suggest a lower incidence of central nervous system metastases as compared to small cell lung cancer. Therefore, routine prophylactic cranial irradiation is not recommended in this population, but may be considered for patients with poorly differentiated neuroendocrine carcinomas of the head and neck or unknown primary (18).

Management of Extensive Disease

The combination of cisplatin and etoposide has been studied in metastatic PD NECAs of the gastrointestinal tract. Moertel reported a response rate of 67% in patients with poorly differentiated neuroendocrine carcinoma with a response duration of 8 months and a median survival of 19 months (19). Mitry also studied this combination in PD NECAs of the gastrointestinal tract and reported a response rate of 42% with a response duration of 9 months and a median survival of 15 months (20). On the basis of these studies, cisplatin in combination with etoposide is recommended as first-line therapy for metastatic PD NECAs. The length of treatment remains unclear and whether treatment beyond four cycles is associated with a survival benefit is debatable.

There is no data for second-line chemotherapy regimens. Retreatment with a platinum and etoposide regimen can be considered in patients who initially responded but then relapsed more than 3 to 6 months after termination of first-line chemotherapy. Other agents with activity in second-line treatment for small cell lung cancer include irinotecan, paclitaxel, docetaxel, vinorelbine, and gemcitabine.

In the case of M.M., a CT scan showed complete remission following six cycles of cisplatin and etoposide, after which he was placed on surveillance with imaging and physical examinations.

REFERENCES

1. Vinik A, O'Dorisio T, Woltering E, Go VL. *Neuroendocrine tumors: a comprehensive guide to diagnosis and management.* Interscience Institute. 2006.
2. Klimstra DS, Modlin IR, Coppola D, Lloyd RV, Suster S. The pathologic classification of neuroendocrine tumors: a review of nomenclature, grading, and staging systems. *Pancreas.* 2010;39(6):707–712.
3. Kulke MH, Anthony LB, Bushnell DL, et al. NANETS treatment guidelines: well-differentiated neuroendocrine tumors of the stomach and pancreas. *Pancreas.* 2010;39(6):735–752.
4. Edge SB, Byrd DR, Compton CC, et al. *AJCC cancer staging handbook: From the AJCC cancer staging manual.* Springer; New York, 2010.
5. Anthony LB, Strosberg JR, Klimstra DS, et al. The NANETS consensus guidelines for the diagnosis and management of gastrointestinal neuroendocrine tumors (NETS): well-differentiated NETS of the distal colon and rectum. *Pancreas.* 2010;39(6):767–774.
6. Rinke A, Müller H, Schade-Brittinger C, et al. Placebo-controlled, double-blind, prospective, randomized study on the effect of octreotide LAR in the control of tumor growth in patients with metastatic neuroendocrine midgut tumors: a report from the PROMID Study Group. *J Clin Oncol.* 2009;27(28):4656–4663.
7. Ehehalt F, Saeger HD, Schmidt CM, Grützmann R. Neuroendocrine tumors of the pancreas. *Oncologist.* 2009;14(5):456–467.
8. Jensen RT, Niederle B, Mitry E, et al. Gastrinoma (duodenal and pancreatic). *Neuroendocrinology.* 2006;84(3):173–182.
9. Metz DC, Jensen RT. Gastrointestinal neuroendocrine tumors: pancreatic endocrine tumors. *Gastroenterology.* 2008;135(5):1469–1492.
10. Kouvaraki MA, Ajani JA, Hoff P, et al. Fluorouracil, doxorubicin, and streptozocin in the treatment of patients with locally advanced and metastatic pancreatic endocrine carcinomas. *J Clin Oncol.* 2004;22(23):4762–4771.
11. Raymond E, Dahan L, Raoil J-L, et al. Sunnitinib maleate for the treatment of pancreatic neuroendocrine tumors. *N Eng J Med.* 2011;364:501–573.
12. Yao JC, Shah MH, Ito T, et al. Everolimus for advanced pancreatic neuroendocrine tumors. *N Eng J Med.* 2011;364:514–523.
13. Allolio B, Fassnacht M. Clinical review: adrenocortical carcinoma: clinical update. *J Clin Endocrinol Metab.* 2006;91(6):2027–2037.
14. Caoili EM, Korobkin M, Francis IR, et al. Adrenal masses: characterization with combined unenhanced and delayed enhanced CT. *Radiology.* 2002;222(3):629–633.
15. Terzolo M, Angeli A, Fassnacht M, et al. Adjuvant mitotane treatment for adrenocortical carcinoma. *N Engl J Med.* 2007;356(23):2372–2380.
16. Berruti A, Terzolo M, Sperone P, et al. Etoposide, doxorubicin and cisplatin plus mitotane in the treatment of advanced adrenocortical carcinoma: a large prospective phase II trial. *Endocr Relat Cancer.* 2005;12(3):657–666.
17. Khan TS, Imam H, Juhlin C, et al. Streptozocin and o,p'DDD in the treatment of adrenocortical cancer patients: long-term survival in its adjuvant use. *Ann Oncol.* 2000;11(10):1281–1287.
18. Strosberg JR, Coppola D, Klimstra DS, et al. The NANETS consensus guidelines for the diagnosis and management of poorly differentiated (high-grade) extrapulmonary neuroendocrine carcinomas. *Pancreas.* 2010;39(6):799–800.
19. Moertel CG, Kvols LK, O'Connell MJ, Rubin J. Treatment of neuroendocrine carcinomas with combined etoposide and cisplatin. Evidence of major therapeutic activity in the anaplastic variants of these neoplasms. *Cancer.* 1991;68(2):227–232.
20. Mitry E, Baudin E, Ducreux M, et al. Treatment of poorly differentiated neuroendocrine tumours with etoposide and cisplatin. *Br J Cancer.* 1999;81(8):1351–1355.

10

Hepatobiliary Cancers

AHMED AWAIS AND PAUL ZHANG

BILIARY TRACT CARCINOMAS

Epidemiology, Risk Factors, Natural History, and Pathology

Biliary tract cancers (BTCs) include both cholangiocarcinoma (CC) and gall bladder cancer (GBC), which are malignant tumors arising from the epithelial lining of the bile duct and gall bladder, respectively. These tumors comprise 3% of all gastrointestinal malignancies. There are approximately 9000 new cases per year in the United States (1), with almost twice as many cases of GBC than CC. High incidence areas of BTC worldwide include Southeast Asia (Thailand and some parts of China), India, and South America (Chile) (2). The incidence of BTC peaks in the sixth and seventh decades of life. A significantly higher proportion of GBC cases occur in women, whereas CC affects men and women equally.

Risk factors for CC include a history of primary sclerosing cholangitis (PSC), congenital biliary cysts, hepatolithiasis, liver flukes (*Clonorchis sinensis* and *Opisthorchis viverrini*), Thorotrast dye, dietary nitrosamines, and chemical agents such as dioxin and asbestos. Recently, an association between CC and hepatitis C infection has been established. PSC is clearly the most established risk factor, with a reported association with CC as high as 40% (3). On the other hand, the most common risk factor for GBC is gallstones, which are identified in 65% to 90% of GBC cases. Other risk factors for GBC include porcelain gall bladder (a sequela of chronic cholecystitis), anomalous pancreaticobiliary duct junction, obesity, and various chemicals. Infections with *Salmonella typhi* and *Helicobacter pylori* have also recently been linked to GBC. These risk factors cause chronic irritation and inflammation of the biliary epithelium, resulting in dysplasia, carcinoma in situ, and eventually, invasive carcinoma. Genetic defects involving *k-ras* and *p53* have been described in a significant number of cases of BTC (4).

More than 90% of BTCs are adenocarcinomas. Anatomically, CC can be divided into intrahepatic (ICC), extrahepatic (ECC), and hilar (i.e., Klatskin tumor) types. The distribution of these tumors is 10% ICC, 20% ECC, and 70% hilar. Hilar CC occurs at the bifurcation of the common hepatic duct and represents the most commonly encountered CC. ICC occurs in the liver and can present a diagnostic challenge due to difficulty in differentiating it radiologically from HCC. ECC originates in the bile duct along the hepatoduodenal ligament. Both HCC and ECC usually present with painless jaundice due to biliary obstruction. Other symptoms may include pruritis, weight loss, dark urine, pale stools, and fever. In contrast, ICC usually presents with dull, right upper quadrant pain without evidence of biliary obstruction. The incidence of ICC has been rising, while the incidence of ECC seems to be declining. Most cases of GBC arise in the fundus of the gall bladder and are often diagnosed incidentally during surgical exploration for cholelithiasis. Frequently, GBC cases are diagnosed in advanced stages and present with many of the symptoms described above.

BTCs are curable, if caught early, with surgical resection; however, only 10% to 20% of patients actually present in an early stage. Even after surgical resection, the recurrence rate can be as high as 50%. The average 5-year survival for this disease remains poor: 5% for GBC and 10% to 20% for CC (3). The majority of patients with unresectable disease die within 6 to 12 months of diagnosis.

Staging

The Cancer Staging System of the American Joint Committee on Cancer (AJCC) is the gold standard classification system used for staging patients. ICC, ECC, and

GBC have independent staging criteria. However, for clinical practice, all patients with BTC may be divided into three distinct groups:

- Localized disease.
- Locally advanced and unresectable disease.
- Metastatic disease.

The surgeon will often request advanced imaging studies and sometimes perform laparoscopy to determine the resectability of the tumor and confirm the clinical stage of the patient. Resectability is the single most important factor in determining the outcome.

The extrahepatic bile duct tumors are further subclassified into perihilar (proximal) and distal groups.

AJCC 7th Edition Staging System for Perihilar (Proximal) Bile Duct Tumors

Stage	Definition
I	Tumor confined to bile duct histologically
II	Tumor invades beyond bile duct wall to adjacent adipose or liver parenchyma
IIIA	Tumor invades unilateral branches of portal vein (PV) or hepatic artery (HA)
IIIB	Regional lymph node metastasis
IVA	Tumor invades main PV or its branches bilaterally; or the HA; or the second-order biliary radicals bilaterally
IVB	Distant metastasis (includes distant lymph nodes)

AJCC 7th Edition Staging System for Distal Bile Duct Tumors

Stage	Definition
IA	Tumor confined to bile duct histologically
IB	Tumor invades beyond bile duct wall
IIA	Tumor invades duodenum, pancreas, gall bladder or other adjacent organs
IIB	Any regional nodal involvement
III	Tumor involves celiac axis or superior mesenteric artery
IV	Distant metastasis

AJCC 7th Edition Staging System for Intrahepatic Bile Duct Tumors

Stage	Definition
I	Solitary tumors, without vascular invasion
II	Multiple tumors or solitary tumors with vascular invasion
III	Tumor perforating the visceral peritoneum or involving the local extrahepatic structures by direct invasion
IVA	Tumor with periductal invasion; or regional lymph node metastasis present
IVB	Distant metastasis present

Case Summaries

Locally Advanced/Unresectable Biliary Tract Cancer

R.T. is a 67-year-old male with no significant past medical history presented with a 5-day history of yellowish discoloration of the skin, darkening of the urine, and pale stools. His wife confirmed a 10-pound weight loss over the last month. Examination revealed icteric sclera and tenderness to deep palpation in the right upper quadrant of the abdomen. The laboratory tests revealed a total and direct bilirubin level of 7.1 and 5.8 mg/dL, respectively. Alkaline phosphatase was elevated at 273 U/L. ALT and AST were within normal limits. An abdominal ultrasound was performed that did not show any evidence of gallstones; however, a suspicious mass was seen in the hilar region. A magnetic resonance imaging (MRI) scan of the abdomen was performed to better characterize the lesion and showed a 3.5 × 4.0 × 3.7 cm T2 hyperintense mass in the region of the confluence of the bile ducts that was suspicious for an HCC. Dilatation of the intrahepatic bile ducts was also noted. The mass was partially infiltrating hepatic segments 4 and 5 and was also invading the porta hepatis, hepatic artery, and portal vein. No extrahepatic biliary ductal dilatation was noted. No other abnormalities were noted in the liver or pancreas, and no regional lymphadenopathy was seen. The CA 19–9 was elevated at 500 U/mL, and the carcinoembryonic antigen (CEA) was normal at 0.5 U/mL.

R.T. was admitted to the hospital for further workup. An endoscopic retrograde cholangiopancreatography (ERCP) revealed a hilar stricture with dilation of the left and right hepatic ducts. Brushings and cytology were obtained, and a stent was placed to relieve the obstruction. An endoscopic ultrasound (EUS) confirmed the presence of the locally invasive mass seen on MRI and the lack of regional lymphadenopathy. EUS-guided biopsy of the mass revealed a cytokeratin (CK) 7 positive and CK 20 negative adenocarcinoma. The cytology from brushings was negative. A chest CT was negative for metastatic disease. According to the AJCC, this tumor was a stage IVA (T4 N0 M0).

Evidence-Based Case Discussion

The differential diagnosis is quite broad for a patient presenting with jaundice and other signs of biliary obstruction. It includes cholelithiasis, benign biliary strictures, PSC, pancreatic tumors, and hepatobiliary malignancies. However, painless jaundice and weight loss are highly suggestive of an underlying hepatobiliary tumor, and the clinician's index of suspicion should be very high. R.T. initially had an ultrasound to assess the biliary tree. An ultrasound is very sensitive for detection of biliary tract dilatation or other obvious biliary pathology, but frequently an MRI or CT scan is required to better characterize the extent of the tumor and to identify regional or distant metastases. The relationship of the tumor to the surrounding structures, including the vasculature, is extremely important when assessing resectability. An early surgical opinion should be obtained, since surgery represents the only chance for cure. In general, stage III and IV disease are not amenable to surgery. Four factors affect tumor resection: (a) the extent of the tumor within the biliary tree; (b) vascular invasion; (c) hepatic lobar atrophy; and (d) metastatic disease. The extensive invasion of this patient's tumor into the porta hepatis, along with involvement of the hepatic artery and portal vein, made this an inoperable tumor. Unresectable disease carries a poor prognosis, and the only remaining options are palliative chemoradiation or chemotherapy alone.

Placement of biliary stents to relieve obstruction is an important intervention. Single or multiple stents can be placed in the hepatic duct, common bile duct, or other points of obstruction in the biliary tree before the initiation of chemotherapy or radiation. On average, the median survival for unresectable CC is approximately 6 months with biliary drainage and 3 months without it (2). Bacterial cholangitis or liver failure are potentially fatal complications. For patients who are expected to live longer and who wish to avoid repeated procedures, surgical bypass may be considered.

Both CEA and CA 19-9 are often checked in patients with suspected biliary tumors, although neither is very specific nor is sensitive for CC. In patients with biliary obstruction, serum CA 19-9 concentrations should be reevaluated once the bilirubin has returned to normal, as elevated CA 19-9 levels may occur due to the obstruction itself. In a recent study, serum CA 19-9 combined with abdominal ultrasound, CT scan, or MRI had a sensitivity of 90% to 100% for detecting CC (5). When CEA and CA 19-9 are evaluated together, the accuracy is greater than either used alone. The sensitivity of brush cytology for diagnosing CC is also quite low due to the desmoplastic reaction associated with the tumor. In a large prospective study, the sensitivity of cytology varied from 9% to 24%, and the specificity varied from 61% to 100% (5).

The clinician can be faced with the challenge of treating locally advanced disease in very diverse situations. The three most commonly encountered scenarios are the following:

- Residual micro- or macroscopic disease after surgery.
- Unresectable disease at presentation (as seen in this patient).
- Recurrent disease in a previous surgical bed.

A comprehensive review analyzed the studies conducted to assess the benefit of chemoradiation in this setting (6). In one of these studies, investigators from the Cleveland Clinic conducted a retrospective analysis of 28 patients with localized, nonmetastatic extrahepatic bile duct cancer. They reported a significantly increased median survival in patients who received external beam radiation therapy (EBRT) after transtumoral dilatation and intubation of the bile duct compared with those patients who underwent surgical decompression alone (12.2 vs. 2.2 months, respectively; $P = 0.05$). In a similar study with a cohort of 55 patients, Tollenaar et al. reported an increase in median survival with the use of EBRT after surgical decompression compared with surgical decompression alone (16 vs. 3 months, respectively). Several other retrospective reports suggest that the addition of brachytherapy (BT) to EBRT has prolonged the median survival in patients with unresectable ECC. A study at the Mayo Clinic reported a median survival of 18.5 months, and 1- and 5-year survival rates of 69% and 7%, respectively, in 14 patients with unresectable ECC who were treated with intraoperative radiation therapy (IORT) and EBRT. In most studies, the use of BT or IORT and EBRT in patients with unresectable ECC resulted in a median survival of 12 to 14 months and a 1-year survival rate of 50% to 70%. Long-term survival is possible in approximately 10% to 20% of highly selected patients. Some studies also demonstrated a benefit from increasing the dose of radiotherapy (XRT); however, other studies showed increased adverse effects and no impact on survival with increased XRT dose.

Patients with known distant metastases should not be subjected to local treatment unless symptomatic relief is required. In such cases, local radiation may help relieve biliary obstruction. Radiosensitizing chemotherapy can also be used. The most extensively studied agent is 5-fluorouracil (5-FU). Capecitabine is fairly well tolerated and may be substituted if needed. Gemcitabine should not be administered concurrently with radiation due to an increased risk of toxicity.

Chemotherapy alone has been used for locally advanced disease when radiation is not an option. A detailed review of chemotherapy is presented in the section on metastatic disease.

R.T. received oral capecitabine (850 mg/m^2) concurrently with 5 weeks of EBRT and tolerated therapy very well. A repeat CT scan 6 weeks after completion of treatment showed stable disease with no obvious progression. A repeat serum CA 19-9 decreased to 100 U/mL. He is followed every 3 months with a history and physical examination, liver function tests, and serum CA 19-9 levels.

The approach to BTC is a multidisciplinary one, and supportive care plays an integral role. Adequate pain control with narcotics, anti-emetics, bowel regimens, and appetite stimulants are essential components of the overall treatment regimen.

Newer therapies, including molecular targeting agents such as erlotinib, are being investigated and have shown some activity in early trials. Photodynamic therapy and orthotopic liver transplant have also been used in some studies with encouraging results; however, they are not yet the standard of care.

Figure 10.1 depicts the general approach to management of cholangiocarcinoma.

Metastatic Biliary Tract Cancer

J.V. is a 77-year-old Hispanic woman with a long-standing history of gallstones presented with 1 month of abdominal pain and 1 week of jaundice, decreased appetite, and 15-pound weight loss. She complained of fatigue and a low energy level but continued to work and perform all her household chores. She also noticed itching of her skin the last few days. Examination revealed icteric sclera and tenderness on palpation in the right upper quadrant of the abdomen. On deep palpation, a firm mass was felt in the same region. Laboratory tests revealed a total and direct bilirubin of 10.1 mg/dL and 8.8 mg/dL, respectively. Alkaline phosphatase was elevated at 373 U/L. Alanine aminotransferase (ALT) and aspartate aminotransferase (AST) were mildly elevated at 75 U/L and 94 U/L, respectively. Carbohydrate antigen 19-9 (CA 19-9) and carcinoembryonic antigen (CEA) level were normal. Hematopoietic and kidney function were well preserved.

Abdominal ultrasound showed a suspicious mass in the gallbladder with small gallstones but no evidence of cholecystitis. Computed tomography (CT) of the abdomen showed a 4.6 × 5.5 × 4.2 cm heterogeneously enhancing, centrally necrotic mass occupying the gall bladder fossa, causing compression of the common bile duct and also associated with intra- and extrahepatic biliary dilatation. An irregular, peripherally enhancing, centrally low-attenuating mass was also visualized in the left lobe of the liver, measuring 4.8 × 7.5 × 8.7 cm. Numerous smaller, peripherally enhancing, low attenuation lesions were seen throughout the liver. Necrotic 1.8-cm para-aortic lymph

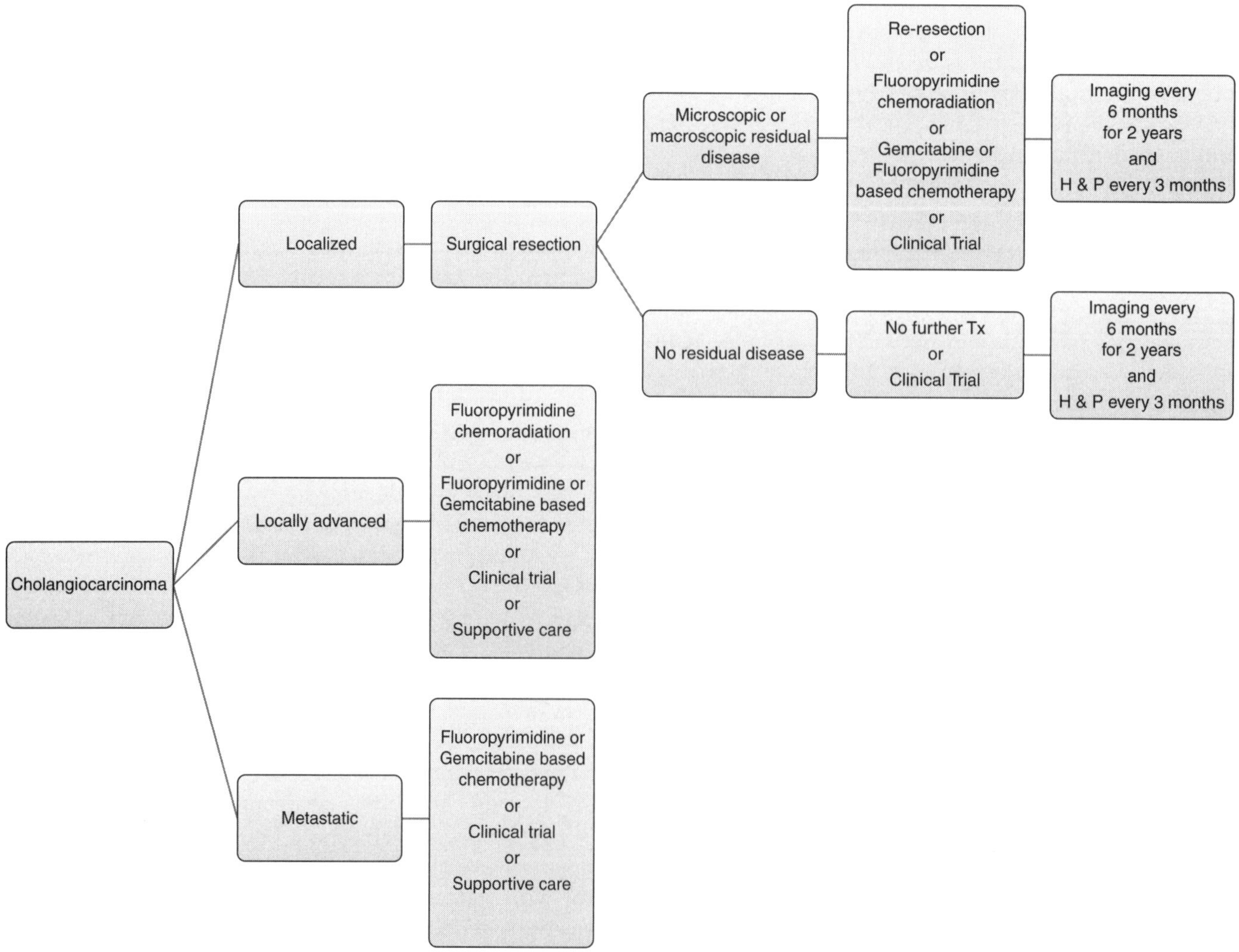

Figure 10.1

Treatment algorithm for cholangiocarcinoma.

nodes were identified, as well as a 2 cm necrotic porta hepatis lymph node. Owing to the tumor's location, a percutaneous CT-guided biopsy of the gall bladder mass was performed. The pathology was consistent with adenocarcinoma of the gall bladder. A metal stent was placed in the common bile duct to relieve the obstruction. The metastases to the liver and lymph nodes resulted in a T3 N1 M1 (stage IV) disease classification.

Evidence-Based Case Discussion

J.V. has advanced GBC with Eastern Cooperative Oncology Group (ECOG) performance status of 0 and was performing daily household chores. Jaundice as a presenting sign in GBC indicates a poor prognosis, and 50% of these tumors are unresectable. The presence of metastases to the lymph nodes and liver does not favor any local treatment modality such as surgery or radiation. In these situations, palliative chemotherapy would be the only option. J.V.'s ECOG performance status is crucial to determining the treatment approach, since patients with poor performance status are not good candidates for chemotherapy and should receive supportive care.

GBC, like CC, is a rare tumor, and most of the evidence for treatment is derived from small retrospective studies or phase II trials of advanced BTC. The survival benefit of chemotherapy over best-supportive care was demonstrated approximately two decades ago in a study that used 5-FU and etoposide in patients with advanced pancreaticobiliary malignancies (6.0 months for the treated patients vs. 2.5 months untreated) (7). The quality of life was also improved with chemotherapy. Historically, 5-FU alone had a response rate of 10%. When combined with other agents such as oxaliplatin and cisplatin, the response rate increased between 25% and 55%, with a median survival of 6 to 12 months (8). Capecitabine showed similar results as 5-FU when used in combination with platinum compounds (9). Later, gemcitabine was found to be active in biliary tract neoplasms and was successful in various combinations, with a median survival of 9 months to 12 months. A recent meta-analysis of 104 trials, including 2810 patients with advanced BTCs (both locally advanced and metastatic), demonstrated an average response rate of 22.8% to various chemotherapy regimens (10). The median times to progression and overall survival (OS) were 4.1 and 8.2 months, respectively. Gemcitabine as a single agent was found to be superior to the fluoropyrimidines. Doublet chemotherapy demonstrated superior response rates (28% vs. 15.3%) and trends toward increased OS (9.3 vs. 7.5 months) compared to single agents. Three or more drug combinations added no extra benefit over two-drug regimens. Gemcitabine and platinum (cisplatin and oxaliplatin) based doublets demonstrated the best response rates, with some as high as 50%. There was a trend toward a longer time to progression with the gemcitabine-platinum doublet compared to the fluoropyrimidine-platinum combination (5.5 vs. 3.7 months).

There are only two phase III trials conducted to date studying chemotherapy for advanced BTC. The first trial compared 5-FU, leucovorin, and etoposide (FELV) to 5-FU, epirubicin, and cisplatin (ECF) (11). However, due to poor recruitment, it was underpowered to detect any difference in OS. The median OS was 9.02 versus 12.03 months for ECF and FELV, respectively, and this was not statistically significant. The overall response rates and nonhematologic toxicities were very similar in both groups. The other phase III trial (ABC-02) recruited 410 patients from 37 centers in the United Kingdom. Half of the patients were assigned to gemcitabine as a single agent, and the other half received a gemcitabine-cisplatin combination (1). The tumor control rate was 81.4% for the combination versus 71.8% for the single agent. Progression-free survival (PFS) and median OS were 8 and 11.7 months, respectively, for the gemcitabine-cisplatin combination. PFS and OS were 5 and 8.1 months, respectively, for the single-agent gemcitabine. There was a nonsignificant increase in the incidence of neutropenia in the gemcitabine-cisplatin group; however, infections were similar in the two groups.

Therefore, in patients with good performance status, the combination of cisplatin and gemcitabine is the chemotherapy of choice. Other commonly used combinations include gemcitabine-oxaliplatin, gemcitabine-capecitabine, and capecitabine-oxaliplatin; however, none has been compared head to head. Single-agent 5-FU, capecitabine, or gemcitabine can be offered in patients who have borderline ECOG performance status of 1 to 2, that is, even those who are able to carry out daily life activities with some difficulty, as long as the patient can tolerate treatment. Chemotherapy is generally continued until there is evidence of disease progression. There is no approved second-line treatment regimen, but the aforementioned chemotherapy drugs may be used if they were not used as part of the first-line treatment.

J.V. in the clinical vignette was started on gemcitabine-cisplatin chemotherapy, which was well tolerated except for some nausea and mucositis. A CT scan performed 8 weeks after the initiation of treatment showed no evidence of progression. She was maintained on the same treatment and continues to follow up in the clinic.

HEPATOCELLULAR CARCINOMA

Epidemiology, Risk Factors, Natural History, and Pathology

Hepatocellular carcinoma (HCC) ranks as the fifth most common cause of cancer-related mortality in the world and is responsible for up to 1 million deaths worldwide

(12). The prevalence of HCC parallels the distributions of hepatitis B (HBV) and hepatitis C (HCV) viral infections, and the incidence of HCC has been on the rise worldwide due to HBV and HCV epidemics (13). Significant improvements in the management of cirrhosis complications have led to increased survival of patients who carry these viruses. High incidence areas for HCC include mainland China, Taiwan, Hong Kong, and sub-Saharan Africa (14).

Most patients with HCC have underlying liver disease, which further complicates the diagnosis and management of HCC. HCC can be distinguished from other tumor types where the organ function is well preserved despite malignant transformation. HCC generally has a progressive course and poor overall prognosis. Surgical resection and ablation of a localized tumor are the only curative options, and less than one third of patients present at this early stage. Overall, the 5-year survival for HCC is approximately 5%.

HCC arises from the liver epithelium, and the morphology can vary from well differentiated to very poorly differentiated. Tumors arise in the context of chronic hepatocyte injury, which results in inflammation and increased hepatocyte turnover. Dysplastic changes and subsequent fibrosis can predispose the patient to develop HCC. In fact, patients with HCC often have underlying fibrotic nodules and hyperplasia that make the diagnostic process more complex. However, up to 10% of patients with HCC have no underlying liver disease. These tumors arise in young people (fibrolamellar variant) and sometimes in the elderly (de novo HCC).

Risk factors for HCC include HBV and HCV infection (80% of all cases) and other causes of cirrhosis such as alcoholism, adult fatty liver disease, hemochromatosis, alpha-1 antitrypsin deficiency, primary biliary cirrhosis, autoimmune hepatitis, and carcinogens such as aflatoxin and Thorotrast. The HBV genome may become integrated into the hepatocyte DNA, leading to mutations and malignant transformation. Male sex and advanced age are also risk factors. Since HCC is largely a preventable disease, surveillance guidelines now incorporate both alpha-fetoprotein (AFP) and ultrasound to screen high-risk populations (14).

Staging

The stage at presentation generally determines the prognosis in solid tumors. In HCC, however, the underlying liver function also affects the outcome, and the Child-Pugh score can be used for this purpose. Many

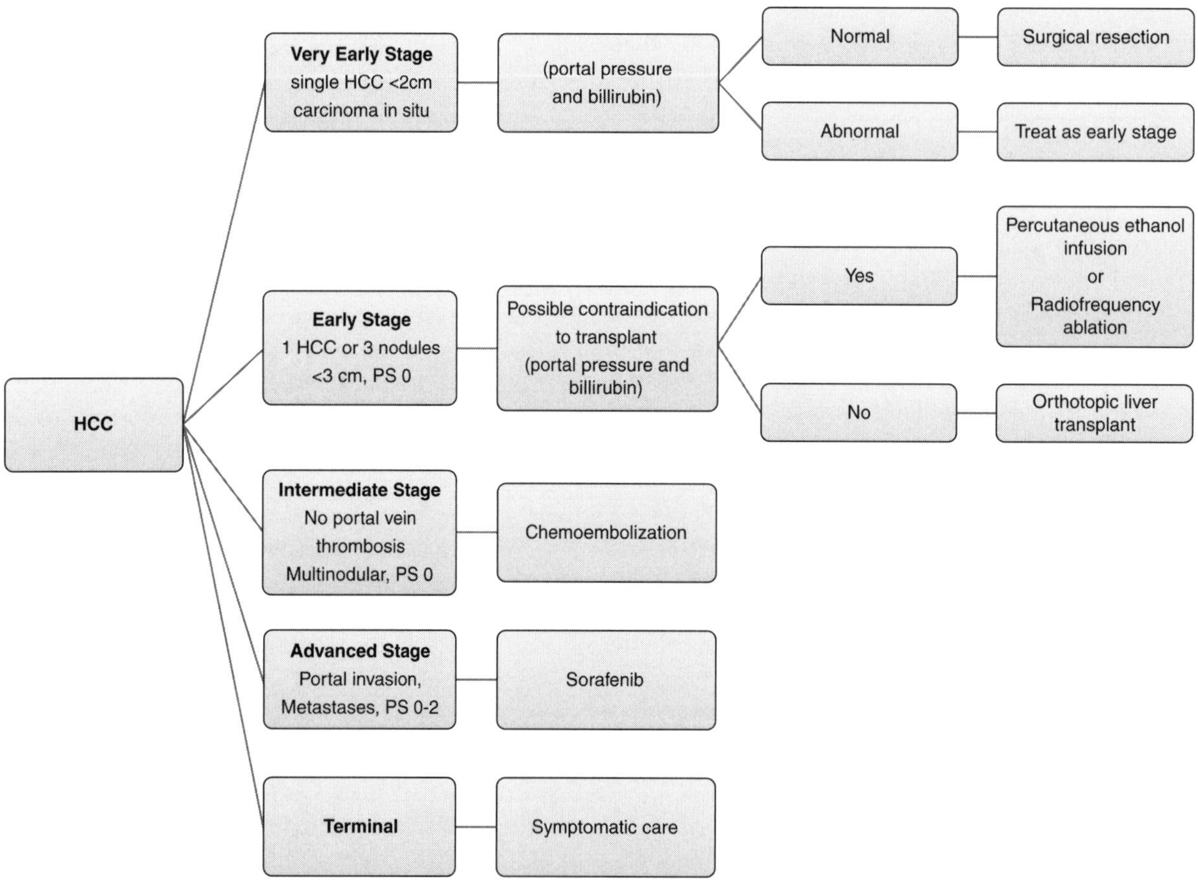

Figure 10.2

The Barcelona Clinic Liver Cancer Scale (BCLC) system and treatment algorithm.

staging systems have been used for HCC, including the Tumor, Lymph Nodes, Metastasis (TNM); Okuda; and Cancer of the Liver Italian Program (CLIP) classifications. The AJCC TNM staging system was recently revised and is the only system that has been validated in patients treated with either surgical resection or transplantation. However, this system does not include liver function. The Barcelona Clinic Liver Cancer (BCLC) system (Figure 10.2) has been chosen as the best staging system by the American Association for the Study of Liver Diseases (AASLD) (13). The BCLC incorporates tumor stage, liver function, physical condition of the patient, and cancer-related symptoms; all of these factors appear to impact the prognosis and the treatment approach.

AJCC 7th Edition TNM Staging System for Hepatocellular Carcinoma

Stage	Definition
I	Solitary tumor without vascular invasion
II	Solitary tumor with vascular invasion or multiple tumors but none >5 cm
IIIA	Multiple tumors >5 cm
IIIB	Single tumor or multiple tumors of any size involving a major branch of the portal vein or hepatic vein
IIIC	Tumor(s) with direct invasion of adjacent organs other than the gall bladder or with perforation of visceral peritoneum
IVA	Regional nodal metastasis
IVB	Distant metastasis

Case Summaries

Locally Advanced Hepatocellular Carcinoma

S.R. is a 53-year-old woman with a history of alcoholic cirrhosis and portal hypertension was seen at an outpatient facility for mild abdominal distension. She denied any history of hepatic encephalopathy but did have an episode of variceal bleeding a few months ago. On examination, she was found to have mild ascites. Labs revealed a platelet count of 105,000/μL, albumin of 3 g/dL, prothrombin time prolonged 4 s beyond normal, and a bilirubin of 1.5 mg/dL. A CT of the abdomen showed an irregular mass measuring 6.6 × 4.3 cm in the lateral segment of the left hepatic lobe. Another mass measuring 5.5 × 2.8 cm was identified in the left hepatic lobe. Both lesions showed arterial enhancement and rapid washout in the venous and delayed phases. There were scattered additional foci of arterial enhancement throughout the liver. The liver had a nodular contour consistent with cirrhosis. Prominent esophageal, gastric, and peri-portal venous collaterals were seen, as well as signs of portal hypertension such as an enlarged portal vein and splenomegaly. No significant intra-abdominal lymphadenopathy was noted. A CT of the chest did not show any metastases. AFP was 500 ng/mL. The ECOG performance status was 0 to 1.

Evidence-Based Case Discussion

S.R. was diagnosed with HCC based on the size of the tumor and the classic findings on imaging. Owing to the presence of multiple tumors >5 cm in diameter, she was classified as stage IIIA according to the TNM classification and was not deemed a candidate for surgical resection or transplant. She was Child-Pugh class B. According to the BCLC system, the classification was stage B, intermediate disease. She was referred to interventional radiology for transarterial chemoembolization (TACE).

TACE is a combination of targeted chemotherapy (chemotherapeutic agents delivered via hepatic arterial infusion through a catheter directly into the HCC) and arterial embolization (selective obstruction of blood flow to the tumor using gelatin sponge particles). The rationale behind this approach is the fact that the hepatic artery is the major source of blood supply to the tumor. Antineoplastic agents can include doxorubicin, mitomycin, and cisplatin. Clinical trials have demonstrated TACE response rates from 16% to 60% (15). The OS benefits of TACE over best-supportive care have been shown in some phase 3 clinical trials (16); however, meta-analyses of several phase III trials by different groups generated conflicting results (15,17). The improvement in survival in patients undergoing TACE ranges from 20% to 60% at 2 years and 20% to 50% at 3 years in prospective trials. Some studies have also documented the success of TACE as an effective bridge to potentially curative treatments such as surgery or liver transplant. Contraindications for TACE are advanced (Child-Pugh Class C) cirrhosis, portal vein thrombosis, hepatic encephalopathy, and biliary obstruction. Performing TACE in such cases may cause hepatic failure. S.R. had no contraindications and was prepared for the procedure with vigorous intravenous hydration and prophylactic antibiotics. The first TACE was uncomplicated; however, the second TACE 4 weeks later was followed by a low-grade fever and abdominal pain. This "postembolization syndrome" occurs in up to 50% of patients and is due to acute hepatic ischemia and tumor necrosis. Characterized by fevers, abdominal pain, and ileus, the syndrome is generally self-limited and can be treated with IV hydration and no oral intake. Major complications from TACE include portal vein thrombosis, hepatic abscess, hepatic artery dissection or thrombosis, and liver failure. S.R. recovered within 2 days and was discharged in stable condition. A CT scan post-TACE showed necrosis of 80% of the tumor, and a repeat AFP level decreased to 200 ng/mL. S.R. continues to be monitored with serial scans.

In recent years, early stages of HCC have been increasingly recognized due to efficient screening guidelines and better imaging techniques. HCC in the early stage can be treated with surgical resection and demonstrates a 5-year survival up to 70% (18). Hepatic resection is a potentially curative option in patients with adequate liver function, those with a solitary mass, no evidence of major vascular invasion and adequate future liver remnant. Interestingly, the size of the tumor may not limit surgical consideration. In some centers, hepatic vein catheterization is performed to assess the hepatic vein pressure gradient prior to surgical planning. Only those patients with a hepatic venous pressure gradient <10 mm Hg and a normal bilirubin level are cleared for surgery. This policy is in accordance with the most recent 2010 AASLD practice guidelines (18). There is currently no role for pre- or postresection therapy; however, in clinical practice, neoadjuvant local techniques are sometimes used to shrink the tumor so that it may become surgically resectable. Also, portal vein embolization may be carried out preoperatively in an attempt to induce hypertrophy of the residual liver segments after surgical resection. This is especially beneficial for those with chronic liver disease who are being considered for major liver resection.

Liver transplant is indicated for patients with underlying portal hypertension and cirrhosis. On the basis of the Milan criteria, any patient with a solitary tumor <5 cm in diameter, or up to three lesions, each <3 cm in diameter, without evidence of vascular invasion or extrahepatic spread, may be eligible for transplantation (19). Patients with HCC within these criteria have posttransplant survival rates of 70% at 5 years. There is level II evidence to support the use of preoperative therapy if the waiting list for transplant exceeds 6 months. This approach helps minimize the risk of progression during the waiting time.

Radiofrequency ablation or percutaneous ethanol injection are local techniques that can be used with curative intent if the patient is not a transplant candidate because the disease burden falls outside the Milan criteria or has other comorbidities. The local control and OS rates for these procedures are very similar to surgical resection (12,18). Even after successful surgery, a high risk of recurrence remains (up to 50% at 5 years). Therefore, the National Comprehensive Cancer Network (NCCN) guidelines recommend patients be followed with serial imaging.

Metastatic Hepatocellular Carcinoma

F.S. is a 50-year-old white man with a long-standing history of chronic HCV infection and liver cirrhosis was admitted to the hospital with abdominal pain and a 20-pound weight loss in the last 3 months. He also noted decreased appetite and fatigue for the last few weeks. He had been treated for HCV infection a few years ago and had been doing fairly well until recently. He denied any history of encephalopathy or admission to the hospital in the past for decompensated cirrhosis. Abdominal examination revealed mild tenderness to palpation in the right upper quadrant. No jaundice or ascites was appreciated. Laboratory testing revealed an albumin of 3.6 g/dL, bilirubin of 1.9 mg/dL, and a prothrombin time within normal limits. A complete blood count and liver chemistry were also within normal limits. A CT scan of the abdomen with contrast was performed and showed several heterogeneous lesions with areas of necrosis in the liver measuring 2 to 6 cm in diameter. The lesions showed arterial enhancement and early venous washout, and there was concern for portal vein invasion. Multiple retroperitoneal lymph nodes were enlarged, which suggested metastatic disease. Serum AFP was 800 ng/mL. His ECOG performance status was zero.

Evidence-Based Case Discussion

F.S. was diagnosed with HCC based on the size of the tumor and the classic findings seen on imaging. The elevated AFP also supported a diagnosis of HCC. The tumor was classified as stage IV according to the TNM classification. The Child-Pugh score was class A. According to the BCLC system, the classification was stage C, advanced disease.

In this case, and many other similar cases seen in clinical practice, tissue biopsy is not required to prove HCC. As per the NCCN guidelines, presence of either classic findings on one imaging study (usually CT or MRI with contrast) or an AFP > 200 ng/mL is diagnostic of HCC when the tumor size is >2 cm. If the AFP < 200ng/mL and there is no classic finding in imaging, biopsy is indicated to establish diagnosis. Once the diagnosis was confirmed in this case, CT of the chest was performed to complete the staging and was negative.

The BCLC system is very useful in this scenario. Four main factors determine the outcome in HCC: (a) stage; (b) tumor aggressiveness; (c) liver function; and (d) performance status of the patient. The BCLC system uses all of these factors, as well as the Child-Pugh score. The BCLC system also links the tumor with the recommended treatment modality and the expected life expectancy based on published responses (18).

The most appropriate treatment for F.S. is systemic therapy; local therapies are not likely to be helpful. Historically, many different treatment strategies have been used in such advanced cases, including doxorubicin chemotherapy, interferon, tamoxifen, and radiation therapy, but none has demonstrated a survival benefit (14). The median survival in untreated patients is usually a few months. The landmark study that significantly impacted clinical practice was the Study of Heart and

Renal Protection (SHARP) trial (20). This was a multicenter, double-blinded, phase III clinical study that proved the efficacy of sorafenib, a multikinase inhibitor that targets vascular endothelial growth factor receptor 2 (VEGFR2), platelet derived growth factor receptor (PDGFR), Raf-1, B-Raf, c-Kit, other tyrosine kinases, and serine threonine kinases. This trial enrolled 602 patients with advanced HCC who were not candidates for local treatment or had progressed after failing local treatment. All patients had an ECOG ≤2, and 97% were classified Child-Pugh Class A. All had adequate renal and hematopoietic function, and were randomized to either sorafenib (400 mg) twice a day or placebo. Overall median survival was significantly longer in the sorafenib group than the placebo group (10.7 vs. 7.9 months). A 31% reduction in the risk of death was noted. The disease control rate was also significantly higher in the sorafenib group than the placebo group (43% vs. 32%). The two most relevant adverse effects of sorafenib were diarrhea and hand-foot syndrome, both of which occurred in 8% of patients.

The other major phase III trial that evaluated sorafenib in HCC patients was the Asia-Pacific study, a randomized, double-blind, placebo-controlled study (21). Compared with the SHARP trial, this trial was smaller, randomizing a total of 226 patients with advanced HCC to receive either oral sorafenib (400 mg twice daily) or placebo. All patients were Child-Pugh Class A. The median OS was significantly longer in the sorafenib group compared with the placebo group (6.5 vs. 4.2 months). Median time to progression was also improved with sorafenib (2.8 vs. 1.4 months). Sorafenib did not produce a significant response rate. The safety profile of sorafenib was similar to that reported in the SHARP trial. As a result, the NCCN and AASLD guidelines now recommend sorafenib as the first-line treatment for advanced disease (extrahepatic spread or portal invasion) not amenable to other modalities in patients with well-preserved liver function (i.e., Child-Pugh Class A).

F.S. was therefore started on sorafenib treatment, which he tolerated well with only mild diarrhea. A dynamic CT scan was repeated 12 weeks after initiation of treatment and showed no change in the size of the liver mass; however, increased necrosis throughout the tumor was observed. Such necrosis is typically seen in patients who respond to sorafenib, and this patient continues to have stable disease after 1 year on sorafenib.

Data on the use of sorafenib in Child-Pugh Class B and C are limited. Survival in this group of patients is limited by the severity of the underlying liver disease. However, if the liver function allows, a low dose of sorafenib can be tried in Child-Pugh Class B patients and titrated up as tolerated. Further studies are ongoing to assess the benefit of sorafenib treatment in this group of patients.

REFERENCES

1. Valle J, Wasan H, Palmer DH, et al. Cisplatin plus gemcitabine versus gemcitabine for biliary tract cancer. *N Engl J Med.* 2010;362(14):1273–1281.
2. Khan SA, Thomas HC, Davidson BR, et al. Cholangiocarcinoma. *Lancet.* 2005;366(9493):1303–1314.
3. Anderson CD, Pinson CW, Berlin J, et al. Diagnosis and treatment of cholangiocarcinoma. *Oncologist.* 2004;9(1):43–57.
4. Wistuba II, Gazdar AF. Gallbladder cancer: lessons from a rare tumour. *Nat Rev Cancer.* 2004;4(9):695–706.
5. Aljiffry M, Walsh MJ, Molinari M. Advances in diagnosis, treatment and palliation of cholangiocarcinoma: 1990–2009. *World J Gastroenterol.* 2009;15(34):4240–4262.
6. Macdonald OK, Crane CH. Palliative and postoperative radiotherapy in biliary tract cancer. *Surg Oncol Clin N Am.* 2002; 11(4):941–954.
7. Glimelius B, Hoffman K, Sjoden PO, et al. Chemotherapy improves survival and quality of life in advanced pancreatic and biliary cancer. *Ann Oncol.* 1996;7:593–600.
8. Hezel AF, Zhu AX. Systemic therapy for biliary tract cancers. *Oncologist.* 2008; 13(4):415–423.
9. Knox JJ, Hedley D, Oza A, et al. Combining gemcitabine and capecitabine in patients with advanced biliary cancer: a phase II trial. *J Clin Oncol.* 2005;23(10):2332–2338
10. Eckel F, Schmid RM. Chemotherapy in advanced biliary tract carcinoma: a pooled analysis of clinical trials. *Br J Cancer.* 2007;96(6):896–902
11. Rao S, Cunningham D, Hawkins RE, et al. Phase III study of 5FU, etoposide and leucovorin (FELV) compared to epirubicin, cisplatin and 5FU (ECF) in previously untreated patients with advanced biliary cancer. *Br J Cancer.* 2005;92:1650–1654
12. Verslype C, Van Cutsem E, Dicato M, et al. The management of hepatocellular carcinoma. Current expert opinion and recommendations derived from the 10th World Congress on Gastrointestinal Cancer, Barcelona, 2008. *Ann Oncol.* 2009;20 Suppl 7:vii1–vii6.
13. El-Serag HB, Marrero JA, Rudolph L, et al. Diagnosis and treatment of hepatocellular carcinoma. *Gastroenterology.* 2008; 134(6):1752–1763.
14. Bartlett DL, Di Bisceglie AM, Dawson LA. Cancer of the Liver. In: DeVita, Hellman, and Rosenberg's Cancer: Principles & Practice of Oncology, Eighth Edition. Lippincott, 2008:1129–1155.
15. Llovet JM, Bruix J. Systematic review of randomized trials for unresectable hepatocellular carcinoma: chemoembolization improves survival. *Hepatology.* 2003;37(2):429–442.
16. Llovet JM, Real MI, Montaña X, et al. Arterial embolisation or chemoembolisation versus symptomatic treatment in patients with unresectable hepatocellular carcinoma: a randomized control trial. *Lancet* 2002;359(9319):1734–1739
17. Geschwind JF, Ramsey DE, Choti MA, et al. Chemoembolization of hepatocellular carcinoma: results of a metaanalysis. *Am J Clin Oncol.* 2003;26(4):344–349.
18. Bruix J, Sherman M. Management of hepatocellular carcinoma: An update. *Hepatology*, July 2010. Previous version published 2005. AASLD practice guideline.
19. Mazzaferro V, Regalia E, Doci R, et al. Liver transplantation for the treatment of small hepatocellular carcinomas in patients with cirrhosis. *New Eng J Med.* 1996 14;334(11):728–729.
20. Llovet JM, Ricci S, Mazzaferro V, et al. Sorafenib in advanced hepatocellular carcinoma. *New Eng J Med.* 2008;359(4):378–390
21. Cheng AL, Kang YK, Chen Z, et al. Efficacy and safety of sorafenib in patients in the Asia-Pacific region with advanced hepatocellular carcinoma: a phase III randomised, double-blind, placebo-controlled trial. *Lancet Oncol.* 2009;10(1):25–34. Epub 2008 Dec. 16.

11

Colorectal Cancer

YVONNE SADA AND BENJAMIN MUSHER

EPIDEMIOLOGY, RISK FACTORS, NATURAL HISTORY, AND PATHOLOGY

Colorectal cancer (CRC) remains the second leading cause of cancer-related mortality in the United States, accounting for 140,000 new cases and 50,000 deaths each year. Although the overall incidence of CRC has been declining, presumably due to excision of premalignant adenomatous polyps during routine screening, emerging data suggest a rising incidence among patients younger than 50 years. Advances in treatment continue to improve 5-year survival rates for both early- and late-stage CRC; however, outcomes among minority populations, in particular African Americans, remain significantly worse because of less access to medical care and perhaps more aggressive tumor biology.

The pathogenesis of CRC involves a well-described evolution from normal colonic epithelium, to adenoma, and ultimately to frank carcinoma. Since this transformation generally requires 10 years, experts recommend colonoscopy every 5 to 10 years in people at "average risk" for CRC. Two distinct processes have been implicated in this adenoma-carcinoma sequence: chromosomal instability and microsatellite instability. Chromosomal instability, which accounts for the majority (80–85%) of cases, occurs when inactivating mutations in genes that regulate DNA replication alter chromosome copy number or function, leading to loss of function of tumor suppressor genes. Loss of function of the *APC* tumor suppressor initiates the process, and the accumulation of additional mutations leads to carcinogenesis. While tumorigenesis typically requires two somatic "hits" (one to each allele of the *APC* gene), carriers of *APC* germline mutations require only one somatic mutation to initiate the adenoma-carcinoma sequence. Thus, in contrast to the 5- to 10-year adenoma-carcinoma sequence observed in average-risk patients, carriers of *APC* germline mutations develop thousands of adenomatous polyps at a young age (familial adenomatous polyposis, or FAP) and are at high risk for CRC by late adolescence.

Microsatellite instability (MSI), which accounts for the remaining 15% to 20% of colorectal cancers, occurs when mutation of one or more of the DNA mismatch repair (MMR) enzymes MLH1, MSH2, MSH6, and PMS2 causes slippage within short repetitive DNA sequences (microsatellites). Epigenetic hypermethylation of the MLH1 promoter, which silences MLH1 expression in tumor tissue only, accounts for 80% of microsatellite unstable CRC. The remaining 20% of MSI-related tumors (accounting for 3–4% of all CRC cases), occur in the context of an underlying germline MMR mutation. Starting at relatively young age, carriers of a germline MMR enzyme mutation are at high risk for colorectal, as well as gastric, small bowel, hepatobiliary, genitourinary, gynecologic, and brain tumors—a syndrome known as hereditary non-polyposis colon cancer, or Lynch syndrome. Although carriers of germline APC or MMR mutations carry the highest known lifetime risk of CRC, other high-risk populations include those with inflammatory bowel disease, family history of CRC without an identifiable germline mutation, or a personal history of adenomatous polyps or colon cancer. More frequent screening should be offered to any individual deemed at higher than average risk for developing CRC.

Currently, only a small minority of colorectal cancers can be attributed to known genetic syndromes. Epidemiologists and scientists have therefore hypothesized that various environmental exposures may alter an individual's risk for developing CRC. Thus far, smoking, diabetes, obesity, and high fat diet have been implicated as risk factors, whereas high-fiber diet, hormone replacement therapy, active lifestyle, and anti-inflammatory use have been identified as protective factors. The precise impact of these factors on CRC risk and how they should influence CRC screening have, however, not yet been identified.

Colon cancer and rectal cancer share histopathological, molecular, and genetic features, but, due to anatomical considerations, their clinical behavior differs. Although large or perforated colonic tumors may spread locally to involve adjacent organs or peritoneum, colon cancer more commonly metastasizes remotely by lymphovascular invasion. Because colonic vasculature drains into the portal venous system, the liver is the most common site of metastases, followed by the lungs, remote lymph nodes, bones, and rarely the central nervous system. Compared to colon cancer, rectal cancer has a greater propensity for local spread and recurrence, due to the absence of a rectal serosa and the rectum's proximity to other pelvic structures. As a result, measures to improve local control, namely total mesorectal excision and chemoradiotherapy, have been incorporated into standard therapy for rectal cancer. Rectal cancer also metastasizes remotely, but due to the rectum's dual portal and systemic venous drainage, it commonly bypasses the liver directly and spreads directly to the lungs.

Colorectal cancer may be diagnosed during routine screening or may present with tumor-related symptoms. Symptoms of early disease include anemia-induced fatigue, gross blood per rectum, crampy abdominal pain, change in stool caliber, or tenesmus. Advanced CRC can present with focal symptoms related to the primary tumor and/or metastases but may also present with generalized weakness, fatigue, and weight loss.

STAGING

Colorectal Cancer Staging

Stage	Description
I	Primary tumor invades no deeper than muscularis propria (T1 or T2), no lymph nodes (N0) or metastases
IIA	Primary tumor invades pericolorectal tissue (T3), no lymph nodes (N0) or metastases
IIB	Primary tumor invades visceral peritoneum surface (T4a), no lymph nodes (N0) or metastases
IIC	Primary tumor invades other organs (T4b), no lymph nodes (N0) or metastases
IIIA	Primary tumor invades no deeper than muscularis propria (T1 or T2), ≤ 2 to 3 regional lymph node involvement (N1a, N1b), no metastases
	Primary tumor invades only submucosa (T1), 4 to 6 regional lymph nodes involved (N2a), no metastases
IIIB	Primary tumor invades muscularis propria or pericolorectal tissue (T2, T3), 4 to 6 regional lymph nodes involved (N2a), no metastases
	Primary tumor invades into pericolorectal tissue or visceral peritoneum surface (T3 or T4a), ≤2 to 3 regional lymph node involvement (N1a, N1b), no metastases
	Primary tumor invades no deeper than muscularis propria (T1 or T2), ≥ 7 lymph nodes involved (N2b), no metastases
IIIC	Primary tumor invades visceral peritoneum (T4a), 4 to 6 regional lymph nodes involved (N2a), no metastases
	Primary tumor invades pericolorectal tissue or visceral peritoneum (T3, T4a), ≥7 lymph nodes involved (N2b), no metastases
	Primary tumor invades adjacent organs (T4b), with any lymph node involvement (N1a, N1b, N2a, N2b), no metastases
IVA	Primary tumor invasion any depth (T1–T4), any lymph node involvement (N0–N2b), metastasis confined to one organ (M1a)
IVB	Primary tumor invasion any depth (T1–T4), any lymph node involvement (N0–N2b), metastasis in ≥1 organ or peritoneum (M1b)

Source: AJCC Cancer Staging Handbook, 7th Edition

CASE SUMMARIES

Unresectable Metastatic CRC

L.L. is a 57-year-old woman who presented with a 2-month history of abdominal pain, thin caliber stools, and weight loss. Laboratory evaluation was significant for a hemoglobin of 6.5 g/dL and ferritin of 3 µg/L, consistent with iron deficiency anemia. A CT scan revealed circumferential thickening of the sigmoid colon and numerous bilateral liver masses, the largest of which measured 10.7 × 7.7 cm. Colonoscopy confirmed the presence of a nonobstructing, circumferential sigmoid mass, and pathology revealed poorly differentiated adenocarcinoma. No *KRAS* mutation was identified. Her serum carcinoembryonic antigen (CEA) was 155 ng/mL. Aside from having well-controlled diabetes and hypertension, L.L. was healthy and extremely functional. She had no family history of cancer.

The patient initially received two cycles of FOLFOX (5-fluorouracil [5FU], leucovorin [LV], oxaliplatin) with bevacizumab, but developed uncontrolled hypertension despite an aggressive antihypertensive regimen. Bevacizumab was therefore discontinued. After six additional cycles of FOLFOX, she developed grade II neuropathy. Restaging CT scans showed a 30% decrease in the size of the liver masses, and the CEA measured 2 ng/mL. Due to her neuropathy, oxaliplatin was discontinued. After 12 additional cycles of 5FU/LV alone (10 months total of systemic chemotherapy), the CEA rose to 11 ng/mL, and CT scans showed new bilateral pulmonary nodules. Since she still complained of neuropathic symptoms, precluding reintroduction of oxaliplatin, her chemotherapy was changed to FOLFIRI (5FU, leucovorin, and irinotecan). After four cycles of FOLFIRI, the CEA was 20 ng/mL, and CT scans confirmed progression of pulmonary disease. Her performance status remained excellent, so further treatment options were considered.

Evidence-Based Case Discussion

L.L. has stage IV colon cancer in the context of unresectable liver metastases. Due to her excellent Eastern Cooperative Group (ECOG) performance status and her *KRAS* wild-type (WT) tumor, she is an appropriate candidate for any of the available systemic therapies for metastatic colorectal cancer (mCRC), including monoclonal antibodies targeting the epidermal growth factor receptor (EGFR). This case illustrates the armamentarium that has become available to clinicians treating mCRC, the sequential approach to using these agents, the factors that guide clinical decision making, and the management of treatment-related toxicity.

Determining the Goals of Therapy

Treatment of mCRC should be guided by the primary goal of care: palliation or long-term survival. Until relatively recently, mCRC was considered uniformly fatal and therefore treated exclusively with palliative intent. With the emergence of aggressive multidisciplinary management, consisting of novel surgical and ablative techniques and modern chemoimmunotherapy, a growing number of patients with mCRC are being treated with curative intent (see the section on "Management of Potentially Resectable or Resectable Metastases"). Nevertheless, most patients with mCRC present with widespread disease and are therefore not candidates for curative therapy. While the primary goal of therapy in these cases is palliation—controlling tumor growth, alleviating tumor-related symptoms, prolonging life, and maintaining quality of life—the possibility of long-term survival should be entertained during the course of treatment in case a dramatic clinical response occurs and/or new local therapies emerge. Owing to the number and distribution of her metastases, L.L. has unresectable disease, and her oncologist should explain unambiguously during the initial visit that the primary goal of therapy is palliation.

Addressing the Primary Tumor in mCRC

Before initiating systemic therapy, the oncologist must decide whether the primary colorectal tumor requires surgical intervention. Prior to the advent of effective chemotherapy for mCRC, the risk of developing bowel obstruction or clinically significant gastrointestinal bleeding during the course of systemic treatment was unacceptably high. Primary tumor resection to prevent local complications therefore became common practice. As more effective chemotherapy for mCRC emerged, it made less sense to expose patients to the risks of major abdominal surgery, which, even without major complications, could postpone the initiation of systemic therapy by several weeks.

To illustrate the safety of forgoing primary tumor resection in the context of mCRC, investigators at Memorial Sloan Kettering retrospectively reviewed 233 patients with mCRC who received combination chemotherapy without initial primary tumor resection. Over the course of treatment, 89% did not experience any primary tumor complication requiring intervention. Four percent required nonoperative palliation with stent placement or radiation, and only 7% required emergent surgery for obstruction or perforation (1). These data indicate that, with modern chemotherapy and palliative interventions, the vast majority of mCRC patients with relatively asymptomatic primary tumors may safely forego primary tumor resection at diagnosis. Patients who present with bowel obstruction should preferably undergo diversion rather than resection so that chemotherapy can be started safely within 1 to 2 weeks. On the other hand, patients with heavy bleeding or bowel perforation may still require surgical resection.

L.L. had thin caliber stools but was not frankly obstructed, so urgent surgical intervention was not required. Even if surgical intervention were required (in the case of complete obstruction), diversion would be preferred over resection in order to expedite initiation of systemic therapy. In addition to starting chemotherapy as soon as possible, the treating oncologist should prescribe an appropriate bowel regimen and remind the patient to call if she develops obstipation, worsening abdominal pain, or uncontrolled vomiting.

Systemic Chemotherapy for mCRC

5-Fluorouracil and Leucovorin

The median survival of mCRC with best supportive care (BSC) alone is approximately 6 months, but advances in chemotherapy, starting with the approval of 5FU in 1957, have significantly improved outcomes. As a single agent, 5FU yields an objective response rate of 15% and a median survival of 10 to 14 months. Adding leucovorin (LV), a reduced form of folic acid that stabilizes the binding of 5FU to thymidylate synthase, improves the response rate to 25%, but does not significantly change median survival.

Numerous studies have addressed the optimal administration of 5FU—bolus, infusional, or oral. The original regimen, devised at the Mayo Clinic, consists of bolus 5FU (b5FU) daily for 5 days, repeated every 4 weeks. The Roswell Park regimen, which consists of weekly b5FU for 6 weeks followed by a 2-week break, causes less myelosuppression and mucositis than its predecessor. The newest regimen, devised by de Gramont et al. (LV5FU2), combines b5FU, LV, and infusional 5FU (i5FU). Having undergone several permutations to date, LV5FU2 is most commonly administered as biweekly b5FU 400 mg/m^2, LV 400 mg/m^2, and i5FU 2400 mg/m^2 over 46 hours. Compared to the Mayo Clinic regimen, LV5FU2 yields a higher response rate (32% vs. 14%), significantly longer progression-free survival (PFS) (28 vs. 22 weeks), and less myelosuppresion, mucositis, and diarrhea (2). On the basis of its favorable efficacy and toxicity profile, the LV5FU2 has become the standard for intravenous administration of 5FU. Capecitabine, an oral pro-drug of 5FU, has also proven to be as effective and more tolerable than b5FU and therefore serves as a reasonable alternative to LV5FU2 for patients who prefer an oral regimen (3,4). Aside from myelosuppression and mucositis, capecitabine can cause hand foot syndrome (HFS), which is generally manageable with supportive care and dose adjustment.

Irinotecan

5-Fluorouracil remained the only available chemotherapeutic agent for CRC until the late 1990s, when the FDA approved irinotecan for second-line therapy, based on randomized data showing that irinotecan improved survival and quality of life over BSC in patients with 5FU-refractory mCRC. Irinotecan was subsequently approved for chemotherapy-naïve mCRC after the combination of irinotecan and 5FU demonstrated superior response rate (49% vs. 31%, $P < .001$), PFS (6.7 vs. 4.4 months, $P < .001$), and overall survival (OS) (17.4 vs. 14.1 months, $P = .031$) over 5FU alone (5). Since both irinotecan and 5FU can cause nausea and diarrhea, gastrointestinal toxicity can be compounded when the agents are used simultaneously.

In order to maximize benefit while minimizing toxicity, clinical trials have tested various regimens that combine 5FU and irinotecan. For example, the BICC-C trial compared LV5FU2 plus biweekly irinotecan (FOLFIRI), b5FU plus irinotecan (modified IFL), and capecitabine plus (CapeIRI). FOLFIRI yielded the best PFS and OS (7.6 months and 23.1 months, respectively), and CapeIRI clearly caused the most gastrointestinal toxicity, with 25% of patients in this arm stopping treatment due to intolerable side effects (6). On the basis of the results from BICC-C and other published data, FOLFIRI (biweekly irinotecan 180 mg/m^2 plus LV5FU2) remains the standard regimen for combining irinotecan and 5FU. Although subsequent trials have shown that CapeIRI may be more tolerable than the BICC-C data indicate, this regimen is not included in commonly referenced guidelines, such as the National Comprehensive Cancer Network (NCCN), and should therefore be avoided altogether or used with extreme caution.

Oxaliplatin

A third-generation antineoplastic platinum derivative, oxaliplatin forms platinum-DNA adducts that appear to be more cytotoxic than those formed by cisplatin and carboplatin. Oxaliplatin has demonstrated cytotoxic synergy with 5FU in cancer cell lines and carries a different side-effect profile than its predecessors, causing considerably less nausea, ototoxicity, and nephrotoxicity than cisplatin, less myelosuppression than carboplatin, and more neurotoxicity than either. As opposed to irinotecan, which has proven antineoplastic activity when used alone or in combination with 5FU, oxaliplatin has only demonstrated benefit when combined with 5FU. In 2002, the FDA approved oxaliplatin plus 5FU/LV for mCRC refractory to 5FU/LV and irinotecan. Two years later, oxaliplatin was approved in the first-line setting based on randomized data showing that FOLFOX (oxaliplatin 85 mg/m^2 plus LV5FU2) yielded a significantly better response rate (50% vs. 21.9%) and PFS (9 vs. 6 months) than LV5FU2 in patients with untreated mCRC. Although FOLFOX was well tolerated, it caused more neutropenia, mucositis, diarrhea, and neuropathy than 5FU/LV alone (7).

The question of whether intravenous 5FU and capecitabine can be used interchangeably with oxaliplatin was addressed by NO16966—a noninferiority trial comparing XELOX (capecitabine 1000 mg/m^2 twice daily on days 1 to 14 and oxaliplatin 130 mg/m^2 on day 1 of a 21-day cycle) to FOLFOX in patients with untreated mCRC (3). Initially, NO16966 included only two arms. However, the trial was amended to a 2 × 2 factorial design (XELOX vs. FOLFOX and bevacizumab vs. placebo) after a phase III data showing a survival benefit of adding bevacizumab to chemotherapy were reported. NO16966 met its goal of noninferiority, with XELOX and FOLFOX yielding similar PFS (8 months) and OS (20 months).

Given that XELOX and FOLFOX appear to be equally effective, clinicians must help patients choose between these regimens based on other factors. XELOX offers patients the convenience of taking pills rather than wearing an infusion pump, and receiving intravenous oxaliplatin every 3 weeks rather than every 2 weeks. On the other hand, it requires strict adherence to an oral medication schedule, raises the possibility of unpredictable drug levels due to variable gut absorption, and causes more HFS and diarrhea than i5FU. FOLFOX does not require adherence to an oral regimen and is not affected by gut absorption, but it requires more frequent visits to an infusion suite and a 46-hour outpatient infusion. Because a Port-a-cath is required for i5FU, patients are exposed to additional risk, primarily infection and thrombosis. FOLFOX causes less gastrointestinal toxicity and HFS than XELOX, but more neutropenia.

Distinguishing between the two neuropathic syndromes associated with oxaliplatin is crucial to proper oncological care. The first syndrome is an acute neurosensory complex that appears during or immediately after infusion and is characterized by cold-induced digital sensitivity and pharyngeal dysaesthesisas. Although bothersome to patients, these symptoms are innocuous, transient, and reversible, generally disappearing by 1 week after oxaliplatin administration. Oncologists should warn their patients about the high likelihood of cold sensitivity and advise them to wear gloves in cold weather, avoid holding cold objects or reaching into the freezer, and drink room temperature beverages until cold-induced symptoms subside. The second syndrome—an insidious, cumulative, and potentially debilitating "stocking and glove" peripheral sensory neuropathy (PSN)—develops with prolonged exposure to oxaliplatin. Clinicians must be particularly sensitive to the onset of true PSN so that oxaliplatin can be appropriately dose reduced or discontinued. Although oxaliplatin should be used cautiously in patients with pre-existing neuropathy, diabetic patients without baseline neuropathy do not carry a higher risk for oxaliplatin-induced neurotoxicity than nondiabetics and should therefore not be denied oxaliplatin based on diabetes alone.

Because worsening PSN can significantly affect quality of life and frequently necessitates oxaliplatin discontinuation before loss of treatment effect, various strategies to decrease oxaliplatin-induced neurotoxicity have been evaluated. OPTIMOX1 tested the hypothesis that using oxaliplatin on a "stop-and-go" basis would optimize duration of benefit by limiting cumulative toxicity. Patients were randomized to FOLFOX until progression or intolerance (control arm) or FOLFOX for six cycles, followed by twelve cycles of "maintenance" 5FU, and reintroduction of FOLFOX for six more cycles ("stop-and-go" approach). All outcome measures (response rate, PFS, and OS) were similar between the two arms. However, since only 40% of patients in the experimental arm were reintroduced to FOLFOX and since 70% of these patients had a response or stable disease, the "stop-and-go" approach may have demonstrated improved survival with stricter protocol adherence. In fact, closer examination of the data confirmed that reintroducing oxaliplatin had a statistically significant impact on OS (HR = 0.56, P = .009). Although there was no overall difference in neurotoxicity between the two groups in the intention-to-treat analysis, there was less grade 3 neurotoxicity in the experimental arm when patients were receiving 5FU alone (8). Taking the "stop-and-go" strategy one step farther, OPTIMOX2 discontinued chemotherapy altogether after an initial induction phase of FOLFOX. The control arm in this study was similar to the experimental arm from OPTIMOX 1 (FOLFOX for six cycles followed by maintenance 5FU until disease progression), but the experimental arm included a complete chemotherapy "holiday" (FOLFOX for six cycles followed by observation until disease progression). Duration of disease control was superior in the control arm (13 vs. 9 months), but median OS was not significantly different (9).

Because oxaliplatin's metabolite oxalate may induce nerve damage by affecting permeability of Ca^{2+}-dependent neuronal voltage-gated Na^{+} channels, two randomized trials have examined whether administering oxalate chelators, namely calcium and magnesium, can reduce the incidence and intensity of oxaliplatin-related neurotoxicity. CONcePT simultaneously investigated two potential solutions to this problem by randomizing patients with untreated mCRC to (a) continuous oxaliplatin (CO) versus intermittent oxaliplatin (IO) and (b) Ca/Mg versus placebo infusions given immediately before and after oxaliplatin. The investigators hypothesized that time to treatment failure (TTF), an endpoint that incorporates efficacy and tolerability, would be longer with IO and Mg/Ca infusions. The second trial, N04C7, randomized patients with resected stage II or III colon cancer receiving adjuvant FOLFOX to Mg/Ca or placebo infusions. When an unplanned interim analysis of CONcePT showed a lower response rate in the group receiving Ca/Mg, both trials were terminated. Although subsequent independent review of CONcePT showed no detrimental effect of Mg/Ca on response rate, neither trial reopened, leaving our interpretation of the data compromised by low accrual numbers.

The results of these trials, although limited by inadequate power, support their primary hypotheses. In CONcePT, IO improved TTF and PFS (5.6 months and 12 months, respectively) over CO (4.2 months and 7.3 months, respectively) while reducing neurotoxicity, as well as oxaliplatin discontinuations, dose reductions, and dose delays. Ca/Mg infusions decreased the incidence of chronic neurotoxicity but had no effect on acute neurotoxicity. N04C7, which only addressed Ca/Mg infusions, used three measures to assess neurotoxicity—the NCIC-CTC scale, the oxaliplatin-specific scale, and patient questionnaires for quality-of-life assessment. The trial accrued 102 of its planned 300 patients, and intention-to-treat analysis showed that Mg/Ca infusion significantly reduced neurotoxicity by all three measures. Whereas the first two measures assessed only chronic neurotoxicity, patient questionnaires showed less acute and chronic toxicity with Mg/Ca compared with placebo.

How can we synthesize the data from the various trials addressing oxaliplatin-induced neurotoxicity? First, based on OPTIMOX1 and CONcePT, a "stop-and-go" approach, that is, stopping oxaliplatin after six cycles and continuing 5FU/LV alone until progression, may reduce the cumulative toxicity of oxaliplatin while maintaining, or even augmenting, its efficacy. Many experts therefore advocate stopping oxaliplatin after an initial induction phase and maintaining patients on 5FU/LV (with a targeted agent if included previously) until documented progression, at which time oxaliplatin can be reintroduced. On the other hand, based on the OPTIMOX2 data, discontinuing chemotherapy altogether after an initial induction phase may be detrimental and therefore cannot be *routinely* recommended. A population of patients with indolent and/or exquisitely chemosensitive disease that may benefit from "chemotherapy holidays" likely exists; however, this cohort has not been clearly defined. Finally, although underpowered due to premature closure, CONcePT and N04C7 suggest a neuroprotective role for Mg/Ca infusions. While this strategy has not been incorporated into routine clinical practice, likely due to incomplete data, Mg/Ca infusions may be appropriate for patients receiving adjuvant chemotherapy or those with mCRC who require continuous oxaliplatin for disease control.

FOLFOX or FOLFIRI as First-Line Treatment in mCRC: Does Order Matter?

FOLFIRI and FOLFOX induce similar response rates and PFS in untreated mCRC, and each regimen is active in mCRC refractory to the other. To assess whether the precise order affects OS, Tournigand et al. randomized 220 patients to FOLFOX followed by FOLFIRI upon progression or vice versa (10). Both arms yielded similar median OS (21 months), time to first progression (8 months), and response rate (55%). Because these approaches appear to be equally effective, oncologists and patients must choose an initial regimen based on convenience and potential toxicity. Patients who suffer from pre-existing neuropathy, who rely on fine motor skills professionally or vocationally, or who cannot avoid cold exposure may prefer FOLFIRI. On the other hand, patients who are particularly concerned about gastrointestinal toxicity or who prefer capecitabine over an infusion pump may opt for an oxaliplatin-containing regimen.

5FU, Leucovorin, Oxaliplatin, and Irinotecan (FOLFOXIRI)

One approach to maximize benefit from available cytotoxic agents is to use them sequentially; another is to combine them into one regimen. An Italian study randomized 244 patients to FOLFOXIRI (biweekly irinotecan 165 mg/m^2, oxaliplatin 85 mg/m^2, LV 200 mg/m^2, i5FU 3200 mg/m^2 over 48 hours) or standard FOLFIRI. FOLFOXIRI yielded a significantly higher response rate (66% vs. 41%, P = .0002), longer PFS (9.8 vs. 6.9 months, P = .0006), and longer median OS (22 vs. 16.7 months, P = .032) than FOLFIRI, and more patients receiving FOLFOXIRI underwent R0 resection of metastases. Not surprisingly, FOLFOXIRI caused more neurotoxicity and neutropenia (11). Thus, while FOLFOXIRI remains a first-line option for mCRC, especially in patients who have borderline resectable metastatic disease, it is more toxic and does not clearly provide a survival advantage over sequential FOLFOX and FOLFIRI.

Vascular Endothelial Growth Factor Inhibitors

Having demonstrated that combination chemotherapy improves survival over 5FU alone, investigators hypothesized that adding rationally designed antineoplastic agents to standard cytotoxic regimens would further improve outcomes without appreciably worsening toxicity. On the basis of laboratory evidence that tumors require a vascular supply to proliferate and clinical evidence that higher serum vascular endothelial growth factor (VEGF) correlates with worse prognosis in mCRC, bevacizumab (a humanized monoclonal antibody that binds VEGF) was the first biological agent tested in mCRC. In 2004, Hurwitz et al. published the results of a pivotal trial that randomized 813 patients to IFL (irinotecan, b5FU, and leucovorin) plus bevacizumab 5 mg/kg or IFL plus placebo. The experimental arm demonstrated superior median OS (20.3 vs. 15.6 months, $P < .001$) and PFS (10.6 vs. 6.2 months, $P < .001$) but more grade 3 hypertension (11% vs. 2.3%). Of note, only 25% of patients received oxaliplatin after progression, raising the possibility that OS in both arms would have improved considerably with appropriate second-line therapy (12).

With bevacizumab's role in untreated mCRC having been established, ECOG 3200 randomized patients with FOLFIRI-refractory disease to FOLFOX/bevacizumab or FOLFOX. The combination arm yielded superior response rate, PFS, and OS (12.9 vs. 10.8 months), thereby establishing a role for bevacizumab in previously treated, bevacizumab-naïve mCRC (13). In contrast, NO16966 added bevacizumab to oxaliplatin-containing chemotherapy in the first-line setting. As discussed previously, this trial was initially designed to compare XELOX and FOLFOX but, after the Hurwitz data was published, was amended to include a second randomization of bevacizumab versus placebo. Comparison of all patients who received bevacizumab with those who received placebo revealed superior PFS in the bevacizumab arm (9.4 vs. 8.0 months), and subgroup analysis demonstrated that improved PFS was maintained whether patients had received XELOX or FOLFOX. Although bevacizumab did not, with statistical significance, improve OS over placebo (21.3 vs. 19.9 months, P = .077), only 29% of patients in the bevacizumab arm were treated with bevacizumab and chemotherapy until disease progression (14), introducing the possibility of an underestimation of survival with this strategy. The Hurwitz trial, E3200, and NO16966 support the use of bevacizumab with first-line chemotherapy or with second-line chemotherapy in bevacizumab-naïve patients, but none addresses whether bevacizumab benefits patients who have already received it with another regimen. While there are no published randomized trials to answer this question, the best available data are those compiled from the BRiTE registry, a community-based, prospective observational study that evaluated the safety and efficacy of bevacizumab with chemotherapy in almost 2000 patients with untreated mCRC (15). Because BRiTE was only observational, decisions regarding the initial regimen, dose reductions/delays, and subsequent therapy beyond progression were left to the discretion of the treating physician.

The inherent bias of such a study notwithstanding, the results from the BRiTE registry are intriguing. The median OS of the nearly 50% of patients who received bevacizumab beyond progression (BBP) was 31.8 months, compared with 19.9 months for those who received chemotherapy without BBP and 12.6 months for those who received no further systemic therapy whatsoever. BBP was associated with improved survival in multivariate analysis (HR 0.48, $P < .001$) and maintained benefit across all examined subgroups. Aside from a slightly higher percentage of patients with ECOG PS ≥ 1 in the no-BBP group, baseline characteristics were remarkably similar, arguing against selection bias as a major contributor to the benefit of BBP. Hypertension requiring medical therapy was the only additional toxicity reported more frequently with BBP, confirming the safety of bevacizumab when used in appropriate patients. Because BRiTE was not a randomized trial, the benefit of continuing BBP has not been definitively established. However, BBP appears to be safe and has sound rationale, that is, augmenting chemotherapy's antitumor activity. Until ongoing randomizing trials addressing this very question are reported, the decision whether to continue BBP should be considered on a case-by-case basis, with the understanding that the data supporting this practice are limited.

Side effects of bevacizumab stem from its mechanism of action and therefore differ from those of traditional cytotoxic chemotherapy. Hypertension, proteinuria, arteriovenous thrombosis, and bleeding are attributed to bevacizumab's impact on normal vasculature whereas gastrointestinal perforation and wound dehiscence likely relate to its effect on tissue regeneration. Because major complications tend to occur in patients with identifiable risk factors, a thorough history and physical examination to select appropriate candidates for therapy is imperative. Blood pressure should be within normal range before starting bevacizumab, with the understanding that antihypertensive therapy may require intensification during treatment. Bevacizumab may exacerbate pre-existing proteinuria, but patients with healthy kidneys at baseline are not likely to develop clinically significant high-grade proteinuria from bevacizumab. Following urinalysis closely during therapy, although frequently done, is therefore of relatively low value in patients without baseline proteinuria.

Although bevacizumab has been used safely in patients with occult or bleeding, it should be used cautiously in patients with any degree of gross active bleeding and is contraindicated in patients with heavy bleeding or untreated brain metastases. Patients with active deep venous thrombosis may safely receive bevacizumab as long as they are receiving effective, stable anticoagulation. Arterial thrombosis, however, poses a bigger concern, as consequences are potentially much more serious. Bevacizumab should therefore be withheld in patients with recent stroke or myocardial infarction, ongoing symptomatic vascular disease, or uncontrolled risk factors for vascular disease. Age in itself is also a risk factor for complications, so bevacizumab should be used cautiously in elderly patients. Finally, because bevacizumab has been shown to increase the incidence of wound dehiscence and gastrointestinal perforation, patients should not receive bevacizumab within 6 weeks of a major abdominal surgery.

EGFR Inhibitors

Cetuximab and panitumumab, monoclonal antibodies that compete with epidermal growth factor by binding the extracellular domain of the EGFR, inhibit signaling through pathways that contribute to the proliferation and survival of colon cancer cells. Because skin, the gastrointestinal tract, and the nephron highly express EGFR, rash, diarrhea, and hypomagnesemia are common side effects of EGFR inhibitors. As opposed to panitumumab, which is fully humanized, cetuximab is chimeric and can therefore cause infusion reactions.

In 2007, the first two randomized trials using EGFR inhibitors were published. NCIC CO.17 demonstrated a small, but statistically significant, survival benefit of weekly cetuximab (400 mg/m^2 initially followed by 250 mg/m^2 thereafter) over BSC alone in patients with chemotherapy-refractory mCRC (median OS 6.1 vs. 4.6 months, $P = .01$) (16). As had been the case with nearly every study testing EGFR inhibitors, regardless of the underlying malignancy, the appearance of a rash strongly correlated with treatment response. In the second trial, which included a similar design and patient population, panitumumab (6 mg/kg every 2 weeks) demonstrated superior PFS but similar OS compared to BSC (17). Whereas both trials met their endpoints of *statistical* significance, implying that EGFR inhibitors do, in fact, exert some degree of antineoplastic activity, the widespread use of these costly agents for a modest *clinical* benefit remained difficult to justify. Investigators therefore began searching for biomarkers that could help select those patients most likely to benefit from anti-EGFR therapy.

The *KRAS* story beautifully illustrates how advances in molecular biology can translate into meaningful improvements in clinical care. The *KRAS* oncogene encodes an intracellular GTPase located downstream from EGFR that, when mutated, becomes constitutively active and leads to unregulated cell signaling and proliferation. *KRAS* is mutated in approximately 40% of CRCs, in the form of single amino acid substitutions at codons 12 or 13, and concordance between metastatic and primary tumors nears 100%. Since an activating *KRAS* mutation would likely nullify any potential benefit of EGFR blockade, *KRAS* biomarker analysis was undertaken for clinical trials involving EGFR inhibitors, starting with NCIC CO.17. Using banked tumor from nearly 70% of the patients enrolled in CO.17, Karapetis et al. identified *KRAS* mutations in 42% of these specimens and reassessed benefit from EGFR inhibitors based on *KRAS* mutational status (18). Their findings were unequivocal. In the cohort of patients with *KRAS* WT tumors, cetuximab yielded a survival benefit over BSC (OS 9.5 vs. 4.8 months, $P < .001$; PFS 3.7 vs. 1.9 months, $P < .001$) much greater than had been reported for the unselected population. Cetuximab provided no survival benefit over BSC in patients with *KRAS* mutated (MT) tumors, and the response rate was only 1% (vs. 13% in the *KRAS* WT group). While *KRAS* mutational status was highly predictive of treatment effect, it was not prognostic, in that it did not affect survival in the BSC group.

Having demonstrated the activity of EGFR inhibitors as single agents, investigators then combined EGFR inhibitors with standard chemotherapy. The BOND trial randomized patients previously treated with irinotecan-containing regimens to cetuximab plus irinotecan or cetuximab alone. The combination of irinotecan with cetuximab yielded a significantly higher response rate (23% vs. 11%) and time to progression (4.1 vs. 1.5 months) but no difference in OS (19). In addition to showing that adding chemotherapy to cetuximab is more effective than cetuximab alone, BOND proved the important principle that biologic agents can resensitize tumor cells to a cytotoxic agent previously deemed ineffective. In the CRYSTAL trial, the first trial using cetuximab with front-line therapy, patients were randomized to FOLFIRI/cetuximab or FOLFIRI alone. Analysis of the entire population showed that adding cetuximab to chemotherapy improved PFS and rate of R0 metastasectomy, but not OS. However, restricting analysis to the *KRAS* WT subgroup revealed that response rate, PFS, and OS were all significantly higher with FOLFIRI/cetuximab compared to FOLFIRI alone (RR 57% vs. 40%, $P < .0001$; PFS 9.9 vs. 8.4 months, $P = .001$; OS 23.5 vs. 20.0 months, $P = .009$). While patients with *KRAS* MT tumors enrolled in CRYSTAL did not benefit from cetuximab, the OPUS trial, which randomized patients to FOLFOX/cetuximab or FOLFOX, suggested that cetuximab may actually harm these patients (20).

Data from the trials combining panitumumab with chemotherapy closely resemble those reported with cetuximab. In patients refractory to oxaliplatin-based chemotherapy and naïve to EGFR inhibitors, the combination of panitumumab and FOLFIRI was compared to FOLFIRI alone. Adding panitumumab significantly increased response rate (35% vs. 10%, $P < .0001$) and PFS (5.9 vs. 3.9 months, $P = .004$) in *KRAS* WT patients but provided no benefit in *KRAS* MT patients (21). Similar findings were observed when panitumumab was added to front-line chemotherapy in the PRIME study, which randomized patients with untreated mCRC to FOLFOX/panitumumab or FOLFOX4. Preplanned analysis of the *KRAS* WT group showed improved PFS and a strong trend toward improved OS with the addition of panitumumab to chemotherapy (PFS 9.6 vs. 8 months, $P = .02$; OS 23.9 vs. 19.7 months, $P = .07$) (22). Similar to the findings of OPUS, adding an EGFR inhibitor to chemotherapy appeared to worsen PFS and OS of patients with KRAS MT tumors.

Combining Targeted Agents in mCRC

Despite phase II data strongly suggesting the benefit of combining VEGF and EGFR inhibitors, two phase III trials have yielded disconcerting results. In CAIRO2, patients were randomized to receive CapeOx/bevacizumab/cetuximab (CBC) or CapeOx/bevacizumab (CB). In the unrestricted population, CBC was associated with shorter PFS and a trend toward worse OS. When outcomes were compared according to *KRAS* status, it appeared that *KRAS* WT patients did not benefit from combining biologics and, more disturbingly, that *KRAS* MT patients were actively harmed, with outcomes clearly worse in CBC arm compared to CB (PFS 8.1 vs. 12.5 months, $P = .003$; OS 17.2 vs. 24.9 months, $P = .03$) (23). These findings could not easily be attributed to toxicity, as grade 3 to 4 nondermatologic toxicity was nearly identical between the treatment arms. Similarly, the PACCE trial, which randomized patients to chemotherapy plus bevacizumab or chemotherapy/bevacizumab/panitumumab showed worse PFS and OS in the experimental arm, regardless of *KRAS* status.

Several important conclusions regarding EGFR inhibition can be drawn from the *KRAS* story. First *KRAS* is mutated frequently (40% of CRC cases) and serves as an excellent negative predictive biomarker, meaning that it reliably identifies patients who will *not* benefit from EGFR inhibition. *KRAS* mutational analysis performed on paraffin-embedded tissue is therefore recommended for all patients with mCRC. However, since the majority of patients with *KRAS* WT tumors still do not respond to EGFR inhibitors, we must search for additional biomarkers to further personalize care. Second, EGFR inhibitors improve response rates, PFS, and OS in patients with *KRAS* WT tumors, whether used alone or combined with chemotherapy. Cetuximab and panitumumab appear to be equally effective and should therefore be regarded as interchangeable. Rash is clearly associated with benefit and should, if possible, be managed with supportive care and dose reduction rather than drug discontinuation. Third, although the optimal time to start EGFR inhibitors (front-line or later in the treatment course) is not well established, their single-agent activity in chemorefractory disease and their potential to resensitize tumor cells to cytotoxic agents makes them particularly attractive for mCRC that has progressed on prior therapy. Fourth, combining EGFR and VEGF inhibitors, while making biological sense, worsens outcomes, especially in patients receiving oxaliplatin-based chemotherapy. Toxicity does not seem to account for this antagonistic effect, and various hypotheses, including stimulation of escape pathways and alteration of chemotherapy metabolism have been proposed. For the time being, such combinations should be avoided outside of research protocols.

Summary

Compared to 15 years ago, patients with mCRC have numerous treatment options, from single-agent 5FU to combination chemoimmunotherapy. Since no formula exists to dictate which regimen best suits an individual patient, clinicians can only make recommendations after considering goals of care, underlying age and comorbidity, side-effect profiles, matters of convenience, and patient preference. Figure 11.1 shows a treatment algorithm for managing unresectable metastatic colon cancer. FOLFOX, XELOX, and FOLFIRI are all standard front-line combination regimens. If FOLFOX or XELOX is chosen, strong consideration should be given to an OPTIMOX-like strategy. If a patient is not a candidate for intensive therapy, single-agent 5FU (preferably LV5FU2) or capecitabine can be used. In the absence of contraindications to VEGF therapy, bevacizumab may be added, as it has been shown to improve PFS and OS in the first-line setting. Observational data suggest that continuing bevacizumab beyond progression improves survival, but there are no randomized data to support this practice. Patients with *KRAS* WT tumors are eligible for EGFR inhibitors, which may be used alone or with cytotoxic chemotherapy. EGFR inhibitors have demonstrated survival benefit in untreated mCRC and chemotherapy-refractory mCRC, but their optimal place in the treatment algorithm has not been well defined. Combining VEGF and EGFR inhibitors may worsen outcomes and should be avoided. Finally, although the prognosis of mCRC has improved considerably over the last few decades, the vast majority of patients ultimately succumb to their disease. Improving accrual to clinical trials during all stages of therapy should therefore remain a high priority.

Because of her excellent performance status and a *KRAS* WT tumor, L.L. was deemed eligible for further treatment. Based on the BOND data, she received FOLFIRI plus cetuximab rather than cetuximab alone. After her first cycle, she developed a grade 2 acneiform rash that responded nicely to oral minocycline. She is now 10 months into FOLFIRI/cetuximab with CT scans and CEA indicating ongoing response.

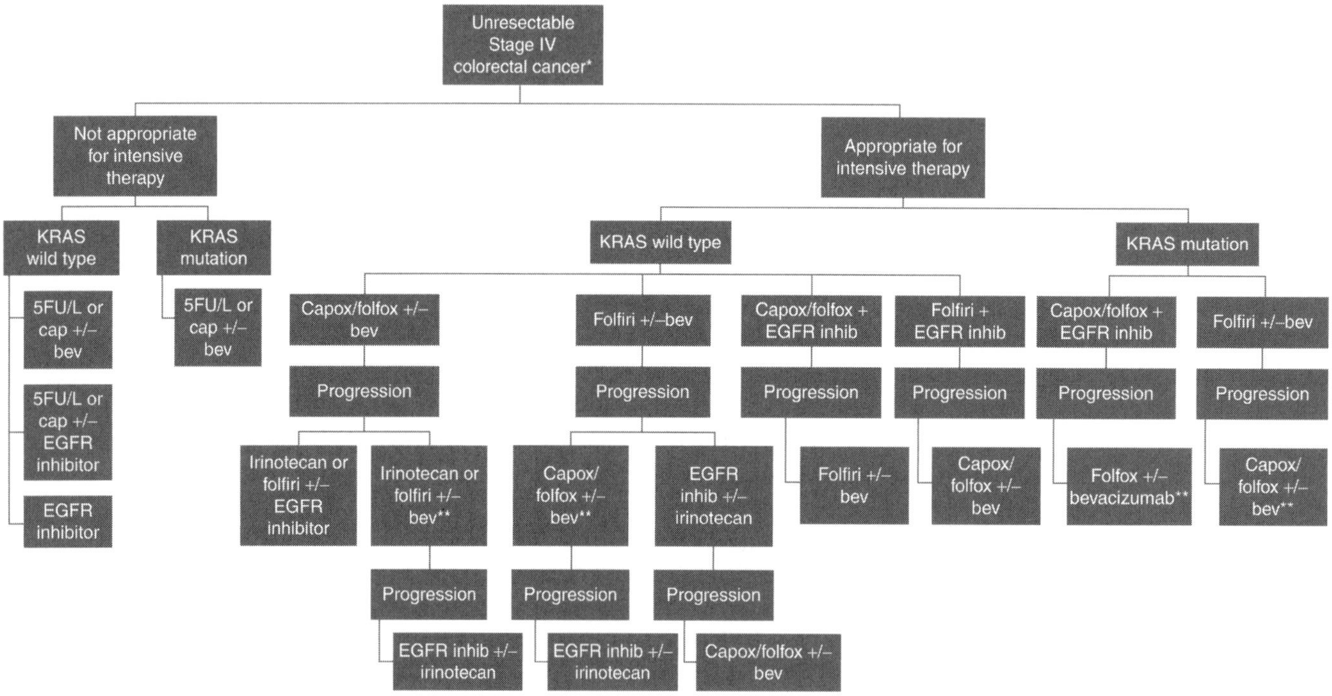

*If response, scans should be assessed for resectability

**Currently no randomized data support continuing bevacizumab after first progression

Figure 11.1

Treatment algorithm for unresectable stage IV colon cancer: 5FU/L, 5FU/leucovorin; Cap, capecitabine; Bev, bevacizumab.

Potentially Resectable or Resectable Metastatic CRC

A.K. is a 51-year-old otherwise healthy male attorney who presented with rectal bleeding and constipation. Colonoscopy with biopsy showed a circumferential adenocarcinoma in the descending colon, and despite near obstruction, the colonoscopy was advanced to the cecum. Staging CT scans showed two masses in the right hepatic lobe measuring 1.3 cm and 1.1 cm and a mass in the left hepatic lobe measuring 1.2 cm. PET/CT showed marked FDG uptake in the colon mass and two right hepatic lobe lesions, but no uptake in the left hepatic lobe or lungs. A left hemicolectomy was performed, and pathological evaluation revealed a T3 N1 adenocarcinoma containing a codon 12 *KRAS* mutation. Intraoperative biopsy of a right liver mass also showed adenocarcinoma. A preoperative CEA was 48 ng/mL and a postoperative CEA was 49 ng/mL. The patient recovered quickly from surgery and was referred to medical oncology to discuss prognosis and further treatment.

Evidence-Based Case Discussion

A.K. has biopsy-proven stage IV colon cancer (T3 N2 M1) with radiographic evidence of two right hepatic metastases and what appears to be a left hepatic lobe cyst. Although his prognosis is worse than that of patients with nonmetastatic colon cancer, the presence of oligometastatic rather than widespread disease raises the possibility of long-term survival with aggressive multidisciplinary management. The treatment approach for A.K. therefore differs significantly from that of the previous patient.

In the 1990s, reports of inducing long-term survival, even cure, with R0 resection of primary colon cancer and its known sites of metastasis began to emerge. Excitement about potentially curative therapy for mCRC was, however, tempered by the following: (a) criteria for resectability were stringent (low burden disease confined to one liver lobe), thereby precluding surgery in the vast majority of patients, and (b) even though 5-year survival rates as high as 50% were reported, 75% of patients relapsed within a few years after surgery, making the actual cure rate very low. As more extensive metastasectomy proved to be safe and as additional interventions, such as radiofrequency ablation and portal vein embolization, were devised to supplement surgical resection, the criteria for resectability liberalized, and the cohort of patients eligible for aggressive therapy expanded. On the other hand, it became clear that intensifying local therapy of known metastases without simultaneously eradicating micrometastatic disease would not further improve treatment outcomes.

Based on the high relapse rate with surgery alone, investigators hypothesized that a multidisciplinary approach of intensive local therapy combined with systemic chemotherapy would improve survival outcomes. Three randomized trials have addressed the issue of supplementing R0 resection of stage IV CRC with chemotherapy. Two European trials randomized patients who had undergone resection of gross disease to observation or six cycles of b5FU/LV. Both trials closed prematurely due to slow accrual, so neither had power to demonstrate differences in disease-free survival (DFS) or overall survival (OS). However, a pooled analysis demonstrated a trend toward improved survival with adjuvant chemotherapy over surgery alone (PFS 27.9 vs. 18.8 months, $P = .058$; OS 62.2 vs. 47.3 months, $P = .095$) (24). The third trial, EORTC 40983, randomized 364 patients with four or fewer resectable liver masses and no extrahepatic disease to metastasectomy alone or metastasectomy with perioperative chemotherapy (3 months of FOLFOX before and after surgery). Because 7% of patients receiving FOLFOX progressed before surgery, more patients in the perioperative chemotherapy arm did not undergo surgery (12% vs. 4%); however, the rate of potentially curative resection was nearly identical (83% vs. 84%). Postoperative morbidity was slightly higher in the chemotherapy arm, but postoperative mortality was 1% in both groups. In the intention to treat population, median PFS was superior in the perioperative chemotherapy arm (18.7 vs. 11.7 months), and among patients who underwent resection, perioperative chemotherapy yielded a 9% improvement in 3-year PFS (25).

Other nonrandomized studies have used perioperative FOLFIRI rather than FOLFOX or have added VEGF or EGFR inhibitors to chemotherapy. Although all regimens approved for mCRC appear to be effective in the setting of resectable oligometastatic disease, the risk for hepatotoxicity and postoperative complications seems to increase significantly with more than 3 months of preoperative oxaliplatin or irinotecan. Based on retrospective data, bevacizumab can be safely added to preoperative chemotherapy, provided that the last dose is not given within 60 days of surgery.

Figure 11.2 outlines the algorithm for treating oligometastatic CRC. First, an experienced surgical oncologist must determine whether the patient is an appropriate candidate for aggressive resection, based on the volume of healthy remnant liver following surgery, the ability to preserve vascular and biliary structures, and the overall health of the patient. Second, the surgical and medical oncologist must decide how to incorporate chemotherapy into the treatment plan. While adding chemotherapy to R0 resection of gross disease is clearly safe and effective, the optimal timing and duration have not been established. Neoadjuvant chemotherapy offers the potential advantages of (a) downsizing borderline resectable metastases to render them frankly resectable, (b) testing the tumor's biology to spare patients with occult, widespread, aggressive disease from surgery that is unlikely to provide long-term benefit, (c) assessing the chemosensitivity of a tumor, which guides postoperative chemotherapy, and (d) serving

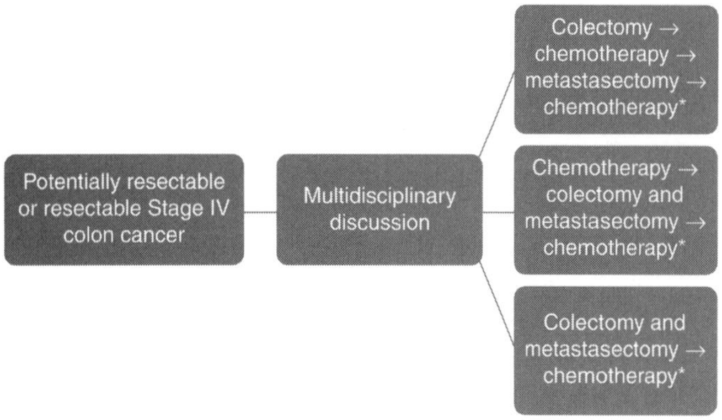

*FOLFOX, FOLFIRI, 5FU/LV, capecitabine, CapOx, or FOLFOXIRI +/– EGFR monoclonal antibody (only in Kras wild type patients) or bevacizumab.
Bevacizumab should not be given within 6 weeks of surgery. Total duration of chemotherapy should be 6 months.

Figure 11.2

Treatment algorithm for potentially resectable or resectable stage IV colon cancer.

as a "stress test" to select out those patients who are not medically fit enough to tolerate surgery. The primary disadvantage of neoadjuvant chemotherapy is the potential for toxicity severe enough to delay or complicate surgical resection.

Aside from cases of metachronous mCRC diagnosed after a lengthy disease-free interval, patients with oligometastatic colon cancer are, with increasing frequency, being treated with the following approach: 3 months of "neoadjuvant" chemotherapy, radiographic assessment, metastasectomy if appropriate, and 3 months of "adjuvant" chemotherapy. The precise sequencing of chemotherapy, primary tumor resection, and metastasectomy depends on various factors, including the urgency of surgical intervention at presentation, the metastatic tumor burden, and the patient's overall health. Due to the complex decision-making process and meticulous coordination of care that such an aggressive approach demands, cases of newly diagnosed oligometastatic CRC should be presented in a multidisciplinary tumor board.

A multidisciplinary tumor board recommended that A.K. undergo neoadjuvant chemotherapy prior to liver resection. He received FOLFOX/bevacizumab for five cycles, followed by an additional cycle of FOLFOX alone to provide at least 6 weeks between the last dose of bevacizumab and surgery. Aside from some transient cold sensitivity following each dose of oxaliplatin, A.K. tolerated treatment well, continuing to work full-time and maintaining a normal diet and active lifestyle. Serum CEA fell from 49 to 3.8 ng/mL, and restaging CT scans showed that both right hepatic lobe lesions had decreased to <1 cm and that the left hepatic lobe lesion, which still appeared to be a cyst, was stable. Approximately 4 weeks after the completion of chemotherapy, he underwent right hepatectomy. Pathological evaluation confirmed R0 resection of two metastases with no other foci of carcinoma. He recovered well from surgery and completed 3 more months of chemotherapy. Due to the onset of peripheral sensory neuropathy after postoperative cycle #4, he received LV5FU2 alone for the last two cycles. He remains without evidence of recurrence 2 years into surveillance.

Stage III Colon Cancer: Adjuvant Chemotherapy

A.M. is a 76-year-old woman who, upon screening colonoscopy, was found to have an adenocarcinoma of the ascending colon. Staging CT scans showed no evidence of distant metastases. A right hemicolectomy was performed, and pathological evaluation revealed a moderately differentiated adenocarcinoma with metastasis to 6 of 20 resected lymph nodes. Her postoperative course was complicated by delayed wound healing, but she quickly regained bowel function and was discharged to her daughter's house on postoperative day 10.

During her initial consultation with medical oncology, A.M. had no major complaints. She was eating a full diet, having normal daily stools, and performing daily activities without compromise. She had multiple comorbidities, including obesity, atrial fibrillation, diabetes with mild sensory neuropathy, and hypertension. She has no family history of colon cancer. She appeared well, and her wound was closed completely without surrounding erythema or drainage. Having been told by the surgeon that she would "need" adjuvant chemotherapy to reduce her risk of cancer recurrence, the patient and her family, although wanting to maximize her chance for cure, are concerned about the potential toxicity of chemotherapy in light of her recent wound infection and her underlying comorbidities.

Evidence-Based Case Discussion

A.M. is an elderly patient who presents for consideration of adjuvant chemotherapy following resection of stage III colon cancer. Despite a complicated postoperative course, she has recovered completely and maintains an excellent performance status. This case raises the various issues that need to be addressed during a patient's initial consultation with medical oncology. The oncologist should explain that, although definitive therapy has been administered, her risk for recurrence without further treatment is 40% to 60% due to microscopic disease beyond the surgical field at the time of resection. And, although assays to detect circulating tumor cells exist, none has yet proven sensitive enough to guide decisions regarding adjuvant therapy. As a result, administration of adjuvant therapy is largely "empiric," that is, it is administered under the *assumption* that micrometastatic disease is both present and sensitive to cytotoxic chemotherapy. If the patient chooses to proceed with chemotherapy, the oncologist must review the various options and discuss timing, logistics, and potential side effects. Keeping this discussion in mind, we will review the data supporting the use of adjuvant therapy for resected colon cancer.

5FU/Leucovorin as Adjuvant Therapy

Hoping to increase the cure rate of resected colon cancer by eradicating micrometastatic disease, investigators started to conduct randomized controlled trials comparing postoperative chemotherapy to observation in the 1980s. Due to the exceedingly high cure rate for resected stage I disease (90% or greater), they focused on stage III and, to lesser degree, stage II disease. Intergroup 0035—which randomized 929 patients with resected stage III colon cancer to 5FU with levimasole for 1 year, levimasole alone for 1 year, or observation—was the first large phase III trial to demonstrate a survival benefit for adjuvant chemotherapy (26). At 3.5 years, 5FU/levimasole yielded superior recurrence-free survival (RFS) and OS over observation alone (RFS 63% vs. 47%, $P < .0001$; estimated OS 71% vs. 55%, $P < .0001$). In two subsequent trials, 5FU/LV was shown to be superior to 5FU/levamisole, thereby establishing LV as the preferred 5FU modulator. Finally, when a pooled analysis of >1500 patients with resected stage II or stage III colon cancer demonstrated that 6 months of 5FU/LV conferred a survival advantage similar to that previously shown with 12 months of 5FU/LV and that the benefit of chemotherapy at 3 years was largely confined to stage III patients (event-free survival, 62% vs. 44%; OS, 76% vs. 64%), 6 months of 5FU/LV became the standard backbone regimen for adjuvant chemotherapy (27).

Combination 5FU-Based Adjuvant Chemotherapy

Having already been approved for use in mCRC, irinotecan and oxaliplatin were logical choices to add to 5FU/LV in the adjuvant setting. PETACC-3 randomized 3278 patients with resected stage II and III colon cancer to LV5FU2 or FOLFIRI. There was no difference in 5-year DFS or median OS between the two arms, and FOLFIRI was associated with more grade 3/4 hematological and gastrointestinal toxicity (28). Two smaller randomized trials—CALGB 89803 and ACCORD—also failed to demonstrate a survival advantage of adding irinotecan to 5FU/LV. Thus, while FOLFIRI has been shown to be superior to 5FU/LV and equivalent to FOLFOX in mCRC, there are no available randomized data to support its use in the adjuvant setting.

On the other hand, two practice-changing trials—MOSAIC and NSABP C-07—demonstrated a statistically significant survival benefit of adding oxaliplatin to 5FU/LV. The MOSAIC trial randomized 2246 patients with stage II (40%) or III (60%) colon cancer to 6 months of LV5FU2 or FOLFOX (29). In the intention-to-treat population, FOLFOX yielded a modest but statistically significant OS benefit at 6 years (78.5% vs. 76%; HR 0.84, $P = .046$). Among the 1247 patients with stage III disease, FOLFOX yielded a more pronounced OS benefit (72.9% vs. 68.7%; HR =0.80; $P = .023$), as well as superior 5-year DFS (66.4% vs. 58.9%; HR 0.78, $P = .005$). FOLFOX was not statistically superior to 5FU/LV among the 899 patients with stage II disease, but subgroup analysis showed that FOLFOX improved DFS in the patients with high-risk stage II disease (82.3% vs. 74.6%; HR = 0.72; *P* not reported). Importantly, 24% of patients receiving FOLFOX had some degree of peripheral sensory neuropathy (PSN) by the end of treatment. Although the prevalence declined over time, 15% of patients examined 2 years after completion of FOLFOX complained of residual PSN (11.9%, 2.8%, and 0.7% with grades 1, 2, 3 PSN, respectively). Nearly identical results were reported from NSABP C-07, which randomized nearly 2500 patients to 5FU/LV (Roswell Park regimen) with or without oxaliplatin. Three-year DFS and OS were superior in the FOLFOX arm, and PSN was still present in 10% of these patients 2 years after completion of adjuvant therapy.

Although adding oxaliplatin to 5FU/LV clearly saves lives when applied to large populations, its potential benefit is modest in any one individual, and its potential long-term neurotoxicity is concerning. In fact, the likelihood that adjuvant FOLFOX will cause chronic PSN (10–12%) is 2 to 3 times greater than its absolute improvement in OS over 5FU/LV alone in stage III disease (4%). In order to identify in *real-time* those patients who will benefit from adjuvant chemotherapy and spare those who will not benefit from its potential toxicity, investigators continue to devise measures to "personalize therapy." Translational researchers are currently testing ultrasensitive peripheral blood assays to detect residual microscopic disease and designing tumor assays to quantify a patient's risk for recurrence and the potential benefit of adjuvant chemotherapy. Meanwhile, clinical researchers continue to devise strategies to prevent or counteract toxicity from available drugs such as oxaliplatin.

One such strategy is the basis for International Duration Evaluation of Adjuvant Chemotherapy (IDEA), an international effort to address the unacceptably high rate of chronic PSN in patients receiving adjuvant FOLFOX. Published data suggest that 3 months of adjuvant 5FU/LV may confer benefit equivalent to that of 6 months (30). Furthermore, since PSN typically appears 4 to 5 months into oxaliplatin therapy, it stands to reason that reducing oxaliplatin exposure by a few months may reduce the likelihood of neurotoxicity. Five ongoing phase III trials (four in Europe and one in North America) are therefore randomizing patients with resected stage III colon cancer to 3 or 6 months of FOLFOX. The North American trial, CALGB 80702, will randomize 2500 patients in a 2 × 2 fashion to (a) 3 or 6 months of FOLFOX and (b) 3 years of celecoxib or placebo with a primary endpoint of DFS (equivalent DFS between 3 and 6 months of FOLFOX and superior DFS with celecoxib compared to placebo). The IDEA investigators will pool the data from all five trials (n = 20,000) to show equivalent DFS between 3 and 6 months of adjuvant FOLFOX.

The results of IDEA's analysis will be much anticipated, and clinicians are strongly encouraged to enroll patients in any of the participating trials. For the time being, without any commercially available biomarkers that can predict which individual patients will benefit from FOLFOX over 5FU/LV alone and without any definitive data to show that a shorter duration of FOLFOX is equivalent to the standard 6 months, clinicians should carefully weigh the risks and benefits of adding oxaliplatin to 5FU/LV and re-evaluate the risk-benefit ratio of continuing oxaliplatin during FOLFOX therapy if PSN arises.

Capecitabine as Adjuvant Therapy

An appropriate substitute for 5FU/LV in mCRC, capecitabine has also been rigorously tested in the adjuvant setting. In the X-ACT trial, Twelves et al. randomized 1987 patients with resected stage III colon cancer to 6 months of 5FU/LV (Mayo Clinic regimen) or capecitabine 1250 mg/m^2 twice daily for days 1 to 14 every 21 days, with the intention of demonstrating equivalent DFS (4). Not only did the study meet its endpoint of noninferiority; capecitabine proved superior to 5FU/LV for DFS (HR 0.87; $P < .001$ for equivalence and $P = .05$ for superiority) and approached superiority for OS (HR 0.84, $P < .001$ for equivalence and $P = .07$ for superiority). Compared to 5FU/LV, capecitabine caused less nausea, vomiting, diarrhea, stomatitis, alopecia, and neutropenia but more hand foot syndrome and hyperbilirubinemia. Approximately, 50% of patients receiving capecitabine required dose reduction.

Building on the results from MOSAIC/NSABP C-07 (which demonstrated superiority of 5FU/LV/oxaliplatin over 5FU/LV in the adjuvant setting) and NO16966 (which demonstrated equivalency of XELOX and FOLFOX in the metastatic setting), investigators set out to demonstrate superiority of XELOX over 5FU/LV in the adjuvant setting. In the multicenter phase III trial NO16968, 1886 patients with resected stage III colon cancer were randomized to XELOX or b5FU/LV. XELOX yielded statistically superior DFS at 5 years (66.1% vs. 59.8%), but OS data have not yet been reported. The benefit of adding oxaliplatin was maintained in patients > 70 years old, reinforcing the recommendation that medically fit older patients should not be denied more aggressive therapy based on age alone.

Targeted Agents as Adjuvant Therapy

Although targeted agents have proven beneficial in mCRC, clinical trials with VEGF and EGFR inhibitors in the adjuvant setting have yielded disappointing results. NSABP C-08 randomized 2672 patients with resected stage II/III colon cancer to 6 months of FOLFOX or 6 months of FOLFOX/bevacizumab followed by 6 months of maintenance bevacizumab. Adding bevacizumab to FOLFOX did not improve DFS at the predefined landmark of 3 years, and the primary endpoint for benefit was therefore not met; however, DFS was clearly superior with FOLFOX/bevacizumab until the 15-month landmark, declining thereafter (31). Bevacizumab therefore appears to have exerted a "static effect" on micrometastatic disease, delaying recurrence with active VEGF inhibition but losing its effect once discontinued. While some investigators advocate designing a clinical trial with longer bevacizumab maintenance, others are concerned that indefinite continuation of bevacizumab would be required to control micrometastatic disease. The latter scenario would not only prove costly, it could also uncover cumulative or delayed toxicity of VEGF inhibition not previously described.

Perhaps more surprisingly, EGFR inhibitors have also failed to improve outcomes when combined with adjuvant chemotherapy. Intergroup N0147, a randomized trial comparing FOLFOX and FOLFOX/cetuximab in patients with resected, *KRAS* WT stage III colon cancer, was prematurely closed after interim analysis showed similar 3-year DFS and a trend toward worse 3-year OS with FOLFOX/cetuximab. PETACC-8, a pan-European trial with a design similar to that of N0147, has finished accruing, but results have not yet been reported. Pending the results from PETACC-8 as well as the three ongoing trials addressing the benefit of bevacizumab in the adjuvant setting—E5202 (FOLFOX vs. FOLFOX/bevacizumab in high-risk stage II disease), AVANT (FOLFOX vs. FOLFOX/bevacizumab vs. XELOX/bevacizumab in stage II/III disease), and QUASAR2 (capecitabine vs. capecitabine/bevacizumab in stage II/III disease)—bevacizumab, cetuximab, and panitumumab should not be administered to patients with resected nonmetastatic colon cancer outside of a research protocol.

Surveillance

Stage III colon cancer patients, regardless of whether they receive adjuvant chemotherapy, should undergo surveillance for 5 years, the period during which disease recurrences generally occur. Guidelines such as those published by NCCN include serial history and physical examination, serum CEA testing, and CT imaging to detect recurrent disease and colonoscopy to screen for second malignancies. While there are no published randomized data to define an optimal schedule for surveillance, large retrospective studies have demonstrated the benefit of intensive surveillance in stage I to III colon cancer, with the rationale that earlier detection of metastatic recurrence may facilitate earlier initiation of systemic therapy and, more importantly, R0 resection of oligometastatic disease. Clinicians should therefore personalize the schedule for surveillance based on an individual's risk of recurrence and whether aggressive treatment would be pursued if, in fact, recurrent disease was uncovered. As long as the endoscopist has visualized the entire colon during the preoperative colonoscopy, the next colonoscopy can be performed 1 year later. If the entire colon has not been visualized (due to obstruction, for example), colonoscopy should be repeated approximately 3 months after surgical resection to rule out a synchronous primary cancer. The findings of each colonoscopy determine the interval until the subsequent one. Finally, with emerging data that strongly link an active lifestyle and healthy diet to lower recurrence rates of CRC, patients should be encouraged to adopt a low-fat, high-fiber diet and to engage in regular exercise.

Summary

Figure 11.3 summarizes the current treatment options for 6 months of 5FU-based chemotherapy following resection of stage III colon cancer. FOLFOX or XELOX are the most aggressive options, significantly decreasing absolute recurrence rates by as much as 20% and improving OS compared to observation alone. However, it is important to remember (a) that most of the benefit conferred by combination chemotherapy is from the 5FU component (absolute benefit 15%), with an additional 5% benefit derived from addition of oxaliplatin, and (b) that the risk of chronic PSN from FOLFOX is up to 15%. Therefore, patients who have pre-existing neuropathy or who are not deemed fit enough to tolerate oxaliplatin, should be offered 5FU/LV or capecitabine, and patients who are deemed fit for combination chemotherapy should be offered FOLFOX or XELOX. Those receiving oxaliplatin should be followed closely for neurological symptoms, with careful attention to distinguish between the acute neurosensory complex and true PSN. At the first sign of PSN, strong consideration should be given to reducing or discontinuing oxaliplatin, given its relatively small marginal benefit over 5FU alone and the possibility that all 12 doses may not be needed to confer benefit. In the case of oxaliplatin discontinuation, 5FU (or capecitabine) should be continued to complete 6 total months of adjuvant therapy. Targeted agents currently have no role in the adjuvant setting outside of a clinical protocol.

Although A.M. is elderly and has multiple comorbidities, her performance status is excellent, and her chance of disease recurrence is appreciable, making her an appropriate candidate for adjuvant chemotherapy. After laying out the rationale for adjuvant chemotherapy, discussing the various chemotherapeutic options, and expressing concern

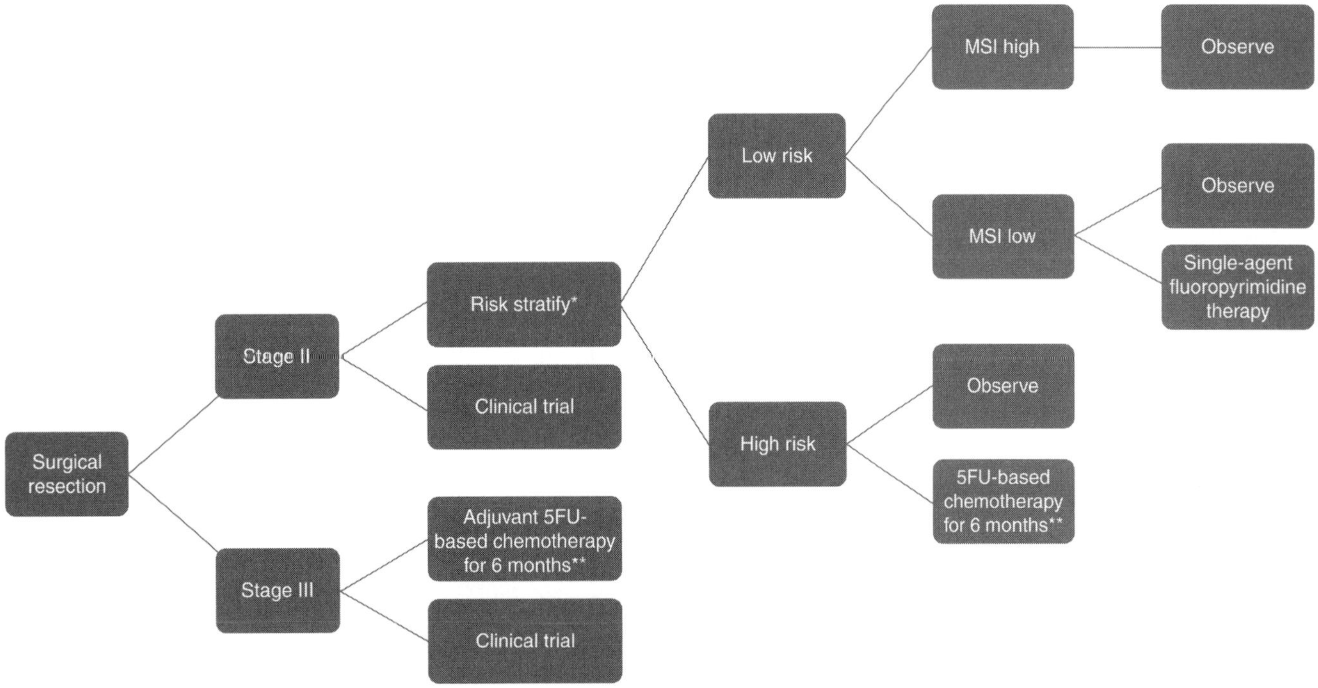

*Poor differentiation, T4, inadequate lymph node dissection (<12 lymph nodes), perforation, obstruction, lymphovascular invasion
** Folfox, Capox, 5FU/leucovorin, capecitabine, or CapOx

Figure 11.3

Treatment algorithm for resected stage II and III colon cancer.

over exacerbating her pre-existing neuropathy with oxaliplatin, we recommended single-agent 5FU therapy. Because the patient did not want a Port-a-cath or infusional pump, she chose capecitabine, which was started at 1000 mg/m^2 twice daily for 14 days of a 21-day cycle. Since she tolerated her first two cycles extremely well, her dose was increased to 1250 mg/m^2 twice daily, and she continued full-dose capecitabine to complete 6 months of adjuvant therapy. Five years of posttreatment surveillance revealed no evidence of recurrence.

Stage II Colon Cancer: Adjuvant Chemotherapy

L.G. is a 38-year-old otherwise healthy woman without any family history of cancer who presented to the emergency room with rectal bleeding. Colonoscopy with biopsy revealed a circumferential, nonobstructing adenocarcinoma in the ascending colon. CT scans showed a right colon mass but no evidence of regional adenopathy or distant metastases. She underwent right hemicolectomy and had no postoperative complications. Pathological evaluation revealed a moderately differentiated adenocarcinoma invading pericolonic adipose tissue; none of the isolated 17 lymph nodes contained carcinoma. The tumor expressed MLH1, MSH2, MSH6, and PMS2 by immunohistochemistry, and molecular analysis demonstrated microsatellite stability. She was referred to medical oncology for an opinion regarding adjuvant therapy.

Evidence-Based Case Discussion

L.G. presents with a resected stage IIA (T3 N0) adenocarcinoma that shows no high-risk histopathological or molecular features (see following sections). Although her chance for tumor recurrence is relatively low (15–20%), she wants to know if adjuvant chemotherapy will further lower her risk for recurrence. This case highlights the controversy surrounding adjuvant chemotherapy in stage II colon cancer, the importance of risk stratification using established factors, and the need for more informative prognostic and predictive biomarkers.

Adjuvant Chemotherapy in Stage II Colon Cancer

Many of the early adjuvant trials comparing chemotherapy to observation included a substantial number of patients with stage II disease. Although subgroup analyses of these trials consistently demonstrated a 15% to 20% lower relative risk for recurrence for stage II patients receiving chemotherapy, attaining statistical significance was difficult due to insufficient sample size and a low absolute risk for recurrence. To generate more statistical power, the IMPACT B2 investigators accumulated clinical data from five randomized trials comparing adjuvant 5FU/LV to observation. Pooled analysis of the 1025 patients with stage II colon cancer demonstrated a strong trend toward superior 5-year event-free survival and OS with chemotherapy (EFS 76% vs. 73%, $P = .061$; OS 82% vs. 80%, $P = .057$) (32). The only large adjuvant trial to enroll primarily stage II patients was QUASAR, which randomized 3239 patients with resected colorectal cancer, 91% of whom had stage II disease, to adjuvant 5FU/LV or observation. Consistent with previously reported data from subgroup and pooled analyses, chemotherapy was associated with a 22% relative reduction of recurrence risk ($P = .001$) and a 3.6% absolute improvement in OS (33). As for the benefit of adding oxaliplatin, subgroup analysis of the 1000 stage II patients in the MOSAIC trial showed no survival advantage of FOLFOX over LV5FU2 (29).

Risk Stratification in Stage II Colon Cancer

Adjuvant 5FU clearly improves survival when applied to large enough groups of patients with stage II colon cancer, but its absolute benefit of 2% to 4% makes an *individual's* chance of deriving benefit exceedingly low. Working under the assumption that stage II patients with a worse prognosis are more likely to benefit from adjuvant therapy, investigators have identified various clinical and pathological features that increase risk for relapse, including bowel obstruction or perforation, invasion of adjacent structures (T4 lesion), poor differentiation, lymphovascular invasion, and inadequate (<12) lymph node dissection. Subgroup analyses of the major trials randomizing patients to 5FU or observation have suggested that patients with stage II colon cancer meeting one or more of these criteria derive benefit from adjuvant therapy greater than the 2% to 4% reported for unselected stage II patients (34). Furthermore, analysis of "high-risk" stage II patients in the MOSAIC trial showed an improvement in DFS (HR 0.72) conferred by FOLFOX over LV5FU2 similar to that seen in stage III patients (HR 0.78) (29). We must, however, keep in mind that these data were generated from post hoc subgroup analyses encompassing small numbers of patients and that the relative contribution of any single-risk factor cannot possibly be quantified. In short, while it is fairly clear that these so-called high-risk features are *prognostic*, their *predictive* role has not been firmly established.

More recently, MSI has emerged as an important risk factor. After pooling data from 1027 patients with stage II and III colon cancer enrolled in six randomized trials comparing adjuvant 5FU to observation, Sargent et al. published compelling data regarding the prognostic and predictive power of MSI. First, they reported that MSI was associated with improved DFS (HR 0.51, $P = .009$) and OS (HR 0.51, $P = .004$) in patients undergoing observation. Second, they showed that patients with stage III, microsatellite stable (MSS) tumors plainly benefit from adjuvant chemotherapy (HR 0.64, $P = .001$) whereas patients with stage III microsatellite unstable (MSI-H) tumors do not (HR 1.01). Finally, they conclusively demonstrated inferior OS in patients with stage II, MSI-H tumors who received chemotherapy compared to those who did not (HR 2.95, $P = .04$) (35). These data therefore establish MSI as positive prognostic factor, as well as a negative predictor of benefit from adjuvant 5FU in stage II patients. ECOG 5202 is an ongoing randomized trial that risk stratifies patients with stage II colon cancer based on the molecular features of MSI and 18q loss of heterozygosity. Low-risk patients will undergo observation whereas high-risk patients will be randomized to FOLFOX or FOLFOX/bevacizumab.

Given the validation and widespread use of Oncotype DX for breast cancer, translational scientists have also developed and tested predictive assays for colon cancer. By analyzing 761 candidate genes from 1851 resection specimens collected during large adjuvant therapy trials, Kerr et al. identified seven genes as being most predictive of recurrence and six genes as most predictive of treatment benefit. The final assay, a multigene RT-PCR that produces a recurrence (prognostic) score and a treatment benefit (predictive) score, was applied to specimens acquired from the QUASAR trial. Although the recurrence score successfully divided patients into low, intermediate, and high risk for recurrence, the differences were not particularly impressive (12%, 18%, and 22%, respectively), and the treatment score did not predict differential benefit from adjuvant chemotherapy. The multigene assay Coloprint yields similar diagnostic information, but has also not been shown to predict benefit from chemotherapy.

Summary

The role of adjuvant chemotherapy for resected stage II colon cancer remains highly controversial. Studies have consistently shown a discernible treatment effect across large groups of patients, but an absolute benefit of no more than 5% makes the number needed to treat (NNT) to prevent one cancer recurrence uncomfortably high. While a cohort of patients who stands to benefit more than others must exist, this population has not yet been identified despite much clinical investigation. Clinicopathological features, while proven to be prognostic, have not proven to predict benefit from chemotherapy. MSI is a strong positive prognostic factor and predicts lack of benefit, even harm, from adjuvant 5FU in stage II disease. However, no predictive effect for patients receiving a fluoropyrimidine plus oxaliplatin has been established. Finally, the Oncotype DX and Coloprint multigene assays provide limited prognostic, but no predictive information.

In light of these inconclusive data, ASCO guidelines do not support the *routine* use of adjuvant chemotherapy in stage II colon cancer. As such, the oncologist and patient can only arrive at an appropriate, informed decision after engaging in a detailed conversation. Specifically, the physician should delineate the known risk factors for cancer recurrence, acknowledging their aforementioned limitations; assess the patient's overall health status and life expectancy; explain the potential benefit of chemotherapy in layman's terms (using absolute benefit and NNT instead of relative benefit or hazard ratios); and review the potential side effects of treatment. If the patient decides to proceed with adjuvant therapy, the clinician must recommend a specific treatment (see Figure 11.3). When considering a fluoropyrimidine-only regimen, the clinician should test the resected tumor for MMR expression (IHC) or MSI (PCR). LV5FU2 and capecitabine are reasonable options for low-risk, MSS disease. However, patients with low-risk, MSI-H tumors should not receive adjuvant therapy due to their excellent prognosis and the potential harm of exposing them to 5FU. Adding oxaliplatin is reasonable for high-risk disease, but it is important to remember that the data supporting this practice were derived from MOSAIC subgroup analysis, which showed improved DFS but not OS of FOLFOX over LV5FU2. Finally, clinicians should encourage their patients to enroll in trials such as E5202 and to donate tumor and blood to research tissue banks.

Because L.G.'s tumor expressed all four MMR enzymes and did not manifest any high-risk clinicopathological features, we explained that her risk of recurrence was approximately 15% and that adjuvant 5FU/LV or capecitabine could reduce her recurrence risk by 3% to 4%. She chose not to undergo adjuvant therapy or enroll in E5202 but agreed to donate blood and her resected tumor to our institutional biorepository.

Stage II/III Rectal Cancer

G.F. is a 72-year-old Caucasian man who presented with a 5-month history of low caliber stools, intermittent rectal bleeding, tenesmus, and weight loss. Colonoscopy with biopsy revealed a friable, circumferential rectal adenocarcinoma, extending proximally from the anal verge to about 12 cm. CT scans of the chest, abdomen, and pelvis showed an irregular rectal mass without perirectal adenopathy or distant metastases. Rectal endoscopic ultrasound (EUS) showed tumor invasion through the muscularis propria into the subserosa, but no lymphadenopathy (uT3 N0). Since G.F. is otherwise healthy with an excellent performance status, he would like to receive the most aggressive treatment warranted to cure his cancer.

Evidence-Based Case Discussion

Because they share cell of origin and pathogenesis, rectal cancer and colon cancer respond to identical chemotherapy regimens are therefore treated similarly when metastatic. However, due to anatomical considerations, treatment of nonmetastatic rectal cancer differs from that of colon cancer. First, because of the rectum's proximity to pelvic structures, rectal cancer carries a high risk for local recurrence while maintaining its potential to metastasize remotely. Thus, lowering the risk for local recurrence, which is particularly morbid and extremely difficult to manage, has become an important focus of rectal cancer therapy. Second, because low-lying rectal tumors approximate or involve the anal sphincter and genitourinary nerves, surgical resection may require permanent colostomy and/or compromise of sexual and urinary function. With these considerations in mind, we will briefly review the management of localized rectal cancer.

Surgical Considerations

Surgery remains the mainstay of treatment for nonmetastatic rectal cancer. Although patients with superficial tumors (T1 and some T2 tumors without nodal involvement) can be treated with local transanal excision, the majority of patients (those with T3/T4 or node-positive tumors) will require more extensive resection. In these circumstances, the distance of the tumor from the anal verge will determine the type of procedure performed. Because the anal sphincter muscle fibers are located within 3-cm proximal of the dentate line, distal rectal tumors frequently require abdominoperineal resection (APR), which leaves the patient with a permanent colostomy. Mid- to high-rectal tumors can generally be removed by low anterior resection (LAR), which spares the anal sphincter. Tumors that are low but not clearly low enough to require an APR may be downsized with neoadjuvant therapy (see the following sections), thereby facilitating resection by LAR instead. Regardless of whether APR or LAR is employed, total mesorectal excision (TME)—removal of the tumor, lymph nodes, rectal mesentery, and autonomic nerves en bloc by sharp dissection—increases the likelihood of negative margins and improves local control.

Neoadjuvant Chemoradiation

Surgical resection of stage II or stage III rectal cancer yields an unacceptably high rate of local relapse, and stage III disease carries a risk for distant relapse similar to that of stage III colon cancer. Therefore, in contrast to colon cancer, both radiation and chemotherapy have been incorporated into the treatment algorithm for stage II to III rectal cancer. Although postoperative radiation has been shown to improve local control but not OS, concurrent 5FU-based chemoradiation (CRT) improves both local control and OS over radiation alone, with i5FU proving to be less toxic and possibly more effective than b5FU. As a result, standard CRT for rectal cancer includes 5 to 6 weeks of radiation (5040 cGy over 5 weeks in 180 cGy fractions) with concurrent 5FU 200 to 250 mg/m^2/day by continuous infusion (CIFU) or capecitabine 800 to 850 mg/m^2 twice daily (36).

Administering preoperative rather than postoperative CRT offers the potential advantages of (a) downsizing the tumor, thereby facilitating sphincter preservation, (b) expanding the number of patients that receive adjuvant therapy (since slow postoperative recovery may delay or preclude further therapy), and (c) reducing postoperative complications. To address the question of how best to sequence CRT in relation to surgery, Sauer et al. randomized 421 patients with stage II/III rectal cancer to preoperative or postoperative CRT. All patients underwent TME and received four cycles of adjuvant b5FU. Although preoperative CRT did not improve OS when compared to postoperative CRT, it improved local control, caused significantly less grade 3/4 toxicity (both acute and chronic), and facilitated more frequent delivery of full-dose chemotherapy and radiation. The rate of sphincter-preserving surgery did not differ between the two groups; however, restricting analysis to the 194 patients determined before randomization to require APR revealed that patients receiving preoperative CRT had higher rates of sphincter-preserving surgery (37). This trial established the standard of care for clinical stage II/III rectal cancer: neoadjuvant CRT followed by TME and adjuvant 5FU-based chemotherapy. Since all patients in this trial received both chemotherapy and CRT, the individual contribution of each modality could not be assessed; both are therefore included in standard therapy. With the publication of the MOSAIC and X-ACT trials, options for adjuvant chemotherapy have been expanded to include FOLFOX, capecitabine, or XELOX.

Despite aggressive treatment with concurrent 5FU and radiation, many patients still experience local and/or distant relapse. While intensifying radiosensitizing chemotherapy has yielded promising results in single-arm trials, two randomized phase III trials—ACCORD 12 and STAR-01—showed that adding oxaliplatin to 5FU-based CRT increased toxicity without improving pathological complete response (38). Ongoing trials are incorporating VEGF and EGFR inhibitors into the chemosensitizing regimen, using short-course radiotherapy instead of the traditional 5- to 6-week course, sequencing chemotherapy and CRT, and assessing whether neoadjuvant chemotherapy alone may be sufficient in selected cases.

Summary

Evaluation of tissue-proven, nonmetastatic rectal cancer should include rigid proctoscopy and precise tumor localization by an experienced colorectal surgeon, as well as endoscopic ultrasound (or pelvic MRI) for local staging. Patients with clinical stage I tumors should undergo surgical resection, followed by adjuvant therapy only if the pathological stage is higher than expected. Since

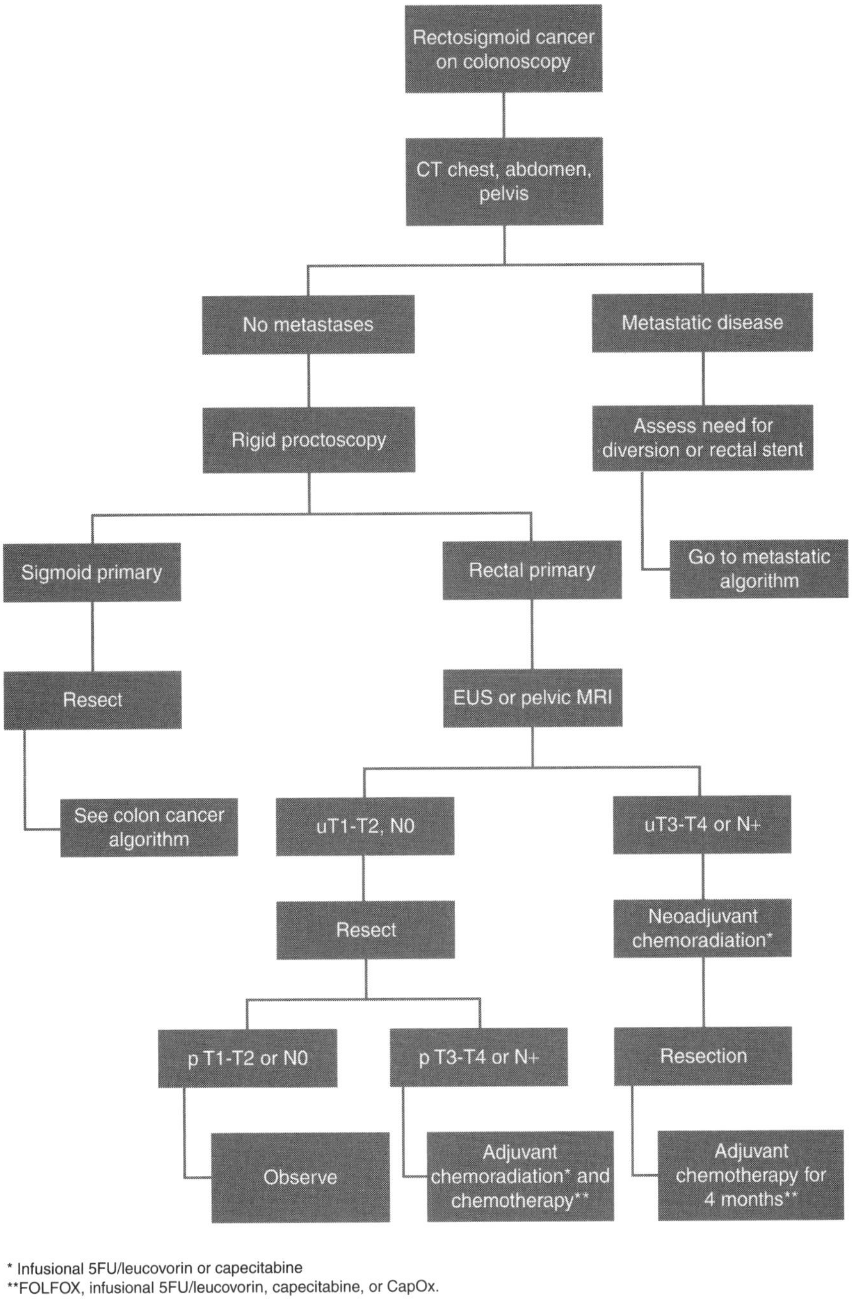

Figure 11.4

Treatment algorithm for rectal cancer.

neoadjuvant CRT improves local control, facilitates higher rates of sphincter preservation, and causes less toxicity than adjuvant CRT, patients with clinical stage II/III tumors (see Figure 11.4) should undergo neoadjuvant chemoradiation (CIFU or capecitabine), surgical resection, and 4 months of adjuvant chemotherapy (LV5FU2, capecitabine, FOLFOX, or XELOX). Surveillance is similar to that of resected colon cancer.

G.F. received neoadjuvant chemoradiotherapy (5040 cGy concurrently with capecitabine) and, aside from mild radiation dermatitis, tolerated treatment well. Six weeks after the completion of CRT, an experienced colorectal surgeon performed an APR (due to the tumor's proximity to the anal verge). Pathological evaluation revealed pT2 N0 adenocarcinoma with evidence of treatment-related tumor necrosis. After an additional 4 months of FOLFOX chemotherapy, surveillance was initiated.

REFERENCES

1. Poultsides GA, Servais EL, Saltz LB, et al. Outcome of primary tumor in patients with synchronous stage IV colorectal cancer receiving combination chemotherapy without surgery as initial treatment. *J Clin Oncol*. 2009;27(20):3379–3384.
2. de Gramont A, Bosset JF, Milan C, et al. Randomized trial comparing monthly low-dose leucovorin and fluorouracil bolus with bimonthly high-dose leucovorin and fluorouracil bolus plus continuous infusion for advanced colorectal cancer: a French intergroup study. *J Clin Oncol*. 1997;15(2):808–815.

3. Cassidy J, Clarke S, Díaz-Rubio E, et al. Randomized phase III study of capecitabine plus oxaliplatin compared with fluorouracil/folinic acid plus oxaliplatin as first-line therapy for metastatic colorectal cancer. *J Clin Oncol.* 2008;26(12):2006–2012.
4. Twelves C, Wong A, Nowacki MP, et al. Capecitabine as adjuvant treatment for stage III colon cancer. *N Engl J Med.* 2005; 352(26):2696–2704.
5. Douillard JY, Cunningham D, Roth AD, et al. Irinotecan combined with fluorouracil compared with fluorouracil alone as first-line treatment for metastatic colorectal cancer: a multicentre randomised trial. *Lancet.* 2000;355(9209):1041–1047.
6. Fuchs CS, Marshall J, Mitchell E, et al. Randomized, controlled trial of irinotecan plus infusional, bolus, or oral fluoropyrimidines in first-line treatment of metastatic colorectal cancer: results from the BICC-C Study. *J Clin Oncol.* 2007;25(30):4779–4786.
7. de Gramont A, Figer A, Seymour M, et al. Leucovorin and fluorouracil with or without oxaliplatin as first-line treatment in advanced colorectal cancer. *J Clin Oncol.* 2000;18(16):2938–2947.
8. Tournigand C, Cervantes A, Figer A, et al. OPTIMOX1: a randomized study of FOLFOX4 or FOLFOX7 with oxaliplatin in a stop-and-go fashion in advanced colorectal cancer—a GERCOR study. *J Clin Oncol.* 2006;24(3):394–400.
9. Chibaudel B, Maindrault-Goebel F, Lledo G, et al. Can chemotherapy be discontinued in unresectable metastatic colorectal cancer? The GERCOR OPTIMOX2 Study. *J Clin Oncol.* 2009;27(34):5727–5733.
10. Tournigand C. FOLFIRI Followed by FOLFOX6 or the Reverse Sequence in Advanced Colorectal Cancer: A Randomized GERCOR Study. *J Clin Oncol.* 2003;22(2):229–237.
11. Falcone A, Ricci S, Brunetti I, et al. Phase III trial of infusional fluorouracil, leucovorin, oxaliplatin, and irinotecan (FOLFOXIRI) compared with infusional fluorouracil, leucovorin, and irinotecan (FOLFIRI) as first-line treatment for metastatic colorectal cancer: the Gruppo Oncologico Nord Ovest. *J Clin Oncol.* 2007;25(13):1670–1676.
12. Hurwitz H, Fehrenbacher L, Novotny W, et al. Bevacizumab plus irinotecan, fluorouracil, and leucovorin for metastatic colorectal cancer. *N Engl J Med.* 2004;350(23):2335–2342.
13. Giantonio BJ, Catalano PJ, Meropol NJ, et al. Bevacizumab in combination with oxaliplatin, fluorouracil, and leucovorin (FOLFOX4) for previously treated metastatic colorectal cancer: results from the Eastern Cooperative Oncology Group Study E3200. *J Clin Oncol.* 2007;25(12):1539–1544.
14. Saltz LB, Clarke S, Díaz-Rubio E, et al. Bevacizumab in combination with oxaliplatin-based chemotherapy as first-line therapy in metastatic colorectal cancer: a randomized phase III study. *J Clin Oncol.* 2008;26(12):2013–2019.
15. Grothey A, Sugrue MM, Purdie DM, et al. Bevacizumab beyond first progression is associated with prolonged overall survival in metastatic colorectal cancer: results from a large observational cohort study (BRiTE). *J Clin Oncol.* 2008;26(33):5326–5334.
16. Jonker DJ, O'Callaghan CJ, Karapetis CS, et al. Cetuximab for the treatment of colorectal cancer. *N Engl J Med.* 2007;357(20): 2040–2048.
17. Van Cutsem E, Peeters M, Siena S, et al. Open-label phase III trial of panitumumab plus best supportive care compared with best supportive care alone in patients with chemotherapy-refractory metastatic colorectal cancer. *J Clin Oncol.* 2007;25(13):1658–1664.
18. Karapetis CS, Khambata-Ford S, Jonker DJ, et al. K-ras mutations and benefit from cetuximab in advanced colorectal cancer. *N Engl J Med.* 2008;359(17):1757–1765.
19. Cunningham D, Humblet Y, Siena S, et al. Cetuximab monotherapy and cetuximab plus irinotecan in irinotecan-refractory metastatic colorectal cancer. N. Engl. J. Med 2004 Jul;351(4):337–345.
20. Bokemeyer C, Bondarenko I, Makhson A, et al. Fluorouracil, leucovorin, and oxaliplatin with and without cetuximab in the first-line treatment of metastatic colorectal cancer. *J Clin Oncol.* 2008;27(5):663–671.
21. Peeters M, Price TJ, Cervantes A, et al. Randomized phase III study of panitumumab with fluorouracil, leucovorin, and irinotecan (FOLFIRI) compared with FOLFIRI alone as second-line treatment in patients with metastatic colorectal cancer. *J Clin Oncol.* 2010;28(31):4706–4713.
22. Douillard J, Siena S, Cassidy J, et al. Randomized, phase III trial of panitumumab with infusional fluorouracil, leucovorin, and oxaliplatin (FOLFOX4) versus FOLFOX4 alone as first-line treatment in patients with previously untreated metastatic colorectal cancer: the PRIME study. *J Clin Oncol.* 2010;28(31):4697–4705.
23. Tol J, Koopman M, Cats A, et al. Chemotherapy, bevacizumab, and cetuximab in metastatic colorectal cancer. *N Engl J Med.* 2009;360(6):563–572.
24. Mitry E, Fields ALA, Bleiberg H, et al. Adjuvant chemotherapy after potentially curative resection of metastases from colorectal cancer: a pooled analysis of two randomized trials. *J Clin Oncol.* 2008;26(30):4906–4911.
25. Nordlinger B, Sorbye H, Glimelius B, et al. Perioperative chemotherapy with FOLFOX4 and surgery versus surgery alone for resectable liver metastases from colorectal cancer (EORTC Intergroup trial 40983): a randomised controlled trial. *Lancet.* 2008;371(9617):1007–1016.
26. Moertel CG, Fleming TR, Macdonald JS, et al. Levamisole and fluorouracil for adjuvant therapy of resected colon carcinoma. *N Engl J Med.* 1990;322(6):352–358.
27. Efficacy of adjuvant fluorouracil and folinic acid in colon cancer. International Multicentre Pooled Analysis of Colon Cancer Trials (IMPACT) investigators. *Lancet.* 1995;345(8955):939–944.
28. Van Cutsem E, Labianca R, Bodoky G, et al. Randomized phase III trial comparing biweekly infusional fluorouracil/leucovorin alone or with irinotecan in the adjuvant treatment of stage III colon cancer: PETACC-3. *J Clin Oncol.* 2009;27(19):3117–3125.
29. Andre T, Boni C, Navarro M, et al. Improved Overall Survival With Oxaliplatin, Fluorouracil, and leucovorin as adjuvant treatment in stage II or III colon cancer in the MOSAIC trial. *J Clin Oncol.* 2009;27(19):3109–3116.
30. Chau I, Norman AR, Cunningham D, et al. A randomised comparison between 6 months of bolus fluorouracil/leucovorin and 12 weeks of protracted venous infusion fluorouracil as adjuvant treatment in colorectal cancer. *Ann Oncol.* 2005;16(4):549–557.
31. Allegra CJ, Yothers G, O'Connell MJ, et al. Phase III trial assessing bevacizumab in stages II and III carcinoma of the colon: results of NSABP Protocol C-08. *J Clin. Oncol* 2011;29(1):11–16.
32. Efficacy of adjuvant fluorouracil and folinic acid in B2 colon cancer. International Multicentre Pooled Analysis of B2 Colon Cancer Trials (IMPACT B2) investigators. *J Clin Oncol.* 1999;17(5):1356–1363.
33. Quasar Collaborative Group, Gray R, Barnwell J, McConkey C, et al. Adjuvant chemotherapy versus observation in patients with colorectal cancer: a randomised study. *Lancet.* 2007;370(9604):2020–2029.
34. Gill S, Loprinzi CL, Sargent DJ, et al. Pooled analysis of fluorouracil-based adjuvant therapy for stage II and III colon cancer: who benefits and by how much? *J Clin Oncol.* 2004;22(10):1797–1806.
35. Sargent DJ, Marsoni S, Monges G, et al. Defective mismatch repair as a predictive marker for lack of efficacy of fluorouracil-based adjuvant therapy in colon cancer. *J Clin Oncol.* 2010;28(20):3219–3226.
36. Krishnan S, Janjan NA, Skibber JM, et al. Phase II study of capecitabine (Xeloda) and concomitant boost radiotherapy in patients with locally advanced rectal cancer. *Int J Radiat Oncol Biol Phys.* 2006;66(3):762–771.
37. Sauer R, Becker H, Hohenberger W, et al. Preoperative versus postoperative chemoradiotherapy for rectal cancer. *N Engl J Med.* 2004;351(17):1731–1740.
38. Gérard J, Azria D, Gourgou-Bourgade S, et al. Comparison of two neoadjuvant chemoradiotherapy regimens for locally advanced rectal cancer: results of the phase III trial ACCORD 12/0405-Prodige 2. *J Clin Oncol.* 2010;28(10):1638–1644.

12

Anal Canal Carcinoma

MUHAMMAD ANAS TARAKJI AND ELIZABETH YU CHIAO

EPIDEMIOLOGY, RISK FACTORS, NATURAL HISTORY, AND PATHOLOGY

Anal canal cancer (ACC) is an uncommon gastrointestinal malignancy and comprises approximately 1.9% of digestive system cancers with an estimated incidence of 5290 new cases in the United States annually (1), resulting in approximately 710 deaths. The disease includes two distinctive histologic subtypes: the squamous cell subtype, which comprises most ACC cases and arises in the transitional or squamous mucosa, and the anal gland adenocarcinoma subtype, which is much less common and is estimated to represent 2.9% to 10% of all ACC (2). Because squamous cell cancer of the anus (SCCA) is by far the most common type of anal cancer, this chapter will focus on SCCA.

Over the last 30 years, the incidence of SCCA has been increasing among men (particularly, among black men) (3). The annual incidence among men and women was similar between 1994 and 2000 (2.04 and 2.06 per 100,000, respectively), which is in contrast to the period between 1973 and 1979 (1.06 and 1.39 per 100,000, respectively). When broken down by race, a remarkable increase was observed among black men going from 1.09 per 100,000 to 2.71 per 100,000 in the same time period (1973–2000) (3).

The incidence has also significantly increased in other specific populations such as HIV-infected homosexual men. This finding is particularly noteworthy because several studies have shown that the incidence of SCCA among HIV-infected men continues to increase despite the widespread utilization of highly active antiretroviral treatment (HAART), indicating that the incidence of SCCA among HIV-infected individuals is unlikely to decrease in the future.

Several risk factors have been implicated in the development of SCCA. Probably, the strongest risk factor for SCCA is human papillomavirus virus (HPV) infection. Previous studies have shown that HPV is associated with up to 93% of SCCA pathology specimens among women (4). In the past, SCCA was thought to develop in sites of chronic local inflammation. However, a recent Danish study failed to confirm such a relation in large series of patients who had inflammatory bowel disease (5).

Chronic immunosuppression, including iatrogenic causes such as solid organ transplant recipients, as well as HIV infection, have been shown to increase the risk of SCCA. A large meta-analysis found that the standardized incidence ratio (SIR) for SCCA was 28.75 (95% CI 21.6–38.3) (6). In addition, a prospective study has shown that the prevalence of anal intraepithelial neoplasia (AIN), an anal cancer precursor lesion, is clearly increased in HIV- infected patients (7). Among renal transplant recipients, the meta-analysis SIR for SCCA was 4.85 (95% CI 1.36–17.3) (6). Sexually transmitted diseases are also associated with a strong risk for SCCA, especially among homosexual men, likely due to an increased risk for HPV infection (8) (Table 12.1). Finally, cigarette smoking is significantly associated with an increased risk of anal cancer (RR 1.9 for 20 pack-years, RR 5.2 for 50 pack-years) (9).

Table 12.1 SCCA Risk Factors Associated With Sexual Behavior

SCCA Risk Factors Associated With Sexual Behavior	Relative Risk
Never married men	8.6
Homosexual men	50
Genital Warts	27
Gonorrhea	17

Adapted from Daling et al. (8).

STAGING

The staging of SCCA, unlike most gastrointestinal malignancies, is not dependent on the degree of tumor tissue penetration but rather on the size of the primary tumor.

AJCC Staging System for Anal Carcinoma

Stage	Definition
I	Tumor confined to anal canal, ≤2 cm (T1)
II	Tumor confined to anal canal, >2 cm <5 cm (T2) or >5cm (T3)
IIIA	Tumor of any size with metastasis to perirectal lymph nodes (N1), or tumor of any size with invasion of adjacent organs (e.g., vagina, urethra, bladder) (T4) without lymph node metastases
IIIB	Tumor invading adjacent organs (T4) and perirectal lymph node metastases (N1) or tumor of any size with metastases to internal iliac and/or inguinal lymph nodes (N2, N3)
IV	Tumor of any size with or without lymph node metastases with distant metastases (e.g., liver, lung, etc.)

The prognosis of SCCA was stratified in a recent cohort of 19,195 patients, which showed that patients with SCCA had a higher risk of death if they were male ≥ 65 years old, black, living in lower median incomes areas, and had more advanced T stage tumors, nodal or distant metastases, or poorly differentiated cancers ($P < .0001$)(10). The 5-year overall survival is shown in Table 12.2.

Table 12.2 Five-Year Overall Survival for SCCA

Stage	Percentage
I	70
II	59
III	41
IV	19

Adapted from Bilimoria et al. (10).

CASE SUMMARIES

Limited Stage Anal Carcinoma

P.G. is a 61-year-old Caucasian HIV-negative female with a past medical history of hypertension and hyperlipidemia. She presented to her local gynecologist complaining of bright red blood per rectum. Digital rectal exam showed nodularity in the anal canal, and subsequent colonoscopy revealed a smooth anterolateral anal canal nodule, which was 1 to 1.5 cm in greatest dimension, and involved the anal sphincter. Biopsies were consistent with invasive squamous cell carcinoma. Staging CT scans of the chest, abdomen, and pelvis were unremarkable for other lesions or lymphadenopathy and the staging at presentation was T1, N0, M0 (stage I).

Evidence-Based Case Discussion

P.G. has stage I squamous anal carcinoma, which was staged clinically by digital rectal examination. Palpation of inguinal lymph nodes is an indication for fine-needle aspiration (FNA) or excisional biopsy to determine if there is inguinal lymph node involvement. A CT scan or MRI of the abdomen and pelvis is generally necessary to evaluate the pelvic nodes for metastases. In addition, chest imaging with chest x-ray or CT scan is also recommended as a part of the initial staging work up. The use of PET scanning is not generally accepted as a routine method for initial staging (11). See Figure 12.1 for a diagnostic and therapeutic algorithm.

HIV testing is recommended because of the increased risk for SCCA among HIV-infected individuals, and measurement of CD4 count and HIV viral load is recommended for all HIV-infected patients. In addition, gynecologic exam and screening for HPV and cervical cancer is suggested for female patients.

The 5-year overall survival for this patient is up to 70% and currently the recommended treatment for patients with stages I to III ACC is concurrent chemotherapy and radiation (XRT) according to the Nigro protocol (12). This regimen consists of 5-fluorouracil (5-FU) (1000 mg/m^2 per day by continuous infusion days 1 through 4 and 29 through 32), mitomycin (10 to 15 mg/m^2 on day 1 only), and intermediate dose XRT (45 Gy) given in 25 fractions over 5 weeks. Patients with stage II or III ACC are treated with the same chemotherapy regimen but with higher XRT doses (55–59 Gy). Surgery with abdominoperineal resection (APR) is only needed in patients who have residual tumor at the time of post-radiation biopsy.

A number of studies have addressed the efficacy and safety of chemotherapy and XRT regimens. A phase III intergroup study done by the Radiation Therapy Oncology Group (RTOG 87-04) showed that patients who received concurrent XRT plus 5-FU and mitomycin had a lower APR rate (9% vs. 22%, $P = .002$), and a higher 4-year disease-free survival (DFS) (73% vs. 51%, $P = .0003$) compared with patients receiving XRT with 5-FU alone (13).

A more recent study done by the intergroup RTOG 98-11 compared the use of cisplatin in place of mitomycin, each along with 5-FU and concurrent XRT, and though there were no differences in primary end points of DFS (54% vs. 60%, $P = .17$) and 5-year overall survival (70% vs. 75%: $P = .10$) between the two regimens, the APR rate in the group that received cisplatin was significantly higher

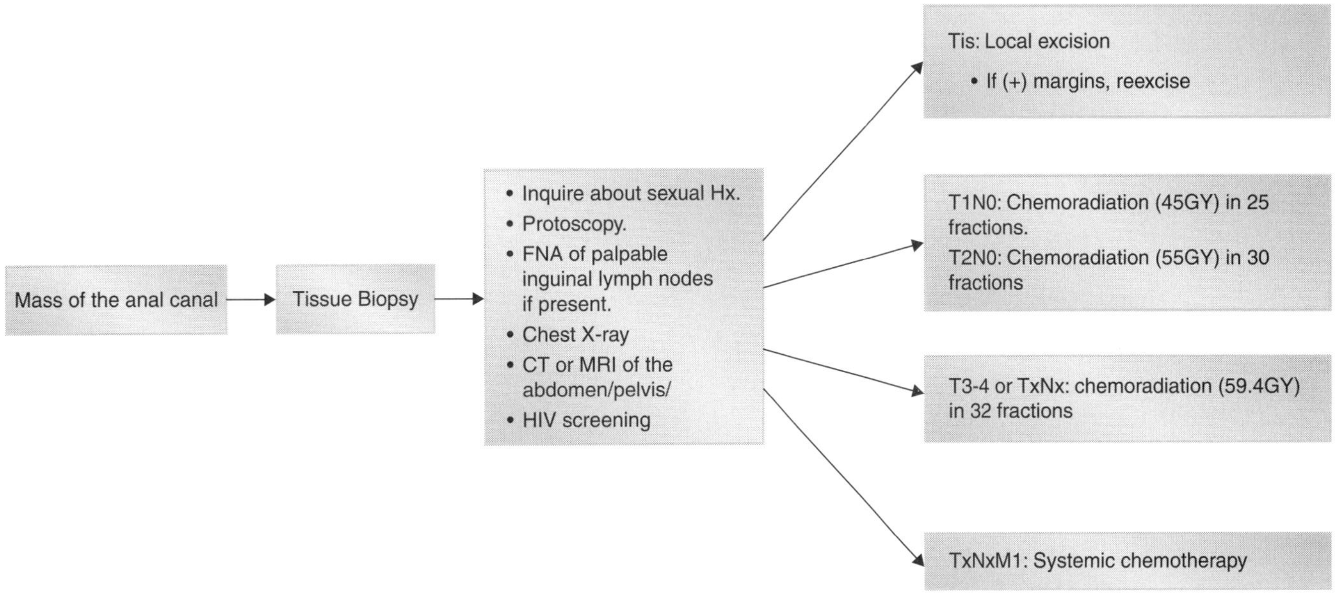

Figure 12.1

Diagnostic evaluation for anal canal mass. Adapted from Ang C. Chapter 17: Anal Cancer. MD Anderson, Manual of Medical Oncology. 2006. The McGraw-Hill Companies INC.

(19% vs. 10%: $P = .02$) (14). Thus, the current standard of care for early-stage SCCA (stages I–III) is concurrent 5-FU plus mitomycin chemotherapy with XRT.

Metastatic Anal Carcinoma

F.A. is a 49-year-old Hispanic male with a history of HIV/AIDS (CD4= 63 cells/μL), hepatitis B, and pulmonary cryptococcosis. He presented with an 8-month history of an enlarging perianal mass that had become increasingly painful over the 2 months prior to presentation. He also reported nonpurulent drainage with subjective fever and was evaluated by general surgery for possible incision and drainage. Anal exam under anesthesia showed an anal abscess, and a hard, palpable, 6-cm nodule associated with severe anal stenosis. Excision of the abscess along with multiple core biopsies was performed and showed pathology consistent with moderately differentiated, invasive squamous cell carcinoma. A CT scan of the chest, abdomen, and pelvis was performed and showed an increased number of enlarged perirectal and unilateral internal iliac lymph nodes in addition to the anal mass. The patient was staged as T3 N2 M0 (IIIB). He was started on fluconazole treatment for his pulmonary cryptococcosis, and on discharge he was referred to an outpatient HIV clinic, where a highly active antiretroviral therapy (HARRT) was initiated. Six weeks later, the patient had an undetectable HIV viral load and was started on the Nigro protocol with concurrent chemotherapy and XRT (59 Gy). The patient tolerated the treatment well without the need for any delays or dose reductions. Anoscopy performed 2 months later showed a complete resolution of the anal mass and CT scanning of the abdomen and pelvis demonstrated no lymphadenopathy, consistent with a complete response to therapy.

A posttreatment surveillance CT scan at 6 months showed a new 6.0 cm hypodense mass in the right hepatic lobe along with the re-appearance of retroperitoneal lymphadenopathy. A liver biopsy was performed and the pathology was consistent with invasive squamous carcinoma. He did not return for any chemotherapy appointments, and was subsequently lost to follow-up.

Evidence-Based Case Discussion

F.A. initially had stage IIIB SCCA and after an initial complete response to therapy subsequently developed stage IV SCCA. Of note, he completed standard dose concurrent chemotherapy and XRT while on HAART despite having a low CD4 count and an opportunistic infection 6 weeks before. This case demonstrates that HIV-infected patients with low CD4 counts can often tolerate standard dose therapy, as long as the patients demonstrate a response to HAART therapy, resulting in an undetectable HIV viral load.

Although concurrent chemotherapy and XRT in the treatment of early stages of SCCA is generally effective, there is up to a 40% rate of locoregional failure (15) and salvage surgery with an APR would be then the next appropriate step unless the recurrence is associated with distant metastasis. The most common sites of metastases outside of the pelvis are the liver, lung, and extrapelvic lymph nodes. For metastatic disease, systemic treatment with cisplatin combined with 5-FU is generally the most active and effective palliative treatment regimen with an overall response rate of approximately 66% (16,17) and a 5-year survival of 19% (Table 12.2).

HIV-infected patients with SCCA should be treated similar to those who are HIV-uninfected. However, patients with active opportunistic infections and/or with poorly controlled HIV as reflected by low CD4 counts or detectable HIV viral loads (due to poor compliance or drug resistance) may not be able to tolerate full doses of mitomycin. In a retrospective study that compared 20 HIV-infected patients versus 24 HIV-uninfected patients, both the objective initial response rate and median overall survival were superior in HIV-uninfected patients (50% vs. 88% and 18 months vs. 28 months, respectively; $P < .01$). However, patients who were HIV-infected had a higher incidence of lymph node metastases (60% vs. 17%, respectively) and were less likely to have received combined-modality therapy (25% vs. 54%, respectively), which likely accounted for the inferior results (18).

A more recent series compared 17 immunodeficient (ID) HIV-infected patients with 19 immune competent (IC) HIV-uninfected patients and concluded that there was no significant relationship between the CD4 count and treatment-related acute toxicities even when CD4 counts were less than 200 cells/μL. In addition, there was also no difference in terms of overall survival, with 3-year overall survival reported as 83.6% (95% CI, 68.2–100) and 91.7% (95% CI, 77.3–100) in the IC and ID group, respectively. The disease-specific survival was 88.2% (95% CI =74.2–100) in the IC group and 91.7% (95% CI = 77.3–100) in the ID group. Finally, APR-free survival was 78.3% (95% CI =61.5–99.5) and 80.9% (95% CI = 63.4–100) in the IC and ID groups, respectively (19).

Other Special Considerations for HIV-Infected Patients

Given the fact that the risk for SCCA is significantly higher among HIV-infected individuals, and the fact that HIV-infected patients who are not on effective HIV therapy may not tolerate chemotherapy and XRT, screening of all new SCCA cases for HIV should be considered as a part of any standard SCCA diagnostic work up (Figure 12.1). Finally, for individuals already known to be HIV-infected, SCCA screening among high-risk patient populations, using anal cytology, has been advocated. In particular, it has been shown that yearly pap testing of HIV-infected men who have sex with men is cost-effective and has a cost per quality adjusted life year (QALY) similar to other accepted cancer screening programs such as colon cancer screening with colonoscopy (20).

REFERENCES

1. Jemal A, Siegel R, Ward E, et al. Cancer statistics, 2009. *CA Cancer J Clin`*. 2009; 59(4):225–249.
2. Abel ME, Chiu YSY, Russell TR, et al. Adenocarcinoma of the anal glands: Results of a survey. *Dis Colon Rectum*. 1993; 36(4):383–387.
3. Johnson LG, Madeleine MM, Newcomer LM, et al. Anal cancer incidence and survival: the surveillance, epidemiology, and end results experience, 1973–2000. *Cancer*. 2004;101(2):281–288.
4. Joseph DA, Miller JW, Wu X, et al. Understanding the burden of human papillomavirus-associated anal cancers in the US. *Cancer*. 2008;113(10 Suppl):2892–2900.
5. Frisch M, Johansen C. Anal carcinoma in inflammatory bowel disease. *Br J Cancer*. 2000;83(1):89–90.
6. Grulich AE, van Leeuwen MT, Falster MO, et al. Incidence of cancers in people with HIV/AIDS compared with immunosuppressed transplant recipients: a meta-analysis. *Lancet*. 2007;370(9581):59–67.
7. Palefsky JM, Holly EA, Ralston ML, et al, Anal squamous intraepithelial lesions in HIV-positive and HIV-negative homosexual and bisexual men: prevalence and risk factors. *J Acquir Immune Defic Syndr Hum Retrovirol*. 1998;17(4):320–326
8. Daling JR, Weiss NS, Hislop TG, et al. Sexual practices, sexually transmitted diseases, and the incidence of anal cancer. *N Engl J Med*, 1987;317(16):973–977.
9. Holly EA, Whittemore AS, Aston DA, et al. Anal cancer incidence: genital warts, anal fissure or fistulsa, hemorrhoids and smoking. *J Natl Cancer Inst*, 1989;81(22):1726–1731.
10. Bilimoria KY, Bentrem DJ, Rock CE, et al. Outcomes and prognostic factors for squamous-cell carcinoma of the anal canal: analysis of patients from the National Cancer Data Base. *Dis Colon Rectum*. 2009;52:624.
11. Winton E, Heriot AG, Ng M, et al. The impact of PET scan on the staging, management and outcome of anal cancer. *Br J Cancer*. 2009;100(5):693–700.
12. Leichman L, Nigro N, Vaitkevicius VK, et al. Cancer of the anal canal. Model for preoperative adjuvant combined modality therapy. *Am J Med*. 1985;78(2):211–215.
13. Flam M, John M, Pajak TF, et al. Role of mitomycine in combination with fluorouracil and radiotherapy, and of salvage chemoradiation in the definitive nonsurgical treatment of epidermoid carcinoma of the anal canal: results of a phase III randomized intergroup study. *J Clin Oncol*. 1996;14:2527–2539.
14. Ajani JA, Winter KA, Gunderson LL, et al. Fluorouracil, mitomycin, and radiotherapy vs. fluorouracil, cisplatin, and radiotherapy for carcinoma of the anal canal. A randomized controlled trial. *JAMA*. 2008;299:1914–1921.
15. Mullen JT, Rodriguez-bigas MA, Change GJ, et al. Results of surgical salvage after failed chemo radiation therapy for epidermoid carcinoma of the anal canal. *Ann Surg Oncol*. 2007:14:478–483
16. Faivre C, Rougier P, Ducreux M, et al. 5-Fluorouracile and cisplatinum combination chemotherapy for metastatic squamous-cell anal cancer. *Cancer*. 1999;86(10):861–865.
17. Tanum G. Treatment of relapsing anal carcinoma. *Acta Oncol*. 1993;32(1):33–35.
18. Vatra B, Sobhani I, Aparicio T, et al. Anal canal squamous-cell carcinomas in HIV positive patients: clinical features, treatments and prognosis, *Gastroenterol Clin Biol*. 2002;26(2):147–149.
19. Seo Y, Kinsella MT, Reynolds HL, et al. Outcomes of chemoradiotherapy with 5-fluorouracil and mitomycin C for anal cancer in immunocompetent versus immunodeficient patients. *Int J Radiat Oncol Biol Phys*. 2009;75(1):143–149.
20. Goldie SJ, Kuntz KM, Weinstein MC, et. al. The clinical effectiveness and cost-effectiveness of screening for anal squamous intraepithelial lesions in homosexual and bisexual HIV-positive men. *JAMA*. 1999;281(19):1822–1829.

13

Prostate Cancer

JINGSONG ZHANG, KATHLEEN A. COONEY, AND MAHA H. HUSSAIN

EPIDEMIOLOGY, RISK FACTORS, NATURAL HISTORY, AND PATHOLOGY

Prostate cancer is the most common nonskin cancer diagnosed among U.S. men with approximately 220,000 new cases annually. It remains the second leading cause of cancer deaths in men resulting in the loss of nearly 32,000 lives in 2010. On the basis of the data collected between 1975 and 2004 from the Surveillance Epidemiology and End Results (SEER), the lifetime risk of developing prostate cancer for American men is 16%, but the risk of dying of prostate cancer is only 2.9%.

Age, race, and positive family history are the most important recognized risk factors for prostate cancer. Approximately 10% of all prostate cancer cases are diagnosed in men less than 55 years of age, and the incidence of prostate cancer increases with age. The incidence of prostate cancer varies tremendously by race with generally lower incidence rates in Asian men and high incidence rates in African American men. African American men also suffer from excess mortality from prostate cancer.

Familial clustering of prostate cancer has been widely reported since the early 1990s. Since then, a number of different studies have been conducted to measure the impact of family history on the risk of prostate cancer. Review of this literature reveals several important factors about family history of prostate cancer that are associated with increased risk of disease, and these include young age at diagnosis, the number of affected relatives, and the degree of relatedness of affected relatives (1). In addition, having an affected brother is associated with a higher risk compared with only having an affected father. Much research has been conducted to identify the genetic basis for familial clustering of prostate cancer, however, to date, no highly penetrant prostate cancer susceptibility genes have been identified that account for disease in a significant number of families.

Prostate-specific antigen (PSA) is a serum protease that became widely used around 1990 to diagnose prostate cancer and monitor disease activity. As a screening test, PSA lacks specificity and a number of algorithms have been developed to enhance its utility including the use of age-specific reference ranges and studies of free versus complexed PSA. Use of PSA in combination with digital rectal examination or DRE provides the ability to diagnose prostate cancer in an asymptomatic period. As a result of widespread use of PSA for diagnosis, there has been stage migration toward more localized stage prostate cancer. In addition, use of PSA testing has contributed to overdiagnosis and overtreatment of low-risk prostate cancers (defined as low-grade/small-volume tumors). Current recommendations regarding prostate cancer screening emphasize the use of patient preferences for specific health outcomes as an important factor.

Over 95% of all prostate cancers are adenocarcinomas. The remaining types of prostate cancer include entities such as mucinous adenocarcinoma, large cell neuroendocrine tumors, small cell carcinoma, and sarcomatoid carcinoma. The Gleason histological grading system provides microscopic evaluation of prostate adenocarcinoma using a five-point grading scale. The Gleason score is based on the sum of the score for the most common or primary pattern followed by the second most common or secondary pattern (e.g., 4 + 3 = 7). Since its introduction several decades ago, the Gleason score has been recognized as one of the most powerful prognostic factors for prostate adenocarcinoma, and it is now incorporated in the current edition of AJCC's (American Joint Committee on Cancer) prostate cancer staging and prognostic grouping.

STAGING

The current (7th Edition) AJCC staging system for prostate cancer that incorporates both the Gleason score and the PSA is shown in the following table.

Prostate Cancer

Stage	Description
I	A clinically inapparent tumor (T1a-c) as an incidental finding from a transurethral resection of the prostate (TURP) or needle biopsy performed for an elevated PSA (<10 ng/mL) with a Gleason score ≤6. OR A tumor confined to one-half of one lobe or less of the prostate (T2a) with a PSA <10 ng/mL and a Gleason score ≤6 OR A T1–2a tumor with an unknown PSA and Gleason score
IIA	A clinically inapparent tumor (T1a-c) with a PSA <20 ng/mL and a Gleason score of 7 OR A T1a-c tumor with a PSA ≥10≤20 ng/mL with a Gleason score of ≤6 OR A tumor confined to one-half of one lobe or less of the prostate (T2a) with a PSA ≥ 10 ≤20 ng/mL with a Gleason score ≤6 OR A T2a tumor with a PSA <20 ng/mL and a Gleason score of 7 OR A tumor involving more than one-half of one lobe of the prostate (T2b) with a PSA <20 ng/mL and a Gleason score of ≤7 OR A T2b tumor with an unknown PSA and Gleason score
IIB	A tumor involving both lobes of the prostate (T2c) with any PSA and Gleason score OR A T1 or T2 tumor with a PSA≥20 ng/mL and any Gleason score OR A T1 or T2 tumor with any PSA and a Gleason score ≥8
III	A tumor with extracapsular extension (T3a) or invasion of seminal vesicles (T3b) with any PSA or Gleason score
IV	A tumor that is fixed or invades adjacent structures other than seminal vesicles (T4) (e.g., bladder neck, rectum, pelvic wall) with any PSA or Gleason score OR Any tumor with metastases to regional lymph nodes (N1) and any PSA or Gleason score OR Any tumor, with or without regional lymph node metastases with distant metastases in other sites (M1) (e.g., bone, nonregional lymph nodes)

CASE SUMMARIES

Locally Advanced, High-Risk Prostate Cancer

A.M. is a 60-year-old African American man who presented to his personal physician with a several month history of urinary hesitancy and dribbling. DRE was notable for bilateral nodularity of the prostate gland and fixation of the gland to the pelvic sidewall. His serum PSA was 6.3 ng/mL and the patient reported no prior PSA tests. The patient's past medical history was significant for coronary artery disease, insulin-dependent diabetes mellitus, hypertension, and obesity with a body mass index (BMI) of 34. His family history was positive for prostate cancer diagnosis in one of his two brothers. A transurethral resection of the prostate (TURP) was performed for symptom management, which revealed adenocarcinoma of the prostate, Gleason score 5 + 5 = 10, extensively involving multiple prostate chips. A staging evaluation including CT scan of the abdomen and pelvis as well as a bone scan failed to reveal evidence of distant metastases. Therefore A.M. was considered to have a clinical stage IV, T4 N0 M0 Gleason 10 adenocarcinoma of the prostate.

After evaluation by urology, medical oncology, and radiation oncology, A.M. was enrolled on RTOG 0521, which is a phase III clinical trial assessing the addition of docetaxel and prednisone to androgen suppression in patients with clinically localized, high-risk prostate cancer treated with three-dimensional conformal radiation therapy or intensity modulation radiation therapy (3DCRT/IMRT). The patient was randomized to receive radiation therapy and androgen suppression without chemotherapy. He received 75.6 Gy of IMRT in 1.8 Gy fractions plus neoadjuvant (8 weeks), concurrent and then adjuvant androgen deprivation therapy (ADT) with leuprolide every 12 weeks for a total of 2 years and the oral antiandrogen bicalutamide.

A.M.'s PSA was less than 0.1 ng/mL when he finished radiation therapy and his PSA remained low when he received the last (eighth) dose of leuprolide. The main complications of treatment experienced by the patient were urinary leakage, fatigue, sexual difficulty, and hot flashes. He maintained his BMI around 34 during the 2 years of ADT. A.M. experienced an acute myocardial infarction after 1 year of ADT, which was followed by a three-vessel coronary artery bypass graft procedure.

Approximately 1 year after completion of androgen deprivation, A.M.'s PSA rose to 1.8 ng/mL therapy and then 7.4 ng/mL after 3 months. Restaging bone scan, chest x-ray, abdomen, and pelvis CT were performed, which showed diffuse axial skeletal metastases. The patient was restarted on combined ADT with leuprolide and bicalutamide but experienced continued rise of his serum PSA indicating presence of castrate-resistant disease.

Evidence-Based Case Discussion

A.M. was at an increased risk for developing prostate cancer because he has a first-degree relative (brother) with prostate cancer and because he is an African American. Based on the lack of clinical trial data that treatment of asymptomatic prostate cancer cases diagnosed by use of serum PSA and/or DRE improves health outcomes, the U.S. Preventative Services Task Force concludes that "the current evidence is insufficient to assess the balance of benefits and harms of prostate cancer screening in men younger than age 75 years" (2). However, other medical organizations recommend that physicians discuss the risks and benefits of participation in prostate cancer early detection strategies beginning at age 50 for men with at least a 10-year life expectancy. For high-risk individuals such as A.M. (African American, positive family history), some groups such as the American Cancer Society recommend considering prostate cancer early detection beginning at age 45. Whether prostate cancer screening beginning at age 45 would have identified A.M.'s cancer at a time when it was localized and therefore amenable to surgery is unknown.

The majority of prostate cancer cases detected by screening with PSA and/or DRE are considered localized and therefore amenable to several different approaches. Men with low-risk prostate cancer (including some/all of the following features: clinical T1c, Gleason score ≤ 6, PSA < 10 ng/mL, fewer than three biopsy cores positive and each less than 50% tumor) may be considered for active surveillance. Men considered to be at higher risk of recurrence based on larger tumors with higher Gleason score (score = 7) and/or higher PSA values (up to 20 ng/mL) are recommended to be treated definitively with external beam radiation therapy (EBRT) or radical prostatectomy (3).

A.M. was diagnosed with stage IV prostate cancer on the basis of the local extension to the pelvic side wall (T4). The cancer involved a significant percentage of the gland as demonstrated in the TURP pathology specimen and was high grade (Gleason 10). Surgery was not possible given the extension to the pelvis side wall, therefore limiting the treatment choices to radiation therapy or hormonal therapy achieved through androgen deprivation. Given the absence of metastatic disease and need for control of local disease, the multidisciplinary approach selected for this patient was radiation therapy with ADT.

Evidence Supports Adding ADT to Radiation Therapy for High-Risk Prostate Cancer

In an analysis of 500 patients treated with radiation therapy alone for clinically localized prostate cancer, Pisansky et al. (4) noted that clinical tumor stage, Gleason score of the diagnostic biopsy, and pretreatment PSA level were all independently associated with clinical relapse. Using these factors, the investigators were able to separate patients into low-, intermediate-, and high-risk groups with distinct relapse-free probabilities at 5 years after radiation therapy (92%, 67%, and 24%, respectively; $P < .0001$). In the most recent National Comprehensive Cancer Network (NCCN) guideline (3) patients with T3b or T4 prostate cancer were separated from the high-risk group and defined as very high risk or locally advanced cancers.

Several phase III clinical trials reported that adding ADT to radiation therapy improved survival of men with localized, high-risk prostate cancer. The RTOG 85–31 study randomized 977 patients with either clinical T3 or T2 prostate cancer with regional lymph node involvement to either EBRT alone versus EBRT with indefinite goserelin starting at the last week of EBRT. When the updated results were published in 2005, the median follow-up time was 7.6 years for all patients and 11 years for living patients (5). The addition of indefinite ADT to EBRT significantly reduced the 10-year disease specific mortality and improved the 10-year absolute survival rates.

In the EORTC study by Bolla et al. (6), 415 patients were randomly assigned to either EBRT alone or EBRT plus 3 years of goserelin starting at the first day of radiation. Cyproterone acetate (150 mg orally) was given for 1 month starting 1 week before the first goserelin injection. Among these patients, 82% had T3 disease, 9% had T4 disease, and rest of the participants had WHO grade 3 T1-T2 disease. When reported at a median follow-up of 5.5 years, adding ADT to EBRT significantly improved the 5-year clinical disease-free survival (primary endpoint) (74% vs. 40%; $P = .0001$) and the 5-year overall survival (secondary endpoint) (78% vs. 62%; $P = .0002$). Extended follow-up with a median of 9.1 years confirmed the improved disease-free and overall survival without an increase in cardiovascular toxicity.

RTOG 92-02 randomized over 1500 patients with clinical T2c to T4 disease to either (a) a 4-month course of combined ADT or (b) ADT (goserelin plus flutamide) given for 2 months prior to and then concurrently with radiation therapy (70.2 Gy) or (c) 4 months of combined ADT plus radiation therapy followed by androgen suppression with goserelin alone for a total of 2 years. In this study, the addition of long-term adjuvant androgen deprivation significantly improved disease-free survival but not overall survival of patients with localized high-risk prostate cancer (7).

Although there is no consensus on the optimal duration of adjuvant ADT, this decision should be tailored to the patients' comorbidities, life expectancy, as well as expected tolerance to treatments. As per the available data, at least three years of ADT is required to improve overall survival. Improving cure rate and survival with minimum toxicity would be the ultimate goal of adjuvant trials. The efficacy and safety of adding adjuvant chemotherapy with docetaxel and prednisone to adjuvant ADT will be determined by the RTOG 0521 study. Until more effective treatment is available, long-term (at least 3 years) adjuvant ADT is considered the standard of care for patients with high-risk prostate cancer who elect radiation therapy.

Recognizing and Managing Side Effects of Long-Term ADT

Although generally less toxic than cytotoxic chemotherapy, prolonged ADT is not without side effects, which include hot flashes, fatigue, loss of libido, and a decline in sexual function. Recently, however, significant focus has been placed on metabolic consequences from ADT. A number of studies in the past two decades have highlighted the increased risk of osteoporosis in men receiving ADT for prostate cancer. ADT has been shown to decrease bone mineral density (BMD) after as early as 6 months of treatment for either localized or metastatic prostate adenocarcinoma (8). Most of the bone loss occurred in lumbar spine, femur neck, and total hip. Loss of BMD serves as a surrogate marker for risks of fracture. Two large retrospective studies directly assessed the risks of fracture in men treated with GnRH agonist. Smith et al. used claims-based cohort of Medicare beneficiaries and demonstrated a significantly increased fracture risk in men with nonmetastatic prostate cancer treated with gonadotrophin releasing hormone (GnRH) agonist (n = 3887) versus those who were not (n = 7774) during a 7-year follow-up (9). Shahinian et al. studied the SEER-Medicare records of 50,613 men with prostate cancer (AJCC stage I to IV) and demonstrated a statistically significant relationship between the number of doses of GnRH agonist received during the 12 months after diagnosis and the subsequent risk of fracture (8).

There are a number of strategies used in the clinic to minimize potential bone loss related to ADT. Bisphosphonates have been shown to inhibit osteoclast activities and several studies have reported the role of bisphosphonates in preventing bone loss. Men on ADT should be assessed for osteoporosis soon after initiating ADT and at regular intervals while continuing on treatment. Unless contraindicated based on other health conditions, routine use of calcium (>1200 mg/day) and vitamin D supplements (800 IU/day) should be considered along with lifestyle modifications (exercise, smoking reduction, etc.). Oral bisphosphonate therapy should be considered for men starting ADT who already have significant evidence of osteoporosis. In a small study of men with severe osteopenia or osteoporosis (T-score of > –2.0) and receiving ADT for prostate cancer, once-weekly 70-mg alendronate significantly improved the BMD and decreased the risk of femoral neck fracture compared to a control group of men who did not receive alendronate (10).

The efficacy of intravenous bisphosphates in preventing bone loss in patients receiving ADT for nonmetastatic prostate cancer was also reported in several randomized placebo-controlled trials. Pamidronate given at 60 mg intravenously every 12 weeks compared to the placebo significantly decreased the loss of BMD in the lumbar spine, trochanter, and total hip, but not in the femoral neck at week 48 (11). Significant increase of BMD in femoral neck, lumbar spine, trochanter, and the total hip were reported with zoledronic acid (4 mg) administered intravenously every 3 months for a total of five doses. Compared to the placebo, the BMD differences at 1 year all reached a P-value of < .001. The effects of annual zoledronic acid was then studied in a 12-month study of 40 men with nonmetastatic prostate cancer who were receiving a GnRH agonist and had T scores more than –2.5. Compared to the pretreatment baseline, single dose of zoledronic acid also led to significant increase in BMD of the lumbar spine, trochanter, and the total hip at 12 months. The increase in BMD at the femoral neck, however, did not reach statistical significance (P = .06). Of note, all of the studies above focus on improving BMD but none has addressed the question of whether use of bisphosphonates decreases the clinically important risk of fracture in men with nonmetastatic prostate cancer on ADT.

Newer options for preventing osteoporosis include denosumab, which is a fully humanized monoclonal antibody that specifically binds to the receptor activator of nuclear factor-κB ligand or RANKL. RANKL is a member of the family of tumor necrosis factors and is a key mediator of osteoclast formation, function, and survival. In a randomized, double-blind phase III study, denosumab at a dose of 60 mg subcutaneously every 6 months compared to placebo significantly increased BMD and reduced the incidence of new vertebral fractures at 36 months (1.5%, vs. 3.9% with placebo, P = .006) among men receiving ADT for nonmetastatic prostate cancer (12). The significant differences in BMD between the two groups were seen as early as 1 month and sustained through 36 months. The adverse events reported at 24 months did not appear to be significantly different in the denosumab arm compared to the placebo arm.

Other complications of ADT relate to the observed decrease in lean body mass and increase in fat mass. These changes appear to be early adverse effects with minimal additional changes in body composition beyond 18 months of treatment. ADT also reduces insulin sensitivity while increasing low-density lipoprotein cholesterol, high-density lipoprotein cholesterol, and triglycerides. These metabolic changes are consistent with an increased incidence of cardiovascular diseases and diabetes mellitus reported by multiple large observational studies. Although no randomized trials have prospectively addressed the risks of cardiovascular diseases and diabetes associated with ADT, none of the prospective randomized trials demonstrated any increase in cardiovascular mortalities in the

ADT arms, and cardiovascular mortalities were found to be nonsignificant in retrospective analyses of randomized trials (13).

A.M. had a BMI of 34 before initiating ADT, which by definition classifies him as obese. He was encouraged to participate in an exercise routine and he maintained his BMI throughout the 2 years of ADT. Note that A.M. suffered an acute myocardial infarction in November 2007 during the leuprolide treatment; however, he had no signs of glucose intolerance even after two years of androgen deprivation.

PSA Recurrence

W.R. is a 65-year-old Caucasian man who was referred to a multidisciplinary urologic cancer clinic for evaluation and treatment of a rising PSA after primary treatment for localized prostate cancer. Previously, at age 58, he was found to have prostate cancer during an evaluation for an elevated PSA of 8, which was determined for screening purposes. His DRE was normal and a biopsy confirmed adenocarcinoma with Gleason 7 (3 + 4) histology. He underwent radical prostatectomy and the pathology report confirmed Gleason 7 adenocarcinoma with evidence of extracapsular extension and positive margins (stage III). Two of the dissected lymph nodes were negative for cancer. His PSA was undetectable 6 weeks after the operation. It was recommended to W.R. that he consider adjuvant radiation therapy but he declined.

W.R. was followed over the next several years and his PSA increased from below 0.1 ng/mL to 0.6 ng/mL. By 5 years after radical prostatectomy, his PSA reached 2.3 ng/mL. Imaging studies including bone scan, abdominal CT, and pelvic CT were negative for metastatic disease. At this time, he underwent salvage radiation therapy (RT) (66.6 gray total) to the prostatic bed. His PSA declined to 1.2 ng/mL, 4 months after completion of radiation; however, 3 months later it increased to 10.7. Radiological imaging for metastatic cancer was again negative. On further evaluation, W.R. remained completely asymptomatic from his prostate cancer. His repeat PSA in 8 weeks stabilized at around 11.0 ng/mL. W.R. expressed concerns about the potential side effects of ADT and he subsequently enrolled into an immunotherapy trial.

Evidence-Based Case Discussion

W.R. was diagnosed with prostate cancer based on elevated screening serum PSA despite the absence of clinical symptoms. The fact that his biopsy Gleason score was 7 placed him in the intermediate-risk category for recurrence. However, it is important to consider that the majority of men who undergo radical prostatectomy are cured (3). Postsurgical monitoring for prostate cancer includes a serum PSA checked every 6 to 12 months for 5 years and then annually. Given the long natural history of prostate cancer, it is currently not known when PSA surveillance can be discontinued.

PSA Recurrence: Definition and Risk Stratification

Serum PSA is very sensitive for detecting recurrence after definitive local treatment for prostate cancer, which leads to the identification of men with a PSA-only or biochemical recurrence. According to the American Urological Association (AUA) guidelines, a biochemical recurrence after radical prostatectomy is defined as a serum PSA > 0.2 ng/mL, with a second confirmatory level of PSA of >0.2 ng/mL. Since some prostatic glandular tissues remain after radiation therapy, serum PSA levels are unlikely to fall to undetectable levels and typically will not reach a nadir until 1 year after completion of radiation therapy. To account for the variable PSA kinetics after different forms of radiation therapy, a consensus committee proposed the "Phoenix Definition" of PSA failure, which is defined as a PSA rise by 2 ng/mL or more above the postradiotherapy nadir.

Several studies have demonstrated that PSA doubling time (PSADT) at the time of PSA recurrence is an important marker to predict prostate-cancer-specific mortality. Using multi-institutional databases, D'Amico et al. analyzed the outcome of 8669 patients treated with radical prostatectomy or radiation therapy for clinical stage T1c-4 NX or N0 M0 prostate adenocarcinoma between 1988 and January 2002. For men with PSADT of less than 3 months, the hazard ratios for the time to prostate-cancer-specific and all-cause mortality were 19.6 and 6.9, respectively (14). Freeland et al. conducted a retrospective study of 379 men who underwent radical prostatectomy at Johns Hopkins Hospital between 1982 and 2000 and confirmed the value of PSADT for time to prostate-cancer-specific mortality (HR of 27.48 for PSADT <3 months and 8.76 for PSADT between 3 and 8.9 months). Recurrence within 3 years of radical prostatectomy and Gleason score of 8 or above were also important predictors of time to prostate-cancer-specific mortality (HR of 3.53 and 2.26 respectively) (15). The role of Gleason score of 8 or above in PCSM was also shown by D'Amico's study of 1159 men who developed PSA failure after initial definitive treatment with surgery or radiation (16).

Adjuvant Radiotherapy for Pathologically Advanced Prostate Cancer

Adjuvant radiotherapy is often considered in men with adverse pathological features, and these include positive surgical margins, extracapsular invasion, and involvement of the seminal vesicles or a combination of these features. Both SWOG 8794 and EORTC 22911 compared radical prostatectomy alone to radical prostatectomy and immediate salvage RT for men with pT3 cancers or with positive surgical margins. Neither study excluded patients with detectable postoperative PSA levels. When the EORTC 22911 trial was reported after a median follow-up of 5 years, 60 Gy adjuvant radiotherapy significantly improved biochemical progression-free survival and local control compared to observation, but not overall survival (17). SWOG 8794 had a longer follow-up and, with a median follow-up of 12.6 years, showed that the adjuvant external beam radiotherapy with 60 to 64 Gy to the prostatic fossa significantly improved both metastasis-free and overall survival compared to observation (18). Notably, only one third of the patients originally assigned to observation received salvage RT at the time of a biochemical recurrence, and these results cannot be used to compare a strategy of adjuvant RT with observation followed by salvage RT at the first sign of PSA recurrence. Adverse effects of radiotherapy include rectal complications (3.3% vs. 0% in observation), urethral strictures (17.8% vs. 9.5%) and total urinary incontinence (6.5% vs. 2.8 %) (19).

Salvage Radiotherapy

For some men with low-level PSA recurrences after radical prostatectomy and life expectancy greater than 10 years, salvage RT can be considered. Salvage RT is typically limited to the prostatic fossa. Based on the available PSA data, W.R. had a PSA recurrence within 3 years of initial radical prostatectomy. Unfortunately, he was not evaluated for salvage radiotherapy until his PSA increased from 0.6 to 2.3. Multiple retrospective studies have shown that PSA level prior to salvage radiotherapy is the most consistent variable associated with the PSA-relapse-free outcome after salvage radiotherapy, that is, the lower the PSA level at the time of salvage RT, the better the treatment outcome. On the basis of the available evidence prior to 1999, the American Society for Therapeutic Radiology and Oncology (ASTRO) consensus panel concluded that the appropriate PSA cut point for salvage radiotherapy "seemed to be 1.5 ng/mL." Stephenson et al. (20) developed a nomogram to predict outcome of salvage radiotherapy based on a pooled cohort of over 1500 patients. Significant variables in the model were PSA level before salvage treatment, prostatectomy Gleason grade, PSA doubling time, surgical margins, ADT before or during salvage RT, and lymph node status. This nomogram has a reported concordance index of 0.69 and is currently available at: http://www.mskcc.org/applications/nomograms/prostate/PostRadicalProstatectomy.aspx

Based on W.R.'s high presalvage radiotherapy PSA, it is not surprising that he experienced a PSA progression shortly after salvage radiotherapy. Fortunately, his PSA stabilized around 10 after the initial rapid rise. The patient was offered ADT for biochemical recurrence but he declined. It is not uncommon to see men refuse ADT when they are asymptomatic and there is no radiological evidence of advanced disease due to the side-effect profile and noncurative potential of this treatment.

Metastatic Prostate Cancer

J.T. is a 62-year-old Hispanic man who was referred to a multidisciplinary urologic cancer clinic for treatment of metastatic prostate cancer. The patient initially presented with a PSA of 39 ng/mL and he was diagnosed with clinical stage IIB, T2c, Gleason 8 (4 + 4) prostate adenocarcinoma. Imaging studies were negative for metastatic diseases. He underwent external beam radiation treatment (78 Gy) with the initial plan of a total of 2 years ADT. His PSA was 3.2 ng/mL 3 months after completing radiation therapy. It then started to increase shortly afterward and J.T. was maintained on continuous ADT. His PSA continued to progress despite the addition of bicalutamide and subsequent bicalutamide withdrawal. He was eventually found to have metastatic cancer to the bone and lymph nodes when his PSA jumped to 220 ng/mL. Clinically, he experienced painful bone metastases and weight loss.

The patient was started on docetaxel at 75 mg/m^2 every 3 weeks, oral prednisone (10 mg/day), and monthly intravenous zoledronic acid. His symptoms significantly improved after two cycles of chemotherapy and his PSA declined from 220 ng/mL to 140 ng/mL after four cycles of therapy. Cycle 5 of therapy was delayed for 3 months due to multiple admissions for atypical chest pain and non-neutropenic fever of unknown source. During the 3-month break from chemotherapy, the patient's PSA increased to 1190 ng/mL. Docetaxel was restarted but he soon developed recurrent diffuse bone pain and intermittent epigastric pain. A repeat CT and bone scan when compared with prechemotherapy scans showed progressive metastatic disease. No apparent source for the epigastric pain was found despite comprehensive workups. He received one dose of samarium^{153} for diffuse bone pain.

Docetaxel and prednisone was restarted at the same dose as before with monthly zoledronic acid. His bone pain had resolved after one cycle of docetaxel and prednisone. His PSA dropped from 1800 ng/mL to 8.5 ng/mL after five cycles of docetaxel and prednisone administered with neulasta support.

Evidence-Based Case Discussion

Castration-Resistant Prostate Cancer: Definition and Treatment Options

Castration-resistant prostate cancer (CRPC) is defined as disease progression evidenced by increasing serum PSA values or progressive disease on radiological imaging studies despite a castrate level of testosterone (<50 ng/dL or 17 nmol/lL). Current treatment options for CRPC include secondary ADT, sipuluecel-T, chemotherapy with docetaxel, or clinical trials. Cabazitaxel is indicated for CRPC post-docetaxel failure and mitoxantrone is an option for post-cabazitaxel (Figure 13.1).

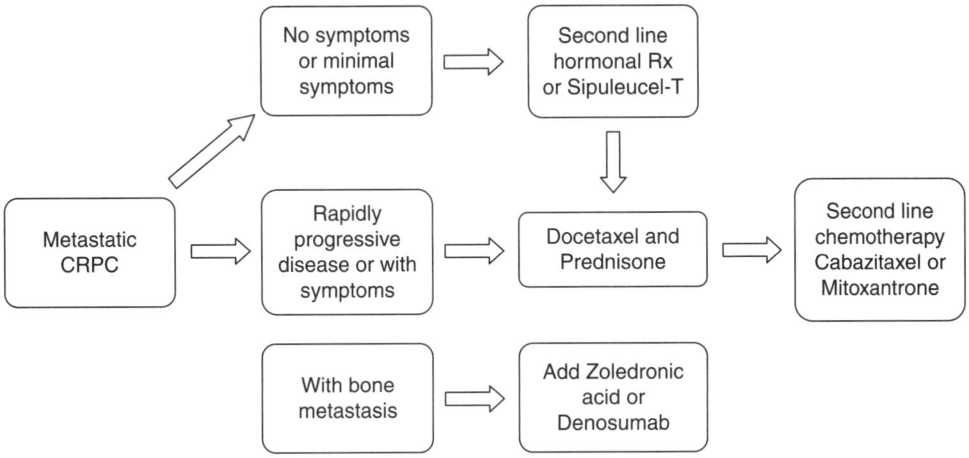

Figure 13.1

Treatment algorithm for the metastatic castration resistant prostate cancer (CRPC).

In men with CRPC who are asymptomatic, antiandrogen withdrawal followed by secondary hormonal therapy with steroids or ketoconazole and hydrocortisone is often attempted. Withdrawal responses have been reported in approximately 20% of men treated with a variety of antiandrogens including both flutamide and bicalutamide. As demonstrated by a phase III CALGB 9583 study, antiandrogen withdrawal and immediate addition of ketoconazole can result in approximately 30% PSA response rate although with no impact on survival (21).

Chemotherapy for Metastatic Castrate-Resistant Prostate Cancer

J.T.'s Gleason 8 prostate adenocarcinoma became castrate resistant within 2 years of diagnosis with a rapid development of symptoms. Docetaxel-based chemotherapy has been shown to improve pain, quality of life, as well as survival in chemotherapy-naive metastatic CRPC patients. In the TAX-327 trial, 1006 men were randomly assigned to docetaxel (75 mg/m^2 every 3 weeks), docetaxel (30 mg/m^2, 5 weeks on 1 week off), or mitoxantrone (12 mg/m^2 every 3 weeks) (22). Among the three treatment arms, docetaxel administered every 3 weeks plus daily prednisone led to superior survival, pain palliation, and quality of life improvement. With 3.5 years of additional follow-up, the survival benefits of docetaxel plus prednisone have persisted with median survival of 16.3 months in the mitoxantrone group, 17.8 months in the weekly docetaxel group, and 19.2 months in the every 3-week docetaxel group (23). Of note, all patients were continued on maintenance androgen suppression and received prednisone 5 mg orally twice a day.

At the time of consultation, several factors would contribute to J.T.'s rapidly progressing disease: aggressive nature of his CRPC, delays in cytotoxic chemotherapy and ADT. The results of phase III studies have shown the utility of the bone-seeking radiopharmaceutical samarium^{153} in palliating pain associated with bone metastases (24,25). Pain relief was observed in 62% to 72% of those who received the 1.0-mCi/kg dose during the first 4 weeks, with marked or complete relief noted in 31% by week 4 (24). Although a phase I study demonstrated the feasibility of combining samarium^{153} with docetaxel chemotherapy, the antitumor efficacy of samarium remains to be determined.

When J.T. demonstrated rapid progression of metastatic cancer during the several month delay of chemotherapy, another strategy would be to change to treatment with cabazitaxel. Cabazitaxel was approved for second-line therapy of CRPC based on the phase III TROPIC trial. In this trial, cabazitaxel plus prednisone resulted in a significantly improved progression-free survival and overall survival compared to mitoxantrone plus prednisone in men with progressive disease during or after treatment with a docetaxel-containing regimen (26). Although J.T.'s post–cycle 5 imaging studies documented progressive diseases compared to his prechemotherapy scans, there was a 3-month delay between cycle 4 and 5 treatments. He had previously demonstrated a significant PSA decline after 4 cycles of docetaxel treatment. Restarting docetaxel and daily prednisone was a reasonable choice for him as demonstrated by the excellent clinical response after re-initiation of this treatment. Since there are several FDA-approved treatment options for CRPC including docetaxel, cabazitaxel, and mitoxantrone, one strategy commonly pursued is to maximize the efficacy of each therapy and save as many treatment options as possible for the future. After all, none of the current systemic therapies has been shown to be curative for metastatic CRPC.

Bone-Targeted Therapy in Metastatic Prostate Cancer

J.T. received monthly intravenous zoledronic acid for metastatic CRPC to the bone. In patients who are asymptomatic or minimally symptomatic from metastatic CRPC to the bone, the administration of zoledronic acid at 4 mg

(N = 214) versus placebo (N = 208) every 3 weeks for 15 months significantly reduced skeletal-related events—which are defined as pathologic bone fractures, spinal cord compression, a change of antineoplastic therapy to treat bone pain, surgery, or radiation therapy to bone (27). Conversely, the combined analysis of two multicenter, double-blind, randomized, placebo-controlled trials with intravenous pamidronate disodium (90 mg) administered every 3 weeks for 27 weeks failed to palliate the bone pain or reduce skeletal-related events compared with placebo in patients with bone pain due to castration-resistant metastatic prostate cancer. Accordingly, zoledronic acid as a more potent bisphosphonate is approved by FDA in patients with metastatic CRPC.

Most recently, subcutaneous denosumab was compared to intravenous zoledronic acid in a phase III noninferiority trial involving 1904 patients with CRPC metastasized to the bone (28). Subcutaneous denosumab 120 mg every 4 weeks was superior to intravenous zoledronic acid 4 mg every 4 weeks in preventing or delaying the first and multiple skeletal-related events. No differences were observed in progression-free survival or overall survival. Compared with zoledronic acid, there were more events of hypocalcemia, but less acute phase reactions with denosumab. Cumulative incidences of osteonecrosis of the jaw during 2 years of therapy were 1% in zoledronic acid and 2% in denosumab.

In addition to inhibiting osteoclast function with bisphosphonates or denosumab, osteoblast function can also be inhibited by inhibitor of endothelin-A receptor A (ETA). Atrasentan is a highly potent, selective ETA receptor antagonist. Atrasentan at 10 mg per day, however, did not delay disease progression (primary endpoint) compared with placebo in a randomized placebo-controlled phase III trial with 809 asymptomatic chemotherapy naïve metastatic CRPC patients (29).

Bone-targeted therapy represents a new strategy in cancer therapy, that is, targeting cancer microenvironment. Despite the promising preclinical data, its efficacy as a single agent in metastatic prostate cancer has not been proven. Combing bone-targeted treatment with cancer directed therapy would likely be the approach to improve endpoints like overall survival or progression-free survival.

REFERENCES

1. Zeegers MP, Jellema A, Ostrer H. Empiric risk of prostate carcinoma for relatives of patients with prostate carcinoma: a meta-analysis. *Cancer.* 2003;97(8):1894–1903.
2. Screening for prostate cancer: U.S. Preventive Services Task Force recommendation statement. *Ann Intern Med.* 2008;149(3): 185–191.
3. NCCN Clinical Practice Guidelines in Oncology—Prostate Cancer. NCCN Guidelines & Clinical Resources Version 1.2011, 2011. http://www.nccn.org/professionals/physician_gls/pdf/prostate.pdf
4. Pisansky TM, Kahn MJ, Rasp GM, et al. A multiple prognostic index predictive of disease outcome after irradiation for clinically localized prostate carcinoma. *Cancer.* 1997;79(2): 337–344.
5. Pilepich MV, Winter K, Lawton CA, et al. Androgen suppression adjuvant to definitive radiotherapy in prostate carcinoma—long-term results of phase III RTOG 85-31. *Int J Radiat Oncol Biol Phys.* 2005;61(5):1285–1290.
6. Bolla M, Van Tienhoven G, Warde P, et al. External irradiation with or without long-term androgen suppression for prostate cancer with high metastatic risk: 10-year results of an EORTC randomised study. *Lancet Oncol.* 2010;11(11):1066–1073.
7. Hanks GE, Pajak TF, Porter A, et al. Phase III trial of long-term adjuvant androgen deprivation after neoadjuvant hormonal cytoreduction and radiotherapy in locally advanced carcinoma of the prostate: the Radiation Therapy Oncology Group Protocol 92-02. *J Clin Oncol.* 2003;21(21):3972–3978.
8. Shahinian VB, Kuo YF, Freeman JL, et al. Risk of fracture after androgen deprivation for prostate cancer. *N Engl J Med.* 2005;352(2):154–164.
9. Smith MR, Lee WC, Brandman J, et al. Gonadotropin-releasing hormone agonists and fracture risk: a claims-based cohort study of men with nonmetastatic prostate cancer. *J Clin Oncol.* 2005;23(31):7897–7903.
10. Planas J, Trilla E, Raventos C, et al. Alendronate decreases the fracture risk in patients with prostate cancer on androgen-deprivation therapy and with severe osteopenia or osteoporosis. *BJU Int.* 2009;104(11):1637–1640.
11. Smith MR, McGovern FJ, Zietman AL, et al. Pamidronate to prevent bone loss during androgen-deprivation therapy for prostate cancer. *N Engl J Med.* 2001;345(13):948–955.
12. Smith MR, Egerdie B, Hernandez TN, et al. Denosumab in men receiving androgen-deprivation therapy for prostate cancer. *N Engl J Med.* 2009;361(8):745–755.
13. Levine GN, D'Amico AV, Berger P, et al. Androgen-deprivation therapy in prostate cancer and cardiovascular risk: a science advisory from the American Heart Association, American Cancer Society, and American Urological Association: endorsed by the American Society for Radiation Oncology. *CA Cancer J Clin.* 2010;60(3):194–201.
14. D'Amico AV, Moul JW, Carroll PR, et al. Surrogate end point for prostate cancer-specific mortality after radical prostatectomy or radiation therapy. *J Natl Cancer Inst.* 2003;95(18): 1376–1383.
15. Freedland SJ, Humphreys EB, Mangold LA, et al. Risk of prostate cancer-specific mortality following biochemical recurrence after radical prostatectomy. *JAMA.* 2005;294(4):433–439.
16. Zhou P, Chen MH, McLeod D, et al. Predictors of prostate cancer-specific mortality after radical prostatectomy or radiation therapy. *J Clin Oncol.* 2005;23(28):6992–6998.
17. Bolla M, van Poppel H, Collette L, et al. Postoperative radiotherapy after radical prostatectomy: a randomised controlled trial (EORTC trial 22911). *Lancet.* 2005;366(9485):572–578.
18. Thompson IM, Tangen CM, Paradelo J, et al. Adjuvant radiotherapy for pathological T3N0M0 prostate cancer significantly reduces risk of metastases and improves survival: long-term followup of a randomized clinical trial. *J Urol.* 2009;181(3):956–962.
19. Thompson IM, Tangen CM, Paradelo J, et al. Adjuvant radiotherapy for pathologically advanced prostate cancer: a randomized clinical trial. *JAMA.* 2006;296(19):2329–2335.
20. Stephenson AJ, Scardino PT, Kattan MW, et al. Predicting the outcome of salvage radiation therapy for recurrent prostate cancer after radical prostatectomy. *J Clin Oncol.* 2007;25(15): 2035–2041.
21. Small EJ, Halabi S, Dawson NA, et al. Antiandrogen withdrawal alone or in combination with ketoconazole in androgen-

independent prostate cancer patients: a phase III trial (CALGB 9583). *J Clin Oncol.* 2004;22(6):1025–1033.

22. Tannock IF, de Wit R, Berry WR, et al. Docetaxel plus prednisone or mitoxantrone plus prednisone for advanced prostate cancer. *N Engl J Med.* 2004;351(15):1502–1512.
23. Berthold DR, Pond GR, Soban F, et al. Docetaxel plus prednisone or mitoxantrone plus prednisone for advanced prostate cancer: updated survival in the TAX 327 study. *J Clin Oncol.* 2008;26(2):242–245.
24. Serafini AN, Houston SJ, Resche I, et al. Palliation of pain associated with metastatic bone cancer using samarium-153 lexidronam: a double-blind placebo-controlled clinical trial. *J Clin Oncol.* 1998;16(4):1574–1581.
25. Sartor O, Reid RH, Hoskin PJ, et al. Samarium-153-Lexidronam complex for treatment of painful bone metastases in hormone-refractory prostate cancer. *Urology.* 2004;63(5):940–945.
26. de Bono JS, Oudard S, Ozguroglu M, et al. Prednisone plus cabazitaxel or mitoxantrone for metastatic castration-resistant prostate cancer progressing after docetaxel treatment: a randomised open-label trial. *Lancet.* 2010;376(9747):1147–1154.
27. Saad F, Gleason DM, Murray R, et al. A randomized, placebo-controlled trial of zoledronic acid in patients with hormone-refractory metastatic prostate carcinoma. *J Natl Cancer Inst.* 2002;94(19):1458–1468.
28. Fizazi K, Carducci M, Smith M, et al. Denosumab versus zoledronic acid for treatment of bone metastases in men with castration-resistant prostate cancer: a randomised, double-blind study. *Lancet.* 2011;377(9768):813–822.
29. Carducci MA, Saad F, Abrahamsson PA, et al. A phase 3 randomized controlled trial of the efficacy and safety of atrasentan in men with metastatic hormone-refractory prostate cancer. *Cancer.* 2007;110(9):1959–1966.

14

Testicular Carcinoma

DIEGO BEDOYA AND MARTHA PRITCHETT MIMS

EPIDEMIOLOGY, RISK FACTORS, NATURAL HISTORY, AND PATHOLOGY

In many ways, testicular cancer represents a break from the common paradigm of solid malignancies. First, as the most common solid malignancy in males between the ages of 15 and 35 years, it usually affects a much younger population. Second, long-term survival is expected even in the presence of advanced disease with less than 400 deaths annually in the United States. Finally, staging of testicular cancer incorporates an additional element to the common Tumor, Node, and Metastasis (TNM) staging system: serum tumor markers.

An estimated 8400 new testicular cancer cases were observed in the United States in 2009 representing 1.1% of all solid tumors in men (1). Testicular cancer is most common in white males, with a lower incidence in Hispanics and the disease is relatively rare in African Americans. Data suggest an increasing incidence of testicular cancer over the last several decades, mostly restricted to seminoma in white males. The reasons for this increase are poorly understood.

Abdominal cryptorchidism is responsible for approximately 10% of testicular tumors (2). Interestingly, malignancy arises in the normally descended testicle in 25% of these cases. Prophylactic orchiectomy is recommended for cases of cryptorchidism presenting after puberty. The cumulative risk of a contralateral testicular cancer in men with a previous diagnosis of testicular cancer is 1.9% at 15 years, whereas the incidence of bilateral tumors at presentation is 1% to 5% (3). Risk is also increased in patients presenting with an extragonadal germ cell tumor especially those with retroperitoneal presentation. The relative risk of testicular cancer increases 6- to 10-fold in first-degree relatives of a patient diagnosed with testicular cancer. Intratubular germ cell neoplasia (carcinoma in situ) is commonly found in patients at risk for testicular cancer; the risk of progression is 50% at 5 years when left untreated. An increased incidence of testicular cancer has also been described in patients with hypospadias, HIV infection (seminomas), testicular microlithiasis, Klinefelter and Down's syndromes, and following exposure to exogenous estrogens in utero.

Most patients present with an incidental finding of a painless mass; however, about one third complain of a heavy sensation in the lower abdomen or perianal area. Acute pain and symptoms secondary to metastatic disease are each reported by about 10% of patients at presentation.

Germ cell tumors (GCTs) account for 95% of testicular cancer. Most of the remainder are sex cord stromal tumors. Other tumor types including lymphoma, leukemia, or plasmacytoma are exceedingly rare and will not be discussed in this chapter. For management purposes, GCTs are divided into seminomas and nonseminomatous germ cell tumors (NSGCTs), each accounting for roughly half of the cases. By definition, seminomas exist only in their pure form, whereas NSGCTs are usually composed of a mixture of different subtypes (including seminomatous components). Table 14.1 summarizes the primary differences between the subtypes. These data highlight the high prevalence of the most specific cytogenetic abnormality in testicular cancer, the gain of 12p-sequences, most commonly through isochromosome formation (i12p) (4). This cytogenetic abnormality has also been shown in some cases of testicular carcinoma in situ, suggesting a role in the early development of this malignancy. Although GCTs are usually differentiated and classified according to their morphology, occasionally immunohistochemical stains are required (Table 14.2) (5).

Unlike other solid malignancies, serum tumor markers have important implications in the diagnosis, management,

Table 14.1 Major Subtypes of Germ Cell Tumors

	Average Age at Diagnosis (years)	Contribution to Mixed NSGCT (%)	Serum Tumor Markers	i12p (%) (1)
Seminoma	40	20	AFP: Normal (2) β-hCG: normal or mildly elevated	50%
Spermatocytic seminoma (3)	>60	0		0%
NSGCT	30			80%
Embryonal carcinoma		85	AFP: normal or mildy elevated. β-hCG: normal or mildly elevated	
Choriocarcinoma (4)		10	AFP: normal β-hCG >1000 IU/L	
Yolk sac tumor		40	AFP: >100 ng/ml (5) β-hCG: normal	
Teratoma		30		

(1) isochromosome of the short arm of chromosome 12. (2) If AFP is elevated, the diagnosis of pure seminoma should be doubted. (3) Accounts for 1–4% of pure seminomas. Shows a different behavior. Good prognosis. (4) Most aggressive subtype. Hematogenous spread occurs early. (5) Levels correlate with disease extent.

Table 14.2 Immunohistochemical patterns of Germ Cell Tumors

				Transcription factors					
	Cytokeratin	CD 30	PLAP (1)	OCT3/4 (2)	NANOG	SOX2 (3)	CD 117 (4)	AFP	β-hCG
Seminoma	+/–	–	++	+	+	–	++	–	+/–
Spermatocytic seminoma	–	–	+/–				+/–	–	
Embryonal carcinoma	++	+	+	+	+	+	+/–	+/–	
Choriocarcinoma	+/–			–	–	–	–		++
Yolk sac tumor	++	+/–	+/–	–	–	–	+/–	+	

(1) Placental-like alkaline phosphatase; (2) Octamer-binding transcription factor; (3) Sex determining region Y-box 2; (4) c-KIT receptor.

prognosis, and monitoring of GCTs. Three serum tumor markers are clinically important: beta human chorionic gonadotrophin (βHCG), alpha-fetoprotein (AFP), and lactate dehydrogenase (LDH) (6). The likelihood of having abnormally increased levels of one or more of these markers increases with tumor volume and the severity of the disease. As a consequence, they have been included as part of the TNM staging system and the International Germ Cell Cancer Collaboration Group (IGCCCG) prognostic model (see the section on Staging). As most patients with suspected GCTs undergo orchiectomy for diagnostic and therapeutic purposes, tumor markers are not routinely used for diagnosis. However, increased levels of βHCG and/or AFP associated with a testicular mass may be highly suggestive of a GCT, especially considering that the causes of false positive elevation of these markers are few and relatively rare (namely hypogonadism for the former and hepatocellular carcinoma in the latter). Nevertheless, in the unusual case in which obtaining tissue for diagnosis is not possible without significant risk for the patient (e.g., primary mediastinal tumor) or the pathologic report is nondiagnostic, serum tumor markers may be used to support the diagnosis and initiate treatment.

More frequently, serum tumor markers are used for monitoring both the response to a given treatment as well as the possibility of relapse after a complete response. It is important to note that βHCG and AFP have different half-lives; that of βHCG is 18 to 36 hours, whereas AFP has a significantly longer half-life of 4 to 5 days. Thus, depending on the initial serum tumor marker values, a 10-fold decrease or normalization of these levels should be evident after 2 weeks and/or 25 to 30 days, respectively, of successful treatment. A slower response is considered unsatisfactory and a likely marker of treatment failure, which may prompt the clinician to consider early salvage therapy. If on the other hand the response is adequate and a complete response is achieved, periodic measurement of the serum tumor markers is of the utmost importance. Indeed, in more than half the cases, an elevation of βHCG and/or AFP is the first and sometimes sole evidence of disease relapse.

STAGING

As previously stated, the American Joint Committee on Cancer (AJCC) TNM staging system for GCTs incorporates serum tumor markers as part of the classification.

AJCC Staging of Germ Cell Tumors

Stage	Definition
I	No regional lymph node involvement or metastasis
IA	Tumor invades up to the tunica albuginea without vascular/lymphatic invasion and normal serum tumor markers
IB	Invasion beyond tunica albugínea or vascular/ lymphatic invasion
IS	Any tumor size and elevated serum tumor markers
II	Any tumor size with regional lymph node involvement but no distant metastasis. Serum tumor markers are normal or only mildly elevated*
IIA	Lymph node mass 2 cm or less
IIB	Lymph node mass more than 2 cm in diameter, but less than 5 cm
IIC	Lymph node mass more than 5 cm in diameter
III	Distant metastasis or significantly elevated serum tumor markers
IIIA	Nonregional nodal or pulmonary metastasis, with normal or only mildly elevated serum tumor markers*
IIIB	Moderate elevation in serum tumor markers† with regional lymph node involvement without distant metastasis, or those with nonregional nodal or pulmonary metastasis regardless or regional lymph node status
IIIC	Similar to stage IIIB but with markedly elevated serum tumor markers ‡ or those with nonpulmonary metastasis.

*LDH < 1.5× upper limits of normal; βHCG <5000 IU/L; AFP < 1000 ng/mL.
†LDH 1.5–10× upper limits of normal; βHCG 5000–50,000 IU/L; AFP 1000–10,000 ng/mL.
‡LDH > 10× upper limits of normal; βHCG > 50,000 IU/L; AFP > 10,000 ng/mL.

It is important to note that the serum tumor marker values to be considered for staging and prognosis purposes are those obtained after orchiectomy and before other treatment begins (surgery, radiation therapy, or chemotherapy), and not those obtained at the time of diagnosis. Briefly, stage I includes those patients with no regional node or metastasis, regardless of the size of the tumor. Stage II includes those with regional node involvement and only a mild elevation in the serum tumor markers, whereas stage III comprises those patients with metastatic disease or those with regional lymph node involvement and a more significant elevation of the serum tumor markers. In addition to the TNM system, GCTs are classified into good, intermediate, or poor prognosis (Table 14.3) on the basis of the validated prognostic model from the IGCCCG (7).

CASE SUMMARIES

Early-Stage Seminoma

D.L. is a 32-year-old business man who presents with lower abdominal discomfort, noticed initially after a long international flight. Physical examination revealed a painless swelling of his right testicle and scrotal ultrasound showed a 6-mm well-defined hypoechoic lesion. No abnormalities were found in the contralateral testicle. LDH, βHCG, and AFP levels were all within normal limits, and chest x-ray (CXR) was unremarkable. A radical inguinal orchiectomy was performed, with pathology confirming the diagnosis of pure seminoma, with no lymphovascular invasion (LVI) but involving the tunica vaginalis. A computed tomography (CT) scan of abdomen was then performed, with no evidence of enlarged lymph nodes. Therefore, the patient was diagnosed with a stage IB pure seminoma.

Evidence-Based Case Discussion

The above-mentioned case describes the initial diagnostic evaluation of any suspected GCT. After a thorough history and physical examination, a scrotal ultrasound should be pursued. Ultrasound can identify intrinsic testicular lesions as small as 1 mm. Seminomas tend to have a more homogeneous appearance on ultrasound with well-defined margins compared to NSGCT, although this is not always the case. Once a mass is confirmed, serum tumor markers should be obtained and patient referred for an inguinal radical orchiectomy. A transscrotal surgery or biopsy (scrotal violation) is contraindicated because of the increased risk of the tumor spreading locally. In general, a biopsy of the contralateral testicle is not indicated unless there is an increased suspicion of synchronous GCT based on ultrasound findings (e.g., a hypoechoic mass or marked atrophy) or in the setting of cryptorchidism. If any of these were present, an open inguinal approach should be elected for the biopsy. Imaging studies should also be obtained as part of the initial workup. These include a CT scan of abdomen and pelvis and a CXR. Although routinely ordered as part of the initial workup by many physicians, the current guidelines recommend that a CT scan of the chest should only be requested if the CXR shows abnormalities or if retroperitoneal lymphadenopathy is apparent on the abdominal CT scan. Similarly, other imaging studies like bone scan or brain MRI are not routinely ordered, unless the symptoms reported by the patient are concerning for metastasis to these sites (8). Finally, serum tumor markers should be repeated postoperatively if they were elevated before the orchiectomy. As mentioned previously, the postoperative values should be used for both staging and IGCCCG prognosis classification.

The overall prognosis of stage I seminoma after orchiectomy is excellent, with almost 100% of patients being cured regardless of the treatment strategy adopted.

Table 14.3 Prognostic Features of Germ Cell Tumors

Prognosis	Percent of Total	Seminoma Features	Seminoma TNM	NSGCT Features	NSGCT TNM	5-Year Survival (%)
Good prognosis	60	No nonpulmonary visceral metastasis	I, II, IIIA, IIIB	Testicular or retroperitoneal primary No nonpulmonary visceral metastasis Normal or mildly elevated serum tumor markers	I, II, IIIA	91
Intermediate prognosis	26	Nonpulmonary visceral metastasis	IIIC	Same as good prognosis but with moderately elevated serum tumor markers	IIIB	79
Poor prognosis	14	N/A		Mediastinal primary Nonpulmonary visceral metastasis Markedly elevated serum tumor markers	IIIC	48

There are three treatment alternatives currently accepted: surveillance, radiation therapy (RT), and chemotherapy (Figure 14.1). One of the main advantages of surveillance is that it avoids unnecessary treatment for a significant percentage of patients. Despite a higher relapse rate with surveillance alone (15–20% compared with less than 5% for both RT and chemotherapy), overall survival (OS) is not affected with this approach since most relapses, if detected early, can be salvaged with RT or chemotherapy. In a pooled analysis of 638 patients from Europe, two factors were found to be predictive of a higher relapse rate in patients managed by surveillance; tumor size >4 cm (HR = 2.0) and invasion of the rete testis (HR = 1.7) (9). However, even in the presence of one or both of these risk factors, surveillance is not contraindicated as long as the patient is motivated and compliant with the surveillance schedule. Unfortunately, there is no absolute consensus regarding the frequency of follow-up. Most relapses will occur within the first 2 years, which justifies a more frequent monitoring during this period. Similarly, given its longer natural history and higher incidence of late relapses compared with NSGCT, most experts agree that follow-up should be extended for at least 10 years. For example, the National Comprehensive Cancer Network (NCCN) guidelines recommend obtaining serum tumor markers and abdominal/pelvic CT scan every 3 to 4 months for the first 3 years, every 6 months from years 4 to 7 and yearly thereafter. Other authors propose a less strict imaging schedule with CT scan every 4 to 6 months for the first 3 years, considering the relatively indolent course of seminomas. The usefulness of frequent serum tumor marker measurement is even more controversial as they are not reliable in detecting disease recurrence in pure seminomas.

Radiation therapy has been historically the adjuvant therapy of choice in stage I seminoma (and it is still the preferred management for stage Is seminoma). However, late toxicity (primarily the development of second malignancies) suggested by the long-term follow-up data, has made surveillance a more attractive option in recent years. In fact, a long-term, worldwide, retrospective analysis of more than 28,000 testicular cancer patients (15,000 with seminoma) treated from 1935 to 1993 showed an increased incidence of solid tumors diagnosed 5 or more years after the diagnosis of testicular cancer (cumulative risk at 25 years of 18.2%). Prior RT was significantly associated with those patients developing bladder, stomach, pancreas, and rectal cancer, as well as kidney cancer (in 20-year survivors) (10). This observation prompted changes in the radiation dose and field with attempts to reduce toxicity while maintaining efficacy (risk of relapse <4%). RT evolved from the "hockey-stick" or "dog-leg" field, which involves radiation to the renal hilum, pelvic lymph nodes, and para-aortic lymph nodes, to the so-called "PA-strip" radiation, which is limited to the para-aortic lymph nodes. This was based on data showing that the other sites included on the hockey-stick field are rarely involved at the time of diagnosis of a stage I seminoma. A direct comparison of these two approaches (Fossa et al., 1999) showed that while pelvic relapses were more common with PA-strip compared with the hockey-stick field (1.7% vs. 0%), the total number of relapses was the same (4% on each arm) and the acute toxicity was less pronounced in the PA-strip group. Moreover, there was no difference in the OS at 3 years (96%). Although the median follow-up on this study (4.5 years) does not allow for an adequate assessment of long-term toxicity, most radiation oncologists currently use the PA-strip as the standard field of choice in stage I seminoma.

Traditionally, a radiation dose of 30 Gy divided in 15 fractions has been used for the treatment of GCTs. However, in a more recent study of 625 men who were randomized to this dose or to 20 Gy in 10 fractions, similar low relapse rates were observed (2% vs. 3%, respectively) after a median of 61 months of follow-up (11). Furthermore, a decrease in acute morbidity variables (mainly lethargy) in patients allocated to receive 20 Gy allowed them to return to work sooner than those receiving 30 Gy. Six patients in this study were diagnosed with a second malignancy (nonGCTs), all of them in the 30 Gy group. However, longer follow-up will be required to assess the effect of dose reduction on the development of second malignancies.

In addition to second malignancies, there are concerns regarding the risk of cardiac toxicity and impaired fertility in those patients receiving RT. Although the data for these risks are either insufficient or conflicting, the use of smaller radiation fields (with no prophylactic radiation to mediastinum) and the use of scrotal shielding to the contralateral testicle (even in those patients receiving PA-strip fields) are likely reducing these risks.

The use of chemotherapy as an alternative to RT in men with stage I seminoma has been evaluated more recently given the success of cisplatin in treating advanced GCTs. Due to the higher risk of toxicity with cisplatin, carboplatin has been used as a single dose (AUC of 7) with excellent results. When compared against RT, carboplatin showed similar relapse rates at 3 years (12). The results at 6.5 years were later updated in the 2008 American Society of Clinical Oncology meeting. Although the relapse rates remained similar, there was a significant difference in the incidence of new contralateral GCTs, favoring carboplatin over RT (0.3% vs. 1.7%). With short follow-up, there was no difference in the incidence of nonGCTs.

Given the excellent and quite similar outcomes, choice is usually based on the individual patient preferences or personal circumstances (Figure 14.1). For example, the patient described in this first case is a businessman who travels frequently making him unable to comply with a tight surveillance protocol. He would likely benefit from either RT or chemotherapy.

Early-Stage Nonseminomatous GCT

R.M. is a 28-year-old man who presented with a painless testicular mass, confirmed with ultrasound. AFP levels were mildly elevated (500 ng/mL) whereas βHCG and LDH were within normal limits. After radical orchiectomy, pathology reported an NSGCT (60% embryonal, 40% yolk sac) invading tunica albuginea with LVI present. A CT scan of the abdomen/pelvis and CXR were unremarkable. AFP levels were markedly decreased 2 weeks after surgery and normalized after 4 weeks.

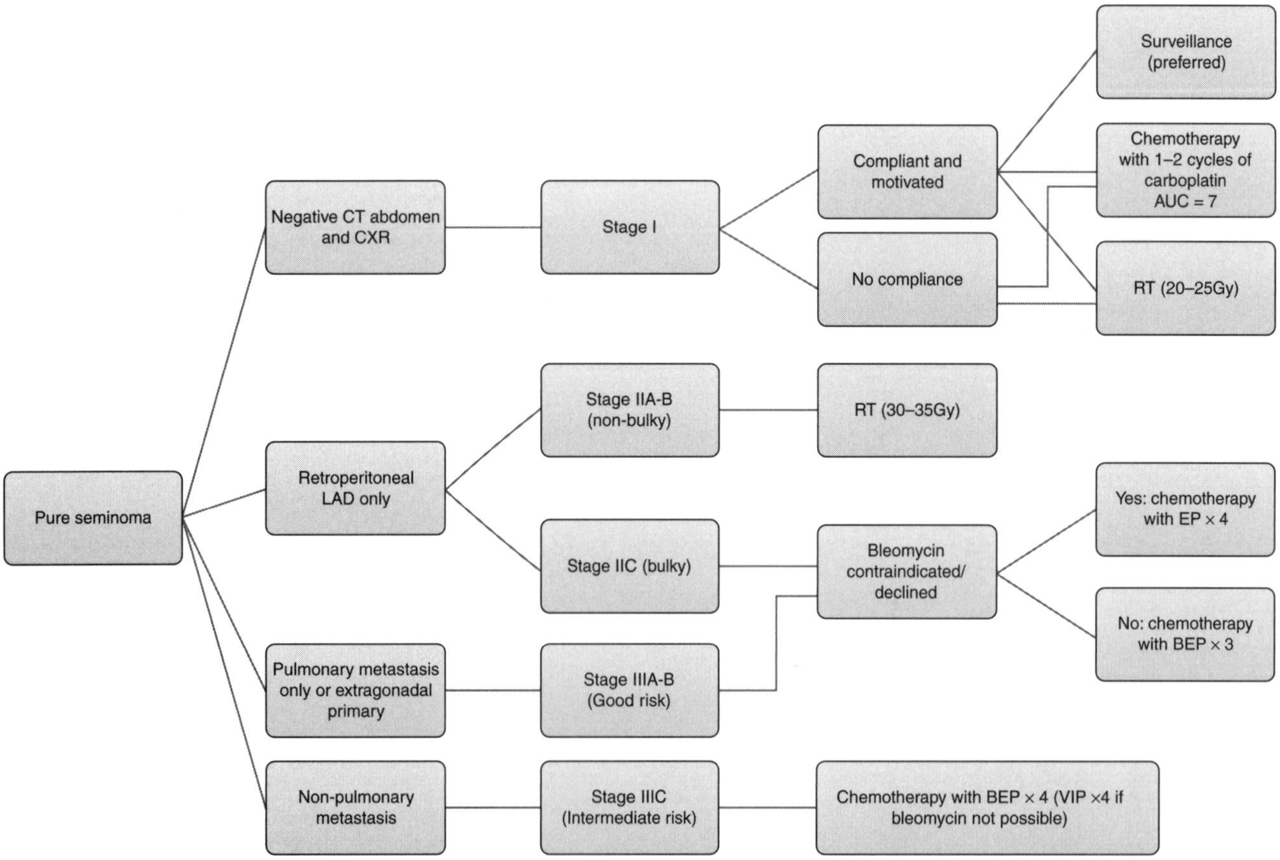

Figure 14.1

Management algorithm for pure seminoma.

Evidence-Based Case Discussion

This patient was also diagnosed with stage I testicular cancer, in this case a NSGCT. The treatment of stage I NSGCT is a contentious topic (Figure 14.2). Like stage I seminoma, surveillance alone is an attractive option in stage I NSGCT as it can potentially prevent unnecessary treatment in a subset of patients. Unlike seminoma, however, the overall chance of relapse in a patient with stage I NSGCT undergoing surveillance is approximately 30%, likely due to undetected micrometastasis at the time of diagnosis. In fact, 30% of patients undergoing retroperitoneal lymph node dissection (RPLND) for clinical stage I disease are eventually upstaged to stage II after this procedure. Also, unlike seminoma, late relapses are not common, with most occurring within the first 2 years. In a large European series, 373 patients with stage I NSGCT were followed by surveillance only (13). A relapse rate of 27% was observed with 80% occurring in the first year (61% in the retroperitoneal nodes and 25% in lungs).

Efforts are underway to define which patients have a higher probability of relapse and are thus more likely to benefit from adjuvant treatment with either RPLND or chemotherapy. Two features from this patient's primary tumor have been demonstrated to be useful in the stratification of patients into low risk and high risk of relapse: the presence of LVI and an embryonal carcinoma component. A retrospective Dutch study showed that the relapse rate in the absence of LVI was 11% compared to 51% when LVI was present (14). In addition, 50% of patients undergoing RPLND in this study were upstaged to stage II disease when LVI was present in the primary tumor (only 26% of those without LVI were upstaged). These results, as well as those in previous studies suggest that LVI is the single most important predictor of relapse in stage I NSGCTs. Similarly, the presence of embryonal carcinoma has been demonstrated to be an independent risk factor for relapse. Recent studies suggest that the predictive power is higher with increasing proportions of embryonal carcinoma, and not its mere presence. A cutoff of 45% has been used in some studies. If both LVI and embryonal carcinoma predominance are present, the risk of relapse increases significantly. When 105 patients with stage I NSGCT where followed at a single institution in the United States (Sogani

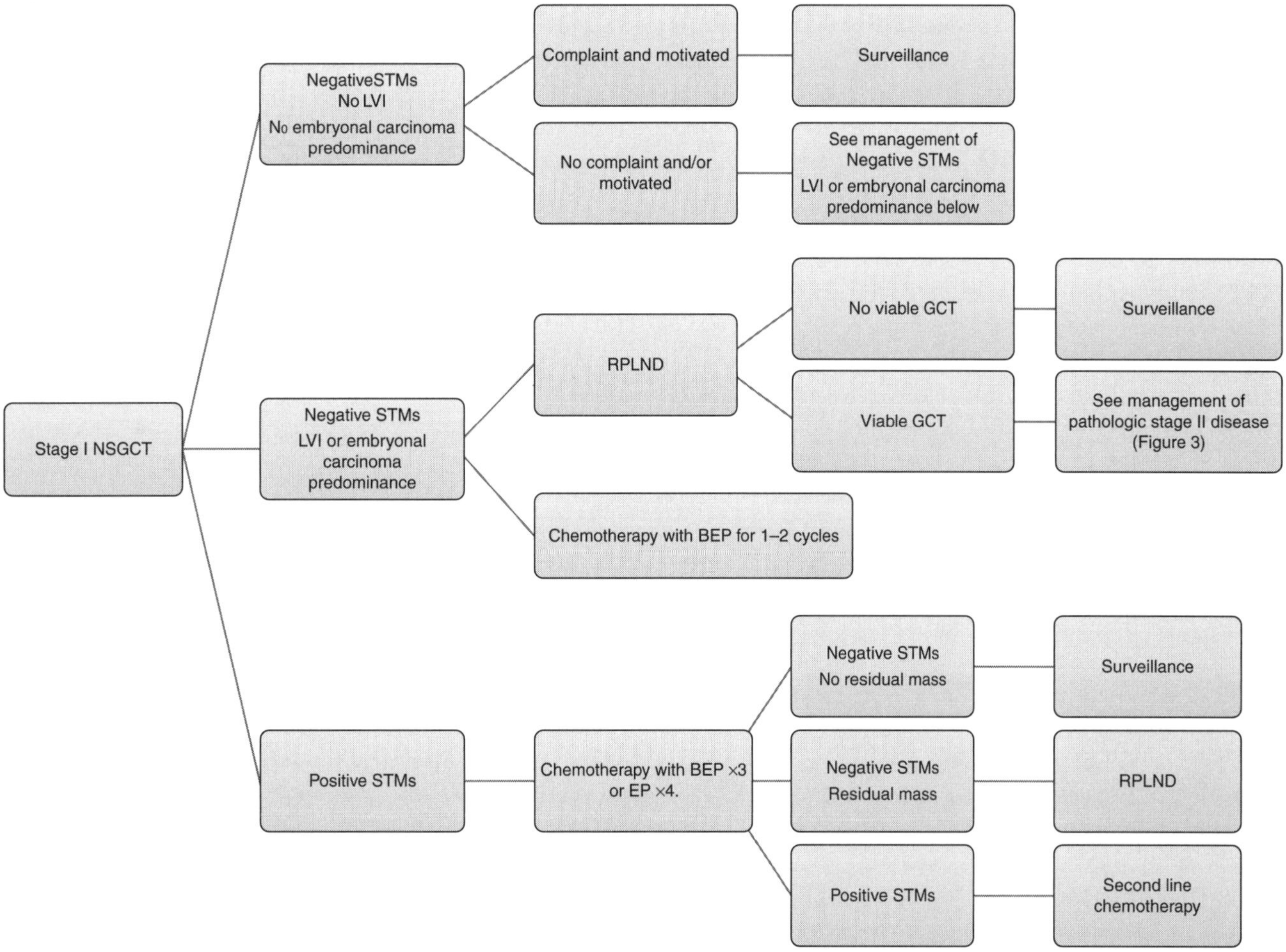

Figure 14.2

Management algorithm for stage I NSGCT.

et al., 1998), the overall relapse rate after 11 years was 25.7%, with three patients dying after relapse (2.8%). The relapse rate was 12% for those patients without LVI or embryonal carcinoma (n = 66), compared with 71% when both factors were present (n = 7).

Other factors linked to a higher risk of relapse are the absence of yolk sac component, tumor size, and the immunohistochemical analyses of proliferative rates of MIB1 antibody. Their overall importance does not seem to be as significant as the presence of LVI or embryonal carcinoma, but may be taken into consideration at the time of counseling a patient.

Although surveillance can prevent unnecessary treatment in 70% to 75% of patients with stage I NSGCT (and close to 90% in low-risk patients), when relapse occurs, these patients are exposed to at least three cycles of chemotherapy. Furthermore, this approach requires close follow-up (especially during the first 2 years) and reliable imaging (CT scan) to decrease the risk of false negative staging. The results of positron emission tomography (PET) scan in this setting had been disappointing and its use for stage I NSGCT is not advocated.

Nevertheless, surveillance is a reasonable approach—and preferred in many centers—for patients with low-risk stage I NSGCT. However, patients with high-risk features could benefit from adjuvant treatment. The choice of optimal treatment in this setting, between RPLND and chemotherapy, is still a matter of controversy.

Proponents of RPLND (the preferred method in the United States) claim that it has therapeutic benefit and allows for accurate staging. In fact, as previously mentioned, almost half of patients with clinical stage I NSGCT with embryonal carcinoma predominance and/or LVI will be upstaged to pathological stage II disease. Many of these men will be cured with RPLND alone. In a retrospective analysis of 292 patients with clinical stage I NSGCT treated with RPLND, 66 (22.6%) had retroperitoneal nodal involvement (Hermans et al., 2000). Thirty-one of these sixty-six patients were followed with surveillance alone, with relapse occurring in seven (23%) patients, compared with no relapses in the group receiving chemotherapy. While the benefits from post-RPLND chemotherapy seem evident, the authors conclude that 77% of patients remained relapse-free with RPLND alone and thus RPLND alone remains an option for patients able to comply with surveillance who want to avoid chemotherapy toxicity. On the basis of these studies, the NCCN consensus guidelines propose that further treatment after RPLND be considered depending on the individual patient's compliance and the extent of the retroperitoneal nodal involvement. Two cycles of BEP (bleomycin, etoposide, cisplatin) chemotherapy are recommended for noncompliant patients with pN1 or pN2 disease (positive nodal involvement up to 5 cm) and three or four cycles of chemotherapy for pN3 disease (more than 5 cm).

Although it can potentially prevent exposure to chemotherapy toxicity, RPLND is not exempt from complications, especially outside centers with extensive experience with this procedure. Among different series, the morbidity rate is 10% to 23%, and the mortality rate is approximately 0.3%. For example, in a retrospective analysis of 239 RPLND procedures performed in seven centers in Germany, minor complications were reported in almost 20% of patients, whereas major complications were seen in 5% (Heidenreich, 2003). Moreover, the frequency of complications was inversely correlated with the number of these procedures performed by each individual surgeon. Laparoscopic RPLND has been advocated by some, given its reported low complication rate and decrease in hospital stay. However, few surgeons have enough experience with this procedure and its efficacy has come into question, particularly due to concerns about inadequate sampling. For this reason, an open nerve-sparing RPLND is still favored by most centers. The major morbidity associated with this procedure is the infertility due to retrograde ejaculation. However, new techniques in experienced hands result in preservation of antegrade function in more than 90% of cases.

Some centers, especially in Europe, advocate the use of chemotherapy as the initial adjuvant treatment after orchiectomy, based on the very low relapse rate (<3%) seen in most studies. Currently, two cycles of BEP is recommended for stage I NSGCT in this setting. This recommendation is based on results of relatively small studies, although more recent studies suggest that only one cycle may have similar efficacy. A risk-stratified approach was used in a study from Scandinavia (Tandstad et al., 2009) in 745 men with stage I NSGCT. Based on the presence of LVI, patients were recommended to receive one cycle of BEP if LVI was present (but patients could opt to receive two cycles or just surveillance) or to undergo surveillance if no LVI was observed (patients could choose to receive chemotherapy). The overall relapse rate on those receiving two cycles (n = 70), one cycle (n = 312), and surveillance (n = 350) was 0%, 2%, and 13%, respectively. In the presence of LVI, the relapse-free survival was significantly better for those patients receiving two cycles and one cycle of adjuvant chemotherapy compared with surveillance (100%, 96.5%, and 58.3%, respectively). A significant difference was observed in patients without LVI receiving chemotherapy (98.6%) versus those on surveillance (86.5%). Similarly, a study randomized 382 patients to receive either one cycle of BEP or RPLND (Albers et al., 2008). Patients who had a pathological stage II disease after RPLND received two cycles of BEP, with no relapses seen in this group. After a median of 4.7 years, two patients randomized to one cycle of BEP relapsed compared with 15 patients in the RPLND group. No mortality was reported. Interestingly, almost half of patients relapsing in the RPLND group had a retroperitoneal relapse, which highlights the potential for suboptimal results when this procedure is performed outside an experienced center.

In summary, stage I NSGCT carries an excellent prognosis regardless of the postorchiectomy strategy, with an OS of 98% since the vast majority of patients that relapse can be cured with salvage treatment. Therefore, the decision of adjuvant treatment should be based on the individual's circumstances including the risk of relapse. In low-risk patients, surveillance is the preferred method, with RPLND or chemotherapy left for noncompliant patients. Surveillance is still an option in high-risk patients (like the patient in our vignette) as long as the patient is willing to accept a 50% risk of relapse. If adjuvant treatment is pursued, RPLND is preferred in those centers with extensive experience that lowers the risk of complications. Otherwise, adjuvant chemotherapy is a good alternative with one cycle of BEP being probably as effective as the two cycles previously recommended (Figure 14.2).

The patient described in our vignette also reflects the most common pattern in stage I disease: the normalization of serum tumor markers after the orchiectomy. Rarely, however, the serum tumor markers will remain persistently high or will increase. Even in the absence of supporting imaging, it should be assumed that metastatic disease is present in these cases and treatment should be given accordingly with three cycles of BEP or four cycles of EP (etoposide and cisplatin).

Locally Advanced Seminoma

B.C. is a 37-year-old man who presents with a painless mass incidentally found in his left testicle. Scrotal ultrasound showed a 23-mm lesion with no abnormalities seen on the contralateral testicle. LDH, βHCG, and AFP levels were all within normal values and CXR was unremarkable. A radical inguinal orchiectomy was performed, with pathology confirming the diagnosis of pure seminoma. A CT scan of abdomen showed enlarged para-aortic lymph nodes, with largest diameter of 6 cm. Patient was diagnosed with a stage IIC pure seminoma. B.C. received three cycles of chemotherapy with BEP. Six weeks after the last cycle, a repeat CT scan of the abdomen showed that the para-aortic lymphadenopathy had decreased in size, and now was 3 cm in diameter.

Evidence-Based Case Discussion

Stage II disease is defined as one limited to regional (retroperitoneal) lymph nodes. Unlike stage I disease, surveillance is not considered an appropriate option for these patients as the majority can expect to be cured with modern RT or chemotherapy. RPLND is not used as primary treatment given the sensitivity of seminoma to both chemotherapy and RT. Although either strategy can be used as adjuvant treatment for stage II seminoma, RT is preferred for those with nonbulky disease whereas chemotherapy is considered as first-line treatment for patients with bulky disease (Figure 14.1). The definition of bulky disease is admittedly artificial and somewhat variable among experts, but the presence of any para-aortic lymph node larger than 5 cm would be considered "bulky" disease by most. Therefore, a patient with stage IIA or IIB disease is considered to have nonbulky stage II seminoma wherease those with stage IIC are classified as having bulky disease.

As stated above, RT is considered the treatment of choice for men with nonbulky disease. A total of 35 to 40 Gy are administered to the infradiaphragmatic areas, including para-aortic lymph nodes and ipsilateral pelvic nodes, with a boost given to affected nodal areas. Scrotal and inguinal node shielding is indicated unless scrotal violation occurred during orchiectomy. Likewise, prophylactic mediastinal radiation is no longer performed. With modern RT, the relapse rate is expected to be between 5% and 15%. However, OS remains >90% given the good response to salvage chemotherapy (15). For patients who do not wish to undergo RT, those with previous radiation to the retroperitoneum or those with a relative contraindication to RT (e.g., horseshoe kidney or inflammatory bowel disease), chemotherapy with four cycles of EP or three cycles of BEP can be given as an alternative (Garcia del Muro et al., 2008). Single-agent carboplatin has also been evaluated given its success in stage I seminoma. However, the German Testicular Study Group reported a relapse rate of 18% after three or four cycles of carboplatin (Krege et al., 2006). Thus, despite the lower toxicity, this approach cannot be recommended.

In men who present with para-aortic lymph nodes >5 cm in diameter, RT alone resulted in relapse rates of 35%, with 5-year OS of 77% after salvage chemotherapy. Although newer RT techniques and improvements in salvage chemotherapy improved these outcomes, these patients fare better with upfront chemotherapy, with cure rates near 90%. Furthermore, several reports suggest that response to chemotherapy is significantly better for patients without prior exposure to radiation. The extent of radiation also seems to affect the outcomes, with patients with more limited exposure having better responses. At this time, either EP × 4 or BEP × 3 are considered the treatment of choice for stage IIC (bulky stage II). Both are consider equivalent for the treatment of stage II as well as for stage IIIA and IIIB seminoma (good-risk disease on the IGCCCG classification, Table 14.3), although most centers will favor BEP given a trend toward improved outcomes when full doses of bleomycin are used. The evolution of this regimen started in the 1970s with the introduction of cisplatin, currently the most active drug for the treatment in GCTs. Cisplatin (20 mg/m^2 from day 1 to 5), was initially combined with bleomycin (30 units weekly) and vinblastine (0.4 mg/kg) for a total of four cycles followed by maintenance vinblastine. While this regimen (PVB) had remarkable results when compared with historical controls, the development of vinblastine induced neuromuscular toxicity was a limiting factor. Eliminating maintenance vinblastine helped reduce this risk without affecting efficacy, but still remained a concern. Around this time, the activity of etoposide against GCTs and its synergism with cisplatin was demonstrated. This led to its use in combination with cisplatin and bleomycin instead of vinblastine. When both regimens were compared head to head (Williams et al., 1987), BEP showed a significantly better response rate, particularly in those with bulky disease. Furthermore, neurotoxicity was significantly more common in those receiving PVB, whereas no difference in myelosuppression was noted. Later, four cycles of BEP were compared to only three cycles in patients with good-risk disease. No differences in OS or disease-free survival was reported; so currently a fourth cycle of BEP is considered unnecessary for patients with good-risk GCTs.

The choice between three cycles of BEP or four cycles of EP depends mostly on the pulmonary function of the individual. Whereas most patients with testicular cancer (usually young patients without comorbidities) are able to tolerate three doses of bleomycin, older patients and those with prior pulmonary damage or who cannot afford the risk of pulmonary toxicity (e.g., certain athletes) may be better served with four cycles of EP. Nevertheless, as stated above, most trials comparing BEP with EP showed a non-significant difference in disease-free survival and mortality favoring BEP. Similarly, dose reductions in bleomycin or etoposide produced inferior results. Therefore, BEP should be the treatment of choice in this setting unless a clear indication to avoid bleomycin is present.

Many patients with stage II seminoma, especially those with bulky disease, will have a residual mass seen on CT scan after chemotherapy. Unlike NSGCT, where any residual mass should be surgically resected, a subset of patients with residual seminoma can be followed by surveillance. Before the advent of PET scan, the distinction between which patients should undergo further treatment and who can be followed up with surveillance alone was based on size parameters, with 3 cm used as cutoff. Several reports showed that many of the masses of less than 3 cm will disappear during surveillance and therefore no further treatment was recommended. Conversely, the risk of disease progression was higher for those patients with a residual mass larger than 3 cm as they frequently would have residual seminoma (Herr et al., 1997). Moreover, the radiographic appearance of the residual mass has been used by some to predict the presence of residual disease. Two distinct radiographic patterns had been described. In the first one, the residual tumor obliterates radiographic planes, merging with great vessels, psoas muscles, and retroperitoneal structures. These are considered unresectable and usually represent fibrotic tissue. The second clinical presentation shows well delineated masses that, especially when larger than 3 cm, have a high incidence of residual seminoma. In those cases, surgical resection is justified although a complete RPLND is frequently not possible.

This led to recommendations of surgical resection of the residual mass for patients with residual masses larger than 3 cm, particularly when well defined on CT scan. Alternative, second-line chemotherapy or RT can be considered. However, in the appropriate setting and selected patients, surveillance alone is a viable option when only size criteria is used. For example, a single institution reported the outcomes of 36 patients with advanced seminoma (Schultz et al., 1989). Twenty-one had residual lymphadenopathy after chemotherapy, nine of which were larger than 3 cm in diameter. Eight of the latter remained disease free at a minimum 2-year follow-up. The authors concluded that observation is a reasonable approach for residual seminoma, with size criteria alone being insufficient to determine which patients have viable seminoma. This led to the study of PET scan in this setting. When performed at least 6 weeks after chemotherapy (to avoid false positives), PET scan has shown to be a better predictor of residual seminoma than size criteria. In the largest multicenter study that included 51 patients, PET scan correctly predicted all 19 cases with residual masses larger than 3 cm, and 35 of the 37 with residual lesions of less than or equal to 3 cm (16). The specificity (100% vs. 74%), sensitivity (80% vs. 70%), positive predictive value (100% vs. 37%), and negative predictive value (96% vs. 92%) all favored PET scan over size criteria.

Therefore, PET scan is currently recommended for those patients with residual mass and negative serum tumor markers after chemotherapy for locally advanced seminoma, like the patient described in the clinical vignette. If PET scan is negative, surveillance is suggested, while further treatment (surgery, second-line chemotherapy, or RT) should be considered for those patients with positive PET scan regardless of the size of the mass. If PET scan is not readily available, patients with a residual mass bigger than 3 cm should be considered for surgery or RT, with surveillance being a reasonable option for selected patients. For a residual mass smaller than 3 cm, surveillance alone is recommended. Patients with growing lymphadenopathy or positive tumor markers should be treated for progressive disease with second-line chemotherapy.

Locally Advanced NSGCT

X.N. is a 29-year-old man who presents with scrotal pain. On physical examination a testicular mass is noted and confirmed with ultrasound. βHCG levels were mildly elevated (4000 IU/L) whereas AFP and LDH were within normal limits. After radical orchiectomy, pathology reports a NSGCT (60% yolk sac, 30% choriocarcinoma, 10% mature teratoma). CT scan of the abdomen and pelvis showed a 1.5-cm pelvic lymph node and the CXR was unremarkable. Serum tumor markers returned to normal baseline after surgery. X.N. is diagnosed with a stage IIA NSGCT. On discussion of further management, he expresses that he does not want to have more children and, moreover, he is concerned about long-term effects of chemotherapy. Based on this, RPLND is performed with plans for surveillance after this. The pathology report confirms presence of NSGCT in seven lymph nodes, with a maximum diameter of 1.8 cm. After being informed of these results, X.N. asks if surveillance is still a reasonable option.

Evidence-Based Case Discussion

This clinical vignette reflects the frequent disconnect between clinical and pathological staging. This patient was classified as stage IIA based on imaging (N1, no lymph node > 2 cm), and received primary RPLND. Given the relapse-free survival of approximately 90% for stage IIA NSGCT after RPLND, this procedure is favored by many, especially if done at a specialized center. Alternatively, three cycles of BEP or four cycles of EP can be used (Figure 14.3). However, the numbers of positive lymph nodes upstages him to a pathologic stage IIB (pN2).

Although surveillance is still a reasonable option after RPLND in stage IIB disease, many argue in favor of adjuvant chemotherapy in this setting based on the higher relapse rate (35% compared with 10–15% in those with stage IIA). Indeed, the choice between surveillance and chemotherapy in patients with pathologic stage II disease depends on the volume of nodal disease burden. In a previous section, the NCCN recommendations for adjuvant chemotherapy for patients upstaged to stage II after RPLND for suspected stage I NSGCT were reviewed. The same principles apply to patients who undergo RPLND for clinical stage II, like the patient in the vignette. Briefly, surveillance is recommended for those with pN0, whereas two cycles of BEP is recommended for pN2 disease and three cycles (or four cycles of EP) for those with pN3. For patients with pN1, either surveillance or two cycles of BEP are considered appropriate, and the decision based on patient's preference or compliance (Figure 14.3). These recommendations are aimed at decreasing the risk of relapse without impacting OS as most patients who relapse during surveillance can be successfully cured with three cycles of chemotherapy. The patient in this vignette could potentially benefit from two cycles of chemotherapy, since this will significantly decrease his risk of relapse. However, if he is motivated, surveillance is not contraindicated as his survival will not be affected.

Primary chemotherapy (BEP × 3 or EP × 4) is favored for patients with stage IIB, especially if there is multifocal involvement in the retroperitoneum. This also applies to patients with stage IIC and patients with positive serum tumor markers after orchiectomy. Similarly, patients with stage IIIA (good-risk disease, Table 14.3) should undergo primary chemotherapy. Relapse-free survival and OS are excellent after chemotherapy. If complete response is seen after chemotherapy, including negative markers, surveillance is considered appropriate.

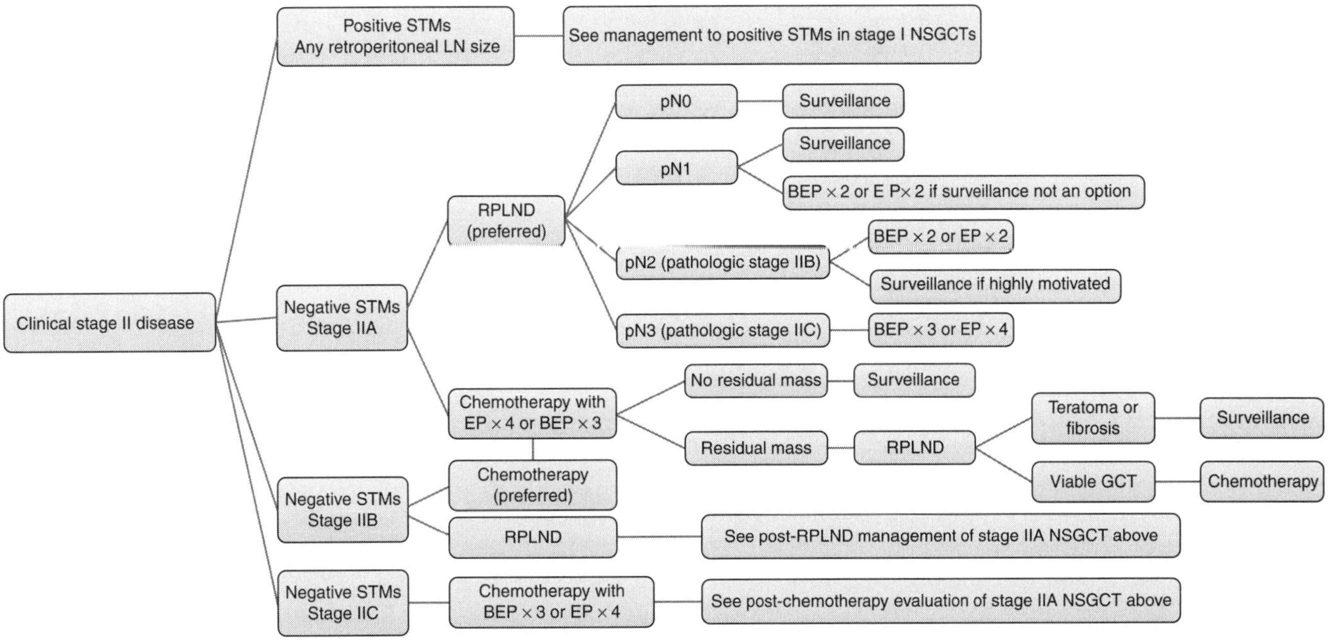

Figure 14.3

Management algorithm for stage II NSGCT.

However, some authors recommend RPLND after chemotherapy regardless of response (i.e., normal postchemotherapy scans). Although this recommendation is somewhat controversial, it may improve outcomes if a teratoma component is present as this is relatively resistant to chemotherapy. In fact, this aggressive surgical approach may decrease the rate of growing teratoma syndrome (GTS), a phenomenon considered to be rare although its true incidence is largely unknown. It was first described almost 30 years ago (Logothetis et al, 1982) and since then it has been described mostly as case reports or case series. In one large retrospective review of 373 patients treated for NSGCT at a single institution over 23 years, 9 patients (2.2%) fulfilled the criteria for GTS (17). It should be suspected in the presence of a metastatic lesion (most commonly retroperitoneal, but has been described in other locations) that increases in size during chemotherapy, while serum tumor markers decline or normalize. Suspicion should also arise when a mixed response to treatment is seen on imaging during chemotherapy or if an isolated mass grows after chemotherapy despite normal serum tumor markers, especially if a teratoma component was present in the primary tumor. Surgery should be considered as soon as this process is suspected and is curative if a complete resection is possible.

If markers return to normal but a residual mass is seen at follow-up CT scan, RPLND should be performed. It should be kept in mind that small lymph nodes are usually detected after chemotherapy with current high-resolution imaging techniques. PET scan does not have a role in this setting as it does in seminoma as it cannot reliably differentiate fibrosis from teratoma. What constitutes a normal size residual lymph node varies from institution to institution, but most centers will perform postchemotherapy RPLND for any residual mass larger than 1 cm. For those with masses smaller than 1 cm, surveillance may be considered as results seem to be excellent as reported by two recent studies. The first study is a retrospective analysis of the long-term outcomes of 141 patients with advanced GCT treated at Indiana University between 1984 and 2005 who achieved CR (normal serum tumor markers and residual mass <1 cm) after chemotherapy alone (18). Median follow-up was 15.5 years. A total of 12 patients relapsed, 6 of the relapses occurred in the retroperitoneum. The disease-free survival was 90% and the OS reached 97% as 8 of the 12 patients showed no evidence of disease (NED) after salvage treatment. Five patients relapsed more than 3 years posttreatment, which reinforces the need for prolonged follow-up in these patients. The authors concluded that patients achieving a CR after chemotherapy alone can be safely monitored without RPLND.

Similarly, another retrospective analysis of 276 patients treated for disseminated NSGCT in British Columbia and Oregon between 1999 and 2007 was recently reported (Kollmannsberger et al., 2010); most of them (84%) presented with low stage, IGCCCG good-risk disease. Of the 276 patients, 187 were treated with chemotherapy alone and of those, 161 achieved a CR. Only ten relapses occurred in this group, eight treated with delayed RPLND for teratoma and two with chemotherapy for serum tumor marker recurrence (one of these received RPLND as well). After a median follow-up of 64 months, all the ten patients who relapsed showed NED.

In those patients in whom postchemotherapy resection is performed, further treatment after surgery is based on pathology findings. In most patients (approximately 85%), teratoma or fibrosis will be reported after residual mass resection. In these patients surveillance can be safely started. Conversely, if residual viable tumor is found, two more cycles of combination chemotherapy are currently recommended. Etoposide/cisplatin (EP), etoposide/ifosfamide/isplatin (VIP), vinblastine/ifosfamide/cisplatin (VeIP) or paclitaxel/ifosfamide/cisplatin (TIP) are all acceptable options in this setting. Similarly, if markers remain positive, patient should be treated with second-line chemotherapy, like the ones mentioned above, for refractory disease.

Intermediate Risk, Advanced NSGCT

T.R. is a 39-year-old man who presented to his primary care physician with 3 weeks history of dry cough, worsening over the previous week. He denied any fever associated with these symptoms. On review of systems, he reported an occasional abdominal discomfort and bloating for the last several months, worse after meals, but otherwise no other symptoms were reported. His past medical history was positive for smoking and obesity. He denied any significant family history. Auscultation of the lungs was unremarkable and abdominal examination did not reveal any tenderness, organomegaly, or masses. His symptoms were attributed to gastroesophageal reflux and a trial of proton pump inhibitors was given. T.R. returned 2 weeks later with a report that his cough was somewhat worse. His physical examination was unchanged. His physician ordered a CXR that showed multiple nodules in both lungs, concerning for malignancy. Laboratory data showed an increased LDH (two times the upper limits of normal), with normal blood counts and basic metabolic panel. A CT scan of the chest, abdomen, and pelvis confirmed multiple lung nodules with the largest measuring 4.5 cm. In addition, bulky lymphadenopathy was noted in the retroperitoneum. Given this presentation, serum tumor markers and a scrotal ultrasound were ordered. The ultrasound showed a 1-cm hypoechoic mass on the right testicle that was missed on physical examination. βHCG and AFP were elevated at 10,000 IU/L and 8,000 ng/mL, respectively. Immediate orchiectomy was performed and pathology confirmed the presence of a GCT with 70% yolk sac tumor, 25% choriocarcinoma, and 5% teratoma.

After surgery, βHCG and AFP levels fell to 5000 IU/L and 2000 ng/mL, respectively. T.R. was diagnosed with stage IIIB NSGCT and received four cycles of BEP. Repeat scans obtained 6 weeks after completion of chemotherapy showed that all pulmonary nodules had resolved except for the largest one, now 1.5 cm, as well as a residual 2.5-cm para-aortic mass. Serum tumor markers were within normal limits.

Evidence-Based Case Discussion

This patient was diagnosed with stage IIIB NSGCT which, along with stage IIIC seminoma, constitutes an intermediate-risk advanced disease (Table 14.3). This case encompasses two important concepts: the use of four cycles of BEP for intermediate-risk disease and the possibility of residual masses in more than one anatomical location, which creates a challenge for both the oncologist and the surgeon.

Currently, four cycles of BEP is considered the treatment of choice for intermediate-risk metastatic disease. With this approach, a disease-free survival between 70% and 80% can be expected. Although this survival could be considered to be quite good, up to 30% of patients will relapse after being exposed to four cycles of chemotherapy including bleomycin. About a third of these patients can be salvaged with an ifosfamide-based regimen. This success led to the study of ifosfamide as a possible first-line agent for the treatment of intermediate-risk and poor-risk disease. Two studies addressing this question were started in the late 1980s. The first was a multicenter study sponsored by the Eastern Cooperative Oncology Group (ECOG), Southwest Oncology Group (SWOG), and the Cancer and Leukemia Group B Study (CALGB). Three hundred and four patients with poor-risk disease were randomized to receive either four cycles of BEP or four cycles of VIP (etoposide, ifosfamide, and cisplatin). Two hundred and eighty four patients were assessable for response and 299 for toxicity. There was no significant difference reported in the efficacy between both treatment groups, with a 2-year OS of 74% in the VIP group versus 71% in the BEP group. While equivalent in efficacy, the incidence of clinically important hematologic and genitourinary toxicity was significantly higher in the ifosfamide group. On the basis of these results, the authors concluded that four cycles of BEP was still the standard of care for advanced disseminated GCTs (19). The second study, which had a very similar design except it recruited patients with intermediate-risk disease, was ended prematurely once the results of the ECOG study became available. This trial, sponsored by the European Organization for Research and Treatment of Cancer (EORTC), randomized 84 patients before closing (de Wit et al, 1998). Again, no significant difference in response or disease-free survival was noted, but the group receiving ifosfamide experienced an increased incidence of myelosuppression when compared with the BEP group (89% vs. 37%, respectively).

Another alternative that had been studied recently is the addition of paclitaxel to BEP. In the initial phase I/II study (de Wit et al., 1999) a complete response in all 13 patients receiving escalating doses of paclitaxel combined with BEP was reported. A phase II/III study (EORTC 30983) comparing these regimens in intermediate-risk prognosis patients had completed enrollment, but results have not been reported yet.

On the basis of these results, four cycles of BEP is still the standard of care for intermediate-risk advanced GCT. Treatment with VIP can be considered as a good alternative in those patients with lung disease or those who can be expected to need an extensive pulmonary resection (Figure 14.4). It is important to mention that the presence of lung metastasis by itself, like in the patient described, is not a contraindication for bleomycin.

A persistent mass after chemotherapy is a relatively frequent occurrence in patients with advanced disease, being more common with higher disease burden at the time of presentation. Whenever possible, resection of all residual masses is recommended after chemotherapy, as long as serum tumor markers return to normal. In patients with metastatic disease, the retroperitoneum is also the most common site for a residual mass. Most commonly, this will represent either necrosis or teratoma. For example, a retrospective chart review of 152 consecutive patients with advanced GCTs treated with postchemotherapy RPLND at two referral centers in Germany revealed that 55% had either necrosis or fibrosis, whereas 30% had mature teratoma and 15% had viable GCT in the surgical sample (Heidenreich et al., 2008). Only eight recurrences and three disease-related deaths were reported at 39 months of follow-up.

In patients with intrathoracic residual masses after chemotherapy, efforts should be aimed toward a complete surgical resection. When this is achieved, good outcomes can be expected as reported in some early studies. The outcomes of 141 patients who underwent thoracic metastasectomy for GCT at a single institution in England from 1980 to 1997 had been described (20). Of these, 104 had lung metastasis at the time of presentation whereas 37 developed them after initial chemotherapy. Eighty-seven percent (123 patients) received chemotherapy prior to surgery. At the time of surgery, 51% had lung-only metastasis, 24% had both lung and mediastinum metastasis, and 24% had residual disease only in the mediastinum. Complete resection was possible in 123 patients (87%). There were two perioperative deaths. Pathological analysis of the resected metastasis revealed necrosis or fibrosis (23%), mature teratoma (45%), and viable malignancy (32%). Sixty-seven patients recurred after surgery, with recurrence being more common in patients with viable GCT (33 of 46; 72%) than in those with fibrosis (10 of 32; 31%) or

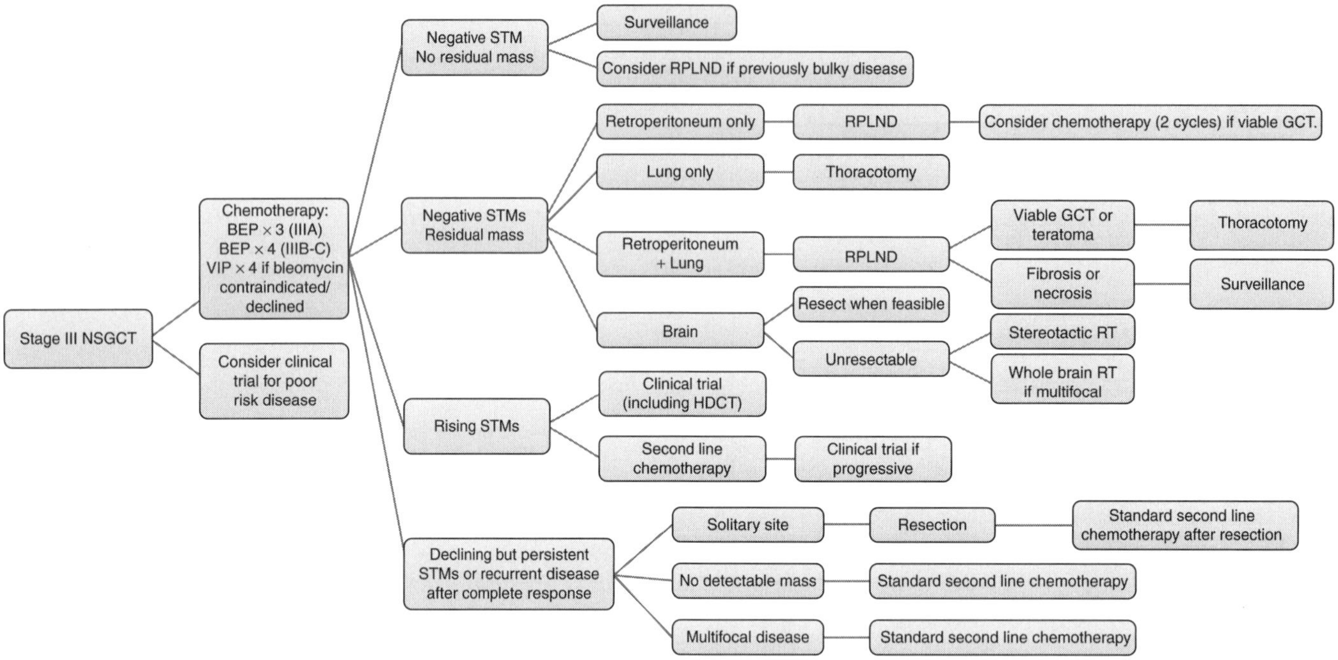

Figure 14.4

Management algorithm for stage III NSGCT and disease relapse.

teratoma (24 of 63; 38%). Many of these patients received a second thoracotomy successfully and the OS was 78% at 5 years after the initial metastasectomy surgery. In a multivariate analysis, a significantly increased risk of death from disease was found for those with viable malignancy in the surgical sample (RR = 5.7), residual disease at resection (RR = 4.0), and multiple metastases (RR = 4.1). It is important to mention that less than half the patients included in this study received the current standard regimen of BEP. With modern therapy, even better outcomes should be expected. Liu and colleagues reflected on their 28-years experience performing pulmonary metastasectomy at MSKCC (Liu et al., 1998). They reviewed the data on 157 patients who underwent this procedure starting in 1967. Survival before 1974 (when cisplatin was introduced) was 41% compared with 65% after that year. For patients diagnosed after 1985, the 5-year survival was 82% after pulmonary resection.

As stated above, close to 50% of patients undergoing thoracotomy for a residual pulmonary mass are found to have fibrosis or necrosis. Since relapse is unusual in these patients, surveillance would have been appropriate for them, avoiding the risks associated with surgery. Unfortunately, imaging alone cannot predict which patients will have residual disease (GCT or teratoma) on resection. As previously stated, PET scan cannot differentiate between teratoma and fibrosis. Attempts to create predictive models led to the observation that histology at RPLND was the most useful predictor of the histology of a residual pulmonary mass. A retrospective, international, multicenter study evaluated the outcomes of 215 patients undergoing thoracotomy after chemotherapy (21). More than half of these patients (54%) had necrosis found after pathology evaluation, while mature teratoma and viable GCTs were found in 33% and 13%, respectively. In addition, when RPLND was performed prior to pulmonary resection, the finding of necrosis in the retroperitoneum predicted necrosis in the pulmonary tissue in 89% of the cases, thus constituting the strongest predictor of pulmonary histology. Conversely, if mature teratoma or persistent cancer was found after RPLND, the probability of finding necrotic tissue only after thoracotomy was 38% and 30%, respectively. Other predictors of necrosis in the residual pulmonary mass were a teratoma negative primary tumor, normal AFP before chemotherapy and the presence of a single, unilateral residual lung nodule. As expected, an increase in size of a lung nodule during chemotherapy predicted a low likelihood of necrosis. The authors concluded that thoracotomy can be reconsidered if RPLND shows necrosis only, especially if other predictive factors of necrosis are present, unless the patient or the treating physician feel that the risk of missing teratoma or active cancer at thoracotomy is too high.

These findings were confirmed by a retrospective review of outcomes in 143 postchemotherapy patients with metastatic GCT who underwent both RPLND and thoracotomy simultaneously (Tognini et al., 1998). A significant concordance was found between the histology in the retroperitoneum and the pulmonary pathology. They reported a correlation of 86% predicting necrosis in those cases considered uncomplicated (standard chemotherapy received, normalization of serum tumor markers). When all cases were considered, this correlation was 77%, while concordance was also present for teratoma (70%) and GCTs (69%). Given these results, a sequential rather than concurrent surgical approach is recommended by most experts when both retroperitoneal and pulmonary residual disease is present after initial chemotherapy. Thoracotomy should be pursued when teratoma or viable carcinoma is found after RPLND. This procedure can be delayed and patient placed in surveillance if only necrosis is found.

Poor-Risk, Advanced GCT With Extrapulmonary Matastases

C.P. is a 31-year-old marathon runner with a past medical history of migraine headaches who noted some heaviness on his lower abdomen during his last race. He had also felt that he was tiring more easily while training over the past 2 months, and was experiencing postprandial epigastric pain. His family history was unremarkable. His physical examination revealed mild tenderness on palpation of right upper quadrant of the abdomen, as well as an enlarged right testicle. Scrotal ultrasound confirmed presence of a mass and CT scan showed diffuse retroperitoneal lymphadenopathy, multiple pulmonary nodules as well as three nodules in the liver ranging in size from 1 to 3 cm. Serum tumor markers revealed an LDH five times the upper limits of normal, a βHCG of 68,000 IU/L and an AFP of 8000 ng/mL. Orchiectomy confirmed the diagnosis of NSGCT (50% embryonal, 30% yolk sac, 20% choriocarcinoma). Tumor markers decreased postoperatively, but did not reach normal values (LDH two times upper limits of normal, βHCG = 53,000 IU/L, AFP = 3500 ng/mL). Chemotherapy options were discussed with C.P. and he refused to receive bleomycin due to concerns of its effect on his lung capacity. Therefore, four cycles of VIP were given without immediate complications. Serum tumor markers returned to normal after the third cycle and remained within normal limits 4 weeks after chemotherapy was completed. CT scan revealed residual masses, with a 1-cm pulmonary nodule, a 1.2-cm pelvic lymph node, as well as a 1.1-cm liver nodule. C.P. underwent an RPLND and resection of the liver nodule. Both masses were reported to contain fibrotic tissue only and the patient chose to begin surveillance of the pulmonary nodule. Repeat CT scans at three and six months showed no changes and serum tumor markers remained within normal limits. C.P. presented for an 8-month follow-up visit and tumor markers revealed a βHCG level of 20,000 IU/L. He denied any new symptoms, but did report that his migraine headaches had become more frequent and less responsive to usual measures. CT scans were ordered, including a head CT scan. CT of chest, abdomen, and pelvis reported no significant changes compared with previous scans, but the CT head showed a 2-cm lesion in the right parieto-occipital region.

Evidence-Based Case Discussion

This vignette focuses our attention on few key issues in the management of GCTs, namely the initial management of patients with poor prognosis, the management of a residual liver mass after chemotherapy, the treatment for relapsing or refractory disease, and the approach to brain metastasis, either at initial presentation or, as in this case, as a manifestation of recurrence. If available, inclusion in a clinical trial should be considered for patients with poor-risk prognosis. The patient described in the vignette was initially offered chemotherapy with BEP (four cycles), which, as described in the previous section, is the standard regimen of choice for intermediate or poor-prognosis patients with advanced GCTs. Owing to concerns of his lung function, VIP was used. As previously described, this is an adequate alternative regimen in this setting, although hematologic toxicity is higher.

In the poor-risk population, the 5-year OS is approximately 50% with conventional chemotherapy. Therefore, more intense regimens have been studied trying to improve survival. Nichols and colleagues hypothesized that increasing the dose of the most active drug, cisplatin, would translate in better outcomes in poor-risk GCTs (Nichols et al., 1991). They randomized 159 patients to standard BEP chemotherapy versus BEP chemotherapy with cisplatin given at a dose of 40 mg/m^2 for 5 days. Toxicity was significantly increased in those receiving the high-dose cisplatin, including four treatment related deaths. After 24 months of follow-up, no differences were noted in disease-free survival or overall survival.

Other studies tried to identify a possible induction regimen that could improve outcomes. An intensive induction-sequential chemotherapy schedule with bleomycin, vincristine, cisplatin followed by etoposide, ifosfamide, cisplatin, and bleomycin (BOP/VIP-B) was compared against four cycles of BEP followed by three cycles of EP in 380 patients (Kaye et al., 1998). Whereas no differences were noted in OS, complete responses, or disease-free survival, toxicity (particularly myelosuppression) was more common in the BOP/VIP-B arm.

More promising was the experience of 54 patients with poor-risk prognosis treated with an intensive 6-weeks induction regimen of CBOP (carboplatin on weeks 2 and 4, cisplatin 40 mg/m^2 on weeks 2 and 4, and 100 mg/m^2 on weeks 1 and 3; vincristine was given weekly until week 6 and bleomycin was also given weekly). This was followed by three cycles of BEP (Christian et al., 2003). Overall survival was 91% at 3 years and 87.6% at 5 years. Whereas these numbers compare favorably with historical data, the sample was relatively small and there was a lack of a control arm. Similarly, the favorable experience (OS = 75% at 3 years) in patients with poor-risk prognosis treated with POMB/ACE (cisplatin, vincristine, methotrexate, bleomycin, actinomycin D, cyclophosphamide, and etoposide) over 20 years at two institutions in England has been described (Bower et al., 1997). Although the results of these two trials may be enticing, a prospective phase III randomized study is needed to confirm the results as none of them had proven to be superior to BEP.

Finally, the use of high-dose chemotherapy (HDCT) with stem cell rescue has been evaluated as a possible first-line treatment for poor-risk patients. Two small noncontrolled studies showed some promising results when compared with historical data. In these studies HDCT was offered to those patients with a suboptimal response to the first two cycles of conventional chemotherapy. In the first study (Motzer et al., 1993) a combination of vinblastine, bleomycin, cyclophosphamide, dactinomycin, and cisplatin (VAB-6) was used as conventional chemotherapy, whereas VIP was used in the second study (Motzer et al., 1997). Both studies used high-dose carboplatin and etoposide as HDCT and showed an OS greater than 50% at 30 months of follow-up. This hypothesis was then tested in a phase III trial using BEP with somewhat disappointing results (22). In this study, 219 patients were randomly assigned to receive four cycles of BEP versus two cycles of BEP followed by two cycles of HDCT with carboplatin and etoposide and stem cell rescue. The primary end point was durable CR at 1 year, which was observed in 52% (HDCT arm) compared with 48% (conventional dose arm), a nonsignificant difference. After a median follow-up of 51 months, no difference in the OS was observed either. A planned subset analysis evaluated the response in those patients with elevated serum tumor markers at baseline. In those who showed an inadequate decline in serum tumor markers prior to the third cycle (early chemotherapy resistance), HDCT provided a significant benefit in durable CR at 1 year (61% vs. 34% in those who received conventional chemotherapy) as well as in OS at 2 years (78% vs. 55%, respectively). This difference was not observed in those who had an adequate decline in their serum tumor markers after the first two cycles of chemotherapy. However, since random assignment did not occur within this subset and the benefit of HDCT in the patients with early chemotherapy resistance was based on a small sample size of 70 patients, data were not considered robust enough to be translated into conventional treatment. The authors concluded that four cycles of BEP remains the standard chemotherapy for this population, but early referral for clinical studies should be considered for patients with a suboptimal decline in serum tumor markers after two cycles of conventional cisplatin-based chemotherapy.

In summary, patients diagnosed with a poor-risk prognosis NSGCT (seminomas are never classified as poor-risk prognosis), should be treated within the scope of clinical trial if available for them. Otherwise, four cycles of BEP (or VIP) is considered the standard to which other regimens should be compared. More intensive treatments, including HDCT, should be considered in those patients with early resistance to chemotherapy as part of clinical studies only (Figure 14.4). However, regardless of the treatment, a significant proportion of patients are expected to relapse.

Therapeutic Options at Relapse

The management of relapsed stage I and stage II disease and the excellent results with standard chemotherapy as salvage modality has been described in a previous section. Conversely, approximately half of patients with intermediate and poor-risk disease are expected to relapse, and only 25% of these will have a prolonged response to standard salvage chemotherapy.

Our patient also reflects the most common type of presentation at relapse. Indeed, the majority of relapses are detected by an increase in the serum tumor markers during routine follow-up (even in patients with normal serum tumor markers at original presentation), and most relapses will occur within 2 years of the original chemotherapy. Patients who experience relapse within 4 weeks of receiving cisplatin-based chemotherapy are considered to have cisplatin-refractory disease that carries a particularly poor prognosis. Likewise, those who relapse after 2 years have a tendency for chemotherapy resistance and a worse prognosis unless aggressive surgical resection of residual masses is possible.

Both paclitaxel and ifosfamide had shown activity as salvage treatment after platinum-based chemotherapy. For this reason, for those patients who relapse within 2 years, standard dose chemotherapy options include VeIP (vinblastine 0.11 mg/kg per day for 2 days, ifosfamide 1200 mg/m^2 per day for 5 days, and cisplatin 20 mg/m^2 per day for 5 days) and TIP (paclitaxel 250 mg/m^2 on day 1 followed by ifosfamide 1500 mg/m^2 per day and cisplatin 25 mg/m^2 per day on days 2 to 5). If etoposide was not given during initial chemotherapy (rare occurrence nowadays), VIP chemotherapy becomes an alternative. For patients who relapse after VIP therapy (like the one described here), second-line therapy is less defined. While TIP is still a reasonable option, regimens including gemcitabine and/or oxaliplatin (both of which have showed activity in cisplatin-refractory disease) have also been utilized.

Loehrer and colleagues evaluated 135 patients who received VeIP for relapsed disease after etoposide- and cisplatin-based chemotherapy. A CR was achieved in 49.6% of patients. At 6 years of follow-up, 23.7% were continuously free of disease (23). A previous study from the same institution (Miller et al., 1997), showed that patients with seminoma have a better response to VeIP as salvage therapy, with 54% of patients (13 out of 24) remaining as long-term survivors (median follow-up of 7 years).

Results with paclitaxel had been even more promising. A small phase I/II study (Motzer et al., 2000) included a selected population of 30 patients with relapsing GCTs with favorable prognostic factor as per MSKCC criteria (testicular primary, less than six previous cycles of cisplatin, and a CR to initial chemotherapy). Paclitaxel was started at a dose of 175 mg/m^2 and increased up to 250 mg/m^2 in a subsequent cohort (24 out of 30 patients received the latter dose). They reported a CR in 77% of the patients, with a durable response in 73% (at 33 months). An extension trial included 16 extra patients, all receiving paclitaxel at a dose of 250 mg/m^2 (24). A total of 29 patients showed a CR after chemotherapy alone with another 3 patients achieving a CR after resection of a residual mass (32/46 patients, 70%). Twenty-nine patients remained disease free at 69 months (63% durable complete response). Results were less encouraging in the 43 evaluable patients included in a multicenter study in England (Mead et al., 2005). This study, however, also included patients with less favorable prognostic factors, used a lower dose of paclitaxel and ifosfamide, and allowed dose reductions based on cytopenias (the studies by Motzer and Kondagunta included the routine use of granulocyte colony stimulating factors after chemotherapy). In the whole cohort, a favorable response (CR or partial response with negative serum tumor markers) was recorded in 60%, but only a 38% failure-free survival (FFS) after 1 year. When only the 26 patients meeting similar good-prognosis criteria as those from the MSKCC study were analyzed, favorable response rate and FFS were somewhat better (73% and 43%, respectively) but still less impressive than those at MSKCC.

On the basis of these results, chemotherapy with TIP (with paclitaxel dose of 250 mg/m^2) or VeIP is the preferred treatment strategy for patients who relapse after initial cisplatin-based chemotherapy and good-risk features (testicular primary, low serum tumor markers and disease volume, and complete response to first line chemotherapy). In centers with adequate expertise, HDCT with stem cell rescue can be considered. Conversely, for those patients with poor-prognosis features, inclusion in a clinical trial should be considered, given the suboptimal results with conventional chemotherapy. If no clinical trial is available, conventional chemotherapy or HDCT should be pursued. Poor-prognosis features include an extratesticular primary, high-volume disease or markedly increased serum tumor markers, as well as patients considered cisplatin-refractory and those with late relapse.

Patients who progress within 4 weeks of receiving a cisplatin-based chemotherapy or during chemotherapy cycles, are defined as refractory and absolute refractory, respectively, and have a distinctly poor prognosis. These patients are candidates for palliative gemcitabine/oxaliplatin-based chemotherapy or HDCT. The former is based mostly in phase II studies that began after gemcitabine and later oxaliplatin had shown single-agent activity against GCTs. When used as a single agent in 32 patients, oxaliplatin showed a response rate of 13% (Kollmannsberger et al., 2002). The same group subsequently reported the use of oxaliplatin in combination with gemcitabine in 35 patients (63% cisplatin-refractory and 89% relapsed after HDCT). The overall response was 46% (16 patients), including three patients with a CR (all of whom remained disease free at the end of follow-up). Seven of the sixteen responders were cisplatin-refractory, including one patient who achieved CR (25). Similarly, Pectasides and colleagues reported their experience with this combination (GEMOX) in 28 patients with refractory (83%) or absolute refractory (17%) disease (Pectasides et al., 2003). A response was seen in nine patients (32%) including four patients who achieved a CR. All of those in CR remained disease free at the end of follow-up (one after salvage surgery), giving a long-term disease-free survival of 14%, an encouraging result in this heavily pretreated group of patients. The combination of paclitaxel with gemcitabine has been evaluated as well (Hinton et al., 2002). Of 28 patients, 6 responded (21.4%) and 3 patients achieved CR. Two of the latter remained disease free at follow-up (15 and 25 months). More recently, paclitaxel was used in combination with both gemcitabine and oxaliplatin by the German Testicular Cancer Study Group (Bokemeyer et al., 2008) in 41 heavily pretreated patients (35% with refractory or absolute refractory disease). An overall response of 51% was observed (5% CR, 34% marker-negative PR and 12% marker-positive PR). The CR rate increased to 17% after resection of residual disease was achieved in five patients. After 5 months, 15% of patients remained in CR, with a median response duration of 8 months. Although each of these regimens is considered palliative for patients with very poor prognosis, a small number of patients may achieve a significant survival.

The Use of High-Dose Therapy With Autologous Stem Cell Support

Another treatment option for advanced GCT involves the use of HDCT regimens followed by stem cell rescue. This strategy has been tested in different settings, and currently HDCT is considered part of the armamentarium of second-line treatment for patients who relapse after initial chemotherapy and a reasonable third-line treatment in those who relapse after conventional dose salvage chemotherapy. Some patients will respond to conventional chemotherapy, and are thus spared from the potential toxicity of HDCT. Identifying patients unresponsive to conventional therapy who are more or less likely to respond to HDCT remains an important challenge. The first attempt to define these prognostic factors came from a multicenter retrospective analysis of 310 patients treated with HDCT for relapsing or refractory disease (26). In a multivariate analysis, progressive disease before HDCT, mediastinal NSGCT primary, refractory disease, and HCG levels before HDCT greater than 1000 IU/L correlated with worse prognosis. These were used to classify patients with good, intermediate, and poor prognoses, with FFS rates at 2 years of 51%, 27%, and 5%, respectively. Subsequent studies validated the Beyer model. A phase II trial (Rick et al., 2001) evaluated 80 patients treated with three cycles of TIP followed by HDCT with carboplatin, etoposide, and thiotepa. Patients with good prognosis as per the Beyer model had an OS of 53% and an FFS rate of 47% at 3 years compared with 23% and 8%, respectively, for those with intermediate prognosis and no long-term survivors among those with poor prognosis.

The appropriate timing for HDCT as well as the choice of agents or whether single versus tandem HDCT should be used had been the focus of several studies over the past two decades. These questions, unfortunately, remain mostly unanswered despite these efforts because of the relatively small numbers, lack of randomization, different regimens used, and differences in the population selected for these studies.

A phase I/II study (Motzer et al., 2000) employing a dose-intensive regimen with two cycles of ifosfamide/paclitaxel (given 2 weeks apart) followed by three cycles of high-dose etoposide and carboplatin (with increasing dose of carboplatin between cohorts) included 37 patients considered unlikely to respond to conventional chemotherapy as second-line treatment. Most of these patients had incomplete response to first-line treatment, and eight patients had mediastinal primary tumors. After 30 months of follow-up, 15 patients (41%) remained disease free, including one patient with mediastinal primary. A different approach was used at Indiana University, where two cycles of HDCT are given upfront and patients with primary mediastinal tumors were excluded. The first retrospective analysis (Bhatia et al., 2000) included the outcomes of 65 patients who underwent two cycles of high-dose carboplatin and etoposide followed by stem cell rescue as initial salvage therapy. Forty-one patients achieved a CR and 15 patients got a PR with negative markers. Of these 57 patients, 20 relapsed after a median follow-up of 39 months. Thus, 37 patients (57%) were continuously disease free by the end of the follow-up period. When analyzed separately, 68% of patients (27/40) in the good-prognosis group were disease free compared with 40% (10/25) of the intermediate- or poor-prognosis group. In addition, nine out of ten patients with seminoma were disease free at the end of the trial. A more recent study from the same institution reported the outcomes of 184 patients using the same regimen (27). At a median follow-up of 48 months, 116 patients from the whole cohort were still in CR (63%). In a subset analysis, 70% of those who received HDCT in first relapse were disease free (94 out of 135) compared with 45% of those receiving it after two or more previous regimens (22 out of 49). Moreover, 18 out of 40 patients with cisplatin-refractory disease were still in CR. The multivariate analysis revealed that the timing of HDCT (best when used as second-line rather than third-line treatment), cisplatin-refractoriness, and IGCCCG poor-risk stage were independent predictors of response. When a scoring algorithm was applied using these factors, different OS curves (low, intermediate, and high risk) were statistically significant.

Less encouraging results were obtained in a European multicenter randomized study (Pico et al., 2005). In this study, 280 patients received either four cycles of VeIP/VIP or three cycles followed by one cycle of high-dose carboplatin with etoposide and cyclophosphamide (CarboPEC) with stem cell transplant as rescue. After 3 years, no significant differences in OS (59% vs. 53% in those receiving conventional salvage chemotherapy) or event-free survival (42% vs. 35%) were observed, whereas more deaths attributed to treatment were seen in those receiving HDCT (7% vs. 3%). However, only 73% of the patients randomized to the HDCT arm received this treatment and up to 20% patients had a nontesticular primary tumor that may explain the inferior results compared with those later reported by Einhorn and colleagues. Whether two cycles of HDCT provides better results than a single cycle can only be answered by a well-designed randomized study.

Management of Brain Metastases

Finally, the patient (C.P.) described in this vignette presented with a single site of recurrence, in this case a solitary brain mass. CNS metastases are a relatively rare occurrence, being diagnosed in about 1% of patients with metastatic GCTs at the time of original presentation, whereas up to an additional 4% will develop them during the course of the disease. Given its rarity, most of our knowledge arises from small retrospective series. These studies identified three subsets with distinct prognosis. First, in patients with brain metastasis as part of their initial presentation, disease-specific survival ranges from 43% to 86% in the different series. A second group comprises those with brain metastasis as a manifestation of relapse after a CR with conventional chemotherapy, and the final group includes those who develop brain metastasis after an incomplete response to chemotherapy and those with additional metastatic sites. Whereas the former can show survival rates between 39% and 44%, the latter group usually has poor outcomes with survival rates between 2% and 26%. Patients with a single metastatic site that is amenable for local therapy tend to have significantly better prognosis that explains the wide range of survival rates reported in the different series.

Owing to the lack of prospective data, the optimal management of brain metastasis in metastatic GCTs is unclear. Currently, most centers and guidelines advocate the use of chemotherapy as an initial step. The rationale of this approach is based on the adequate penetration through the brain-blood barrier, in the presence of macroscopic intracerebral metastasis, of the most common chemotherapy agents used for treatment of GCTs, including cisplatin. Moreover, the majority of these patients present with additional metastatic foci, either as part of the initial presentation or as relapse, therefore requiring adequate systemic treatment. Patients who are chemotherapy-naïve tend to have better responses to chemotherapy, hence the better survival rates seen in this group. The development of chemotherapy resistance within clinically silent brain metastases during initial conventional chemotherapy may explain the inferior outcomes of chemotherapy when used in patients with brain lesions as a manifestation of relapse. Whether HDCT could overcome the development of these resistant clones is debatable. A small series from Germany (Kollmannsberger et al., 2000) used HDCT in 22 patients with brain metastasis during the initial presentation. Patients received a median of four cycles of HDCT, with a radiation boost given to 12 patients with residual disease. The PFS and OS were quite impressive with 72% and 81%, respectively, after 2 years of follow-up. Further studies are needed to confirm these results.

The appropriate approach after chemotherapy is controversial. Whole brain radiation (WBXRT) has been used as part of the management of brain metastases in a variety of malignancies. However, given the usual young age of onset and the possibility of long-term survival in patients with GCTs, concerns of late toxicity are a priority. Five cases of delayed CNS toxicity consistent with progressive multifocal leukoencephalopathy among 30 patients considered cured after being treated with WBXRT for metastatic GCT were recently reported (Doyle and Einhorn, 2008), concluding that this treatment is not innocuous for young patients. Furthermore, questions had arisen regarding its usefulness in the absence of multifocal residual disease as surgical resection seems to provide similar results without delayed toxicity. A small study (Gremmer et al., 2008) reported the outcomes of 22 patients treated at a single institution comparing WBXRT after resection of easily accessible solitary brain lesions against a more aggressive surgical approach without WBXRT. They concluded that cure can be achieved with induction chemotherapy and aggressive surgery without WBXRT. Similarly, a retrospective pooled analysis of 139 patients treated for brain metastasis between 1979 and 1995 in Europe showed that the use of WBXRT did not translate into good prognosis in those patients with brain metastasis found at the initial presentation, but did seem to benefit those receiving it as part of relapse treatment (28). Delayed toxicity was not addressed in this study.

Given these questions, many centers had abandoned the routine use of postchemotherapy WBXRT, with further treatment now being given according to the response to chemotherapy. If no residual disease is seen, a careful surveillance approach is adopted. Conversely, if limited residual disease is noted on postchemotherapy imaging, local therapy is used, which includes surgical resection and focal RT. The use of WBXRT is reserved for those patients with more extensive residual disease or those who failed to respond to chemotherapy. There is however, no absolute consensus in this matter and current guidelines still include RT as part of the initial treatment of brain metastasis after chemotherapy.

In summary, C.P. would benefit from inclusion in a clinical trial for management of relapsed disease, including the possibility of HDCT. If no trial is available, conventional salvage chemotherapy with VeIP or TIP should be given. Despite the seemingly limited disease at the time of relapse, systemic chemotherapy should be given initially, especially considering his increased serum tumor markers. After completing chemotherapy, repeat imaging studies should be obtained. If a residual mass is present, surgical resection (or focal radiation if surgery is contraindicated or not feasible) should be pursued. This can be followed by WBXRT (especially in the relapse setting, more likely to be chemotherapy resistant) or surveillance (Figure 14.4).

Extragonadal NSGCT

E.N. is a previously healthy 22-year-old college student who presents to the free clinic during the fall with 3 weeks of dyspnea and cough. Initially he thought he had contracted a common cold from his niece on a recent trip home, but symptoms worsened and he now reports fever and night sweats. He is unsure about weight loss. He is up-to-date with his vaccinations and he is a lifelong nonsmoker. Physical exam is unremarkable and he is given a short course of antibiotics with no improvement in symptoms. A CXR showed a wide mediastinum. A CT of the chest showed a 7-cm mass in the anterior mediastinum. No other masses were found on imaging. Laboratory data were within normal limits except for increased serum tumor markers: AFP (2943 ng/mL), βHCG (11 IU/L), and LDH (523 IU/L). Scrotal ultrasound was unremarkable. These results strongly suggested a GCT and tissue obtained from the mediastinal mass confirmed the diagnosis of extragonadal NSGCT, with predominance of yolk sac tumor. E.N. received four cycles of VIP (etoposide, ifosfamide, cisplatin) with serum tumor markers returning to normal. CT scan images showed a partial response, with mediastinal NSGCT now measuring 4 cm. Surgical resection was then performed, with the pathology report showing necrosis and elements of teratoma with negative margins. Serum tumor markers and CT scans remained within normal parameters on the subsequent follow-up visit. Seven months after the initial diagnosis, he returned to the clinic complaining of weight loss, progressive weakness, and easy bruising. A CT scan did not show any evidence of recurrence and serum tumor markers were again normal but routine laboratory data showed pancytopenia (hemoglobin 8.1 g/dL, platelets 16,000 and WBC 4.1 × 10^9). Bone marrow biopsy was consistent with acute megakaryoblastic leukemia and fluorescence in situ hybridization (FISH) analyses demonstrated the presence of an isochromosome 12p (i12p). He received induction chemotherapy but limited response was seen. He died 3 weeks later due to complications of neutropenic fever.

Evidence-Based Case Discussion

This patient was diagnosed with an extragonadal germ cell tumor (EGCT). These tumors represent up to 5% of all GCTs, and are usually found in the midline on the body, mostly in the mediastinum or retroperitoneum, with other locations such as the pineal gland being much less common. The histogenesis of these tumors is unclear. It has been hypothesized that they may derive from germ cells that fail to complete their migration along the urogenital ridge during the embryonal development or that they may represent transformed testicular germ cells that undergo reverse migration (29). In some cases testicular calcifications can be seen in scrotal ultrasound, leading to the theory that EGCT are really metastatic GCTs with a "burnt-out" testicular primary. However, the fact that testicular GCT rarely metastasize to the anterior mediastinum and the reported association between mediastinal NSGCT with Klinefelter syndrome as well as the increased incidence of hematological malignancies (not seen with testicular primary tumors) support an independent origin. There is, nevertheless, an increased risk of developing a metachronous testicular GCT, especially in cases with a retroperitoneal primary.

There are no significant differences in the histology of these tumors compared with their gonadal counterparts, but there is a difference in their relative frequencies. Teratomas are the most common mediastinal GCT (60–70%), with mature teratomas being more common than immature. Pure seminomas represent less than a third of the remainder of EGCTs, and there is a higher incidence of yolk sac tumor among the nonseminomatous EGCTs. Features of GCT or teratoma are usually clearly defined in biopsy samples, but occasionally only a poorly differentiated tumor is reported. Serum tumor markers are elevated in 85% of patients, with more pronounced AFP levels. Elevations of βHCG are usually less marked. In rare instances, some centers will treat a poorly differentiated mediastinal tumor as GCT based on the concurrent elevation of serum tumor markers in a young male. As with testicular primary tumors, cytogenetic analyses frequently reveal an isochromosome i(12p).

Unlike primary testicular mature teratomas, which have some degree of metastatic potential and malignant transformation, mediastinal mature teratomas have a rather benign behavior and are frequently found incidentally unless symptoms related to compression of surrounding structures occur first. Resection is almost always curative. On the other hand, immature teratomas have a poor prognosis overall and are frequently incurable unless a complete resection is possible.

Most patients with either seminoma or nonseminomatous EGCTs are symptomatic at the time of diagnosis. Dyspnea, cough, chest pain, or discomfort are usual complaints among patients with mediastinal tumors, with weight loss, superior vena cava syndrome, fever, and nausea being less frequent, but reported presentations. Patients with retroperitoneal primaries will frequently present with abdominal and/or back pain.

Pure extragonadal seminomas are rare, with most data coming from relatively small series. Both mediastinal and retroperitoneal seminomas occur with rather similar frequencies, although mediastinal primaries had been considered more common by some series. They tend to grow slowly, and are usually bulky or metastatic by the time they cause symptoms and are diagnosed. Nevertheless, prognosis is still excellent for both mediastinal and retroperitoneal primaries, with no significant differences in PFS or OS between these two presentations (approximately 92% and 88% at 5 years, respectively). Primary chemotherapy is the treatment of choice in extragonadal seminoma. On the basis of the presence or absence of nonpulmonary metastasis, these tumors will have a good- or intermediate-risk prognosis (Table 14.3). The choice of agents and number of cycles to be used in good- and intermediate-risk disease had been previously described. In the case of mediastinal primaries, however, the use of bleomycin is sometimes avoided as there is a chance that thoracic surgery to remove residual masses may be required following chemotherapy. When residual masses are resected after treatment of extragonadal seminoma, necrosis is usually found. For this reason, as with stage II seminoma, many will observe masses of less than 3 cm, especially if resection is technically difficult. However, size criteria alone is even less reliable in this setting compared to those with gonadal primaries, so this recommendation is controversial. The use of PET scan is not yet recommended since false positives seem to be an issue. Occasionally, after resection, teratoma is found that may indicate the presence of nonseminomatous elements in the original tumor. Frequently used in the past as initial treatment for extragonadal seminoma, RT has fallen out of favor against primary chemotherapy. Since most of the times bulky disease is present at the time of the initial diagnosis, the use of RT results in high relapse rates (approximately 30%). Furthermore, patients initially treated with radiation may have a decreased response to subsequent chemotherapy.

Unlike seminomas, patients with extragonadal NSGCT carry a worse prognosis (30). This is particularly true for those with a mediastinal primary who are classified in the poor-risk prognosis group regardless of the serum tumor marker levels or the absence of distant metastases. Before the cisplatin era, survival rates for these patients were usually less than 5%. With the current chemotherapy regimens plus aggressive surgical management of residual masses, survival rates around 50% are common.

Patients with relapsing extragonadal mediastinal primary tumors have dismal responses to salvage therapy, including HDCT. In fact, many centers will exclude these patients from HDCT trials. In general, survival rates of approximately 10% are expected for this population. Although long-term survival had been reported, this usually occurred in cases where complete resection of the mass was achieved. This highlights the important role surgery has in the salvage treatment of these patients even in the presence of increased tumor markers.

Although the prognosis of patients with retroperitoneal primaries is not as poor as those with mediastinal primaries, they usually have worse survival rates than their gonadal counterparts when matched by the IGCCCG prognostic classification, especially for those with good or intermediate prognosis. In the largest retrospective series to date, which included 283 patients with retroperitoneal primary tumors, the survival rate for those with good or intermediate prognosis was 61%, a result clearly inferior compared to those expected in those groups. The authors suggested that these patients may benefit from four cycles of chemotherapy instead of the standard recommendation of three cycles. This study also showed that patients with a retroperitoneal primary who relapsed after chemotherapy had similar long-term salvage rates to those reported for patients with relapsed metastatic gonadal GCT.

The patient described in the vignette was successfully treated with four cycles of chemotherapy for a mediastinal primary GCT. However, he died shortly afterward due to acute leukemia. The short period between chemotherapy and the development of leukemia argues against treatment toxicity, since chemotherapy-induced second malignancies usually take years to develop. Hematologic disorders associated with EGCTs, especially in the megakaryocytic line, had been described in the literature with relative frequency. These had been reported almost exclusively in association with mediastinal NSGCT, with an incidence in this subset of patients as high as 6%. These disorders are usually diagnosed within months of the diagnosis of mediastinal GCT (median time to onset of 6 months), and sometimes are diagnosed concurrently. They follow a rather aggressive course with a poor response to treatment, with a median survival time of 5 months. Cytogenetic analysis of leukemic cells frequently reveals an isochromosome i(12p), which suggests a common carcinogenesis pathway with the original GCT.

REFERENCES

1. Jemal A, Siegel R, Ward E, et al. Cancer statistics, 2009. *CA Cancer J Clin.* 2009;59;225–249.
2. Oh J, Landman J, Evers A, et al. Management of the postpubertal patient with cryptorchidism: an updated analysis. *J Urol.* 2002;167:1329.
3. Fossa SD, Chen J, Schonfeld SJ, et al. Risk of contralateral testicular cancer: a population-based study of 29,515 U.S. men. *J Natl Cancer Inst.* 2005; 97:1056.
4. Bosl GJ, Ilson DH, Rodriguez E, et al. Clinical relevance of the i(12p) marker chromosome in germ cell tumors. *J Natl Cancer Inst.* 1994; 86:349.
5. Ulbright, TM. Germ cell tumors of the gonads: a selective review emphasizing problems in differential diagnosis, newly appreciated, and controversial issues. *Mod Pathol.* 2005;18(Suppl 2):S61.
6. Bosl GJ, Motzer RJ. Medical progress: testicular germ-cell cancer. *N Engl J Med.* 1997;337:242.
7. International Germ Cell Cancer Collaborative Group. International germ cell consensus classification: a prognostic factor-based staging system for metastatic germ cell cancers. J *Clin Oncol.* 1997;15:594–603.
8. National Comprehensive Cancer Network. NCCN clinical practice guidelines in oncology: testicular cancer V.1.2011. http://www.nccn.org/professionals/physician_gls/ f_guidelines.asp.
9. Warde P, Specht L, Horwich A, et al. Prognostic factors for relapse in stage I seminoma managed by surveillance: a pooled analysis. *J Clin Oncol.* 2002;20:4448.
10. Travis LB, Curtis RE, Storm H, et al. Risk of second malignant neoplasms among long-term survivors of testicular cancer. *J Natl Cancer Inst.* 1997;89:1429.
11. Jones WG, Fossa SD, Mead GM, et al. Randomized trial of 30 versus 20 Gy in the adjuvant treatment of stage I Testicular Seminoma: a report on Medical Research Council Trial TE18, European Organisation for the Research and Treatment of Cancer Trial 30942 (ISRCTN18525328). *J Clin Oncol.* 2005;23:1200.
12. Oliver RTD, Mason MD, Mead GM, et al. Radiotherapy versus single-dose carboplatin in adjuvant treatment of stage I seminoma: a randomized trial. *Lancet* 2005;366:293–300.
13. Read G, Stenning SP, Cullen MH, et al. Medical Research Council prospective study of surveillance for stage I testicular teratoma. Medical Research Council Testicular Tumors Working Party. *J Clin Oncol.* 1992;10:1762–1768.
14. Spermon JR, Roeleveld TA, van del Poel HG, et al. Comparison of surveillance and retroperitoneal lymph node dissection in stage I nonseminomatous germ cell tumors. *Urology.* 2002;59:923–929.
15. Classen J, Schmidberger H, Meisner C, et al. Radiotherapy for stages iia/b testicular seminoma: final report of a prospective multicenter clinical trial. *J Clin Oncol.* 2003;21:1101–1106.
16. De Santis M, Becherer A, Bokemeyer C, et al. 2–18 Fluoro-deoxy-d-glucose positron emission tomography is a reliable predictor for viable tumor in postchemotherapy seminoma: an update of the prospective multicentric SEMPET trial. *J Clin Oncol.* 2004;22: 1034–1039.
17. Spiess PE, Kassouf W, Brown GA, et al. Surgical management of growing teratoma syndrome: the M. D. Anderson Cancer Center experience. *J Urol.* 2007;177(4):1330–1334.
18. Ehrlich Y, Brames MJ, Beck SDW, et al. Long-term follow-up of cisplatin combination chemotherapy in patients with disseminated nonseminomatous germ cell tumors: is a postchemotherapy retroperitoneal lymph node dissection needed after complete remission? *J Clin Oncol.* 2010;28(4):531–536.

19. Nichols CR, Catalano P, Crawford ED, et al. Randomized comparison of cisplatin and etoposide and either bleomycin or ifosfamide in treatment of advanced disseminated germ cell tumors; an Eastern Cooperative Oncology Group, Southwest Oncology Group, and Cancer and Leukemia Group B study. *J Clin Oncol.* 1998;16:1287–1293.
20. Cagini L, Nicholson AG, Horwich A, et al. Thoracic metastasectomy for germ cell tumors: long term survival and prognostic factors. *Ann Oncol.* 1998;9:1185–1991.
21. Steyerberg EW, Keizer HJ, Messemer JE, et al. Residual pulmonary masses after chemotherapy for metastatic nonseminomatous germ cell tumor. Prediction of histology. ReHiT Study Group. *Cancer.* 1997;79:345–355.
22. Motzer RJ, Nichols CJ, Margolin KA, et al. Phase III randomized trial of conventional-dose chemotherapy with or without high-dose chemotherapy and autologous hematopoietic stem-cell rescue as first-line treatment for patients with poor-prognosis metastatic germ cell tumors. *J Clin Oncol.* 2007;25(3):247–256.
23. Loehrer PJ Sr, Gonin R, Nichols CR, et al. Vinblastine plus ifosfamide plus cisplatin as initial salvage therapy in recurrent germ cell tumor. *J Clin Oncol.* 1998;16:2500–2504.
24. Kondagunta GV, Bacik J, Donadio A, et al. Combination of paclitaxel, ifosfamide, and cisplatin is an effective second-line therapy for patients with relapsed testicular germ cell tumors. *J Clin Oncol.* 2005;23:6549–6555.
25. Kollmannsberger C, Beyer J, Liersch R, et al. Combination chemotherapy with gemcitabine plus oxaliplatin in patients with intensively pretreated or refractory germ cell cancer: a study of the German testicular cancer study group. *J Clin Oncol.* 2004;22:108–114.
26. Beyer J, Kramar A, Mandanas R, et al. High-dose chemotherapy as salvage treatment in germ cell tumors: a multivariate analysis of prognostic variables. *J Clin Oncol.* 1996;14:2638–2645.
27. Einhorn LH, Williams SD, Chamness A, et al. High-dose chemotherapy and stem-cell rescue for metastatic germ-cell tumors. *N Engl J Med.* 2007;357(4):340–348.
28. Fossa SD, Bokemeyer C, Gerl A, et al. Treatment outcome of patients with brain metastases from malignant germ cell tumors. *Cancer.* 1999;85:988–997
29. Bokemeyer C, Nichols CR, Droz JP, et al. Extragonadal germ cell tumors of the mediastinum and retroperitoneum: results from an international analysis. *J Clin Oncol.* 2002;20:1864–1873.
30. Vuky J, Bains M, Bacik J, et al. Role of postchemotherapy adjunctive surgery in the management of patients with nonseminoma arising from the mediastinum. *J Clin Oncol.* 2001;19:682–688.

15

Kidney Cancer

JENNY J. KIM AND BRUCE G. REDMAN

EPIDEMIOLOGY, RISK FACTORS, NATURAL HISTORY, AND PATHOLOGY

Renal cell carcinoma (RCC) comprises approximately 2% to 3% of all malignancies with an expected 58,240 new cases and 13,040 deaths in the United States in 2010. It is the seventh most common malignancy in U.S. men and the eighth most common malignancy in U.S. women. The median age at diagnosis of RCC is 60 years. Although the gap is narrowing, there is a male predominance in incidence with a male:female ratio of 2:1. Over the last 50 years, the number of new cases of RCC has also steadily increased, largely due to noninvasive imaging studies that permit detection of small, organ-confined disease amenable to definitive therapy. The incidence of advanced disease has also increased over the same period, although the reason for this increase remains unclear.

Several risk factors have been implicated in the development of RCC. Smoking has been shown to double the risk of developing RCC. Obesity (specifically increased body mass index) is also associated with an increased risk of RCC, although specific dietary associations are not well defined. Exposure to chemical carcinogens such as cadmium, asbestos, and petroleum by-products is linked to an increased risk of RCC as well. Furthermore, individuals with end-stage renal disease and acquired renal cystic disease have a higher risk of developing RCC as compared to the general population. Despite these associations, most patients with RCC are without clearly identifiable environmental and/or lifestyle risk factors.

Kidney cancer can also be a feature of several recognizable genetic syndromes and approximately 5% of all RCC cases may be considered to have a strong heritable component. For example, hereditary papillary renal carcinoma is an autosomal dominant hereditary syndrome marked by the occurrence of multifocal, bilateral kidney tumors with a papillary histology. This syndrome has been shown to be due to mutations in the MET proto-oncogene (1). Another well-recognized genetic syndrome is von-Hippel Lindau (VHL) disease, which is an autosomal dominant disorder with a wide spectrum of vascular tumors including hemangioblastomas of the central nervous system, retinal angiomas, serous cystadenomas and neuroendocrine tumors of the pancreas, as well as clear cell RCCs. Renal cell tumors associated with VHL syndrome tend to be early onset and multifocal. VHL is caused by mutations in the VHL tumor suppressor gene on chromosome 3p25 (2). The incidence of VHL syndrome is approximately 1 in 36,000 births.

The prognosis of RCC depends largely on the extent of disease (see AJCC staging system below), nuclear differentiation (Fuhrman grade), and clinical factors (performance status). Several prognostic models have been developed over the years, including the UCLA Integrated Staging System (UISS) the mostly widely and extensively studied model which takes into account several factors mentioned earlier in predicting patients' long term outcome (3) (Table 15.1).

RCC consists of several histologic subtypes, with the clear cell subtype comprising approximately 80% of all RCC. Other histological subtypes include papillary, chromophobe, oncocytic, collecting-duct, unclassified, and medullary, each with its distinct genetic, histological, and clinical characteristics (4,5) (see Figure 15.1).

Table 15.1 UCLA Integrated Staging System (UISS)

UISS Stage	1997 TNM Stage	Fuhrman Grade	ECOG PS	2-Year Survival (%)	5-Year Survival (%)
I	I	1,2	0	96	94
II	I	1,2	≥1	89	67
	I	3,4	Any		
	II	Any	Any		
	III	Any	0		
	III	1	≥1		
III	III	2–4	≥1	66	39
	IV	1,2	0		
IV	IV	3,4	0	42	23
		1–3	≥1		
V	IV	4	≥1	9	0

	Clear cell	Papillary	Chromophobe
Histology			
Frequency	70–80%	10–15%	3–5%
Genetic abnormalities	• Deletions of chromosome 3p segments • Inactvation of *VHL* gene by mutation and promoter hypermethylation • Gain of chromosome 5q • Loss of chromosomes 8p, 9p, and 14q	• Trisomy of chromosomes 7 and 17 • Loss of chromosome Y in men • Gain of chromosomes 12, 16, and 20 • Rare mutations of Met proto-oncogene	• Loss of chromosomes Y, 1, 2, 6, 10, 13, 17, and 21
Characteristics	• Compact nests of tumour cells with clear cytoplasm separated by delicate vasculature • Several architectural patterns, including solid, alveolar, and acinar	• Microscopically variable proportions of papillae, tubulopapillae, and tubules • Type I: papillae lined with one layer of tumour cells with scant pale cytoplasm and low-grade nuclei • Type II: abundant eosinophilic cytoplasm and large pseudostratified nuclei with prominent nucleoli	• Cells are large, polygonal with finely reticulated cytoplasm, distinct cell borders, and atypical nuclei with perinuclear halo • Cells can have intensely eosinophilic cytoplasm

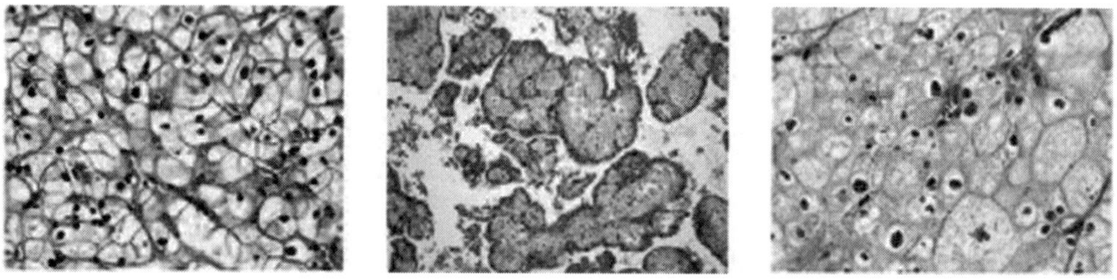

Figure 15.1

Major histological subtypes of RCC. (see color insert)

STAGING

Staging System for Renal Cell Carcinoma

Stage	Description
I	Tumor ≤7 cm in greatest dimension, limited to the kidney
II	Tumor >7 cm in greatest dimension, limited to the kidney
III	Tumor limited to kidney with ONE regional lymph node (LN) involvement OR Tumor extends into major veins or perinephric tissues but NOT into the ipsilateral adrenal gland and NOT beyond Gerota's fascia with or without regional LN involvement
IV	Tumor involves ipsilateral adrenal gland and/or extends beyond Gerota's fascia OR Involvement of more than one regional lymph nodes OR Presence of distant metastasis

Source: AJCC Cancer Staging Handbook, 7th Edition

CASE SUMMARIES

Limited Stage RCC

P.A. is a 42-year-old Caucasian man with no significant past medical history who presented to his local emergency department with left flank pain and gross hematuria. He had a history of kidney stones, thus a CT scan of the abdomen and pelvis was performed to rule out a recurrence. The CT scan showed a 7.7 × 6.7 cm enhancing interpolar left renal mass. A CT of the chest revealed no evidence of metastatic disease. P.A. underwent left radical nephrectomy that showed a 7.5 × 6.6 × 4.3 cm RCC, clear cell type, Fuhrman nuclear grade 3 out of 4. The perirenal and renal sinus fat as well as soft tissue resection margins were free of tumor. No angiolymphatic invasion was identified. The pathologic staging was pT2a N0 M0. No additional treatment was recommended and the patient was followed every 6 months by her surgeon without clinical or radiological evidence of disease recurrence.

Evidence-Based Case Discussion

The classic triad of symptoms of RCC includes flank pain, hematuria, and a palpable mass in the abdomen. However, fewer than 10% of patients with kidney cancer have all three features, which are typically associated with more advanced disease. Notably, P.A. had hematuria that suggests invasion of the tumor into the collecting system. Staging is mainly accomplished by CT imaging where contrast enhancement correlates with malignant disease in about 80% of cases. Chest imaging is also recommended as part of the initial staging evaluation. Further staging including brain MRI and bone scan are indicated only if there is clinical suspicion of metastases to these sites. This patient has stage II disease, and according to the UISS model, has a 60% to 70% probability of 5-year survival (Table 15.1). Currently, the recommended treatment for stage I to III RCC is surgical resection (6). Traditional surgical management of RCC is radical nephrectomy that includes resection of the kidney, perirenal fat, regional lymph nodes, and ipsilateral adrenal gland. However, more recent approaches aim to achieve adequate tumor control while minimizing removal of structures unlikely to be involved with cancer. For example, the National Comprehensive Cancer Network (NCCN) Kidney Cancer panel recommends adrenal gland resection only when involvement is suspected by preoperative CT or in the presence of a large upper pole tumor (6). Other contemporary trends in resection of kidney cancer includes an increased use of partial nephrectomy (also known as "nephron sparing surgery") using open as well as laparoscopic and robotic approaches, thereby maximally preserving the patients' renal function.

Radiation therapy to the nephrectomy site as well as systemic immunotherapy with interferon (IFN) or interleuken-2 (IL-2) have been evaluated in the adjuvant setting, but have demonstrated no significant impact on relapse or survival. The recent success of anti-VEGF therapy in advanced disease has also led to evaluation of these agents in the adjuvant setting. At present, however, there are no data to support routine use of local or systemic adjuvant therapy. Thus, outside of a clinical trial, postsurgical observation remains the standard of care.

Recommended clinical monitoring following primary therapy for RCC should be individualized according to patient factors as well as specific features of the tumor, including grade and stage as they relate to the risk of recurrence (Table 15.1). The majority of recurrences are detected within 3 years of surgery. According to NCCN guidelines, patients should be evaluated at least every 6 months for 2 or 3 years and then annually.

Locally Advanced RCC

T.D. is a 56-year-old Caucasian man who presented to his physician with vague left flank pain of 1-week duration. His physical examination was unremarkable. Urine analysis showed microscopic hematuria without evidence of urinary tract infection. A CT scan of the abdomen showed a 10-cm heterogeneous left renal mass with retroperitoneal lymphadenopathy, the largest of which was 2.5 cm in diameter. A CT scan of the chest was negative for evidence of metastatic disease. T.D. underwent a radical nephrectomy with lymph node dissection, and pathology review showed a 9.5-cm clear cell RCC, Fuhrman grade 3/4 with tumor involvement of the renal vein, and 1 of 10 lymph nodes.

Evidence-Based Case Discussion

Renal vein invasion of the primary tumor and 1 lymph node positivity denote pT3 N1, and therefore a stage III disease. In localized disease, routine lymphadenectomy is not generally recommended as evidenced by the EORTC 30881 trial that randomized 772 patients to nephrectomy with or without regional lymphadenectomy. After 12 years of follow up, there was no difference in disease-specific mortality with lymphadenectomy (7). However, only 4 % of the patients in the lymphadenectomy group had positive lymph nodes on pathology review, suggesting that majority of patients enrolled in the study may have been low-risk patients who likely did not need lymphadenectomy. Currently, however, patients with suspected lymph node involvement on preoperative imaging studies are candidates for extended lymph node dissection, which may provide a survival advantage in this subset of patients. As in the previous case of localized RCC, standard of care after nephrectomy is surveillance. The potential benefit of adjuvant therapy using targeted agents is currently under investigation in ongoing clinical trials as mentioned in the previous case.

Advanced RCC

T.M. is a 67-year-old Caucasian woman who presented with left lower quadrant pain. Diverticulitis was suspected. However, a CT scan of the abdomen and pelvis revealed an 8-cm left renal mass suspicious for RCC. CT of the chest showed no evidence of metastatic disease. T.M. underwent a left radical nephrectomy that revealed a 7.7 cm, Fuhrman grade 2/3 clear cell RCC. She embarked on surveillance postoperatively and remained free of recurrence. Two years postnephrectomy, however, the patient complained of right buttock discomfort and a surveillance CT scan revealed a 7.7 × 5.6 cm lesion in the right ilium. A CT-guided biopsy of the right iliac bone confirmed metastatic RCC. A bone scan showed increased uptake in the right iliac bone and in the left proximal femur suggestive of metastases. A CT scan of the chest showed multiple bilateral lung nodules. Aside from elevated alkaline phosphatase at 296 IU/L, all laboratory studies including hemoglobin, platelet count, and absolute neutrophil count, along with serum calcium, albumin, and LDH, were normal. Her Karnofsky performance status was 90%.

Evidence-Based Case Discussion

T.M. has metastatic clear cell RCC with lesions in the ilium, left femur, and lung after definitive nephrectomy 2 years earlier. With regard to prognosis, a large retrospective multivariate analysis from Memorial Sloan Kettering Cancer Center (during a time period when cytokines were often used in the treatment of metastatic RCC) defined the following negative prognostic variables in advanced RCC patients (8):

- A Karnofsky performance status (KPS) of <80%
- Serum lactic dehydrogenase (LDH) level >1.5 times the upper limit of normal
- Corrected serum calcium >10 mg/dL (2.5 mmol/L)
- Hemoglobin concentration below the lower limit of normal
- Absence of nephrectomy (i.e., no disease-free interval)

These prognostic factors subdivide patients into three risk groups: a favorable-risk group (no risk factors), an intermediate-risk group (1 or 2 risk factors), and a poor-risk group (3 or more risk factors). Survival rates at 1 year for favorable-risk, intermediate-risk, and poor-risk patients are 71%, 42%, and 12%, respectively, and at 3 years are 31%, 7%, and 0%, respectively.

Prognostic factors for survival of advanced RCC in the targeted therapy era have also been reported. A multivariate analysis of baseline characteristics seen in 645 patients who were treated with sunitinib, sorafenib, or bevacizumab also confirmed the relevance of KPS <80, time from original diagnosis to treatment of less than 1 year, hemoglobin less than the lower limit of normal, and elevated serum calcium. Two other laboratory parameters including neutrophil count and platelet count greater than the upper limit of normal were also significantly related to prognosis. These prognostic factors may be helpful in patient care and counseling as well as proper patient stratification and selection in clinical trial design in the targeted therapy era (9).

In the past, treatment options for patients with advanced RCC were limited to cytokine therapy or participation in a clinical trial. Importantly, high-dose IL-2 still remains the only modality of therapy that can result in long-term disease remission in a small, but select group of patients with advanced clear cell RCC. Favorable patient characteristics for high-dose IL-2 include a clear cell histology, good performance status (ECOG 0–1), minimal disease burden and lung only disease. Recently updated data reported in a single arm phase II study (SELECT) confirmed the association between an improved response outcome and these patient selection criteria—results that were reported at the ASCO 2010 Annual Meeting (10).

Furthermore, an improved understanding of the biology of renal cell cancer (including distinctive characteristics such as VHL silencing and resulting hypoxia-induced factor accumulation and a heavy dependence on angiogenesis for viability and progression) has provided the mechanistic rationale for the development and recent FDA approval of six new agents for the treatment of RCC (Table 15.2). These agents target the vascular endothelial growth factor (VEGF) pathway (sunitinib, sorafenib, bevacizumab, and pazopanib) and the mammalian target of rapamycin

Color Insert

	Clear cell	Papillary	Chromophobe
Histology	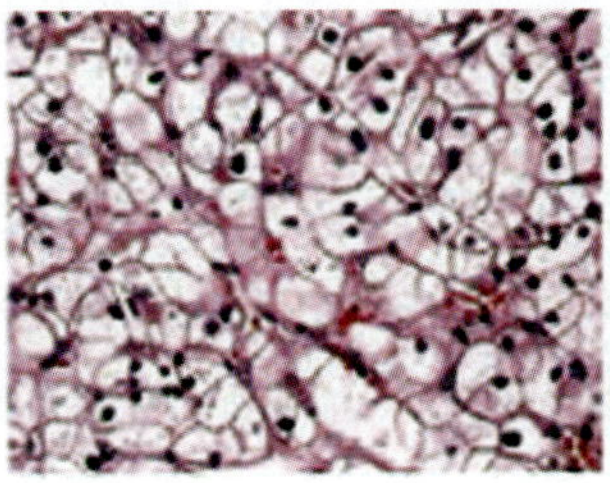	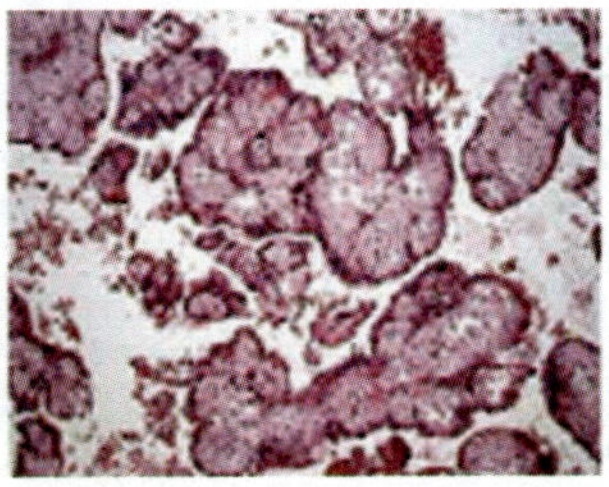	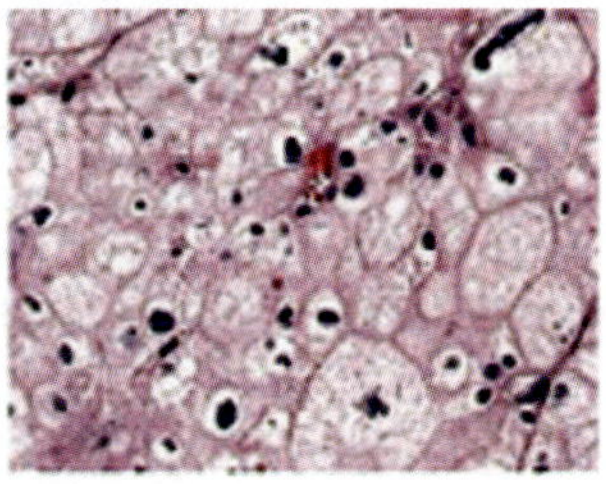
Frequency	70–80%	10–15%	3–5%
Genetic abnormalities	• Deletions of chromosome 3p segments • Inactvation of *VHL* gene by mutation and promoter hypermethylation • Gain of chromosome 5q • Loss of chromosomes 8p, 9p, and 14q	• Trisomy of chromosomes 7 and 17 • Loss of chromosome Y in men • Gain of chromosomes 12, 16, and 20 • Rare mutations of Met proto-oncogene	• Loss of chromosomes Y, 1, 2, 6, 10, 13, 17, and 21
Characteristics	• Compact nests of tumour cells with clear cytoplasm separated by delicate vasculature • Several architectural patterns, including solid, alveolar, and acinar	• Microscopically variable proportions of papillae, tubulopapillae, and tubules • Type I: papillae lined with one layer of tumour cells with scant pale cytoplasm and low-grade nuclei • Type II: abundant eosinophilic cytoplasm and large pseudostratified nuclei with prominent nucleoli	• Cells are large, polygonal with finely reticulated cytoplasm, distinct cell borders, and atypical nuclei with perinuclear halo • Cells can have intensely eosinophilic cytoplasm

Figure 15.1

Major histological subtypes of RCC.

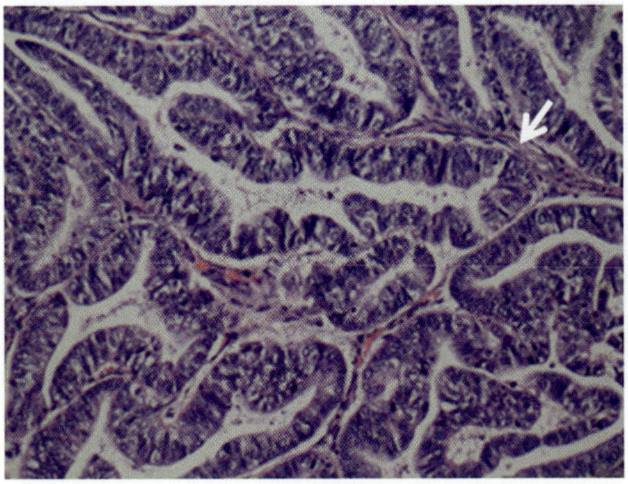

Figure 18.1

Endometrial adenocarcinoma. Uterine cancers are characterized by abnormal gland formation (arrow), diminished or absent stroma between glands, disordered chromatin distribution, nuclear enlargement, increased mitoses, and necrosis. The severity of these features is used to grade tumors and is associated with risk of metastasis and prognosis.

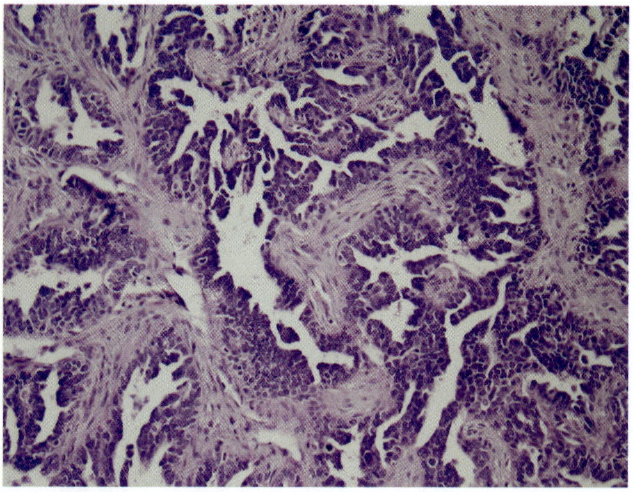

Figure 19.1

Serous epithelial ovarian cancer. Hematoxylin and eosin stain demonstrating the microscopic features characteristic of this tumor type. Papillae are noted as well as slit-like spaces. Stromal invasion and resultant desmoplastic response are common.

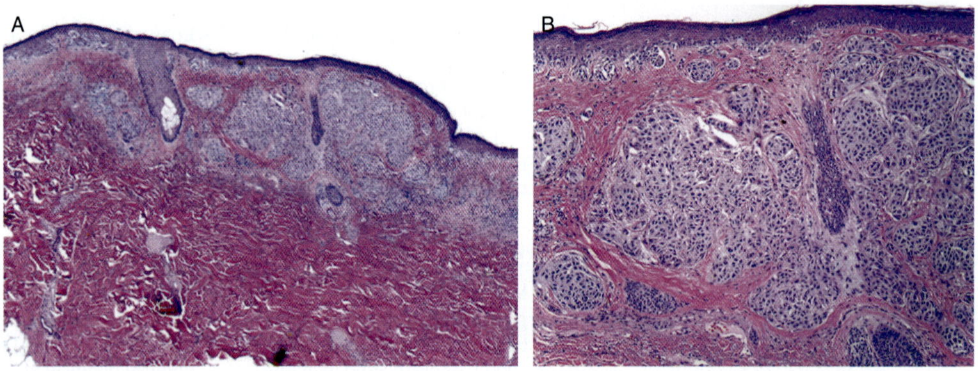

Figure 20.1

A. Invasive superficial spreading type melanoma (low power view, hematoxylin and eosin stain). Nodular areas of dense accumulations of malignant cells noted in the dermis. B. Magnified view (10×) of same melanoma. Aggregates of uniformly, large, atypical melanocytes with abundant cytoplasm evident. Scant melanin pigment dispersed throughout the lesion.

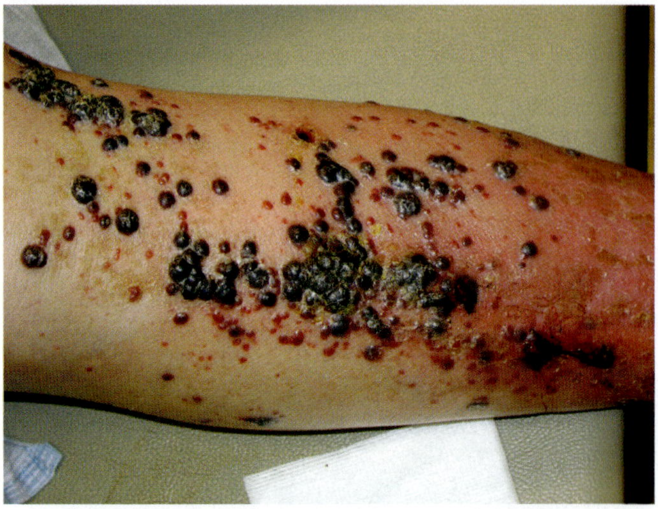

Figure 20.2

Representative photograph of multiple cutaneous and subcutaneous nodules of melanoma on an extremity of a patient.

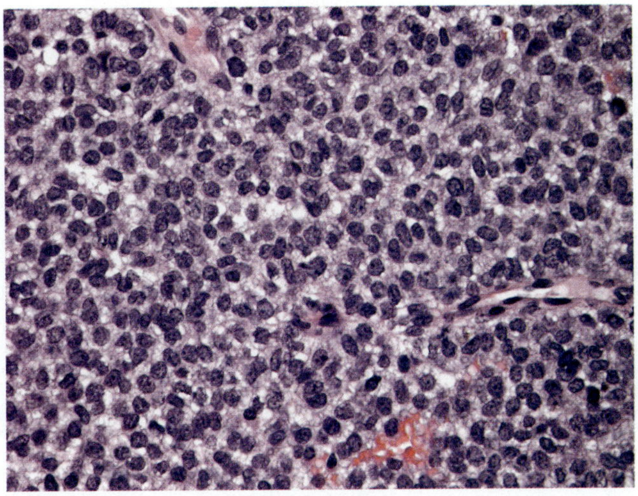

Figure 21.3

Photomicrograph of hematoxylin and eosin stained Ewing's showing finely granular chromatin and cytoplasmic vacuolization caused by glycogen accumulation (400×).

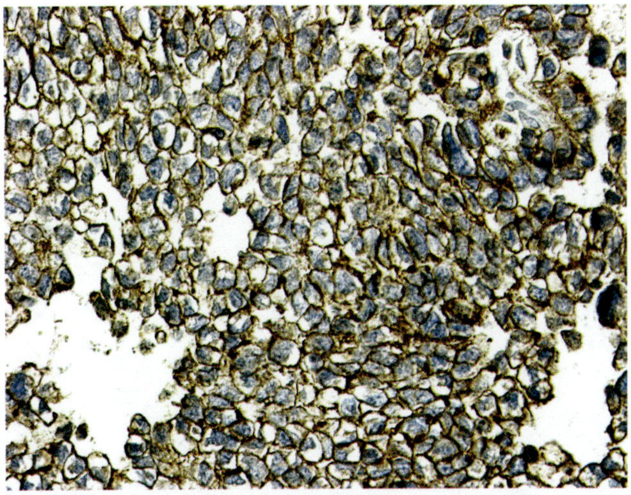

Figure 21.4

Photomicrograph of CD99 immunohistochemical stained Ewing's sarcoma showing intense cytoplasmic membrane staining (immunoperoxidase, 400×).

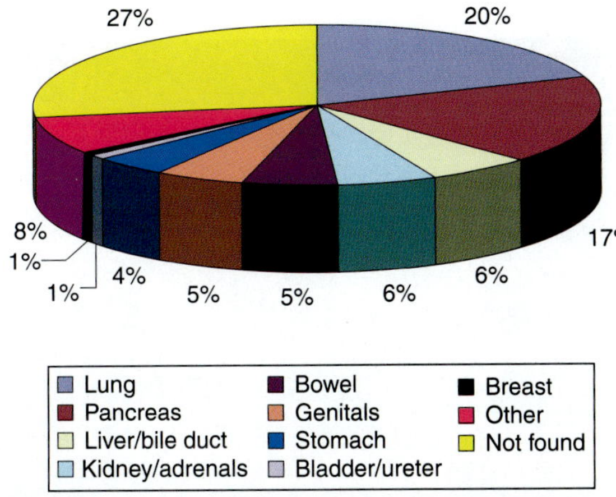

Figure 24.1

Distribution of sites of origin in cancer of unknown primary. Used with permission from Pentheroudakis et al. (4).

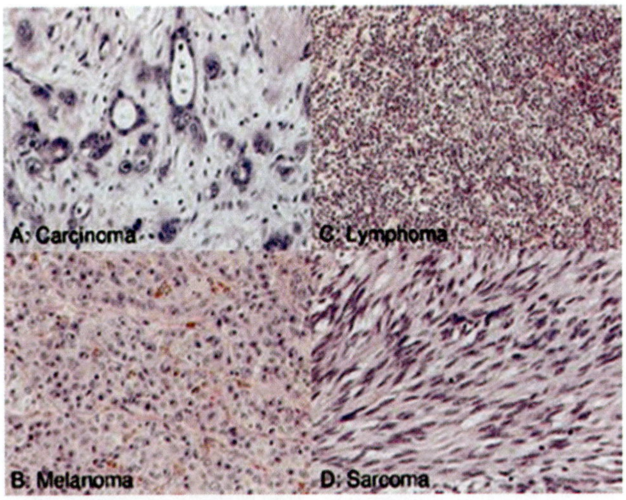

Figure 24.2

Microscopic appearance of cancer types.Carcinoma, as seen in (A), can be described as cohesive cells with a cuboidal or columnar shape, lying in tubules and glands. Melanoma, as seen in (B) with cohesive cells with large nuclei, prominent nucleoli and abundant brown melanin pigment. Lymphoma (C) has uniform small round lymphoid cells with little cytoplasm. Sarcoma (D) has cells with an elongated spindle shape, lying in sheets. The figures are used with permission from Oien (7).

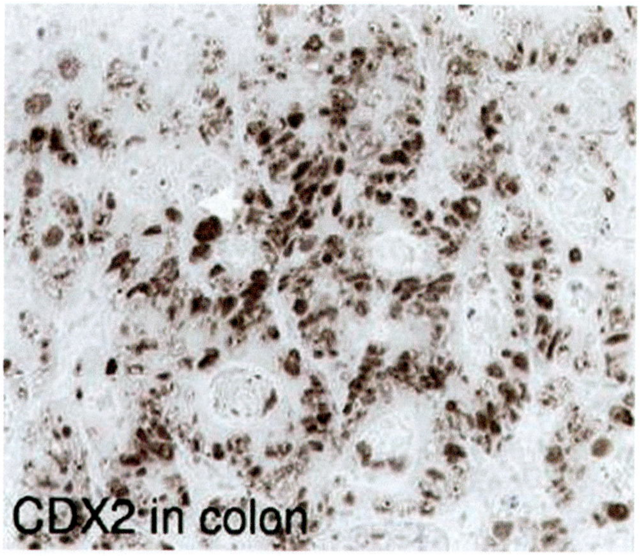

Figure 24.5

CDX-2 positivity in colon cancer. Used with permission from Oien (7).

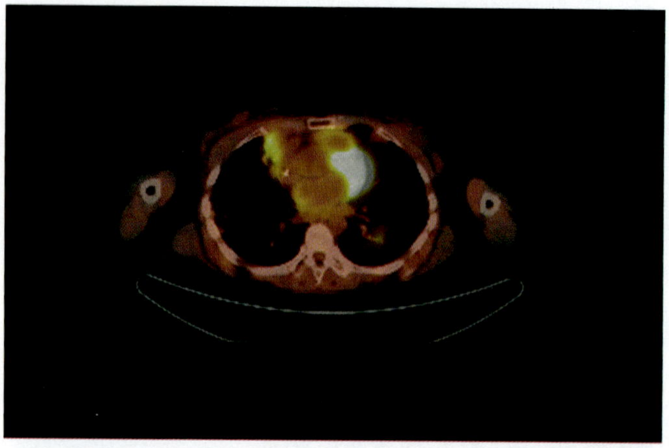

Figure 25.2

PET scan showing residual FDG-avid disease in the mediastinum.

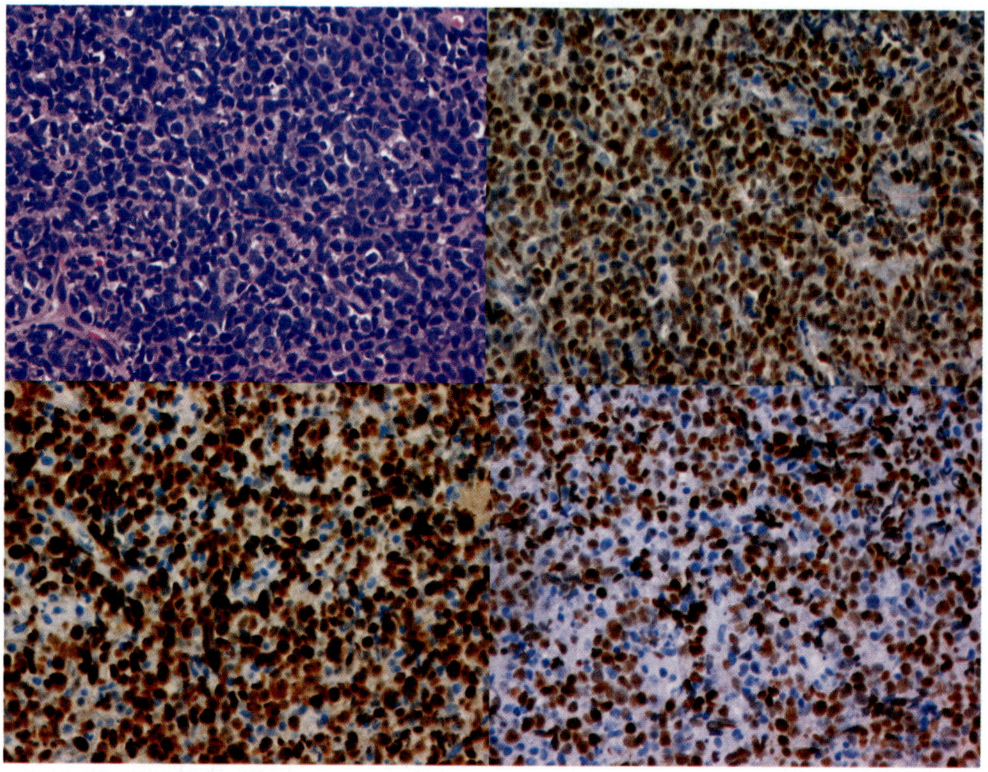

Figure 26.1

Diffuse large B-cell lymphoma. Upper left—H&E, 200 × magnification; upper right—bcl-6 positive, 200 × magnification; bottom left—MIB1 80% positive, 200 × magnificaton; bottom right—MUM1 positive, 200 × magnification.

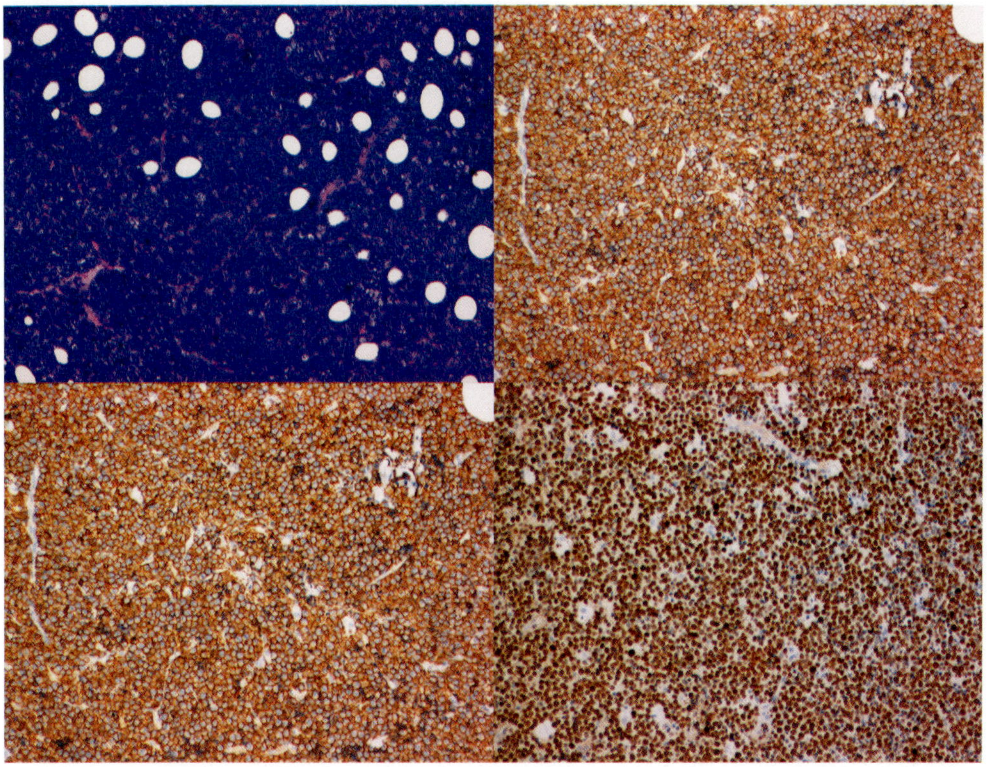

Figure 26.3

Burkitt lymphoma. Upper left—H&E, 40 × magnification; upper right—CD20, 100 × magnification; bottom left—CD10, 100 × magnification; bottom right—MIB1 with >95% positivity, 100 × magnification.

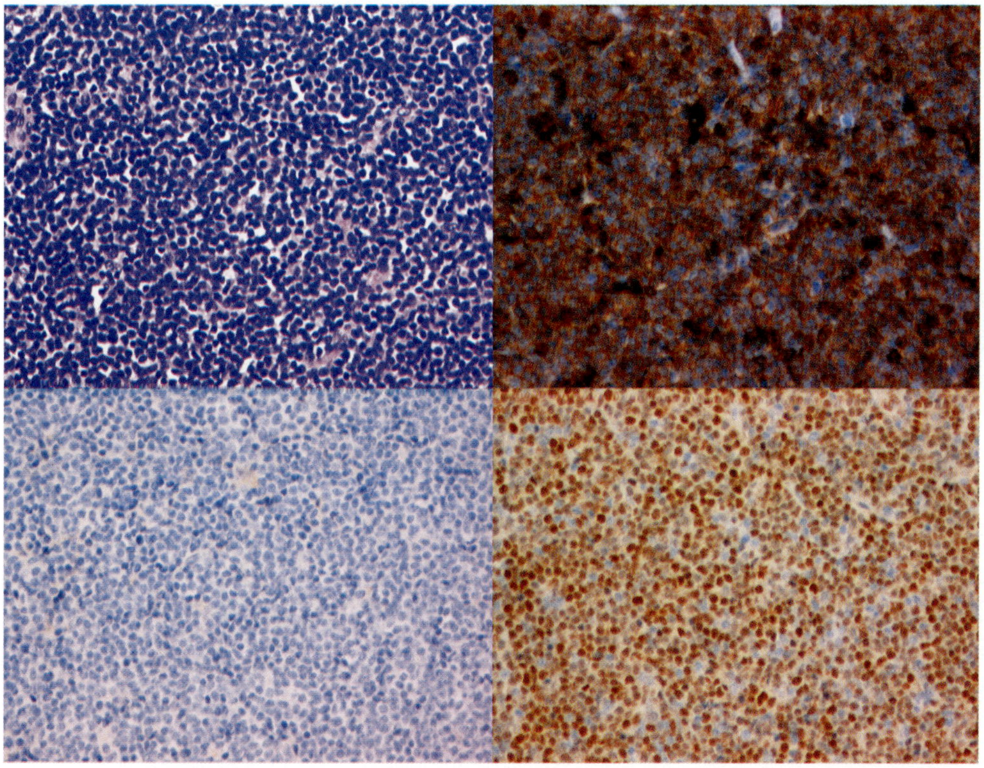

Figure 26.6

Mantle cell lymphoma. Top left—H&E, 100 × magnification; top right—CD5, 100 × magnification; bottom left—CD10, 100 × magnification; bottom right—Cyclin D1, 100 × magnification.

Table 15.2 Targeted Therapy in Advanced RCC

Agent	PFS (Months)	OS (Months)	Setting
Sunitinib (11)	11 vs. 5	26.4 vs. 21.8	First line vs. IFN-α
Sorafenib (12)	5.5 vs. 2.8	17.8 vs. 15.2	Second line vs. placebo
Pazopanib (13)	9.2 vs. 4.2	22.9 vs. 20.5	First line vs. placebo
Bevacizumab + IFN-α (14, 15)	10.2 vs. 5.4	23.3 vs. 21.3	First line with IFN-α vs. IFN-α alone
	8.5 vs. 5.2	18.3 vs. 17.4	
Temsirolimus (16)	5.5 vs. 3.1	10.9 vs. 7.3	First line, poor-risk pts. vs. IFN-α
Everolimus (17)	5.5 vs. 1.9	14.8 vs. 14.4	Second line vs. placebo

PFS, progression-free survival; OS, overall survival; IFN-α, interferon-alpha.

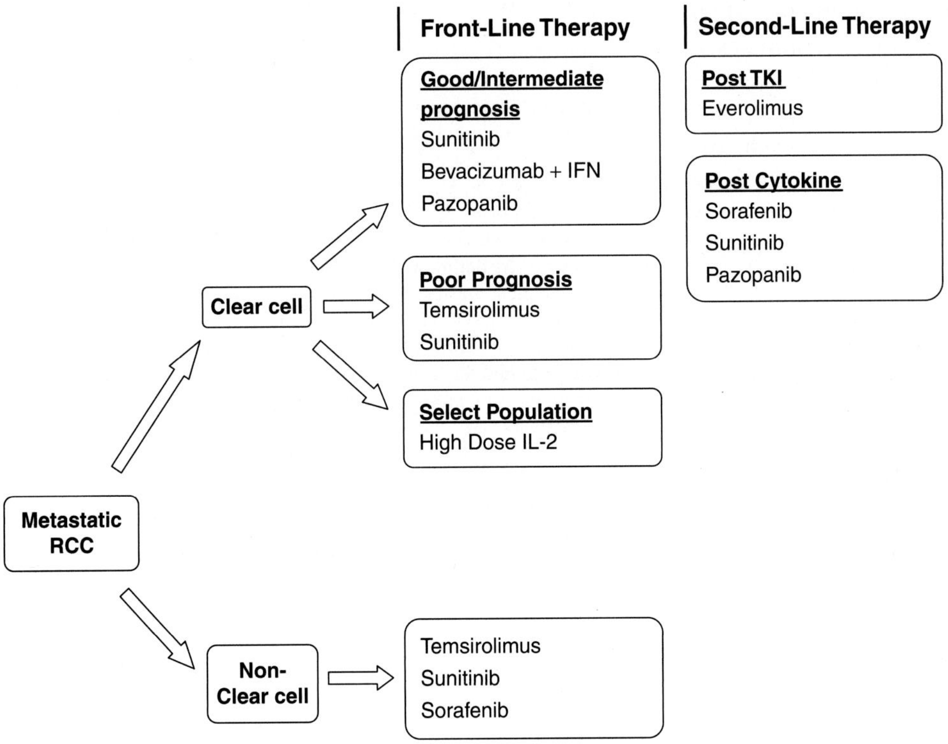

Figure 15.2

Treatment algorithm for the management of metastatic RCC.

(mTOR) pathway (temsirolimus and everolimus), both of which have been described to be critical pathways in tumor survival, proliferation, and angiogenesis in not only renal cell cancer but also several other solid tumors. Most of these agents have been tested in good- and intermediate-prognosis clear cell renal cell cancer patients and have shown proven superiority in progression-free survival relative to interferon (IFN), a standard frontline therapy in the past. Currently, sunitinib, pazopanib, or the combination of bevacizumab plus IFN represent optimal choices as frontline agents in the treatment of patients with good and intermediate prognosis clear cell metastatic RCC, assuming they are not candidates for high-dose IL-2 (11,13–15). Understandably, due to the crossover design employed in the large phase III frontline trials, survival advantage of any of these regimens has been difficult to elucidate. Temsirolimus, an mTOR inhibitor, is the only agent to have been tested in poor prognosis patients, and remains the only agent to have shown a significant survival benefit among all the targeted agents approved to date (16).

Everolimus (Afinitor), another mTOR inhibitor, is the agent of choice in patients with disease refractory to VEGF pathway targeting agents based on a large phase III randomized trial conducted against placebo (17). Nevertheless, several retrospective studies have shown lack of complete resistance among the existing targeted agents, leading to a recent research focus on elucidating the optimal sequential use of currently available agents.

Unfortunately, most of the nonclear cell histological subtypes tend to have a poorer prognosis as compared to the clear cell subtype, and furthermore, therapeutic recommendations for this subset of patients are less well characterized. Temsirolimus is the first-line agent of choice based on the result of the subanalysis of the randomized phase III trial that showed its activity across all histologies, although response as well as progression free survival benefit are modest at best. Alternatively, sunitinib and sorafenib also have been shown to exhibit modest activity as shown in retrospective analyses from expanded access trials (18,19). Further research and therapeutic options are much to be desired in this subset of patients at this time. Figure 15.2 represents a current treatment algorithm for the management of metastatic RCC.

Whereas recent advances in the development of targeted agents have greatly expanded the therapeutic options for the treatment of metastatic RCC, nevertheless durable responses still remain elusive. Participation in clinical trials evaluating new investigational therapies continues to remain an important option for patients with advanced RCC.

It is important to mention the role of cytoreductive nephrectomy in metastatic disease. Data from the interferon era support the use of debulking nephrectomy to improve survival in selected patients with metastatic disease (20). However, similar confirmatory data are lacking in the targeted therapy era. Prospective clinical trials are ongoing to address the issue of cytoreductive nephrectomy in the setting of targeted therapy in metastatic disease

REFERENCES

1. Schmidt L, Duh FM, Chen F, et al. Germline and somatic mutations in the tyrosine kinase domain of the MET proto-oncogene in papillary renal cancers. *Nat Genet.* 1997;16(1):68–73.
2. Latif F, Tory K, Gnarra J, et al. Identification of the von Hippel-Lindau disease tumor suppressor gene. *Science.* 1993;260(5112):1317–1320.
3. Zisman A, Pantuck AJ, Dorey F et al. Improved prognostication of renal cell carcinoma using an integrated staging system. *J Clin Oncol.* 2001;19(6):1649–1657.
4. Rini BI, Campbell SC, Escudier B. Renal cell carcinoma. *Lancet.* 2009;373:1119–1132.
5. Linehan WM, Wlather MM, Zbar B. The genetic basis of cancer of the kidney. *J Urol.* 2003;170: 2163–2172
6. National Comprehensive Cancer Network Guidelines™ Kidney Cancer. Version 2.2011 (http://www.nccn.org/professionals/physician_gls/pdf/kidney.pdf)
7. Blom JH, van Poppel H, Maréchal JM, et al. EORTC Genitourinary Tract Cancer Group. Radical nephrectomy with and without lymph-node dissection: final results of European Organization for Research and Treatment of Cancer (EORTC) randomized phase 3 trial 30881. *Eur Urol.* 2009;55(1):28–34.
8. Motzer RJ, Mazumdar M, Bacik J, et al. Survival and prognostic stratification of 670 patients with advanced renal cell carcinoma. *J Clin Oncol.* 1999;17(8):2530–2540.
9. Heng DY, Xie W, Regan MM, et al. Prognostic factors for overall survival in patients with metastatic renal cell carcinoma treated with vascular endothelial growth factor-targeted agents: results from a large, multicenter study. *J Clin Oncol.* 2009;27(34):5794–5799.
10. McDermott D.F., et al. The high-dose aldesleukin (HD IL-2) "SELECT" trial in patients with metastatic renal cell carcinoma (mRCC): ASCO annual meeting proceedings. *J Clin Oncol.* 2010;28:15s, 2010 (suppl; abstr 4514)
11. Motzer RJ, Hutson TE, Tomczak T, et al. Sunitinib versus interferon alfa in metastatic renal-cell carcinoma. *N Engl J Med.* 2007;356:115–124.
12. Escudier B, Eisen T, Stadler WM, et al. Sorafenib for treatment of renal cell carcinoma: final efficacy and safety results of the phase III treatment approaches in renal cancer global evaluation trial. *J Clin Oncol.* 2009;27:3312–3318
13. Sternberg CN, Davis IN, Mardiak J, et al. Pazopanib in locally advanced or metastatic renal cell carcinoma: results of a randomized phase III trial. *J Clin Oncol.* 2010;28:1061–1068
14. Escudier B, Bellmunt J, Negrier S, et al. Phase III trial of bevacizumab plus interferon alfa-2a in patients with metastatic renal cell carcinoma (AVOREN): final analysis of overall survival. *J Clin Oncol.* 2010;28:2144–2150.
15. Rini BI, Halabi S, Rosenberg JE, et al. Phase III trial of bevacizumab plus interferon alfa versus interferon alfa monotherapy in patients with metastatic renal cell carcinoma: final results of CALGB 90206. *J Clin Oncol.* 2010;28:2137–2143.
16. Hudes G, Carducci M, Tomczak, P, et al. Temsirolimus, interferon alfa, or both for advanced renal-cell carcinoma. *N Engl J Med.* 2007;356:2271–2281.
17. Motzer RJ, Escudier B, Oudard S et al. Phase 3 trial of everolimus for metastatic renal cell carcinoma: final results and analysis of prognostic factors. *Cancer.* 2010;116(18):4256–4265.
18. Gore ME, Szczylik C, Porta C, et al. Safety and efficacy of sunitinib for metastatic renal cell carcinoma: an expanded-access trial. *Lancet Oncol.* 2009;10:757–763.
19. Stadler WM, Figlin RA, McDermott DF, et al. Safety and efficacy results of the advanced renal cell carcinoma sorafenib expanded access program in North America. *Cancer.* 2010;116: 1272–1280.
20. Flanigan RC, Salmon SE, Blumenstein BA, et al. Nephrectomy followed by interferon α-2b compared with interferon α-2b alone for metastatic renal-cell cancer. *N Engl J Med.* 2001;345: 1655–1659.

16

Bladder Cancer

COLIN J. MOONEY AND DAVID C. SMITH

EPIDEMIOLOGY, RISK FACTORS, NATURAL HISTORY, AND PATHOLOGY

Carcinoma of the bladder continues to pose a significant challenge to physicians and patients who attempt to balance the toxicity of overtreating highly curable lower-risk disease while avoiding undertreating lethal high-grade lesions. Over 70,000 patients are expected to be diagnosed with bladder cancer in 2010 whereas nearly 15,000 will ultimately die from their disease (1). The median age of presentation is approximately 70 years, with rare occurrences in individuals less than 40. Three out of four patients will be male; bladder cancer is the fourth and eleventh most common cause of cancer in men and women, respectively, in the United States. The incidence of bladder cancer in Caucasian men is twice that of African American men; however, African Americans are more likely to die of the disease.

Environmental exposures are implicated in the majority of bladder cancers. In the Western world, tobacco exposure strongly correlates with bladder cancer risk contributing to 66% of diagnoses in men and 30% in women. Smoking cessation results in an immediate decrease in cancer risk; however, even after 25 years the risk does not reach that of never-smokers. Occupational exposures account for approximately 20% of bladder cancer diagnoses and affect many groups including painters, truck drivers, aluminum workers, leather and textile workers, and others exposed to industrial chemicals. Several medications, such as chronic oral cyclophosphamide, have been implicated in increased risk of bladder cancer. Prolonged exposure to bladder irritants results in an increased incidence of squamous cell carcinoma (SCC) of the bladder rather than transitional cell carcinoma (TCC). Infectious and noninfectious chronic cystitis, often due to a chronic indwelling catheter, renal calculus, or neurogenic bladder, results in a 25-fold increased risk of SCC bladder cancer. Outside of the United States and Western Europe, schistosomiasis has been correlated with SCC and is considered a major public health issue.

The classic presentation of bladder cancer as painless microscopic or, more often, gross hematuria still occurs in the majority of patients. Hematuria is typically intermittent and occurs throughout micturation. All patients with gross hematuria require a urologic evaluation. Approximately a quarter of patients present with irritable bladder symptoms such as frequency, urgency, and dysuria; this is particularly common in those with carcinoma in situ of the bladder. Unfortunately, these symptoms may inaccurately be ascribed to benign disorders (urinary tract infections, prostatitis, and passage of renal calculi) resulting in a delay of diagnosis. Advanced disease may present with bladder outlet obstruction from the tumor mass or clot, pelvic or flank pain from ureteral obstruction, or lower extremity lymphedema or deep venous thrombosis due to pelvic lymphatic involvement. Occasionally, advanced disease presents with constitutional symptoms such as weight loss or a symptomatic metastatic focus.

According to the World Health Organization/International Society of Urologic Pathology (WHO/ISUP), urothelial cancer is divided into low or high grade based on degree of nuclear anaplasia and architectural abnormalities; invasive urothelial cancer is almost always high grade. Bladder cancer comprises a heterogenous group of histologic entities with a vast majority of epithelial origin. In Western countries, 90% to 95% of these are urothelial, also known as transitional cell carcinoma (TCC). TCC originates from the urinary bladder in 90% of cases, but may also arise from the renal pelvis, ureters, and proximal two thirds of the urethra. SCC accounts for 3% to 5% of bladder cancer in the United States, but it may represent

75% of diagnoses in areas endemic with schistosoma hematobium infection. Of the remaining subtypes, adenocarcinoma and small cell (neuroendocrine) carcinoma account for 2% and 1%, respectively. TCC with mixed histologies often occur; these should be treated as urothelial carcinomas, with the exception of small cell neuroendocrine cancer, which should be treated with a small cell regimen. Chemotherapy regimens most often used for TCC may be ineffective for pure nontransitional cell entities.

STAGING

Clinically, bladder cancer is divided into three categories: non-muscle-invasive (superficial), muscularis propria-invasive, and metastatic disease, each with differing clinical behavior, approach to management, and prognosis.

AJCC Tumor, Node, Metastasis (TNM) Staging System for Bladder Cancer (7th Edition, 2010)

Stage	Definition
0a	Noninvasive papillary carcinoma (Ta), usually low grade
0is	Carcinoma in situ (Tis)
I	Subepithelial connective tissue invasion without muscle involvement (T1)
II	Invasion of the muscularis propria superficially (T2a) or deep (T2b)
III	Microscopic direct perivesicular adipose invasion (T3a) OR Macroscopic direct perivesicular adipose invasion (T3b) OR Direct pelvic organ invasion: prostatic stroma, uterus, or vagina (T4a)
IV	Direct extension to pelvic/abdominal walls or organ outside pelvis (T4b) OR Metastasis to regional nodes; ≤2 cm (N1), >2 cm but ≤5 cm (N2), >5 cm (N3) OR Distant metastasis (M1)

CASE SUMMARIES

Non-Muscle-Invasive Tumors (Ta, Tis, T1)

M.R., a 71-year-old male nonsmoker without a history of occupational exposure, developed gross hematuria but did not initially seek medical attention, attributing this to the warfarin he took for atrial fibrillation. The bleeding resolved spontaneously, but returned with progression to clot formation and irritable bladder symptoms. M.R.'s primary care physician initiated ciprofloxacin empirically for treatment of a presumed bacterial cystitis, but also ordered a urine cytology. This revealed atypical epithelial cells, and since his symptoms persisted, he was referred to a urologist.

The dysuria resolved on completion of the antibiotic course and review of urinary symptoms was otherwise negative. M.R.'s medical history was notable for cardioversion of atrial fibrillation, hypertension, noninsulin-dependent diabetes mellitus, dyslipidemia, obstructive sleep apnea, and morbid obesity. Other than a remote 20-pack-year smoking history, his social and family histories were unremarkable. Physical examination was limited due to significant obesity but was otherwise unrevealing. Laboratory evaluation was unremarkable with normal renal, liver, and hematopoietic function. Office cystoscopy revealed visual bladder tumors. Computed tomographic (CT) urogram showed eccentric wall thickening in the right aspect of the urinary bladder, encompassing the right ureterovesicular junction without hydronephrosis or hydroureter. Staging workup showed no lymphadenopathy or evidence of hepatic or pulmonary metastases. Warfarin was held and cystoscopy and bimanual examination under anesthesia was performed with transurethral resection of the bladder tumor (TURBT). A large solitary, sessile tumor was visualized on the right lateral wall. A complete resection was attempted. Pathology revealed invasive high-grade pure papillary urothelial carcinoma without angiolymphatic invasion. Muscularis propria was present in the sample but without invasion. Adjacent carcinoma in situ as noted.

M.R. underwent a restaging cystoscopy and TURBT ten weeks after his initial diagnosis which revealed recurrent high-grade T1 TCC. The tumor was fully resected. The optimal therapy for his cancer was determined to be cystectomy with neobladder formation to prevent the development of muscle-invasive disease. Unfortunately, the risks of complications of the surgery for this patient with multiple comorbidities were felt to out-weigh the benefit. After long deliberation with the patient, the decision was made to treat with 6-weeks of bacillus Calmette-Guerin (BCG) intravesical immunotherapy. Repeat TURBT revealed recurrent T1 disease. Consideration of cystectomy was again entertained but the risk of surgical complications remained too great. He underwent intravesicular BCG with interferon re-induction. Follow-up cystoscopy and random biopsies demonstrated no malignant disease. A course of maintenance BCG therapy was completed and he followed with close observation without evidence of recurrence to date.

Evidence-Based Case Discussion

The patient described above is representative of the average bladder cancer patient; an older man with multiple medical problems initially presenting with hematuria that, after thorough evaluation, revealed a T1 urothelial cancer. Though the term "superficial" is used for Ta, Tis, and T1 tumors, this is a misnomer as T1 lesions invade the submucosa or lamina propria; "non-muscle-invasive" is a more precise description. This group of tumors (Ta, Tis, T1) represent 70% of all new TCC diagnoses.

Cystoscopy with full evaluation of the bladder mucosa and urethra is the initial diagnostic test for bladder cancer detection. If the appearance of the mass on cystoscopy suggests a tumor that is high grade, solid, or muscle invasive, a CT scan of the abdomen and pelvis with and without contrast is recommended prior to TURBT. This allows evaluation of the local tumor extent and abdominal lymph node involvement as well as synchronous or metachronous upper-tract tumors that occur in 1% to 4% of patients. Following visualization of a mass, TURBT is required to confirm the diagnosis and extent of disease. Determining gross invasion and differences between well and poorly differentiated cancers may be apparent to an experienced cystoscopist; however, pathologic confirmation of a resected specimen is required.

An outline of the treatment of non-muscle-invasive bladder cancer is shown in Figure 16.1. The cornerstone of all non-muscle-invasive bladder cancer therapy is transurethral resection (TUR), utilized to diagnose, stage, and often cure. An inadequate TUR may lead to faulty decision making, undertreatment, and a poorer clinical outcome. Muscularis propria must be included in the resected tumor for the TUR to be considered adequate and complete. For low-grade Ta and low-risk T1 tumors, TUR alone may be sufficient. Large tumors (>3 cm), multifocal lesions, adjacent carcinoma in situ, and recurrence within 2 to 3 months of initial resection are all associated with a poor prognosis. Carcinoma in situ (CIS) is a high-grade intra-urothelial neoplasia confined to the epithelium growing in a flat, disordered pattern that may be focal, multifocal, or diffuse. CIS increases the risk of subsequent muscle-invasive disease whether found alone or associated with a resected superficial tumor. In T1 disease, repeat TUR is recommended because up to 30% will be understaged even when initial resection appeared complete. Recurrence rates of T1 disease at 1, 3, and 5 years from TUR can be as high as 50%, 80%, and 90%, respectively. Though initially limited to the mucosa, Ta tumors may recur locally multiple times prior to eventually becoming invasive. Close observation with repeat cystoscopy initially every 3 to 6 months is recommended.

Intravesical therapy is used adjuvantly after TUR for noninvasive (high grade Ta, Tis) or minimally invasive (T1) disease to reduce the risk of recurrence. With direct infusion therapy into the bladder, high local concentrations of medication can be achieved without systemic side effects. This may eliminate residual and undetected disease, though reduced progression to more invasive cancer has not been demonstrated. Treatments historically have included cytotoxic and immune-mediated agents.

Studies investigating appropriate intravesical therapy tend to be flawed due to poor trial design, small patient numbers, heterogenous populations, and poorly defined outcomes. A meta-analysis was performed reviewing published clinical trials that compared TUR alone to TUR plus one cycle of immediate instillation of chemotherapy (2). Seven trials, totaling 1476 patients with low-risk papillary disease (Ta or T1 without Tis) were reviewed; chemotherapies received included epirubicin, mitomycin C, thiotepa, or pirarubicin. A decreased risk of recurrence from 48% to 37% was noted in the treatment group (odds ratio 0.61). No difference was noted based on agent selected. Patients with multifocal disease also benefitted from intravesical chemotherapy, but the risk of recurrence was still high after treatment (62.5% for multifocal disease vs. 35.8% for a single focus tumor). Single-dose intravesical chemotherapy is insufficient for multifocal tumors. Theoretically, delivering therapy within 24 hours of resection interferes with the implantation process and is more commonly being applied clinically. In the United States, mitomycin C is most frequently used due to limited systemic absorption resulting in a preferred side-effect profile.

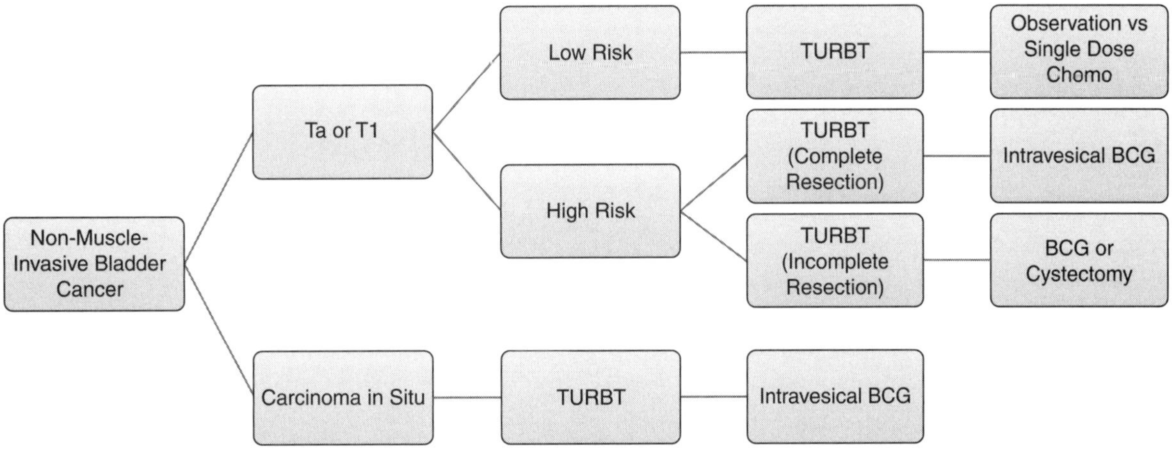

Figure 16.1

Treatment of non-muscle-invasive bladder cancer.

For high-risk, non-muscle-invasive tumors (CIS, multifocal, and recurrent disease), the treatment of choice is immunotherapy with BCG, a live attenuated strain of *Mycobacterium bovis*. Though the mechanism of BCG treatment is not clear, intravesical therapy triggers a variety of local immune responses that correlate with antitumor activity. The dose and schedule most commonly used is 120 mg intravesical weekly for 6 weeks. In a randomized trial of TUR versus TUR plus BCG involving patients with recurrent superficial disease, Herr and colleagues demonstrated a significant decrease in need for cystectomy and a 10-year survival advantage of 75% compared with 55.2% with the addition of BCG immunotherapy (3). Maintenance BCG for those with a complete response to induction, dosed weekly for 3 weeks every 6 months over 2 to 3 years, was superior to induction alone and trials showed that BCG was superior to mitomycin C (4). Although serious complications such as systemic infections and sepsis are rare, a self-limited localized BCG cystitis with increased urinary frequency, low-grade fever, and hematuria occur in most patients for approximately 24 hours after infusion. Symptoms persisting beyond 48 hours raise the concern for systemic infection. Rarely, deaths have occurred secondary to overwhelming BCG sepsis.

Surveillance in early-stage bladder cancer permits organ preservation. Low-grade, noninvasive papillary tumors may be managed with repeat TUR, even in recurrent disease. Early radical cystectomy remains an appropriate option for patients with high-grade histology, multiple tumors or frequent recurrences despite appropriate treatment with intravesical BCG. Patients considered high risk are likely to benefit from earlier cystectomy prior to the development of T2 or greater disease (5). Failures to control carcinoma in situ with TUR and adjuvant BCG therapy or recurrence of T1 tumor 6 to 12 months after appropriate treatment are indications for cystectomy.

Muscle-Invasive Disease (T2 or T3 or T4a)

J.K. is a 49-year-old healthy man who visited his primary care physician after an episode of painless, gross hematuria. An abdominal CT showed a calcified bladder mass. Urology was consulted for cystoscopy and TURBT, which yielded a high-grade papillary urothelial carcinoma invading the lamina propria with tumor adjacent to but not invading muscle. CIS was noted within the resected specimen but there was no angiolymphatic invasion. Re-resection was not completed at that time; instead the patient received six doses of BCG immunotherapy. Urine cytology was suspicious for urothelial carcinoma following treatment and repeat cystoscopy revealed persistent disease on the left bladder wall. CT urogram confirmed a 6- to 7-cm exophytic mass with associated hydronephrosis but no evidence of metastatic disease. Chest radiographs were normal. Repeat TURBT and bimanual examination under anesthesia demonstrated a large palpable muscle-invasive TCC; no attempt at complete resection was made. Clinically, J.K. was felt to have a stage III (cT3, Nx, M0) tumor due to hydronephrosis seen on CT.

J.K. was referred to medical oncology for consultation. Review of systems was positive only for urinary frequency, nocturia, and gross hematuria. The patient was well appearing with an excellent performance status, mild hypertension, and an otherwise unremarkable physical examination. Laboratory evaluations were normal including renal function, alkaline phosphatase, and blood counts.

J.K. underwent three cycles of neoadjuvant chemotherapy with methotrexate, vinblastine, doxorubicin, and cisplatin (MVAC) followed by radical cystectoprostatectomy, bilateral pelvic lymph node dissection, and creation of an ileal neobladder. Pathology revealed a complete response within the bladder and incidental Gleason 3 + 3 = 6, pT2b, N0 prostate adenocarcinoma. His post-op course was complicated by left lower extremity deep venous thrombosis. The urine cytology, CT abdomen, chest radiographs, and physical examination remain unrevealing for metastatic disease on follow-up.

Evidence-Based Case Discussion

J.K. is a relatively young, otherwise healthy man without medical comorbidities who presents with muscle-invasive bladder cancer without evidence of metastatic disease. He is therefore a candidate for aggressive treatment. Unfortunately for many patients, the advanced age and common comorbidities that share risk factors for bladder cancer, such as smoking, often complicate management and limit treatment options. The large mass palpable under anesthesia with hydronephrosis makes this a high-risk tumor; however, the pure urothelial histology and normal alkaline phosphatase predict a more favorable prognosis.

Figure 16.2 shows a treatment algorithm for treating muscle-invasive bladder cancer. For decades, the standard of care for muscle-invasive bladder cancer has been bilateral pelvic lymphadenectomy, radical cystectomy, and urinary diversion. In men, a radical cystectomy involves radical cystoprostatectomy and potentially a urethrectomy if the prostatic urethra is involved. Women undergo anterior exenteration that includes excision of the bladder, urethra, uterus, adnexa, and ventral vaginal wall. Options for urinary diversion include an ileal conduit, internal urinary reservoir with drainage to the abdominal wall or urethra, and orthotopic diversion or neobladder that more closely mimics a native bladder.

Though radical cystectomy is the most efficacious treatment to locally control bladder cancer, it is associated with high morbidity. Historically, postoperative mortality rates reached 40% to 50%, a number now reduced to 1%

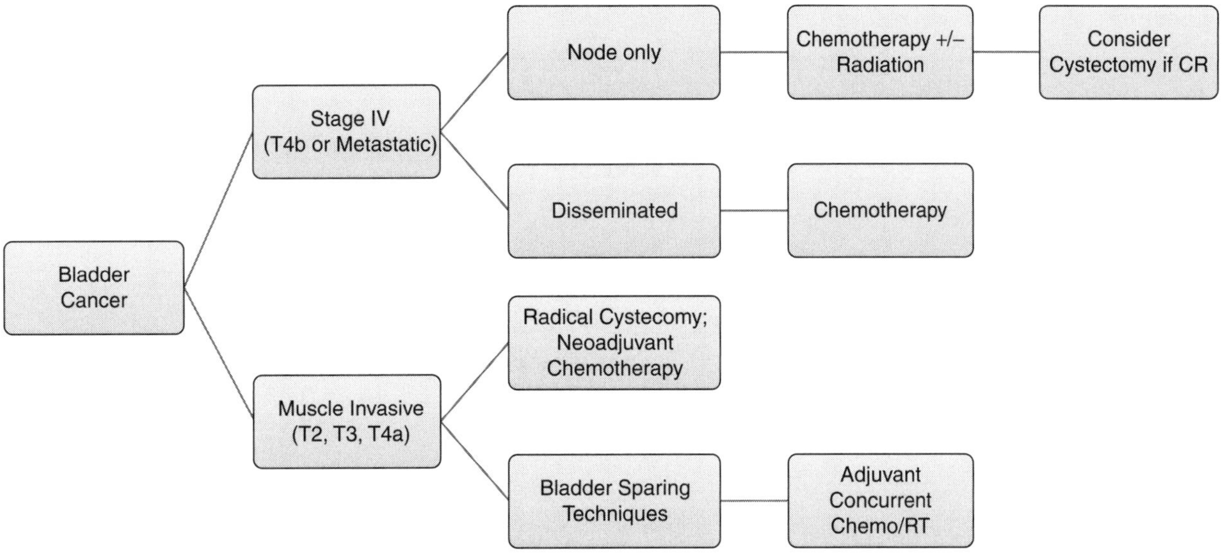

Figure 16.2

Treatment of muscle invasive bladder cancer.

to 3%. Mortality in older patients (>80 years old) is 2 to 3 times higher than for younger patients. Overall 5-year survival status postcystectomy is 50%, but this clearly varies with clinical stage. Organ-confined tumors (≤T2b) have a significantly better prognosis than extravesical disease (≥T3a). At a minimum, lymphadenectomy should include bilateral dissection of common, internal and external iliac and obturator nodes. A metastatic lymph node deposit predicts a much higher recurrence risk; however, cure remains possible especially after completion of an adequate lymph node dissection. Surgical factors negatively influencing survival following radical cystectomy include positive margins and fewer than ten nodes removed (6).

Alternatives to radical cystectomy for those with significant comorbidites, advanced age, or strong desire for organ preservations may be considered, including partial cystectomy, radical transurethral resection, and radiation techniques. Many consider these techniques inferior to radical cystectomy though limited direct comparisons exist. If the group considered for these procedures are carefully selected, outcomes may approach those of the more aggressive approach. Optimal patients include those only with urothelial histology, T2 and T3a tumors with a limited disease burden.

Partial cystectomy, removal of only a portion of the bladder wall to maintain bladder function, may be considered for patients with a T2 solitary lesion without Tis. Only 5% of patients considered for cystectomy will be candidates for this procedure. For this minority of patients, 5-year survival approaches 50%, similar to that of radical cystectomy. Importantly, even in this limited surgery, a bilateral pelvic lymphadenectomy is still required. The role of partial cystectomy is diminishing, given improved orthotopic neobladder formation.

Other options to radical cystectomy include aggressive TUR alone or TUR followed by chemotherapy, radiation, or concurrent chemoradiation. These options are especially appealing for patients who are medically unfit for more aggressive surgeries. A major limitation of TUR is the inability to determine with certainty the completeness of tumor resection. Intensive, long-term cystoscopic follow-up is mandatory due to the high risk of recurrent tumors. TUR followed by single modality radiotherapy is only indicated for those unable to tolerate cystectomy or chemotherapy because of medical comorbidities. Similarly, chemotherapy alone is not adequate to control local disease.

Aggressive TUR followed by concurrent chemoradiation therapy with cisplatin is considered the standard for bladder preservation. Shipley (7), the most heavily published author on this topic, advocates for neoadjuvant chemotherapy prior to concurrent chemoradiation, though this is debated. His regimen includes two cycles of neoadjuvant chemotherapy with cisplatin, methotrexate, and vinblastine (CMV) followed by concurrent chemoradiation. Patients are evaluated during treatment and those with a complete response as documented by transurethral cystoscopy and biopsies go on to complete concurrent therapy. One hundred ninety patients with T2-T4a urothelial bladder cancer were treated prospectively on sequential trials led by Shipley with this basic protocol strategy after completion of optimal TURBT (7). The 5- and 10-year survival rates reached 54% and 36%, respectively. Of the surviving patients, 73% were able to maintain bladder preservation at 5 years. Assessment for complete response is critically important; if unable to achieve a CR due to chemo/radiation insensitive disease, the patient must go to immediate cystectomy barring contraindication. The most common approach to concurrent therapy following complete TURBT is cisplatin dosed weeks 1 and 4 plus 40 Gy external beam radiotherapy followed by cystoscopy with biopsy. If malignant disease is detected, the patient undergoes cystectomy; if biopsies are negative (T0), an additional 25 Gy of radiation and a third dose of cisplatin are delivered. Other chemosensitizing agents that may be considered include 5-FU or paclitaxel in combination with cisplatin or as single agents. Cystectomy may be difficult in patients who recur after receiving the full course of pelvic radiation.

Half of the patients with localized muscle-invasive disease will develop metastatic disease despite optimal surgical management including cystectomy. Given the high responses of TCC to chemotherapy (up to 75% to cisplatin-based regimens with 20% CR), adjuvant and neoadjuvant therapy have been explored to reduce this recurrence rate. The best evidence is for neoadjuvant chemotherapy. Theoretical advantages of this approach include the ability to assess the chemotherapy responsiveness of the tumor, immediate treatment of microscopic metastatic disease rather than waiting for postoperative healing, and better tolerance of therapy preoperatively allowing more chemotherapy to be delivered. In muscle-invasive urothelial cancer, neoadjuvant chemotherapy demonstrates a survival advantage. The largest neoadjuvant chemotherapy trial was a phase III collaborative group study including the Medical Research Council, the European Organization for Research and Treatment of Cancer (EORTC) (8). A total of 976 patients with cT2 to cT4a, N0 to Nx transitional cell carcinoma were randomized to receive neoadjuvant CMV versus no chemotherapy, both followed by institutional choice of radical cystectomy or radiation therapy. The absolute survival benefit of neoadjuvant CMV at 3 years was 5.5% (55.5% vs. 50%; $P = .075$). Though initially not significant, an update published with median follow-up of 7 years at the 2002 American Society of Clinical Oncology (ASCO) meeting demonstrated a significantly superior survival in those randomized to neoadjuvant chemotherapy compared with those with local treatment alone. Further supporting these results, the INT 0080 trial reported by Grossman, a phase III SWOG trial of 317 patients with cT2 to cT4a urothelial carcinoma randomized to either three cycles of methotrexate, vinblastine, doxorubicin, and cisplatin (MVAC) followed by cystectomy versus cystectomy alone (9). The patients receiving neoadjuvant chemotherapy had an improved median overall survival (77 vs. 46 months; $P = .06$) and 5-year overall survival (57% vs. 43%; $P = .06$). Not surprisingly, there was a significant increase in pT0 status at the time of cystectomy from 15% in the cystectomy alone group to 38% in the neoadjuvant group. Patients generally tolerated neoadjuvant therapy well without any treatment-related deaths. Several large meta-analyses have been performed that likewise determined a significant absolute 5-year overall survival advantage of greater than 5% in patients treated with neoadjuvant cisplatin-based chemotherapy followed by radical cystectomy versus surgery alone.

Multiple studies have investigated the use of adjuvant chemotherapy in locally advanced bladder cancer but no statistically significant survival advantage has been demonstrated. The theoretical advantage of this approach is the immediate local control followed by therapy for those with high risk based on pathologic criteria. Trials investigating this issue have been plagued by small sample size, difficult accrual, and methodologically flawed trial designs. The Advanced Bladder Cancer Meta-Analysis reviewed six available randomized controlled trials of 491 individual patients comparing adjuvant cisplatin-based chemotherapy to local treatment alone in invasive urothelial cancer (10). The authors found a significant relative reduction of 25% ($P = .019$) of death in the adjuvant chemotherapy group, but serious methodological flaws limit the interpretation of their results. In spite of the limitations of this trial and others, the data suggest it is reasonable to consider adjuvant therapy if no neoadjuvant therapy was delivered especially in higher-risk disease (T3-T4 tumors or positive nodes).

Unresectable (T4b) or Metastatic Disease (N1-3 or M1)

F.T. is a 50-year-old woman who presented to her primary care physician complaining of dysuria and dyspareunia. Her symptoms failed to resolve after a course of antibiotics for treatment of a presumed urinary tract infection. She then noted a vaginal mass. F.T. was referred to a urologist for cystoscopy and a TURBT revealed high-grade muscle-invasive TCC. A biopsy of the vaginal mass at the time of this procedure was positive for TCC confirming a T4a bladder cancer. A CT scan of the chest, abdomen, and pelvis revealed a tiny right middle lobe pulmonary nodule of uncertain significance, a large bladder mass, and a 2-cm ovoid soft tissue mass right and posterior to the bladder. A pelvic MRI confirmed the large bladder mass and questionable right perivesicular lymph node seen on CT. A bone scan had no evidence of metastatic disease. F.T. was referred to Medical Oncology for consideration of neoadjuvant chemotherapy.

At the clinic visit, F.T. complained of mild fatigue, slight fever, and decreased appetite with some weight loss. She also noted persistent dysuria, pelvic pain, and mild nausea. Past medical history was remarkable for idiopathic polyneuropathy and she was a 30-pack-year current smoker. Physical examination was remarkable only for mild right lower quadrant tenderness to deep palpation noted on examination. The possible pelvic lymph node discovered on imaging suggested possible stage IV disease and she was enrolled on a clinical trial of neoadjuvant paclitaxel, carboplatin, and gemcitabine.

Cisplatin was considered but withheld due to her history of neuropathy. She completed three cycles of neoadjuvant therapy requiring minimal dose reductions and growth factor support due to cytopenias. A follow-up CT scan revealed a partial response without evidence of distant metastatic disease.

F.T. eventually underwent a radical cystectomy, hysterectomy, partial vaginectomy, bilateral pelvic lymph node dissection, and ileal neobladder reconstruction. She tolerated the procedure well. Pathology revealed a residual 20 × 15 mm high-grade urothelial tumor with extensive clear cell features. Margins were negative but angiolymphatic invasion was identified. Four of eight pelvic lymph nodes were involved bilaterally (pT3a, N2) confirming metastatic, locally advanced disease. There was no evidence of distant metastatic disease. Further therapy was considered for this patient with advanced, aggressive disease even though all visible disease had been resected. Her oncologist elected to administer three cycles of adjuvant carboplatin, paclitaxel, and gemcitabine.

F.T. remained without disease following her chemotherapy for almost a year when she developed low-grade fevers, night sweats, and new pelvic pain. She underwent biopsy of an isolated pelvic mass which was consistent with a local recurrent TCC. Doublet therapy with cisplatin and gemcitabine was initiated resulting in tumor shrinkage. However, F.T. developed a progressive neuropathy and treatment was discontinued after five cycles. She had a 10-month progression-free interval off therapy and was eventually enrolled in a clinical trial at the time of further disease progression.

Evidence-Based Case Discussion

F.T. is a relatively young woman with locally advanced bladder cancer and regional lymph node involvement who had only a partial response despite aggressive neoadjuvant chemotherapy. Findings of angiolymphatic invasion, multiple lymph node involvement, lack of complete response to neoadjuvant chemotherapy, and partial clear-cell histology are consistent with an aggressive, poor prognosis tumor. All macroscopic disease had been resected at the time of her surgery. Due to her very high-risk disease, adjuvant chemotherapy therapy was considered despite lack of evidence for increased survival.

Though response rates are high with urothelial carcinoma compared to other solid tumors, the median survival of patients with metastatic disease remains only 14 months even with aggressive chemotherapy and only 15% of patients are alive at 5 years. Poor performance status and visceral organ metastases correspond to shortened survival. More interest in molecular markers have demonstrated increased resistance to methotrexate, vinblastine, doxorubicin, and cisplatin (MVAC), and other cisplatin-based chemotherapy in tumors with *p53* mutations and high excision repair cross-complementing 1 (ERCC1) levels.

First-line chemotherapy in the setting of metastatic disease is MVAC. Historically, cisplatin had been recognized as the most active agent in bladder cancer with objective remissions as high as 40%. Based on promising preliminary results, Loehrer and colleagues compared MVAC (methotrexate 30 mg/m^2 days 1, 15, and 22; vinblastine 3 mg/m^2 2 days 2, 15, and 22; doxorubicin 30 mg/m^2 and cisplatin 70 mg/m^2 on day 2) to single-agent cisplatin (70 mg/m^2) in 226 randomly assigned patients with advanced urothelial carcinoma (11). As expected, the multidrug combination had more toxicities than cisplatin alone including cytopenia, neutropenic fever, sepsis, mucositis, nausea, and treatment-related mortality. There were five (4%) deaths in the combination arm and none with cisplatin alone. Despite this, the MVAC group did significantly better than the single-agent group in response rates (39% vs. 12%; $P < .0001$), progression-free survival (10.0 vs. 4.3 months) and overall survival (12.5 vs. 8.2 months). Multiple regimens have been compared to MVAC to determine a more effective or less toxic alternative. Compared directly to another combination regimen, cisplatin, cyclophosphamide, and doxorubicin (CISCA), in a phase III clinical trial, MVAC had a superior response rate (65% vs. 46%) and overall survival time (median 11 months vs. 10 months) (12). In an attempt to increase response rates, MVAC was compared to fluorouracil, interferon alpha-2b, and cisplatin (FAP) in a phase III trial (13). MVAC had a superior response rate and complete response (24% vs. 10%), but identical overall survival times (12.5 months) and toxicity profile. Other trials evaluating high-dose MVAC with GCSF support failed to demonstrate superiority of standard MVAC. Based on these studies and previous phase II trials, MVAC emerged as the standard of care for metastatic transitional cell carcinoma.

Preliminary studies of the combination gemcitabine and cisplatin (GC) demonstrated promising activity in metastatic urothelial cancer in chemotherapy-naïve patients with less toxicity than seen with other regimens; this led to a phase III study directly comparing GC to MVAC in locally advanced or metastatic TCC (14). Four hundred and five treatment-naïve patients were randomized equally to either GC (gemcitabine 1000 mg/m^2 days 1, 8, and 15 and cisplatin 70 mg/m^2 day 2) or standard MVAC. The overall response rate (47% vs. 46%), time to progression (both 7.4 months), and median survival (13.8 vs. 14.8 months) were very similar in GC and MVAC arms, respectively. With the exception of grade 3 or 4 anemia and thrombocytopenia, the toxicity profile of GC was superior with more patients able to complete six cycles of chemotherapy without dose reductions and fewer treatment-related deaths (1% vs. 3%). This trial was not powered to demonstrate equivalency, but given the similar 5-year overall survival results (GC 13%, MVAC 15%) and a better safety profile and tolerability, many consider GC as the standard first-line regimen for patients with advanced TCC rather than MVAC.

Various other treatment combinations have been evaluated in an attempt to improve response rates and median survival. Taxanes have demonstrated promising single-agent activity in bladder cancer, though double-agent therapy of paclitaxel with cisplatin did not appear superior to standard therapy in subsequent studies. In a randomized phase III trial of 627 patients, the triplet PCG (paclitaxel 80mg/m^2 day 1 and 8, cisplatin 70 mg/m^2 day 1, gemcitabine 1000 mg/m^2 days 1 and 8 of a 21-day cycle) was evaluated against standard GC (15). Overall (57.1% vs. 46.4%) and complete responses (15% vs. 10%) were significantly better in PCG compared with GC; however, the trend toward superiority of PCG to GC for median survival (15.7 vs. 12.8 months) was not statistically significant (P = .10). Both treatments were well tolerated with increased thrombocytopenia and febrile neutropenia in the triplet arm.

Standard salvage therapy in recurrent urothelial carcinoma is not defined. Multiple drugs demonstrate single-agent activity in bladder cancer with response rates of 20% or less in the second-line setting. These drugs include paclitaxel, docetaxel, gemcitabine, ifosfamide, and oxaliplatin. Biologic therapies are currently under investigation. Epidermal growth factor receptor (EGFR) and angiogenesis pathways have demonstrated upregulation in urothelial cancers, and trials are ongoing to assess the incorporation of these targeted agents into standard regimens.

REFERENCES

1. Jemal A, Siegel R, Xu J, et al. Cancer statistics, 2010. *CA Cancer J Clin*. 2010;60(5):277–300.
2. Sylvester RJ, Oosterlinck W, van der Meijden AP. A single immediate postoperative instillation of chemotherapy decreases the risk of recurrence in patients with stage Ta T1 bladder cancer: a meta-analysis of published results of randomized clinical trials. *J Urol.* 2004;171(6 Pt 1):2186–2435.
3. Herr HW, Schwalb DM, Zhang ZF, et al. Intravesical bacillus Calmette-Guerin therapy prevents tumor progression and death from superficial bladder cancer: ten-year follow-up of a prospective randomized trial. *J Clin Oncol.* 1995;13(6):1404 –1408.
4. Malmstrom PU, Sylvester RJ, Crawford DE, et al. An individual patient data meta-analysis of the long-term outcome of randomized studies comparing intravesical mitomycin C versus bacillus Calmette-Guerin for non-muscle-invasive bladder cancer. *Eur Urol.* 2009;56(2):247–256.
5. Lee CT, Dunn RL, Ingold C, et al. Early-stage bladder cancer surveillance does not improve survival if high-risk patients are permitted to progress to muscle invasion. *Urology.* 2007;69(9):1068–1072.
6. Herr HW, Faulkner JR, Grossman HB, et al. Surgical factors influence bladder cancer outcomes: a cooperative group report. *J Clin Oncol.* 2004;22(14):2781–2789.
7. Shipley WU, Kaufman DS, Zehr E, et al. Selective Bladder preservation by combined modality protocol treatment: long-term outcomes of 190 patients with invasive bladder cancer. *Urology.* 2002;60(1):62–67.
8. EORTC. Neoadjuvant cisplatin, methotrexate, and vinblastine chemotherapy for muscle-invasive bladder cancer: a randomized controlled trial. *Lancet.* 1999;254(9178):533–540.
9. Grossman HB, Natale RB, Tangen CM, et al. Neoadjuvant chemotherapy plus cystectomy compared with cystectomy alone for locally advanced bladder cancer. *N Engl J Med.* 2003;349(9):859–866.
10. Advanced Bladder Cancer (ABC) Meta-analysis Collaboration. Adjuvant chemotherapy in invasive bladder cancer: a systemic review and meta-analysis of individual patient data Advanced Bladder Cancer (ABC) Meta-analysis Collaborative. *Eur Urol.* 2005;48(2):199–201.
11. Loehrer PJ Sr, Einhorn LH, Elson PJ, et al. A randomized comparison of cisplatin alone or in combination with methotrexate, vinblastine, and doxorubicin in patients with metastatic urothelial carcinoma: a cooperative group study. *J Clin Oncol.* 1992;10(7):1066–1073.
12. Logothetis CJ, Dexeus FH, Finn L, et al. A prospective randomized trial comparing MVAC and CISCA chemotherapy for patients with metastatic urothelial tumors. *J Clin Oncol.* 1990;8(6):1050–1055.
13. Siefker-Radtke AO, Millikan RE, Tu SM, et al. Phase III trial of fluorouracil, interferon alpha-2b, and cisplatin versus methotrexate, vinblastine, doxorubicin, and cisplatin in metastatic or unresectable urothelial cancer. *J Clin Oncol.* 2002;20(5): 1361–1367.
14. von der Maase Hansen SW, Roberts JT, Dogliotti L, et al. Gemcitabine and cisplatin versus methotrexate, vinblastine, doxorubicin, and cisplatin in advanced or metastatic bladder cancer: results of a large, randomized, multinational, multicenter, phase III study. *J Clin Oncol.* 2000;18(17): 3068–3077.
15. Bellmunt J, von der Maase H, Mead GM, et al. Randomized phase III study comparing paclitaxel / cisplatin / gemcitabine and gemcitabine / cisplatin in patients with locally advanced or metastatic urothelial cancer without prior systemic therapy; EORTC30987 / Intergroup Study. *Am Soc Clin Oncol Annu Meet*, 2007; Abstract LBA5030.

17

Cervical Cancer

SHAN GUO, MARIAN YVETTE WILLIAMS-BROWN, AND CONCEPCION R. DIAZ-ARRASTIA

EPIDEMIOLOGY, RISK FACTORS, NATURAL HISTORY, AND PATHOLOGY

Cervical cancer is the second most common cause of cancer-related morbidity and mortality among women worldwide. Internationally, 500,000 new cases are diagnosed each year and 250,000 deaths occur each year, corresponding to a 50% mortality rate. In the United States, cervical cancer is relatively uncommon; the incidence of invasive cervical cancer has declined steadily over the past few decades due to its widely available screening program. It is estimated in 2010 that 12,200 cases of invasive cervical cancer were diagnosed and that 4210 women died of the disease in the United States. Race and ethnicity are some of the many complex interacting biological and social risk factors for cervical carcinoma in the United States. African Americans, Hispanics, Native Americans, and Vietnamese Americans have a higher risk of death from cervical cancer than white Americans. The mean age for cervical cancer is 51.4 years.

High-risk human papillomavirus (HPV) infection is the carcinogenic trigger of over 99% of cervical cancers. There is a growing list of carcinogenic strains of HPV. Over 65% of healthy volunteers have evidence of past or present infection with HPV. A persistent HPV infection may develop into high-grade cervical intraepithelial neoplasia (HGCIN), the cancer precursor. Annually, in the United States, there are an estimated 400,000 cases of HGCIN and 12,000 cases of invasive cancer. Therefore, an infection with the carcinogenic HPV is only the first step in a series of events that leads to invasive carcinoma. Integration of HPV DNA into the host cellular genome and overexpression of the viral *E6* and *E7* oncogenes leads to cervical carcinogenesis. The *E6* and *E7* proteins bind and inactivate tumor suppressors *p53* and retinoblastoma protein, thereby affecting multiple biologic processes that lead to increased cellular proliferation. HGCIN usually occurs in the transformation zone of the cervix at the squamocolumnar junction. The most common genotypes of HPV associated with cervical cancer are 16, 18, 45, and 56.

Other risk factors for cervical intraepithelial neoplasia (CIN) and cervical carcinoma include a past medical history of abnormal pap smears or CIN, lack of participation in pap smear screening, early onset of sexual activity, multiple sexual partners, a high-risk sexual partner, history of sexually transmitted diseases, high parity, immunosuppression, low socioeconomic status, prolonged use of oral contraceptives, and previous history of anogenital dysplasia. Smoking is associated with an increased risk of squamous cell carcinoma but not with adenocarcinoma of the cervix (1).

CIN is graded based on the extent of the atypical cellular changes in the stratified squamous epithelium. Mild dysplasia (CIN 1) refers to atypical cellular changes involving the basal third of the epithelium. Moderate dysplasia (CIN 2) is considered a high-grade lesion characterized by atypical cellular changes extending to the basal two thirds of the epithelium. Severe dysplasia (CIN 3) is also considered a high-grade lesion with atypical cellular changes encompassing greater than two thirds of the epithelial thickness, and includes full-thickness intraepithelial lesions. Most CIN 1 lesions regress spontaneously or persist, whereas 10% progress to CIN 2 and 3 over 2 years. If untreated, CIN 3 ultimately progresses to cancer over a prolonged period of time, typically 8 to 13 years without any symptoms. Therefore, it is recommended that any CIN 2 and 3 is treated by ablation or excision.

Patients with advanced cervical cancer typically present with abnormal vaginal bleeding. Postcoital bleeding is the pathogonomonic symptom, although the bleeding can also be intermenstrual or postmenopausal. Patients can also present with a vaginal discharge due to an infected necrotic tumor or pelvic pain due to extension of the disease to the surrounding structures. In the presence of pelvic sidewall involvement, the patient can present with the triad of leg edema, pain, and hydronephrosis. In countries where women are screened routinely such as the United States, the most common presentation is an abnormal Pap smear. These asymptomatic patients usually have smaller tumors at an earlier stage of disease.

Cervical cancer spreads primarily by direct extension to surrounding structures such as the vagina, parametria, uterosacral and cardinal ligaments, and the bladder or rectum. Cervical cancer is also characterized by early lymphatic metastasis. The obturator lymph nodes are the primary drainage of the cervix. From there, the lymphatic metastases follow the afferent lymphatics up the iliac nodal chain to the para-aortic lymph nodes, then ultimately to the scalene nodes via the thoracic duct. Hematogenous metastases to the lung, mediastinum, bone, and liver are found late in the disease process.

Histologically, most cervical cancers are squamous cell carcinomas (70%), followed by adenocarcinomas (25%), and adenosquamous carcinomas (3–5%). Rarely neuroendocrine or small cell carcinomas can arise primarily from the cervix. Treatment strategies for adenocarcinoma and adenosquamous carcinoma are similar to that of squamous cell carcinoma. This chapter will focus on squamous cell carcinoma.

STAGING

FIGO staging system is the widely used staging system for cervical cancer and was most recently updated in 2009.

Cervical Cancer

Stage	Description
I	Carcinoma is strictly confined to the cervix; extension to the uterine corpus would be disregarded.
IA	Invasive carcinoma diagnosed only by microscopy. Stromal invasion with a maximum depth of 5.0 mm measured from the base of the epithelium and a horizontal spread of 7.0 mm or less. Vascular space involvement, venous or lymphatic, should not alter the staging.
IA1	Measured invasion of the stroma is 3 mm or less in depth and 7 mm or less in horizontal spread.
IA2	Measured invasion of stroma is more than 3 mm but less than 5 mm and 7 mm or less in horizontal spread.
IB	Clinically visible lesions confined to the cervix or preclinical lesions greater than stage IA. IB1: Clinically visible lesions 4 cm or less in size. IB2: Clinically visible lesions more than 4 cm in size.
II	Carcinoma that extends beyond the uterus but has not extended to the pelvic sidewall or to the lower third of the vagina.
IIA	No obvious parametrial involvement.
IIA1	Clinically visible lesions 4 cm or less in size.
IIA2	Clinically visible lesions more than 4 cm in size.
IIB	Obvious parametrial involvement but not to the pelvic sidewall.
III	Carcinoma that has extended to the pelvic sidewall and/or involves the lower third of the vagina. On rectal examination, there is no cancer-free space between the tumor and the pelvic sidewall. All cases with a hydronephrosis or nonfunctioning kidney should be included, unless they are known to be due to other causes.
IIIA	No extension to the pelvic sidewall but involvement of the lower third of the vagina.
IIIB	Extension to the pelvic sidewall and/or hydronephrosis or nonfunctioning kidney.
IV	Carcinoma that has extended beyond the true pelvis or has involved (biopsy proven) the mucosa of the bladder and/or rectum.
IVA	Spread of the tumor to adjacent pelvic organs.
IVB	Spread to distant organs.

CASE SUMMARIES

Early-Stage Cervical Cancer

C.T. is a 32-year-old G1P1 woman who was referred to the gynecology service for a 6-month history of abnormal vaginal bleeding. The vaginal bleeding was initially postcoital, but then progressed to almost daily bleeding. She also reported generalized fatigue. She denied abdominal pain associated with bleeding. Her last pap smear was 4 years previously. She had no history of sexually transmitted diseases. On pelvic examination she was found to have a 1 cm × 1.5 cm exophytic, friable mass at the posterior lip of the cervix without gross involvement of vaginal walls, parametria, or pelvic sidewall. Biopsy of the mass was consistent with invasive squamous cell carcinoma. MRI imaging of the pelvis showed a 1.5-cm posterior cervical mass with no evidence of involvement of surrounding structures or lymph nodes. A chest x-ray showed no evidence of distant metastasis. Her performance status was 0, and her baseline lab work showed mild anemia with a hemoglobin of 9.2 g/dL. She had normal renal and liver function tests.

Evidence-Based Case Discussion

C.T. has stage IB1 squamous cell carcinoma of cervix. Early-stage cervical cancers include FIGO stages IA, IB1, and selected IIA1 disease. Treatment options for early-stage IA1 carcinoma without lymphovascular space invasion may include simple hysterectomy that can be performed via laparotomy, vaginally, or laparoscopically. For patients who strongly desire to preserve their fertility, an alternative treatment is conization alone, if they are fully informed of the risks for disease recurrence and the need to be carefully followed (Figure 17.1).

Treatment options for stage IA2 to IIA1 lesions include radical hysterectomy with pelvic lymphadenectomy and para-aortic lymph node biopsy, or definitive concurrent chemotherapy and pelvic radiation therapy (which always includes brachytherapy) (the rationale for concurrent chemoradiation therapy is presented in the evidence-based discussion for locally advanced disease). An alternative therapy for those interested in fertility preservation is the radical trachelectomy with pelvic lymphadenectomy where the cervix is removed radically while sparing the uterine body in order to allow for pregnancy (Figure 17.2).

The major difference between a radical hysterectomy and a radical trachelectomy is that in the latter there is preservation of the upper cervix and uterine body allowing for future pregnancy. The major difference between a simple hysterectomy or trachelectomy and a radical procedure is the removal of the parametrial tissue. The parametria is the connective tissue immediately around the cervix that includes the cardinal and uterosacral ligaments. It contains the vascular supply and lymphatics of the cervix well as the distal ureter en route to the bladder. In both the radical trachelectomy and radical hysterectomy, after mobilization of the ureters, the parametria is removed as part of the radical resection of the cervical tumor in order to assure adequate margins of resection.

The role of parametrectomy is currently being investigated. Several retrospective studies have shown that less than 1% of patients with early-stage cervical cancer with favorable pathologic characteristics have parametrial involvement (2). Patients with favorable characteristics include those with lesions less than 2 cm in size without lymphovascular space involvement. However, the long-term oncologic outcome of patients without a parametrectomy has not been evaluated.

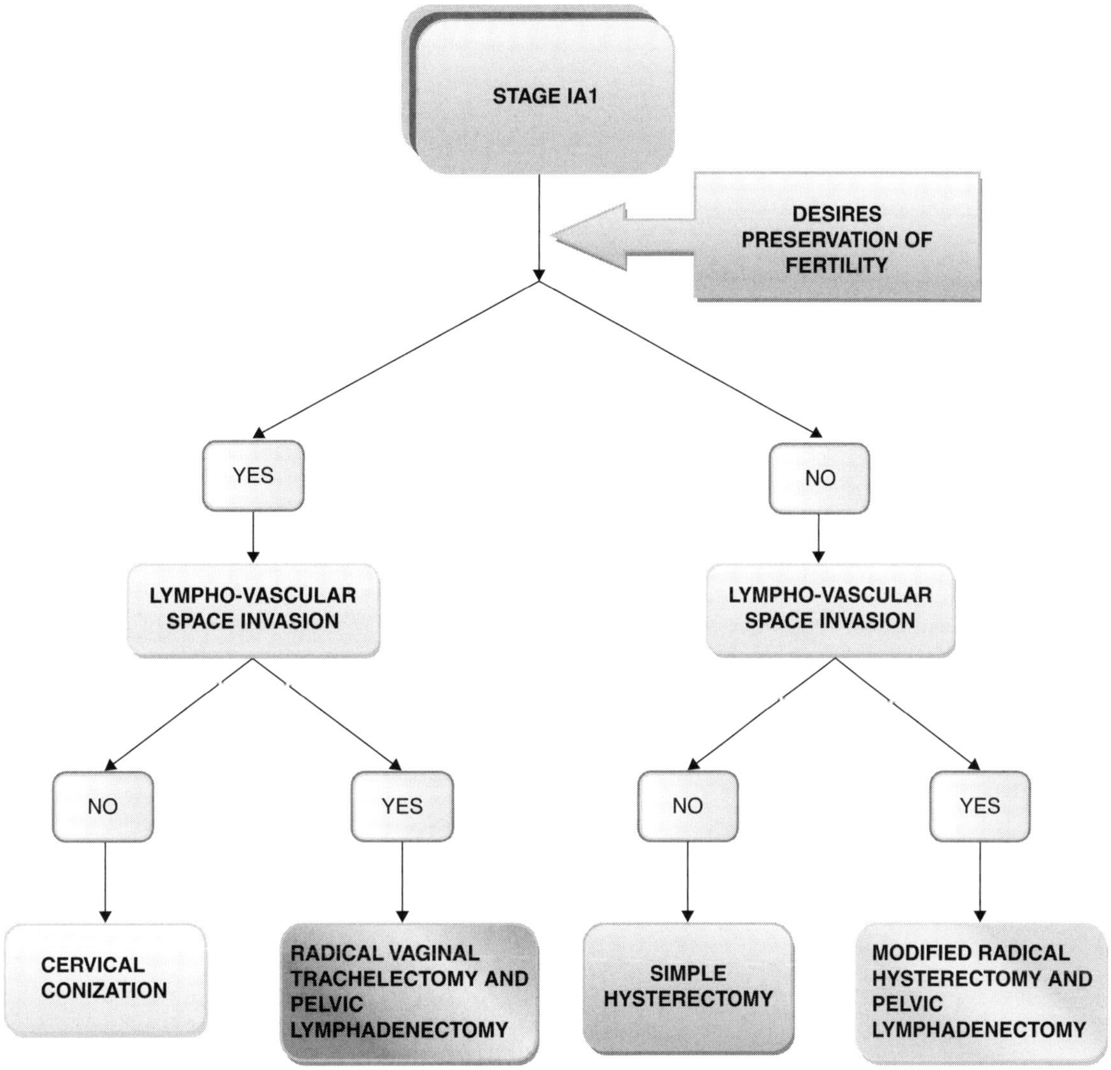

Figure 17.1

Algorithm for the treatment of Stage IA1 cervial carcinoma.

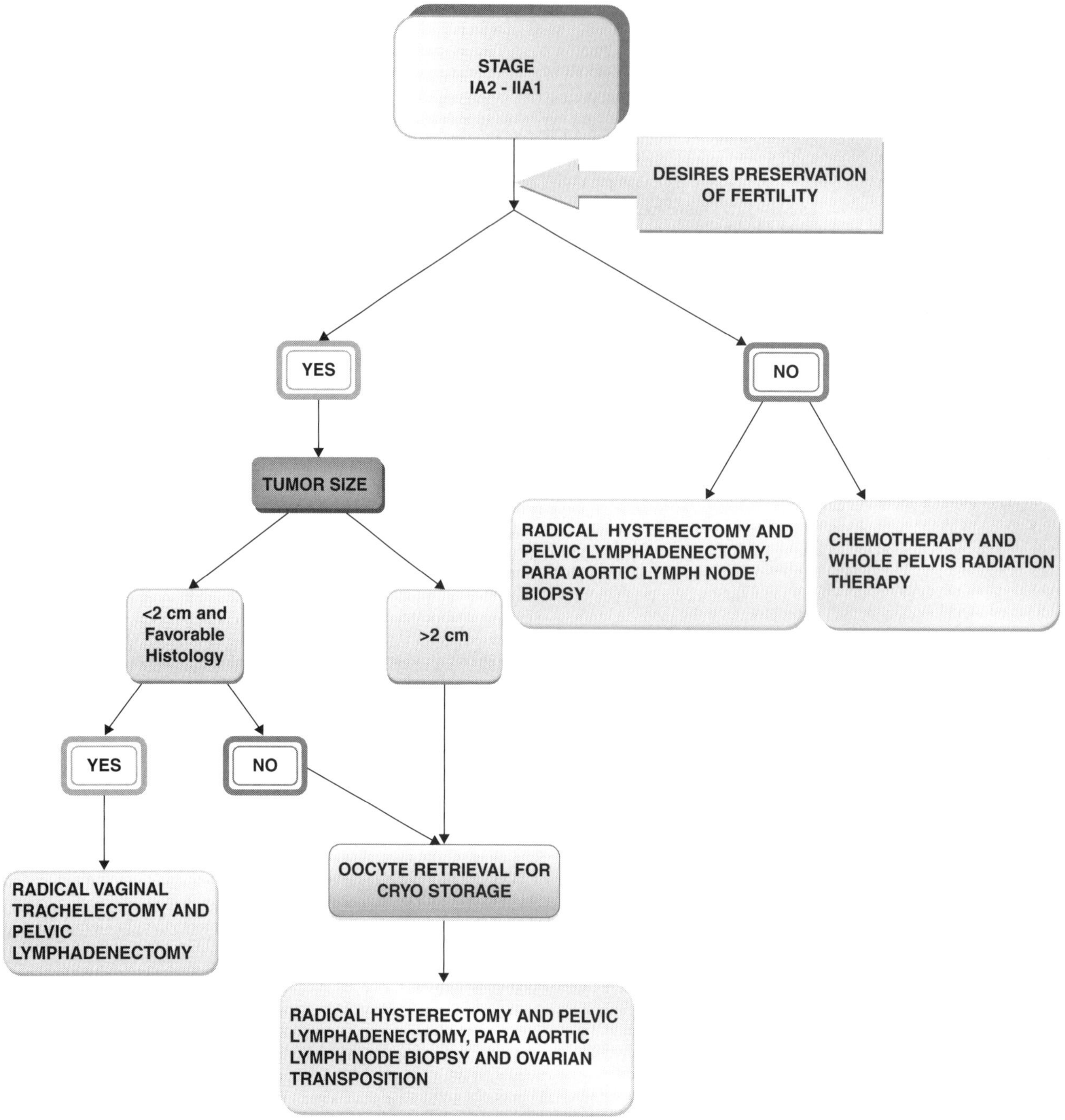

Figure 17.2

Algorithm for the treatment of Stage IA2-IIA1 cervical carcinoma.

Surgery and radiation therapy are equally effective for early-stage disease, resulting in cure rates of 75% to 80% (3). Landoni et al. conducted a randomized clinical trial involving 343 women with stages Ib to IIa cervical cancer in which 172 underwent surgery and 171 received radiation therapy. After a median follow-up of 87 months, the 5-year overall survival (OS) and progression-free survival (PFS) were identical in the surgery and radiation therapy groups (83% and 74%, respectively, for both groups). Twenty-eight percent of women in the surgery group had severe morbidity as compared to 12% in the radiation therapy group (4). Treatment decisions are usually based on patient factors and available local expertise. The advantages of surgery include preservation of ovarian and vaginal function. However, if poor prognostic factors are identified in the surgical specimen, such as positive lymph nodes, positive margins, deep stromal invasion, and lymphovascular space invasion, then adjuvant radiation therapy is recommended. If adjuvant pelvic radiation therapy is indicated postoperatively, the ovaries can be transposed to the upper abdomen out of the pelvic radiation therapy field. Primary surgery also allows for the resection of bulky metastatic lymph nodes, which may be of therapeutic benefit. The downside of a surgical approach is the inherent surgical and anesthesia risks, especially in the patient with other comorbidities. In patients who require postoperative concurrent chemotherapy and radiation therapy, there is the added morbidity associated with triple modality therapy.

C.T. desired to have another child and inquired about treatment options that would preserve her fertility. This is not an uncommon scenario since 42% of cases of cervical cancer are diagnosed in women prior to age 45 (5).

As outlined above, vaginal radical trachelectomy (VRT) with laparoscopic pelvic lymphadenectomy and preservation of the uterine body is an option for a well-selected group of patients who desire to preserve fertility. Selection criteria includes no clinical evidence of impaired fertility, stage IA2 to IB1, lesion size less than 2 cm, limited endocervical involvement as evidenced by direct visualization of the lesion by colposcopy or by MRI, squamous carcinoma or adenocarcinoma histology and no evidence of lymph node metastasis (6). Meeting all of these criteria, C.T. is a candidate for radical trachelectomy with laparoscopic lymphadenectomy.

MRI of the pelvis is useful before surgery to best define the endocervical tumor extension and determine the endocervical margin of resection. The initial surgical step is sentinel lymph node detection with lymphocyntigraphy and isosulfan blue dye lymphatic mapping. If the sentinel lymph node is negative, a complete laparoscopic pelvic lymph node dissection is completed before proceeding with the VRT. A permanent cerclage is sutured in the remaining cervical stump and uterine body as prophylaxis for cervical incompetence in any future pregnancy. Other potential adverse effects of radical trachelectomy include premature labor, chronic vaginal discharge, irregular bleeding, dysmenorrhea, cerclage erosion, amenorrhea, and cervical stenosis (7). Approximately 10% to 12% of these patients are found to have more extensive disease or lymph node metastasis on intraoperative frozen section, contraindicating the fertility-preserving procedure (8).

In the young woman who remains interested in fertility but is not a candidate for radical trachelectomy with preservation of the uterine body, oocyte retrieval for future fertilization and implantation into a surrogate uterus can be offered. In these circumstances, the best option is preoperative ovarian stimulation with retrieval of mature oocytes for immediate fertilization with donor sperm. These early embryos are cryopreserved for implantation into a surrogate uterus at a later time. If immediate in vitro fertilization is not acceptable to the patient, cryostorage of mature oocytes after ovarian stimulation for fertilization at a later time may be an alternative with a limited success rate in comparison to cryostorage of the fertilized embryos. Unfortunately, ovarian stimulation for harvesting mature oocytes requires 3 to 6 weeks of preoperative delay. If this delay in cancer treatment needs to be avoided, newer alternatives include cryostorage of immature oocytes for later in vitro maturation and fertilization as well as cryopreservation of ovarian tissue for later autotransplantation (9,10).

Locally Advanced Cervical Cancer

L.S. is a 39-year-old G2P2 otherwise healthy woman who presented with painful periods for 8 months. She took ibuprofen with some initial relief, but the pain progressed and she also developed vaginal bleeding between periods. Her last Pap smear was done approximately 10 years previously and was reported as normal. She denied a history of sexually transmitted diseases. Speculum exam showed blood clots in vaginal vault and an ulcerative lesion replacing the cervix, extending to the upper third of vagina. Bimanual exam confirmed an ulcerative lesion replacing the cervix and extending to the upper vagina circumferentially and to the parametrial tissues bilaterally. Biopsies of the cervical and upper vaginal lesion were consistent with invasive squamous cell carcinoma of the cervix.

A CT scan of the chest, abdomen, and pelvis showed irregular cervical margins and prominent parametrial strands suggesting parametrial involvement. Mild left hydronephrosis and diffuse bilateral pelvic lymphadenopathy was noted. No para-aortic lymphadenopathy or distant metastasis was identified on CT. As part of the staging procedure, cystoscopy and proctoscopy were performed and both were negative.

Evidence-Based Case Discussion

L.S. has stage IIIB cervical cancer, which is categorized as locally advanced disease (stages IB2 to IVA). Since squamous cell carcinoma of the cervix is both radiation and chemotherapy sensitive, the treatment of choice for locally advanced cervical cancer is concurrent chemotherapy and radiation therapy. Five landmark randomized clinical trials, involving nearly 1900 women, demonstrated a clear survival advantage for the use of cisplatin-based chemotherapy when administered concurrently with radiation therapy. Three of these trials demonstrated the benefit of cisplatin-based regimens when given concurrently with definitive radiation therapy. In a GOG/SWOG phase III trial, Whitney et al. (11) randomized 368 women with stages IIB, III, or IVA cervical carcinoma to receive either pelvic radiation therapy along with oral hydroxyurea (the control group) or the same radiation therapy with intravenous cisplatin and 5-FU (PF). After a median follow-up of 8.7 years, the group receiving PF had a significant improvement in both PFS and OS (risk of death reduced by 21% and 26%, respectively) with the median survival time in the PF arm not met (as compared to 59.8 months for the control group). In a similar GOG trial targeted to stage IIB to IVA disease, Rose et al. (12) compared three study groups involving a total of 526 women who were randomly assigned to receive pelvic radiation therapy along with concurrent chemotherapy consisting of cisplatin alone, hydroxyurea alone, or a combination of cisplatin, 5-FU, and hydroxyurea. After a median follow-up of 35 months, the two treatment groups who received cisplatin had a higher rate of PFS and OS as compared to the group who received hydroxyurea alone, with a relative risk reduction of death of 39% to 42% in the cisplatin-containing arms as compared to the hydroxyurea arm. In the third study, Morris et al. (13) randomly assigned 386 women with IB2 to IVA cancers to receive either radiation therapy to the pelvis and para-aortic lymph nodes or to receive radiation therapy limited to the pelvis along with concurrent cisplatin and 5-FU. For both PFS and OS, the results at 43 months of follow-up favored the PF chemotherapy arm: the estimated 5-year survival rate for women receiving combined pelvic radiation therapy and chemotherapy was 73% as compared to 58% for those treated with extended field radiation therapy ($P = .004$). Two studies examined the role of concurrent therapy prior to hysterectomy or as adjuvant treatment after primary surgery. Keys and his GOG colleagues (14) randomized 369 women with stage IB2 disease to receive pelvic radiation therapy with or without concurrent cisplatin, and showed that both the PFS and OS was significantly better (relative risk of 0.51 and 0.54, respectively) for those receiving combined modality treatment prior to adjuvant hysterectomy. In the adjuvant setting after radical hysterectomy and pelvic lymphadenectomy, 243 women who were found to have positive margins, lymph node metastases, or parametrum involvement were randomized to receive either radiation therapy alone or with concurrent PF (15). At 4-years' follow-up, the concurrent radiation therapy/PF arm was associated with a superior PFS and OS: 80% versus 63% and 81% versus 71%, respectively.

The role of pelvic lymphadenectomy to resect bulky lymphadenopathy before chemoradiation is controversial. In addition to providing accurate treatment planning, lymphadenectomy also has the potential therapeutic survival benefit by resecting the bulky nodes that do not respond well to chemoradiation (16,17). For patients with histologically confirmed para-aortic nodal involvement, extended field radiation therapy to include both pelvic and para-aortic nodes is recommended. For patients with locally advanced cervical carcinoma, disease stage is the most important prognostic factor, followed by lymph node status. Outcomes are worse for women with para-aortic lymph node metastasis.

Neoadjuvant chemotherapy followed by radiation therapy has not been shown to provide any advantage compared to radiation therapy alone. The role of neoadjuvant chemotherapy followed by surgery, however, is unclear. Currently, there are two ongoing phase III trials comparing neoadjuvant chemotherapy followed by surgery versus definitive chemoradiation (EORTC 55994 and NCT00193739).

Distant Metastatic Cervical Cancer

N.S. is a 40-year-old woman, G6P5, who emigrated from her home country in Central America 5 years ago never having had a Pap smear. She presented with episodes of heavy vaginal bleeding for 1 year and with a 4-month history of lower abdominal pain that extended to her back and radiated down her right leg. A pelvic exam revealed a 4.5 × 3.5 cm ulcerated cervical lesion extending down to the lower 1/3 of the vagina, into both parametria and reaching the right pelvic sidewall. Biopsy of the cervical lesion was consistent with moderately differentiated invasive squamous cell carcinoma. A CT showed extensive pelvic and para-aortic lymph node enlargement, mild bilateral hydronephrosis, lytic lesions at right iliac wing, and pulmonary nodules. Biopsy of a pulmonary nodule was consistent with metastatic squamous cell carcinoma of the cervix. Laboratory studies showed severe anemia with a hemoglobin of 6.5 g/dL and mildly impaired renal function. Her performance status was 2.

Evidence-Based Case Discussion

N.S. has disseminated stage IVB cervical cancer that is rare at initial diagnosis in the United States but common in developing countries. The most common sites of metastasis are lymph nodes followed by lung, liver, and bone. Treatment for stage IVB is focused on pallation of symptoms. For example, if vaginal bleeding is the main concern, an abbreviated course of pelvic radiation therapy at a higher dose per fraction can be administered to control acute bleeding. This pelvic palliative treatment can be followed by targeted radiation therapy to symptomatic lesions and/or chemotherapy to treat the systemic disease. Several chemotherapeutic drugs have shown activity in metastatic cervical cancer. Single-agent cisplatin has been used to treat recurrent and metastatic cervical cancer with a response rate of approximately 20%. A Gynecologic Oncology Group (GOG) phase III trial demonstrated a higher response rate (36% vs. 19%) and improved median PFS (4.8 vs. 2.8 months) in the treatment arm that received combination regimen with cisplatin and paclitaxel as compared to cisplatin alone; however, the OS was similar (18). Another phase III trial compared four cisplatin doublet regimens and found a trend in response rate, PFS, and OS that favored a cisplatin/paclitaxel combination.

Specifically, response rates for cisplatin with either vinorelbine, gemcitabine, or topotecan was 25%, 22%, and 23%, respectively, which were not superior to cisplatin and paclitaxel with a response rate of 29% (19).

Another agent currently being studied is bevacizumab, a monoclonal anti-VEGFR agent. It has shown some promising results in a recent GOG phase II trial, and a phase III randomized study is ongoing (20). For patients whose performance status is poor, single-agent chemotherapy or best supportive care can be offered. In the case of N.S., a reasonable approach would be palliative pelvic radiation therapy to control symptomatic bleeding, followed by single-agent cisplatin chemotherapy.

REFERENCES

1. Berrington de, Gonzalez A, Green, J. Comparison of risk factors for invasive squamous cell carcinoma and adenocarcinoma of the cervix: collaborative reanalysis of individual data on 8,097 women with squamous cell carcinoma and 1,374 women with adenocarcinoma from 12 epidemiological studies. *Int J Cancer.* 2007;120:885–891.
2. Schmeler KM, Frumovitz M, Ramirez PT. Conservative management of early stage cervical cancer: Is there a role for less radical surgery? *Gynecol Oncol.* 2011;120:321–325.
3. Eifel PJ, Burke TW, Delclos L, et al. Early stage I adenocarcinoma of the uterine cervix: treatment results in patients with tumors less than or equal to 4 cm in diameter. *Gynecol Oncol.* 1991;41(3):199–205.
4. Landoni F, Maneo A, Colombo A, et al. Randomised study of radical surgery versus radiotherapy for stage Ib-IIa cervical cancer. *Lancet.* 1997;350:535–540.
5. Roy M, Plante M. Pregnancies after radical vaginal trachelectomy for early-stage cervical cancer. *Am J Obstet Gynecol.* 1998;179:1491–1496.
6. Alexander-Sefre F, Chee N, Spencer C, et al. Surgical morbidity associated with radical trachelectomy and radical hysterectomy. *Gynecol Oncol.* 2006;101:450–454.
7. Plante M, Renaud MC, Harel F, Roy M. Vaginal radical trachelectomy: an oncologically safe fertility-preserving surgery. An updated series of 72 cases and review of the literature. *Gynecol Oncol.* 2004;94:614–623.
8. Burghardt E, Baltzer J, Tulusan AH, et al. Results of surgical treatment of 1028 cervical cancers studied with volumetry. *Cancer.* 1992;70:648–655.
9. Smitz JE, Thompson JG, Gilchrist RB. The promise of in vitro maturation in assisted reproduction and fertility preservation. *Semin Reprod Med.* 2011;29(1):24–37.
10. Donnez J, Silber S, Andersen CY, et al. Children born after autotransplantation of cryopreserved ovarian tissue. A review of 13 live births. *Ann Med.* 2011 Jan 13 [Epub ahead of print]
11. Whitney CW, Sause W, Bundy BN, et al. A randomized comparison of fluorouracil plus cisplatin versus hydroxyurea as an adjunct to radiation therapy in stages IIB-IVA carcinoma of the cervix with negative para-aortic lymph nodes: a Gynecologic Oncology Group and Southwest Oncology Group Study. *J Clin Oncol.* 1999;17:1339–1348.
12. Rose PG, Bundy BN, Watkins EB, et al. Concurrent cisplatin based chemoradiation improves progression free and overall survival in advanced cervical cancer: results of a randomized Gynecologic Oncology Group Study. *N Engl J Med.* 1999;340:1144–1153.
13. Morris M, Eifel PJ, Lu J, et al. Pelvic radiation with concurrent chemotherapy versus pelvic and para-aortic radiation for high-risk cervical cancer: a randomized Radiation Therapy Oncology Group clinical trial. *N Engl J Med.* 1999;340:1137–1143.
14. Keys HM, Bundy BM, Stehman FB, et al. A comparison of weekly cisplatin during radiation therapy versus irradiation alone each followed by adjuvant hysterectomy in bulky stage IB cervical carcinoma: a randomized trial of the Gynecologic Oncology Group. *N Engl J Med.* 1999;340:1154–1161.
15. Peters WA III, Liu PY, Barrett RJ, et al. Cisplatin and 5-fluorouracil plus radiation therapy are superior to radiation therapy as adjunctive in high-risk early stage carcinoma of the cervix after radical hysterectomy and pelvic lymphadenectomy: report of a phase III intergroup study. *J Clin Oncol.* 2000;18:1606–1613.
16. Hacker NF, Wain GV, Nicklin JL. Resection of bulky positive lymph nodes in patients with cervical carcinoma. *Int J Gynecol Cancer.* 1995;5:250–256.
17. Marnitz S, Kohler C, Roth C, et al. Is there a benefit of pretreatment laparoscopic transperitoneal surgical staging in patients with advanced cervical cancer? *Gynecol Oncol.* 2005;99:536–544.
18. Moore DH, Blessing JA, McQuellon RP, et al. Phase III study of cisplatin with or without paclitaxel in stage IVB, recurrent, or persistent squamous cell carcinoma of the cervix: a Gynecologic Oncology Group study. *J Clin Oncol.* 2004;22:3113–3119.
19. Monk BJ, Still MW, McMeekin DS, et al. Phase III trial of four cisplatin-containing doublet combinations in stage IVB, recurrent, or persistent cervical carcinoma: a Gynecologic Oncology Group study. *J Clin Oncol.* 2009;27:4649–4655.
20. Monk BJ, Sill MW, Gray HJ, et al. Phase II trial of bevacizumab in the treatment of persistent or recurrent squamous cell carcinoma of the cervix: a Gynecologic Oncology Group study. *J Clin Oncol.* 2009;27:1069–1074.

18

Uterine Cancer

ATISHA MANHAS AND MATTHEW L. ANDERSON

EPIDEMIOLOGY, RISK FACTORS, NATURAL HISTORY, AND PATHOLOGY

Uterine cancer is the most common female genital tract malignancy in the United States (1) and includes both endometrial cancers as well as more rare cancers arising in the myometrium, such as leiomyosarcoma.

Endometrial cancers are most commonly diagnosed in women 50 to 65 years of age. Seventy-five percent of patients are postmenopausal. For many women, the pathogenesis of endometrial cancer appears to be related to prolonged exposure of unopposed estrogen, which promotes endometrial growth and ultimately causes poorly understood changes in endometrial glands. Early-estrogen-induced changes in the endometrium can lead to simple hyperplasia, which is typically reversible with hormonal treatment and not considered to be a premalignant condition. However, more disorganized lesions, such as complex atypical hyperplasia, are now recognized to have significant malignant potential. Hormonal interventions for complex atypical hyperplasia may be less effective and, as a result, many women diagnosed with one of these lesions may be treated with hysterectomy. The molecular basis of complex or atypical endometrial hyperplasia is poorly understood. About 25% of women with complex atypical hyperplasia will eventually develop an invasive endometrial cancer (2). Surgical excision of premalignant lesions is almost always successful in preventing uterine cancer, although a significant proportion of women who undergo hysterectomy for complex endometrial hyperplasia will actually be found to harbor an endometrial cancer when surgical specimens are closely examined.

Hormonally driven cancers are now categorized as type I endometrial cancers. Risk factors for developing type I endometrial cancer and hyperplasia include estrogen therapy use (without concomitant use of progestins), obesity, nulliparity, late menopause, complex atypical hyperplasia, and tamoxifen use. Women taking tamoxifen have an approximately three- to seven-fold higher risk of developing endometrial cancer than women not taking the drug (3). Hereditary non-polyposis colon cancer (HNPCC) syndrome is also a risk factor, associated with a 20% to 60% lifetime risk of endometrial cancer. Factors that decrease the risk of type I endometrial cancer include combined oral contraceptive use, early menopause, multiparity, and smoking (likely through an antiestrogenic effect).

The vast majority (80%) of patients with type I endometrial cancer and traditional risk factors have stage I disease at diagnosis. These cancers often present with postmenopausal bleeding. For these women, office endometrial biopsy often establishes the diagnosis, allowing patients to be triaged to appropriate surgical management. Endometrial cancer is surgically staged. Initial clinical management should include hysterectomy with bilateral salpingo-oophorectomy and a thorough examination of the entire abdominopelvic cavity. Suspicious lesions identified at the time of laparotomy should be thoroughly sampled to establish the presence or absence of carcinoma. Historically, surgical staging procedures such as pelvic washings and pelvic and para-aortic lymph node dissections have been performed once size, grade, and depth of myometrial invasion are established by intraoperative frozen section. However, a number of investigators have recently advocated thorough surgical staging regardless of whether poorly differentiated tumor histology, deep myometrial invasion, or lymphovascular invasion are noted on frozen section. A second, ongoing issue is the extent of lymphadenectomy necessary to adequately surgically stage endometrial cancers. Historically, many gynecologic oncologists have advocated lymph node sampling rather than the more complete lymphadenectomy performed for ovarian cancer. However, increasing retrospective data suggest that thorough lymphadenectomies can not only identify para-aortic lymph node metastases in ~20% of women with no radiographic evidence of metastases in their pelvic lymph nodes, but also that more extensive pelvic and para-aortic lymph node dissections may have therapeutic benefit. Further work is necessary to more precisely resolve these issues.

Type I endometrial cancers are histologically similar to their tissue of origin and are categorized as endometrioid adenocarcinoma. More recently, a second category of endometrial cancers (type II) has been defined and includes less common, but clinically more aggressive cancers such as uterine papillary serous carcinomas (UPSCs). Despite accounting for fewer than 10% of all uterine cancers, UPSC accounts for more than 40% of all uterine cancer deaths that occur each year in the United States. UPSC and other type II uterine cancers are found more frequently in African-American women and are less likely to be associated with obesity or hormonal exposure. In large part, the mortality related to type II cancers is due to their propensity to metastasize early. Whether poorly differentiated endometrioid endometrial cancers should be grouped with UPSC as a form of type II uterine cancer is currently a topic of active debate. However, there is increasing appreciation that type II uterine cancers arise via a distinct endometrial precursor known as endometrial intraepithelial neoplasia (EIN). The molecular events leading to EIN are at present poorly defined.

Five-year survival for endometrial cancer varies by stage: 83% for patients with stage I disease, 73% for those with stage II disease, 52% for those with stage III disease, and 27% for those with stage IV disease. Features associated with a poorer prognosis are higher grade, alternate histology (type II), older age, and vascular invasion.

Rare histologic subtypes of uterine cancer include adenosarcomas and mixed mesodermal cancers (carcinosarcomas). Uterine cancers originating in components of the uterus other than the endometrium account for only about 4% of all uterine cancers and are best exemplified by uterine leiomyosarcoma.

In addition, several malignant conditions exist that may arise in the uterus but are derived from gestational trophoblastic tissue. Collectively, these are defined as malignant gestational trophoblastic disease (malignant GTD). These cancers commonly develop after molar pregnancy but may develop after nonmolar pregnancy as well. The diagnosis is typically confirmed by levels of serum beta-human chorionic gonadotrophin (β-hCG) that fail to fall appropriately or plateau following uterine evacuation, or by histologic evaluation of evacuated contents. An initial β-hCG greater than 100,000 mIU/mL, a history of prior GTD, and age greater than 40 all increase the risk of malignant GTD following molar pregnancy. Subtypes of malignant GTD are quite heterogeneous in clinical behavior and include persistent/invasive gestational trophoblastic neoplasia (GTN), choriocarcinoma, and placental site trophoblastic tumor (PSTT). Persistent/invasive GTN follows approximately 20% of complete molar pregnancies and is rarely metastatic at presentation (4). Conversely, choriocarcinoma is a highly aggressive tumor, and the majority of patients have metastatic disease at diagnosis, most commonly to the lung. Fifty percent of choriocarcinomas develop after molar pregnancies, and 50% follow nonmolar pregnancies (which include normal pregnancies, spontaneous abortions, and ectopic pregnancies). Finally, PSTT is a rare form of malignant GTD that develops from the intermediate cytotrophoblast and presents months to years after a term gestation. These tumors secrete only small amounts of β-hCG and are not as sensitive to chemotherapy as persistent/invasive GTN and choriocarcinoma. Outcomes for these women are typically much more guarded. Staging of malignant GTD has evolved to include both traditional staging, which defines anatomic extent of disease, and the WHO scoring system, which incorporates other prognostic factors. Under this system, patients are given a number score and placed into "low-risk" or "high-risk" categories based on multiple factors including age, interval from antecedent pregnancy, and pretreatment β-hCG. The WHO prognostic score can not only assess risk, but can also predict which patients will respond poorly to single-agent chemotherapy and thus require combination chemotherapy. Fortunately, with the exception of PSTT, even high-risk metastatic malignant GTD is highly sensitive to combination chemotherapy. With standard treatment, cure rates of over 90% are achieved (5).

STAGING

2009 FIGO Staging System for Endometrial Cancer (6)

Stage	Definition
I	Primary tumor is confined to the corpus uteri
IA	Tumor limited to endometrium or invades less than half of the myometrium
IB	Tumor invades one half or more of the myometrium
II	Primary tumor invades cervical stroma, but does not extend beyond uterus*
III	Local and/or regional spread of tumor is present
IIIA	Tumor invades serosa of the corpus uteri and/or adnexae**
IIIB	Vaginal and/or parametrial involvement is present**
IIIC	Metastasis to pelvic and/or para-aortic lymph nodes is present**; IIIC1 to pelvic nodes; IIIC2 to para-aortic nodes ± pelvic node
IV	Tumor invades bladder mucosa and/or bowel, or distant metastasis is present
IVA	Tumor invades bladder mucosa and/or bowel
IVB	Distant metastasis is present

*Endocervical glandular involvement is considered Stage I and no longer is Stage II **Positive peritoneal cytology should be reported separately and does not change the stage.

WHO Prognostic Scoring Index for Gestational Trophoblastic Tumors (7)

Prognostic Factor	Risk Score			
	0	1	2	4
Age	<40	≥40		
Antecedent Pregnancy	Hydatidiform mole	Abortion	Term pregnancy	
Interval months from pregnancy	<4	4–6	7–12	>12
Pretreatment serum β-hCG (IU/mL)	<1000	1000 to <10,000	10,000 to <100,000	
Largest tumor size, including uterus (cm)	<3	3–5	>5	
Site of metastases	Lung	Spleen, kidney	GI tract	Brain, liver
Number of metastases identified		1–4	5–8	>8
Previous failed chemotherapy			Single drug	Two or more drugs
Total score	<6 = Low risk, ≥7 = High risk			

CASE SUMMARIES

Early-Stage Endometrial Cancer

L.C., a 67-year-old retired accountant who was menopausal since age 59, presented to her gynecologist with a 2-week history of vaginal bleeding. She described her bleeding as mild and intermittent, occurring one to two times daily. She also reported an increase in clear vaginal discharge. She denied abdominal pain or weight loss. Her medical and surgical history were remarkable for hypertension, osteoporosis, and a right hip replacement 3 years earlier. She had 3 children from three pregnancies. She had not taken hormone replacement therapy, had no history of cancer in her family, and had smoked 1 pack of cigarettes daily for 40 years. General physical examination was significant for obesity. On pelvic examination there were no external genital or vaginal lesions, the uterus was normal in size and nontender, and the cervix was smooth without lesions. The adnexae were neither tender nor enlarged.

The patient underwent office endometrial biopsy. Results of the endometrial biopsy revealed grade 2 moderately differentiated adenocarcinoma without invasion of the cervical stroma. Chest x-ray and CT scan of the abdomen and pelvis showed no evidence of metastatic disease. The patient underwent total abdominal hysterectomy, bilateral salpingo-oophorectomy, and pelvic and para-aortic lymph node sampling. Final pathology showed a moderately differentiated endometrioid adenocarcinoma with more than 50% invasion of the myometrium (including the outer third) and lymphovascular invasion (Figure 18.1). All lymph nodes were negative for malignancy. She was referred to an oncologist for recommendations regarding adjuvant therapy.

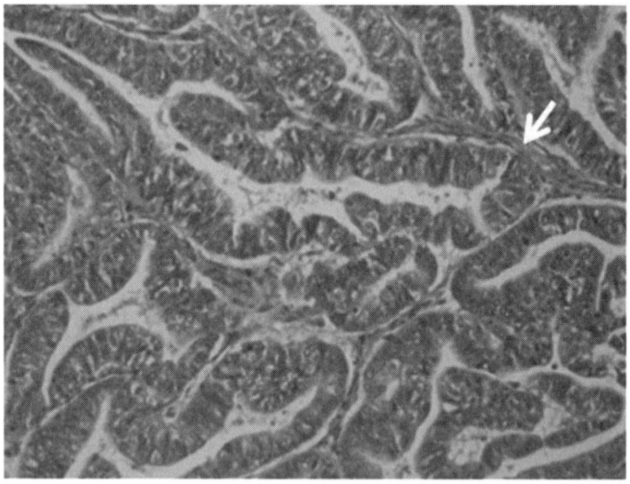

Figure 18.1

Endometrial adenocarcinoma. Uterine cancers are characterized by abnormal gland formation (arrow), diminished or absent stroma between glands, disordered chromatin distribution, nuclear enlargement, increased mitoses, and necrosis. The severity of these features is used to grade tumors and is associated with risk of metastasis and prognosis. (see color insert)

Evidence-Based Case Discussion

Using updated FIGO criteria, this patient's tumor is classified as a stage IB endometrial cancer, since her cancer is localized in the corpus uteri and involves greater than 50% of the myometrium. Under the previous version of FIGO staging, she would be considered to have stage IC disease. Her risk factors for endometrial cancer include obesity and late menopause. The patient has a history of smoking; however, smoking is not a risk factor, as it is actually associated with a lower risk of endometrial cancer.

Approaches to adjuvant therapy in early-stage endometrial cancer have been defined by several randomized trials investigating the role of adjuvant pelvic radiation. The GOG-99 study compared adjuvant pelvic radiation with observation alone in 400 patients with stage I, IB, IC, and II disease (8). There was no difference in overall survival between the two groups; however, local pelvic and/or vaginal recurrences occurred at a lower rate in the pelvic radiation group (3% vs. 12%). The PORTEC trial from the Netherlands, which randomized 714 patients with stage I disease to pelvic radiation or observation, also showed a decrease in local recurrence rate with pelvic radiation, but again, there was no difference in overall survival (9).

To determine which patients may benefit from adjuvant radiation, Creutzberg and colleagues have used data from GOG-99 to define subgroups for "low" risk and "high-intermediate" risk for local recurrence (10). Patients with stage IA or IB and grade 1 or 2 tumors are defined as "low" risk, with a 6% chance of local recurrence; thus, no adjuvant therapy is recommended. In patients with stage IC tumors (or grade 3 tumors in stage IA/IB), risk factors were used to determine "high-intermediate" risk patients who would benefit from radiotherapy. Factors that increase risk include age, grade 2 or 3 tumors, outer third invasion of the myometrium, and lymphovascular invasion. "High-intermediate" risk patients were determined by the following criteria: patients older than 70 years with one other risk factor, older than 50 years with two other risk factors, or any age with all three risk factors. Given that this patient has three risk factors, she would be classified as "high-intermediate" risk for recurrence and should be considered for adjuvant radiation therapy.

In terms of radiation modality, vaginal brachytherapy appears to be equivalent to pelvic radiation in high-intermediate risk, stage I endometrial cancer. This was suggested by the PORTEC-2 trial, which showed no significant difference in local recurrence rates in patients assigned to either modality (11). Because of this equivalence and lower toxicity, vaginal brachytherapy has become the standard modality in adjuvant radiation for high-intermediate risk patients with stage I endometrial cancer.

The role of adjuvant chemotherapy in early-stage endometrial cancer remains undefined and is being evaluated in clinical trials, including a large GOG trial. In a preliminary Japanese GOG trial, which randomized stage IC patients to pelvic radiation versus chemotherapy with cyclophosphamide, doxorubicin, and cisplatin (CAP), there was a higher overall survival rate in the chemotherapy arm for the high-intermediate risk patients (90% vs. 74%) (12).

In summary, patients with stage IA and grade 1 or 2 cancers are considered low risk, and no adjuvant treatment is recommended. For all other patients with stage I disease, risk factors should be evaluated. Those patients deemed to be high-intermediate risk (patients older than 70 with one risk factor, older than 50 with two risk factors, or any age with three risk factors) should be considered for adjuvant radiation therapy. Figure 18.2 outlines a suggested algorithm for the management of stage I disease.

The treatment of stage II endometrial cancer is more complex, due to involvement of the cervical stroma. If surgeons are aware of cervical invasion prior to hysterectomy, one option potentially associated with improved outcome is to perform a radical hysterectomy rather than the more standard simple extrafascial hysterectomy. Postoperatively, physicians have employed a number of different treatment strategies, including primary radioactive implants followed by hysterectomy as well as hysterectomy followed by radiation. Patients with stage II disease

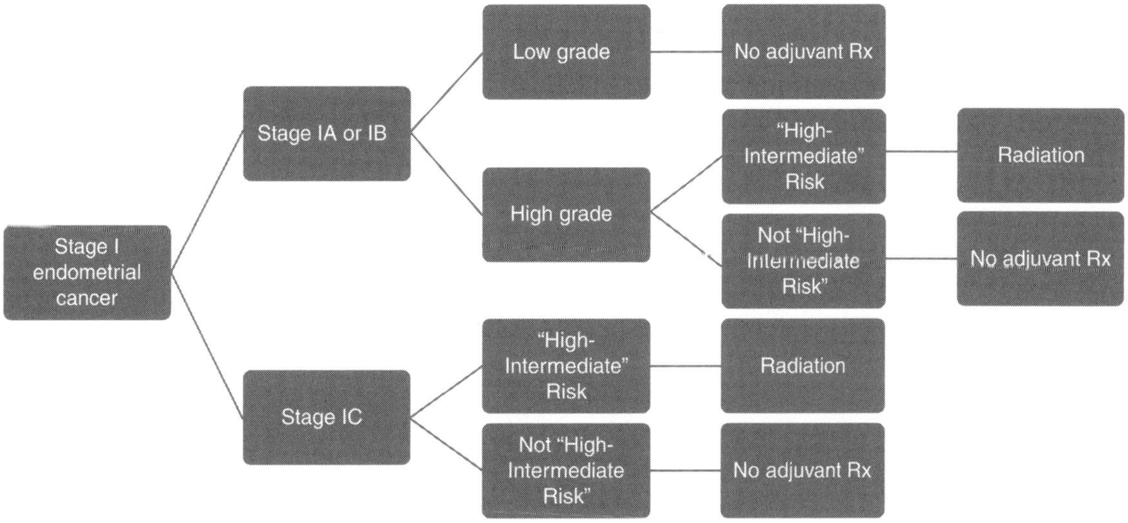

Figure 18.2

Treatment algorithm for early-stage endometrial carcinoma. Adjuvant treatment for early-stage uterine cancer is determined by the histologic features of each cancer and other risk factors for recurrence. Factors that increase risk include age, increasing histologic (≥2) grade, the presence of tumor in the outer third of the myometrium, and lymphovascular invasion. "High-intermediate" risk patients are defined by patients older than 70 years with one other risk factor, older than 50 years with two other risk factors, or any age with all three risk factors.

should be encouraged to enroll in clinical trials evaluating these various treatment approaches.

Locally Advanced Endometrial Cancer

Y.R. is a 48-year-old woman who presented to her gynecologist's office with a complaint of abnormal vaginal bleeding for 3-months' duration. She noted intermittent, mild bleeding between each menstrual cycle, as well as abnormally heavy menses for 3 months. Prior to this, she had had increasing menstrual irregularity for 1 year, but no abnormally heavy menses or spotting. In addition, she noted the development of a dull pain in her left abdomen 1 week prior to presentation. She had experienced a 10-pound weight loss over the last 3 months, but had no other constitutional symptoms. Her medical history was remarkable for type II diabetes and mild peripheral neuropathy. She had never been pregnant. She did not smoke, and her only medication was metformin. Her family history was unremarkable for cancer or gynecologic diseases. On general examination, she was noted to be overweight but had no other abnormalities. Pelvic examination revealed no external genital lesions, no vaginal lesions, a smooth cervix without lesions, and nontender, nonenlarged uterus and adnexae. Transvaginal ultrasound showed an endometrial thickness of 6 mm. Endometrial biopsy was done, and results revealed endometrial adenocarcinoma.

Chest x-ray showed no abnormalities, but CT scan of the abdomen and pelvis revealed an isolated enlarged left pelvic lymph node (Figure 18.3). There was no para-aortic lymphadenopathy. The patient underwent surgical resection and staging, consisting of total abdominal hysterectomy, bilateral salpingo-oophorectomy, and lymph node dissection. Pathology revealed a grade 2 endometrioid adenocarcinoma, with two pelvic lymph nodes positive for malignancy. Peritoneal cytology was also positive for malignancy.

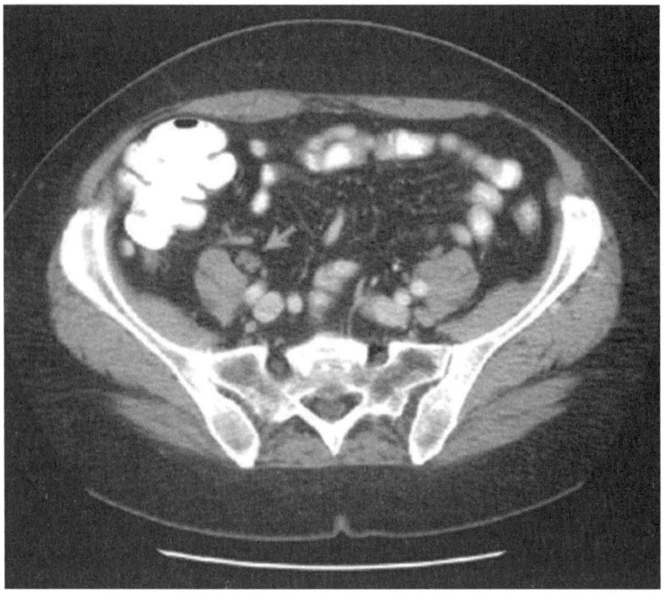

Figure 18.3

Imaging of lymphatic metastasis. An isolated pelvic lymph node metastasis (arrow) was visualized by computed tomography in a patient with endometrial carcinoma.

Evidence-Based Case Discussion

This patient has locally advanced, stage III endometrial cancer. Specifically, she has stage IIIC disease, due to involvement of adjacent pelvic lymph nodes. Although the patient had positive peritoneal cytology, this finding does not contribute to the surgical stage, according to updated 2009 FIGO staging guidelines. Patients with positive peritoneal cytology are no longer automatically defined as stage III, as opposed to previous staging guidelines. This patient's case highlights the fact that endometrial cancer frequently affects perimenopausal women, in addition to women who have already undergone menopause. Younger women of reproductive age can also develop endometrial cancer. In fact, women younger than age 50 constitute 10% to 15% of all endometrial cancer cases (1).

Many patients with stage III endometrial cancer (and select patients with stage IV) are considered to have surgically resectable disease, with an estimated 50% to 80% chance of long-term survival. Randall and colleagues evaluated data from recent studies with the goal of defining prognostic features in patients with surgical stage III and IV disease (13). Favorable characteristics include isolated adnexal or serosal involvement (stage IIIA) and isolated pelvic lymph node involvement with surgically confirmed negative para-aortic lymph nodes. Unfavorable features included the presence of gross residual tumor after surgery, para-aortic lymph node involvement, multiple sites of extrauterine spread, high histologic grade, lymphovascular invasion, peritoneal spread, and high-risk histologies of papillary serous and clear cell carcinoma. These high-risk patients are at greater risk for both local failure and distant metastasis.

Optimal adjuvant treatment for surgically resected, advanced-stage endometrial cancer is a work in progress. Radiation therapy and chemotherapy have both been studied in clinical trials. Initial approaches used whole abdominal radiation (WAI) alone. Smith and colleagues reviewed outcomes for 22 patients with surgical stage III and stage IV endometrial carcinoma (excluding patients with clear cell and papillary serous cancers) treated with WAI and found 5-year disease-free survival and overall survival of 79% and 89%, respectively (14). Gibbons and colleagues reviewed 56 high-risk patients who received WAI and found 7-year disease-free survival of 58% and 25% for stage III and IV patients, respectively (15).

However, in GOG 94, a large phase II trial evaluating WAI in 180 patients with stage III or stage IV disease, 3-year recurrence-free survival rates were much lower, at 29% and 27% for typical and high-risk histologies, respectively (16). Half of the recurrences consisted of distant relapses. These results underscore the need to evaluate adjuvant systemic therapy to improve patients' chances for long-term survival.

The role of chemotherapy in adjuvant treatment of stage III was supported in 2006 by the pivotal GOG 122 trial. This trial evaluated WAI versus chemotherapy with doxorubicin and cisplatin in patients with surgical stage III or IV endometrial cancer with < 2-cm gross residual disease. Chemotherapy consisted of doxorubicin 60 mg/m^2 and cisplatin 50 mg/m^2 every 3 weeks for seven cycles, followed by one cycle of cisplatin. The chemotherapy arm demonstrated greater 5-year progression-free survival (50% vs. 38%) and overall survival (55% vs. 42%). As a result of this trial, chemotherapy is now a mainstay of adjuvant treatment of advanced, surgically resectable endometrial cancer (17). However, the local recurrence rate in the trial was higher in the chemotherapy arm than in the radiation arm (32% vs. 29% of all recurrences), suggesting that radiation should still play a role in these patients.

Many clinicians will combine radiation with chemotherapy for patients who are thought to be at high risk for pelvic recurrence; however, this approach has not yet been validated. Two large trials are currently evaluating combination therapy, which is either given concomitantly (GOG 99-07) or sequentially (GOG 99-08). The optimal chemotherapy regimen that should be used under these circumstances remains to be defined. Although the GOG 122 used doxorubicin and cisplatin, the TAP regimen (doxorubicin 45 mg/m^2 on day 1, paclitaxel 160 mg/m^2 on day 2, and cisplatin 50 mg/m^2 on day 1) is utilized by many clinicians due to a survival benefit seen in advanced or recurrent unresectable endometrial cancer.

In summary, although optimal adjuvant treatment for stage III and IV endometrial cancer is evolving, the current standard of care is chemotherapy. Clinicians often incorporate radiation as part of the treatment plan for women thought to be at high risk for local failure, although this approach is still under investigation. In the case of the 48-year-old patient with stage IIIC endometrial cancer involving pelvic lymph nodes, the recommended adjuvant treatment would be chemotherapy. Her peripheral neuropathy would preclude use of a taxane, so a reasonable regimen for her would be doxorubicin and cisplatin as per the GOG 122 protocol. Her isolated pelvic lymph node metastases place her in a favorable risk group, since her para-aortic nodes were unaffected. Thus, she is not at particularly high risk for local failure, and radiation may not offer additional benefit.

Recurrent and Metastatic Endometrial Cancer

A 72-year-old postmenopausal woman, C.G., presented to her primary care provider with intermittent vaginal bleeding of 6-months' duration. Initially the bleeding was scant, but had increased in frequency during the past 3 weeks. She also described fatigue and dizziness on standing as well as a 9-pound unintentional weight loss over 3 months. She had no ongoing medical problems, took no medications, and did not smoke. She was a retired businesswoman but still volunteered fairly actively in her community. General physical examination was remarkable for slight abdominal fullness, but no discrete mass. Pelvic examination showed no external or vaginal lesions and a smooth cervix without lesions. However, the right adnexae were markedly tender. Transvaginal ultrasound showed increased endometrial thickness and an enlarged right ovary. Endometrial biopsy was done in the office, and the pathology revealed endometrial adenocarcinoma, grade 2. CT scan of the abdomen and pelvis showed a thickened uterus as well as discrete metastatic deposits on the right ovary and bladder, peritoneal implants, and three hypo-attenuating lesions in the liver. Image-guided biopsy of one of the liver lesions was consistent with endometrial adenocarcinoma.

Evidence-Based Case Discussion

The patient presented with endometrial cancer with widespread metastases. She has stage IVB disease based on distant metastasis to the liver. For patients presenting with widely metastatic disease, several recent retrospective studies have examined the potential utility of debulking surgery. Results of these studies have been generally favorable, suggesting improved survival with optimal debulking of metastatic disease at initial presentation. Patients with metastatic or recurrent endometrial cancer have several different treatment options, depending on the extent of disease. For patients with isolated vaginal or pelvic relapse, radiation offers an approximately 50% chance for long-term survival, as shown by several studies. In the PORTEC trial, 3-year survival rates in patients with local relapse were 51% for those who received radiation and 19% for those who did not (9). For those patients who have already undergone pelvic radiation, surgery can also provide an opportunity for long-term survival. Bristow and colleagues found that of the 35 patients who underwent surgery for locally recurrent endometrial cancer at one institution, 54% of women who underwent a complete resection were alive at 3 years, as opposed to none in the group of patients with residual disease following resection (18). Patients with isolated pelvic recurrence after RT may also be considered for pelvic exenteration. Despite its associated morbidity, exenteration with complete tumor resection offers a 20% to 45% chance of long-term survival.

Widely metastatic disease may be treated with systemic therapy, including hormone therapy and chemotherapy. In the 1950s, hormone therapy with progestational agents was found to induce responses in endometrial cancer. Several different agents have been shown to produce clinically significant responses, including megestrol acetate, hydroxyprogesterone caproate, and medroxyprogesterone acetate. Objective response rates for women receiving high doses of these agents are typically between 10% and 30%. Although the average duration of response is 4 months, some patients remain progression free for over 2 years. The likelihood of a response is highly dependent on estrogen and/or progesterone-receptor expression. Progesterone-receptor negative tumors have very low response rates to progestins; thus, a progestin is recommended as initial therapy only in women who have progesterone-receptor positive tumors. Tamoxifen has also shown response in patients with hormone-receptor-positive cancers, although it is not clear whether the drug is beneficial in patients who have failed progestational agents. In general, low-grade histology and a long disease-free interval between initial diagnosis and development of metastatic disease are associated with increased likelihood of a response (19).

Chemotherapy is the treatment of choice for patients with metastatic disease who have PR-negative tumors or have failed hormonal therapy, and it is often considered for many patients, regardless of hormone receptor status. Doxorubicin, cisplatin, carboplatin, and paclitaxel are all active agents, with response rates of up to 30%, and each may be used as monotherapy. Combination chemotherapy has also been studied with some success. The combination of cisplatin and doxorubicin was associated with higher progression-free-survival compared with doxorubicin alone (5.7 months vs. 3.8 months) for 281 patients with advanced unresectable disease (20). However, there was no overall survival benefit. In a large 2004 phase III trial comparing a paclitaxel-containing regimen (TAP, or paclitaxel, doxorubicin, and cisplatin) with doxorubicin and cisplatin, the paclitaxel-containing combination showed an improvement in median survival (15.3 months vs. 12.3 months). However, this was at the cost of added toxicity (21). Another treatment option is paclitaxel and carboplatin, which, when compared with doxorubicin and cisplatin in a French study of 67 patients, was found to improve progression-free survival (35% vs. 24%) and overall survival (41% vs. 27%) at 15 months without added toxicity (22).

To summarize, patients with locally recurrent endometrial carcinoma can potentially be salvaged with radiation. For those patients who have had radiation previously, have an isolated vaginal recurrence, and can undergo a complete resection, surgical salvage is an option. Select patients with isolated pelvic recurrence may undergo pelvic exenteration. Progestational agents should be considered if the tumor expresses progesterone receptors. Otherwise, palliative chemotherapy should be employed. The most effective regimens appear to be paclitaxel-doxorubicin-cisplatin and paclitaxel-carboplatin. Figure 18.4 provides a treatment algorithm for recurrent or metastatic disease. In the case of the patient with disease metastatic to the liver, hormone receptor testing of the tumor specimen is indicated. If the tumor shows positivity for the progesterone receptor, a progestational agent could be considered as initial therapy; if the tumor is progesterone-negative, then palliative chemotherapy should be preferentially started. Despite her old age, the patient discussed appears to have

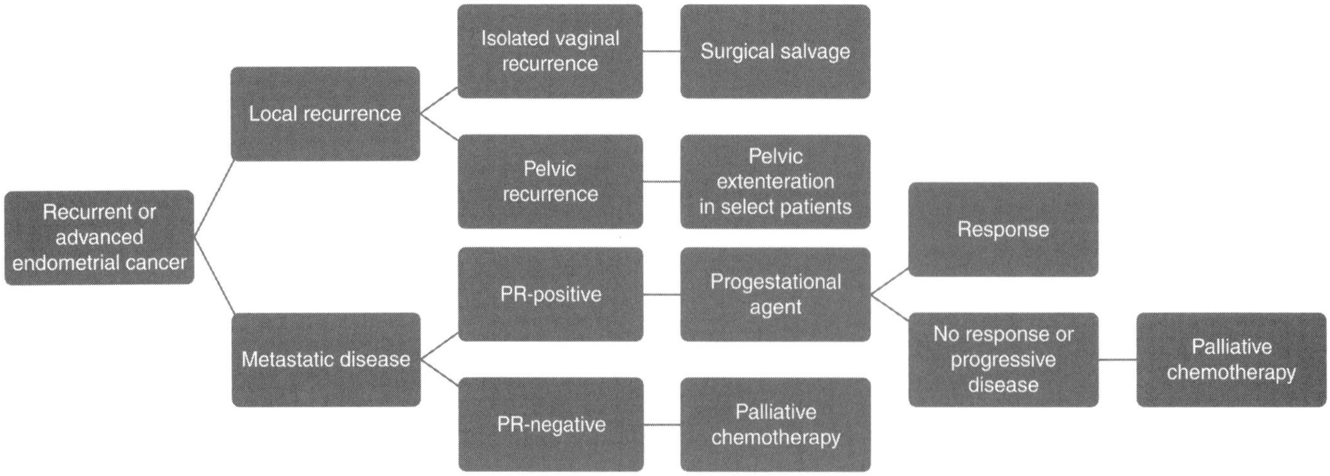

Figure 18.4

Treatment algorithm for metastatic endometrial carcinoma. Salvage can not infrequently be achieved for patients with isolated recurrences of endometrial cancer with surgery and/or radiation. For more widespread disease, multimodality therapy can also be considered for palliation of symptoms and treatment, although cure is less likely.

excellent functional status, so a reasonable approach would be standard chemotherapy with paclitaxel-carboplatin or TAC, with close monitoring for toxicity.

High-Risk Malignant GTD

T.R. is a 16-year-old woman, G_1P_0, who initially presented for evaluation of irregular menses. Four months earlier, she had experienced the onset of irregular vaginal bleeding. The patient described episodes of heavy vaginal bleeding that occurred 3 to 4 times per month, each lasting as long as 4 days. Several weeks earlier, she had started oral contraceptives and iron supplements prescribed by a local primary care physician with little improvement in her symptoms. For several days prior to her initial evaluation, she had also been having problems with lightheadedness and shortness of breath, particularly upon standing. The patient reported one pregnancy slightly more than a year earlier. This pregnancy had ended spontaneously in the first trimester. No uterine evacuation had been performed afterwards and she had recovered uneventfully. She denied any sexual activity since her miscarriage.

Physical examination revealed the patient to be uncomfortable and dyspneic with a blood pressure of 104/70, resting heart rate of 116, and oxygen saturation by pulse oximetry of 93%. Of note, her pulse rate jumped to 160 upon standing, with no significant change in her blood pressure. Breath sounds were normal bilaterally, there was no dullness to chest percussion, and abdominal examination was unremarkable. Pelvic examination revealed scant dark blood in the vaginal vault. The patient's cervix was visually closed and of normal consistency to palpation. Her uterus was normal in size. A urine pregnancy test was performed and found to be positive. Subsequently, a quantitative β-HCG was markedly elevated at 1,316,600 mIU/mL. Hemoglobin was 6.8 gm/dL. Pelvic ultrasound revealed minimal thickening of the endometrial stripe to 2 cm and a large ovoid mass arising from the left side of the uterus, most consistent with a leiomyoma. The adnexae were otherwise normal, and no evidence of an ectopic pregnancy could be found. A chest radiograph was performed, which revealed numerous solid lesions throughout the patient's lung fields bilaterally, some as large as 3 cm. TSH was markedly suppressed at < 0.01 mIU/mL. Testing for anti-thyroglobulin and anti-TPO were negative.

The patient was diagnosed with metastatic GTD and admitted to the hospital. She was successfully transfused with 4 units of PRBCs, after which her hemoglobin rose to 10.2 gm/dL. Because of her metastatic disease (WHO score of 12), she was started on a course of chemotherapy with etoposide, methotrexate, actinomycin D, cyclophosphamide, and vincristine (EMA-CO). On day #2 of her first infusion of this regimen, she experienced the acute onset of worsening shortness of breath. Pulse oximetry was 80% on room air. Oxygen was administered, and a chest radiograph was obtained. This revealed acute pulmonary edema, which was successfully treated with a single dose of intravenous furosemide. Intravenous hydration was held. Thereafter, her oxygen status improved quickly and returned to baseline. She experienced no further complications or issues associated with her chemotherapy infusion. During her initial hospital admission, she was also started on depot medroxyprogesterone for contraception.

The patient successfully went on to receive a total of 5 cycles of the EMA-CO regimen. Immediately prior to her second cycle of chemotherapy, her serum β-hCG dropped to 108 mIU/mL and had completely normalized prior to her 3rd cycle. She received an additional two cycles of EMA-CO after normal serum β-hCG levels had been achieved. The pulmonary lesions noted at the time of her diagnosis resolved completely. The patient has now been followed for nearly a year and has remained healthy. Serum β-hCG levels have remained <5 mIU/mL and her thyroid function tests have remained normal. Her menses have returned and are currently regular.

Evidence-Based Case Discussion

For women diagnosed with malignant GTD, treatment with the goal of cure should be initiated in a timely fashion. The WHO scoring system is used to assess risk and triage patients to appropriate levels of treatment following the diagnosis of this disease. For most women, the diagnosis is established by uterine evacuation, which also serves a therapeutic role, or by tissue biopsy. However, due to this young woman's precarious medical condition, treatment with chemotherapy was initiated without a tissue biopsy to establish the diagnosis. There were several reasons for this decision. First, the uterus was normal in size, and no evidence of retained products of conception or GTD were identified by imaging within her uterus. The value of endometrial biopsy or D&C under these circumstances was thought to be questionable. Second, percutaneous tissue biopsies were thought to be particularly risky, given the propensity of metastases from this disease to bleed severely when disturbed.

Serum β-hCG is typically a sensitive and highly reliable marker for GTD, although not necessarily diagnostic. Thyroid function studies are also characteristically abnormal in patients with GTD. β-hCG has thyroid-stimulating activity due to its structural homology to TSH, and levels of β-hCG correlate directly to levels of free T4. High levels of β–hCG make hyperthyroidism a common complication of GTD. However, subclinical cases do not require treatment with thyroid suppression.

Single-agent regimens of either methotrexate or actinomycin D have been reported to be highly effective for curing low-risk GTD using the WHO scoring system. Although many clinicians prefer methotrexate, either agent can be used with similar efficacy, following serial serum β-hCG until resolution of disease. Both the evidence of diffuse pulmonary metastases as well as this patient's WHO score (WHO = 12) indicated that neither single-agent regimen would have been sufficient to adequately treat the extent of this young woman's disease. This score represents both the number of pulmonary lesions noted, the extremely high serum β-hCG levels found at initial diagnosis as well as the long interval between the patient's antecedent pregnancy and her diagnosis. Each of these characteristics is a poor prognostic feature. For this reason, she was started on EMA-CO, a combination regimen that has now emerged as the treatment of choice for metastatic GTD. Initiation of this regimen resulted in a rapid and impressive resolution of the patient's pulmonary lesions, with improvement in her ability to breathe comfortably as well as rapid quantitative improvement in her serum β-HCG levels. In general, EMA-CO is well tolerated; modest depression of bone marrow function is often accepted with the goal of maintaining dose intensity with few complications such as neutropenic fever. A number of studies indicate that response rates for women diagnosed with high-risk GTD should be favorable, with a cure possible for the majority of patients (5,23,24). For patients who fail to respond to EMA-CO, a number of therapeutic regimens have been examined, including EMA-EP, PVB, and BEP (25–27). Salvage rates for women with GTD who fail EMA-CO are much more guarded; however, durable remission rates of up to 80% have been reported with EMA-EP (25).

Once normal β-HCG levels have been achieved, treatment for an additional two cycles "past normal" has emerged as the standard of care. On completion of chemotherapy, women are followed monthly to bimonthly for 6 to 12 months, regularly checking serum β-HCG levels.

An important aspect of care for women diagnosed with malignant GTD is contraception. Fertility typically returns following the successful treatment of this disease. However, subsequent pregnancy can significantly complicate posttreatment care by causing elevations in serum β-hCG under circumstances where it can often be difficult to distinguish between a normal pregnancy or disease recurrence. For women with high-risk disease, recurrence rates are estimated to range from approximately 15% to 25%, but decline significantly after remaining disease free for at least 1 year (5,23). Options for contraception should be discussed with all patients and a reliable method for birth control selected that can be realistically achieved. Typically, many clinicians recommend that contraception be continued for at least 6 months following the conclusion of therapy.

REFERENCES

1. Lu K, Slomovitz BM. Neoplastic diseases of the uterus: Endometrial hyperplasia, endometrial carcinoma, sarcoma: Diagnosis and management. In: V K, ed. *Comprehensive Gynecology*. Fifth Edition. Philadelphia, PA: Mosley Elsevier; 2007.
2. Kurman RJ, Kaminski PF, Norris HJ. The behavior of endometrial hyperplasia. A long-term study of "untreated" hyperplasia in 170 patients. *Cancer*. 1985;56:403–412.
3. Fisher B, Costantino JP, Redmond CK, et al. Endometrial cancer in tamoxifen-treated breast cancer patients: findings from the National Surgical Adjuvant Breast and Bowel Project (NSABP) B-14. *J Natl Cancer Inst*. 1994;86:527–537.
4. Lu K, Slomowitz BM. Gestational trophoblastic disease. In: V K, ed. *Comprehensive Gynecology*. Fifth Edition. Philadelphia, PA: Mosley Elsevier; 1997.
5. Lurain JR, Singh DK, Schink JC. Primary treatment of metastatic high-risk gestational trophoblastic neoplasia with EMA-CO chemotherapy. *J Reprod Med*. 2006;51:767–772.
6. Creasman W. Revised FIGO staging for carcinoma of the endometrium. *Int J Gynaecol Obstet*. 2009;105:109.
7. Edge SB, Byrd DR, Compton CC, et al. *AJCC Cancer Staging Manual*, Seventh Edition. New York: Springer, 2010:437.
8. Keys HM, Roberts JA, Brunetto VL, et al. A phase III trial of surgery with or without adjunctive external pelvic radiation therapy in intermediate risk endometrial adenocarcinoma: a Gynecologic Oncology Group study. *Gynecol Oncol*. 2004;92:744–751.
9. Creutzberg CL, van Putten WL, Koper PC, et al. Surgery and postoperative radiotherapy versus surgery alone for patients with stage-1 endometrial carcinoma: multicentre randomised trial. PORTEC Study Group. Post Operative Radiation Therapy in Endometrial Carcinoma. *Lancet*. 2000;355:1404–1411.
10. Creutzberg CL. GOG-99: ending the controversy regarding pelvic radiotherapy for endometrial carcinoma? *Gynecol Oncol*. 2004;92:740–743.
11. Nout RA, Smit VT, Putter H, et al. Vaginal brachytherapy versus pelvic external beam radiotherapy for patients with endometrial cancer of high-intermediate risk (PORTEC-2): an open-label, non-inferiority, randomised trial. *Lancet*. 2010;375:816–823.
12. Susumu N, Sagae S, Udagawa Y, et al. Randomized phase III trial of pelvic radiotherapy versus cisplatin-based combined chemotherapy in patients with intermediate- and high-risk endometrial cancer: a Japanese Gynecologic Oncology Group study. *Gynecol Oncol*. 2008;108:226–233.
13. Randall ME, Reisinger S. Radiation therapy and combined chemo-irradiation in advanced and recurrent endometrial carcinoma. *Semin Oncol*. 1994;21:91–99.
14. Smith RS, Kapp DS, Chen Q, et al. Treatment of high-risk uterine cancer with whole abdominopelvic radiation therapy. *Int J Radiat Oncol Biol Phys*. 2000;48:767–778.
15. Gibbons S, Martinez A, Schray M, et al. Adjuvant whole abdominopelvic irradiation for high risk endometrial carcinoma. *Int J Radiat Oncol Biol Phys*. 1991;21:1019–1025.
16. Sutton G, Axelrod JH, Bundy BN, et al. Whole abdominal radiotherapy in the adjuvant treatment of patients with stage III and IV endometrial cancer: a gynecologic oncology group study. *Gynecol Oncol*. 2005;97:755–763.
17. Randall ME, Filiaci VL, Muss H, et al. Randomized phase III trial of whole-abdominal irradiation versus doxorubicin and cisplatin chemotherapy in advanced endometrial carcinoma: a Gynecologic Oncology Group Study. *J Clin Oncol*. 2006;24:36–44.
18. Bristow RE, Santillan A, Zahurak ML, et al. Salvage cytoreductive surgery for recurrent endometrial cancer. *Gynecol Oncol*. 2006;103:281–287.
19. Lentz SS. Advanced and recurrent endometrial carcinoma: hormonal therapy. *Semin Oncol*. 1994;21:100–106.
20. Thigpen JT, Brady MF, Homesley HD, et al. Phase III trial of doxorubicin with or without cisplatin in advanced endometrial carcinoma: a gynecologic oncology group study. *J Clin Oncol*. 2004;22:3902–3908.
21. Fleming GF, Brunetto VL, Cella D, et al. Phase III trial of doxorubicin plus cisplatin with or without paclitaxel plus filgrastim in advanced endometrial carcinoma: a Gynecologic Oncology Group Study. *J Clin Oncol*. 2004;22:2159–2166.

22. Weber B. What is the best chemotherapy regimen in recurrent or advanced endometrial carcinoma? *Proc Am Soc Clin Oncol.* 2003;2003:453a.
23. Bower M, Newlands ES, Holden L, et al. EMA/CO for high-risk gestational trophoblastic tumors: results from a cohort of 272 patients. *J Clin Oncol.* 1997;15:2636–2643.
24. Newlands ES, Bagshawe KD, Begent RH, et al. Results with the EMA/CO (etoposide, methotrexate, actinomycin D, cyclophosphamide, vincristine) regimen in high risk gestational trophoblastic tumours, 1979 to 1989. *Br J Obstet Gynaecol.* 1991;98:550–557.
25. Newlands ES, Mulholland PJ, Holden L, et al. Etoposide and cisplatin/etoposide, methotrexate, and actinomycin D (EMA) chemotherapy for patients with high-risk gestational trophoblastic tumors refractory to EMA/cyclophosphamide and vincristine chemotherapy and patients presenting with metastatic placental site trophoblastic tumors. *J Clin Oncol.* 2000;18:854–859.
26. Gordon AN, Kavanagh JJ, Gershenson DM, et al. Cisplatin, vinblastine, and bleomycin combination therapy in resistant gestational trophoblastic disease. *Cancer.* 1986;58:1407–1410.
27. Lurain JR, Nejad B. Secondary chemotherapy for high-risk gestational trophoblastic neoplasia. *Gynecol Oncol.* 2005;97:618–623.

19

Ovarian Cancer

KAREN MCLEAN AND RONALD J. BUCKANOVICH

EPIDEMIOLOGY, RISK FACTORS, NATURAL HISTORY, AND PATHOLOGY

Ovarian cancer is the fifth leading cause of cancer death in women, and the most lethal gynecologic malignancy. It is estimated by the American Cancer Society that in 2010 there were almost 22,000 new ovarian cancers diagnosed and almost 14,000 ovarian cancer deaths. For sporadic epithelial ovarian cancers, the average age at diagnosis is 59.

Multiple risk factors for ovarian cancer have been identified, including reproductive factors, genetic factors, and environmental factors. The theory of "incessant ovulation" postulates that a woman's risk of ovarian cancer increases with the number of lifetime ovulatory cycles. This is supported by epidemiologic data demonstrating that oral contraceptives, increased parity, and breastfeeding all decrease a woman's risk of ovarian cancer, while nulliparity and infertility are associated with increased ovarian cancer risk. The cellular damage occurring during the wound-repair cycle of the ovarian epithelium at the time of follicle rupture and ovulation may explain the correlation between ovulatory cycles and risk of ovarian cancer.

Genetic factors also clearly play a role in the risk of developing ovarian cancer. Although the risk is 1 in 70 in the general population, this rises to approximately 1 in 25 when one first-degree relative is affected and 1 in 15 when two first-degree relatives are affected. Overall, 10% of ovarian cancers arise in the setting of a hereditary cancer syndrome. These include the hereditary breast-ovarian cancer syndrome (HBOC) and the hereditary non-polyposis colorectal cancer (HNPCC) syndrome, also known as Lynch II syndrome. The majority of cases of the hereditary breast-ovarian cancer syndrome are due to mutations in either the *BRCA1* or *BRCA2* genes, two tumor suppressor genes that play a role in the repair of DNA double-strand breaks. Studies have demonstrated a genotype-phenotype correlation, with the specific mutation within either *BRCA1* or *BRCA2* altering the risk of ovarian cancer in mutation carriers. The risk for *BRCA1* mutation carriers ranges from 10% to 60% and the risk for *BRCA2* mutation carriers ranges from 20% to 40%. Reports suggest that patients with ovarian carcinoma arising in the setting of a *BRCA* mutation have improved survival as compared to those patients with nonhereditary ovarian cancer. HNPCC is a genetic syndrome resulting from a mutation in one of a number of genes, all of which have a protein product that functions in DNA mismatch repair, including *MSH2*, *MLH1*, *MSH6*, *PMS1*, and *PMS2*. Patients with HNPCC have an approximately 10% lifetime risk of developing epithelial ovarian cancer, in addition to their increased risk of colon and other cancers. Several additional gene loci that are associated with increased ovarian cancer susceptibility have recently been reported and hopefully these loci will add to our understanding of the genetic etiology of ovarian cancer. In addition, a variant of the *KRAS* oncogene has been shown to be associated with over 25% of ovarian cancer cases and a marker for increased risk of ovarian cancer in nonaffected individuals. This study also identified the presence of the *KRAS* variant in over 60% of hereditary ovarian cancer pedigrees that did not harbor *BRCA* mutations. This has led to FDA approval of the PreOvar test to assess for the presence of this gene variant.

Whereas it is not possible to change one's genetics, it is possible to reduce an individual's ovarian cancer risk even in the setting of genetic mutation. Several recent studies have reported that prophylactic oophorectomy can reduce ovarian cancer risk by 90% to 95% in *BRCA* mutation carriers (1). Environmental factors are potentially more easily modifiable risk factors for cancer development.

Unfortunately, none has clearly been linked as causative. The finding that tubal ligation decreases the risk of ovarian cancer has led to the hypothesis that there may be retrograde factors increasing the risk of ovarian cancer. However, it has also been suggested that tubal ligation may reduce ovarian cancer risk by decreasing blood flow to the ovary and/or the development of epithelial carcinomas that are actually arising in the fallopian tube. Vitamin D deficiency has been correlated with increased ovarian cancer risk in some, but not all studies. Obesity and high-fat diet are associated with higher rates of ovarian cancer in industrialized nations, but a causative association remains unproven.

The vast majority of epithelial ovarian cancers are diagnosed at advanced stage, because early-stage disease is often asymptomatic. When patients do ultimately develop symptoms, they are usually vague symptoms related to disease spread, including abdominal, pelvic or back discomfort or pain, bloating, and urinary symptoms. Increasing data suggest that persistent nonspecific symptoms are correlated with an increased risk of malignancy (2), and the use of a symptom index to screen women has been proposed. In patients with multiple symptoms, it is recommended that ovarian cancer be considered as a possible etiology. Typically the patient should undergo a pelvic ultrasound and CA125 testing. Recently, the FDA has approved the OVA1 test, a blood test that combines the results of five immunoassays to give a likelihood of ovarian cancer in someone with an ovarian mass. This test has application in helping triage patients who should be referred to a gynecologic oncologist for further management. Several studies indicate that ovarian cancer patients who have surgery performed by gynecologic oncologist, as compared to a general gynecologist or a surgical oncologist, are more likely to be appropriately staged and optimally debulked, resulting in better patient outcomes.

In patients with ovarian cancer, standard therapy includes surgical debulking followed by chemotherapy for all but the earliest stage, and overall survival is dependent on both the stage at the time of debulking and the degree to which optimal surgical debulking is obtained. Overall, prognosis remains poor largely due to advanced stage at diagnosis and the development of chemoresistant disease; overall 5-year survival is currently approximately 45%.

There are many histological subtypes of ovarian cancer based on their cell of origin: coelomic epithelial cell, mesenchyme (stromal and sex-cord), and germ cell. More than 90% of ovarian tumors are epithelial, and these will be the focus of this chapter. For practical purposes, fallopian tube carcinoma and primary peritoneal carcinoma are considered "epithelial ovarian carcinoma"; tumors arising from these sites share coelomic epithelial embryonal origins and have similar staging, management, and prognosis. In fact, increasing data suggest that some "ovarian cancers" may actually originate in the fallopian tube.

Within the subtype of epithelial ovarian cancer, there are several histological variants. Serous histology represents the vast majority of cases (over 70%), followed in descending order of frequency by endometrioid, mucinous, and clear cell histologies. Tumors with endometrioid histology typically portend a better prognosis, whereas clear cell histology predicts a poorer outcome. Although the vast majority of ovarian tumors are invasive, 15% of ovarian cancers are of low malignant potential (LMP). LMP tumors can spread within the peritoneum and even metastasize to lymph nodes; however, they do not invade tissue stroma. LMP tumors generally demonstrate low mitotic activity, rendering them largely chemoresistant. Therefore, even advanced stage LMP tumors are typically treated with surgical debulking alone, and repeat surgery in the setting of recurrent disease. Given that LMP tumors pose fewer clinical dilemmas than invasive epithelial ovarian cancers and have a generally favorable prognosis, they will not be further discussed in this chapter.

STAGING

Ovarian cancer is surgically staged, with the staging system defined by the International Federation of Gynecology and Obstetrics (FIGO).

Ovarian Cancer Staging

Stage	Definition
I	Limited to one or both ovaries
IA	Involves one ovary; capsule intact; no tumor on ovarian surface; negative washings
IB	Involves both ovaries; capsule intact; no tumor on ovarian surface; negative washings
IC	Tumor limited to ovaries with any of the following: capsule ruptured, tumor on ovarian surface, positive washings
II	Pelvic extension or implants
IIA	Extension or implants onto uterus or fallopian tube; negative washings
IIB	Extension or implants onto other pelvic structures; negative washings
IIC	Pelvic extension or implants with positive peritoneal washings
III	Extension out of the pelvis
IIIA	Microscopic metastases
IIIB	Macroscopic peritoneal metastases beyond the pelvis less than or equal to 2 cm in size
IIIC	Peritoneal metastases beyond the pelvis greater than 2 cm in size or lymph node metastases
IV	Distant metastases to the liver parenchyma or outside the peritoneal cavity, pleural effusion with positive cytology

CASE SUMMARIES

Early-Stage Disease

D.N. is a 43-year-old premenopausal woman who presents to her gynecologist for an annual examination, and on bimanual examination is noted to have an 8-cm, freely mobile left adnexal mass. She is sent for an ultrasound that demonstrates a left ovarian mass measuring 8 cm with two thick septations and a 1 cm nodular area. Imaging also demonstrates a 3 cm cystic structure on the right adnexus. She is counseled to undergo surgical resection. Preoperative CA125 is 26.3 U/mL (normal < 35 U/mL) and chest x-ray is unremarkable. Laparoscopic left salpingo-oophorectomy is performed and pelvic washings are obtained. Intraoperative pathology frozen section demonstrates serous invasive epithelial ovarian carcinoma (Figure 19.1). She therefore undergoes comprehensive surgical staging consisting of hysterectomy, bilateral salpingo-oophorectomy, bilateral pelvic lymphadenectomy, para-aortic lymphadenectomy, staging biopsies, diaphragm scrapings, and omentectomy. Final pathology demonstrates grade 3 serous ovarian cancer in both ovaries, without surface involvement, and no other disease spread. Pelvic washings are negative for cancer cells.

Evidence-Based Case Discussion

D.N. has stage IB, grade 3 serous ovarian adenocarcinoma. From a surgical standpoint, her 8-cm mass had a less than 5% chance of resolving spontaneously, and by ultrasound it demonstrated multiple concerning findings, including septations and nodularity. CA125 is elevated in approximately 55% of early-stage disease, and plays a limited role in triaging premenopausal patients with an adnexal mass. Likewise, CT imaging is not necessary in the preoperative setting in this case. It was appropriate to proceed with the surgical staging and debulking procedure. Although fertility sparing surgery can be safely performed in the setting of the earliest stage disease (stage IA, grade 1), a complete staging procedure is recommended whenever possible. Up to 30% of patients with apparent early-stage disease will be upstaged with appropriate surgery and over 20% are upstaged to stage III disease. Serous tumors are bilateral in up to one third of cases at the time of diagnosis.

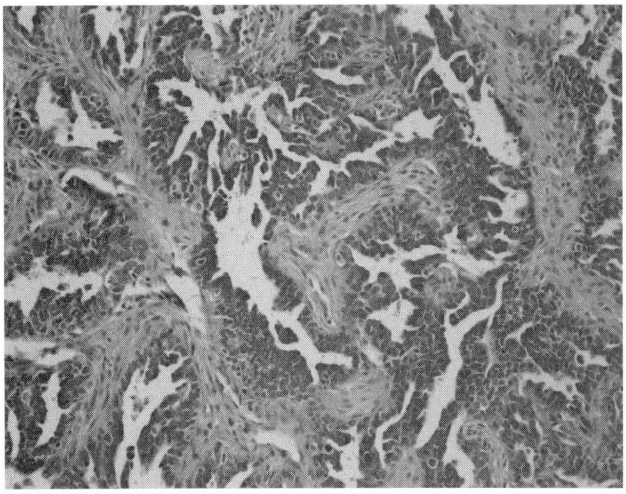

Figure 19.1

Serous epithelial ovarian cancer. Hematoxylin and eosin stain demonstrating the microscopic features characteristic of this tumor type. Papillae are noted as well as slit-like spaces. Stromal invasion and resultant desmoplastic response are common. (see color insert)

For patients with early-stage disease (stage I or II), it is important to determine if they have high-risk or low-risk disease. Although the number of observational studies is limited, the primary risk factors for recurrent disease appear to be tumor grade (grade 2 or 3) and the presence of extra-ovarian disease (stage IC or stage II). Patients with stage IA or IB grade 1 tumors, who have had appropriate surgical treatment, have an estimated 5-year overall survival of 90% to 95%. Thus the lack of a need for chemotherapy in these patients is generally well accepted (3). In fact, an Italian study concluded that for patients with low-risk disease, adjuvant therapy and salvage therapy were equally effective.

For patients with high-risk early-stage disease, treatment guidelines are based primarily on two large trials, the EORTC ACTION trial and ICON1, which investigated the benefit of adjuvant platinum-based chemotherapy in women with high-risk early-stage ovarian cancer. Both trials had limitations with regard to how the patient populations were defined and the quality of surgical staging. However, both trials suggested a nonstatistically significant trend favoring overall survival in the women receiving adjuvant platinum-based chemotherapy. When the results of the two studies were combined, the outcomes suggested a statistically significant absolute increase in 5-year overall survival of 8% (4). Serial phase III clinical trials performed by the Gynecologic Oncology Group (GOG) have established the efficacy of platinum and taxane chemotherapy for epithelial ovarian cancer, with the standard intravenous regimen now consisting of carboplatin and paclitaxel. Given the increased risk of recurrence with increasing tumor grade, it is reasonable and preferred by these authors to administer adjuvant chemotherapy in the setting of all early-stage disease other than stage IA, grade 1 and stage IB, grade 1 disease.

The number of cycles of adjuvant therapy necessary for the treatment of early-stage ovarian cancer was addressed in the GOG Trial 157 that compared three versus six cycles of adjuvant carboplatin and paclitaxel for this patient population. This study concluded that six cycles increased toxicity without significantly altering recurrence risk (5). However, there was a nonstatistically significant trend for a 5% improvement in 5-year overall survival in the group receiving six cycles of adjuvant therapy. Subsequent subset analysis of this patient data set, in the effort to identify specific factors suggesting higher risk of recurrence for which six cycles of chemotherapy would be indicated, suggested that patients with serous histology who received six cycles of carboplatin and paclitaxel had a statistically significant decrease in recurrence-free survival, but no difference in overall survival (6). Although recent data suggest a role for intraperitoneal (IP) chemotherapy in the adjuvant setting for optimally debulked, advanced stage ovarian cancer (7, discussed in further detail later), currently no randomized, controlled studies exist for IP chemotherapy in stage I or II disease. Taken together, it would be our recommendation that the patient in this case, with stage IB, grade 3 disease, receive three cycles of intravenous carboplatin and paclitaxel chemotherapy.

Advanced Stage Disease

K.H. is a 56-year-old who presents to the emergency department with persistent nausea and vomiting. She reports a 2-month history of progressive bloating and abdominal distension. She is otherwise healthy with no significant past medical or surgical history. In the emergency department, she undergoes a CT scan (Figure 19.2), with findings including an adnexal mass, omental cake, and ascites. Her CA125 is 3221 U/mL. She is consented for surgery and undergoes exploratory laparotomy, total abdominal hysterectomy, bilateral salpingo-oophorectomy, omentectomy, staging biopsies, and argon beam tumor ablation, with optimal tumor debulking to microscopic residual disease. An IP port is placed at the time of her surgery.

Evidence-Based Case Discussion

K.H.'s presentation is typical of many ovarian cancers. She presented with vague abdominal symptoms, and imaging demonstrates a large burden of disease consistent with advanced stage. The patient undergoes optimal surgical debulking, with findings demonstrating stage IIIC papillary serous ovarian cancer. The fundamental components of ovarian cancer treatment are surgical debulking and chemotherapy. Therefore, following her surgery, adjuvant chemotherapy is advisable.

The first management decision in this case is actually whether to attempt surgical debulking or to proceed with neoadjuvant chemotherapy followed by surgery. Currently there are no good preoperative predictors of which patients will be optimally debulked at the time of surgery. A preoperative CA125 should be obtained, since the value has prognostic implications as well as utility in tracking disease response and recurrence. However, preoperative CA125 has not been shown to predict patients in whom optimal debulking can be achieved. In the absence of specific contraindications to initial surgical debulking, such as medical comorbidities, current data support an attempt at surgical debulking. In settings in which this is not possible, one can begin with neoadjuvant chemotherapy followed by a debulking surgery if the patient demonstrates a good disease response. The majority of data support improved patient outcomes with surgery first and then adjuvant chemotherapy rather than neoadjuvant chemotherapy (8).

For the past decade, the standard of care for epithelial ovarian cancer chemotherapy had been a two drug regimen consisting of a platinum and a taxane (Figure 19.3). The efficacy of carboplatin and paclitaxel has been

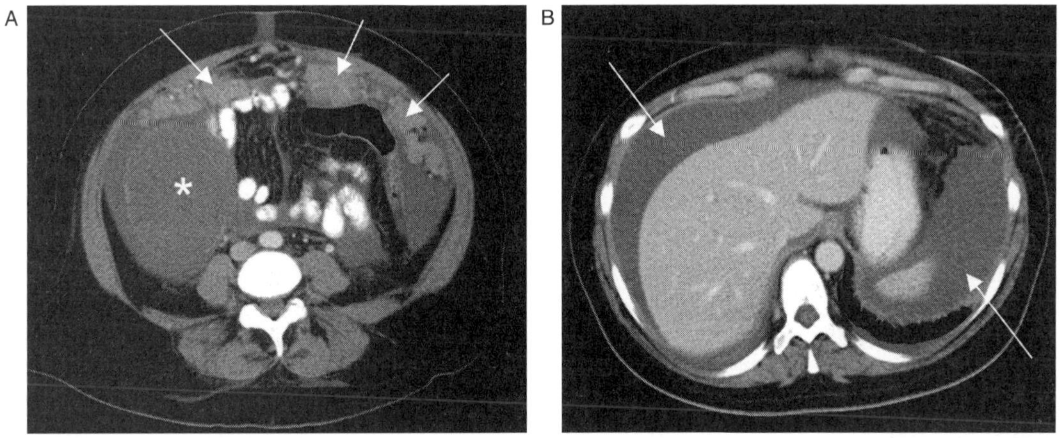

Figure 19.2

CT imaging. (A) Right adnexal mass and omental cake. CT scan in the mid-pelvis reveals a cystic mass in the right adnexa measuring 9 × 10 × 11.7 cm (indicated by the asterisk), as well as omental caking (indicated by white arrows) and mesenteric nodularity. (B) Ascites. CT imaging high in the abdomen demonstrates ascites (indicated by white arrows), particularly evident around the liver.

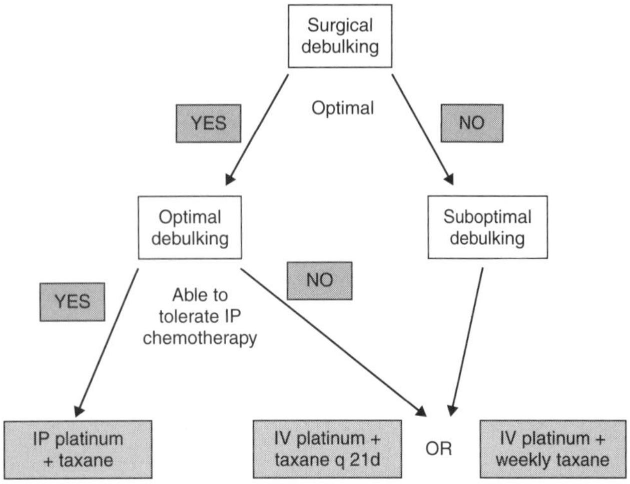

Figure 19.3

Decision analysis for adjuvant chemotherapy in advanced epithelial ovarian cancer. Adjuvant chemotherapy in advanced epithelial ovarian cancer consists of a regimen containing both a platinum drug and a taxane. The choice of specific regimen is dependent on whether optimal surgical cytoreduction was achieved as well as the performance status of the patient.

demonstrated in randomized, controlled trials, with lower toxicity than earlier regimens. In these regimens, paclitaxel and carboplatin are given intravenously on day 1 of a 21-day cycle, for six cycles. However, several studies have reported that IP chemotherapy can increase overall survival when compared to intravenous chemotherapy. Most recently, GOG Trial 182 randomized patients with optimally debulked stage III ovarian cancer to receive either intravenous cisplatin and paclitaxel (day 1 of a 21-day cycle for six total cycles) or to receive intravenous paclitaxel over a 24-hour period followed by IP cisplatin day 2 and IP paclitaxel on day 8 of a 21-day cycle. GOG 182 demonstrated that IP chemotherapy resulted in an 8% improvement in progression-free survival at 5 years, and a greater than 10% improvement in overall survival at 5 years (7); this is the most dramatic improvement in survival for ovarian cancer patients since the discovery of paclitaxel. IP treatment in this trial was associated with increased toxicity, with only 42% of patients able to complete the planned six cycles due to side effects, including port complications, pain, fatigue, and gastrointestinal, hematologic, and neurologic toxicities. However, several single institution studies have reported modifications to the IP chemotherapy protocol to reduce side effects. These modifications include the addition of hematologic growth factor support, aggressive anti-emetic regimens, preventative intravenous hydration, and the use of intravenous docetaxel instead of paclitaxel to reduce neurotoxicity. With these modifications, more than 85% of patients can successfully complete all six cycles of IP chemotherapy (9). It is possible that with a reduction in side effects and more patients capable of completing IP chemotherapy, even greater improvements in patient survival may be seen. Thus, with judicious patient selection with regard to risk of toxicities, IP chemotherapy represents an excellent adjuvant chemotherapy approach and one that we would favor in the patient in this case study.

The IP chemotherapy trials have included patients with optimal tumor debulking at the time of surgery, but this route of chemotherapy administration has not been validated in patients with suboptimal surgical debulking. Conceptually, the IP approach could be less effective due to decreased penetration of the chemotherapy into large tumor deposits. Therefore, alternative approaches must be considered in the patient with suboptimal tumor debulking. A recent study from the Japanese Gynecologic Oncology Group investigated a regimen of dose-dense chemotherapy in which carboplatin is given on day 1 and paclitaxel is given weekly on a 21-day cycle. This study included suboptimally debulked patients and reports an 11-month increase in progression-free survival as well as an increase in overall survival with this regimen (10). This is one alternative regimen that may have a role in patients who would not be treated with IP chemotherapy. A decision analysis schema for adjuvant chemotherapy in advanced stage epithelial ovarian cancer is shown in Figure 19.3.

Finally, recent clinical studies are supporting a role for targeted biologic therapies in the treatment of some epithelial ovarian cancers. The anti-vascular endothelial growth factor (VEGF) antibody bevacizumab has shown promise in clinical trials. GOG 218 investigated outcomes when bevacizumab is added to carboplatin and paclitaxel during the initial six cycles of adjuvant chemotherapy and then either continued or not for an additional 12 months of consolidation. In data published only in abstract form to date, patients who received bevacizumab both with their adjuvant chemotherapy and for consolidation showed a 4-month improvement in progression-free survival. Unfortunately, overall survival data has not yet been reported. It is also important to note that bevacizumab is a very expensive drug, raising questions with regard to the relative cost versus benefit in ovarian cancer. In the absence of a clear overall survival advantage, and given the side effects of the drug and its extreme cost, at this time we do not support the use of bevacizumab in the adjuvant therapy of ovarian cancer. Another targeted biologic therapy currently under investigation is poly-ADP ribose polymerase (PARP) inhibitors, such as olaparib. These inhibitors block the PARP enzyme that functions in DNA repair, and data suggest that this inhibition may be particularly effective in patients that have germline mutations in a *BRCA* gene that normally functions in DNA repair. PARP inhibitors are currently under active investigation in the clinical setting.

Recurrent Disease

K.H. from the case above completes six cycles of adjuvant chemotherapy using an outpatient IP regimen, with normalization of her CA125 before the fifth cycle. She undergoes a CT scan after completion of therapy that shows no evidence of disease, and her CA125 is 12.4 U/mL. She returns to the office every 3 months for surveillance visits with a physical examination and CA125. Nine months after completion of chemotherapy, her CA125 had risen to 30.6 U/mL. She is asymptomatic. She therefore has her CA125 checked again 1 month later, with levels now increased to 124.3 U/mL, and she is starting to have vague abdominal pain. She undergoes a CT scan to assess for recurrent disease, with the finding of liver metastases (Figure 19.4). She elects to restart chemotherapy.

Evidence-Based Case Discussion

Unfortunately, despite initial responses to chemotherapy, recurrent disease is common in epithelial ovarian cancer, and with few exceptions is incurable. The next step in treatment is dependent on disease-free interval following the completion of initial adjuvant chemotherapy. If the interval is 6 months or longer, the patient has platinum-sensitive disease, and is typically retreated with a platinum-based regimen, most commonly carboplatin and paclitaxel, based on results of the ICON4 trial (11). For patients with late disease recurrences, more than 1 year since completion of chemotherapy, an interval debulking procedure could be considered (see below). If a patient develops recurrent disease in less than 6 months, they are categorized as having platinum-resistant disease and are therefore typically treated with nonplatinum-based regimens.

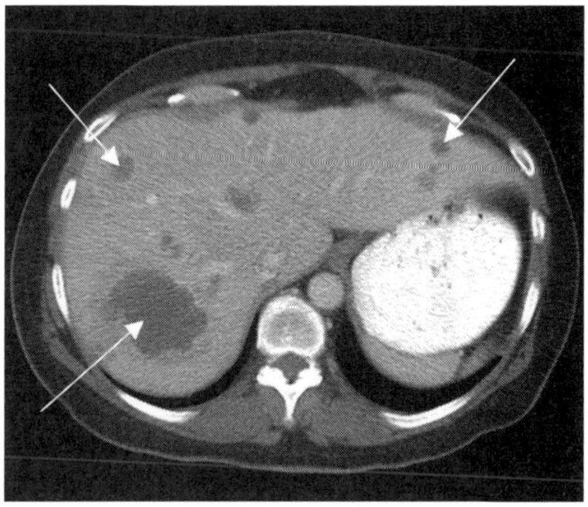

Figure 19.4

CT imaging demonstrating liver metastases. Areas of decreased signal intensity are noted within the liver, consistent with parenchymal metastatic disease (indicated by white arrows). Hepatomegaly is also appreciated on this image.

Multiple studies have investigated the role of CA125 during chemotherapy. A rapid fall in the CA125 level during chemotherapy has been correlated with a more favorable prognosis in the majority of studies (12). In patients in whom the CA125 is not falling during initial adjuvant chemotherapy, an earlier change in chemotherapy regimens may be indicated. The role of CA125 in monitoring patients in the surveillance setting is currently disputed. In the United States, standard practice is to check a CA125 level at every surveillance visit, whereas in Europe CA125 is not routinely checked. A recent European trial reports that women who restart chemotherapy based on an asymptomatic rise in CA125 do not live longer than women who wait until the development of symptoms before the reinitiation of chemotherapy (13). The clinical use of CA125 for monitoring recurrent disease and triggering reinitiation of chemotherapy remains an area of active investigation.

Before reviewing chemotherapy options for recurrent epithelial ovarian cancer, it is important to address the role of surgical exploration and secondary cytoreduction. Secondary cytoreduction has only been shown to have potential benefit in select patients with platinum-sensitive recurrent disease. Factors predicting a survival benefit for secondary cytoreduction include disease-free interval greater than 12 months, few recurrence sites, a lack of ascites, and surgical debulking to less than 0.5 cm on secondary cytoreduction (14). Given our patient in this case study has cancer that recurred in less than 12 months with multifocal disease including liver lesions, she would not be a good candidate for attempted secondary cytoreduction.

The chemotherapy regimen of choice for patients with platinum-sensitive recurrent disease is carboplatin and paclitaxel (Figure 19.5). This is based on results of the ICON4 trial, which compared treatment of these patients with carboplatin alone versus carboplatin and paclitaxel (11). In this study, patients treated with carboplatin and paclitaxel had a 7% absolute increase in overall survival at 2 years. Response rates were approximately 65%. If paclitaxel side effects such as persistent neuropathy limit the use of this agent in the recurrent disease setting, an alternative regimen would be carboplatin and pegylated liposomal doxorubicin. In the CALYPSO trial, this drug combination demonstrated improved progression-free survival compared to carboplatin and paclitaxel in patients with platinum-sensitive recurrent disease, but overall survival outcomes have yet to be reported (15). Alternatively, carboplatin and gemcitabine also have been shown to have significant activity, although it is not clear this is equivalent to carboplatin and paclitaxel.

Patients with recurrent platinum-sensitive disease are typically treated with systemic therapy. In addition to cytotoxic chemotherapies, as discussed above, there is also a role for hormonal agents such as tamoxifen and aromatase inhibitors in the treatment of recurrent ovarian

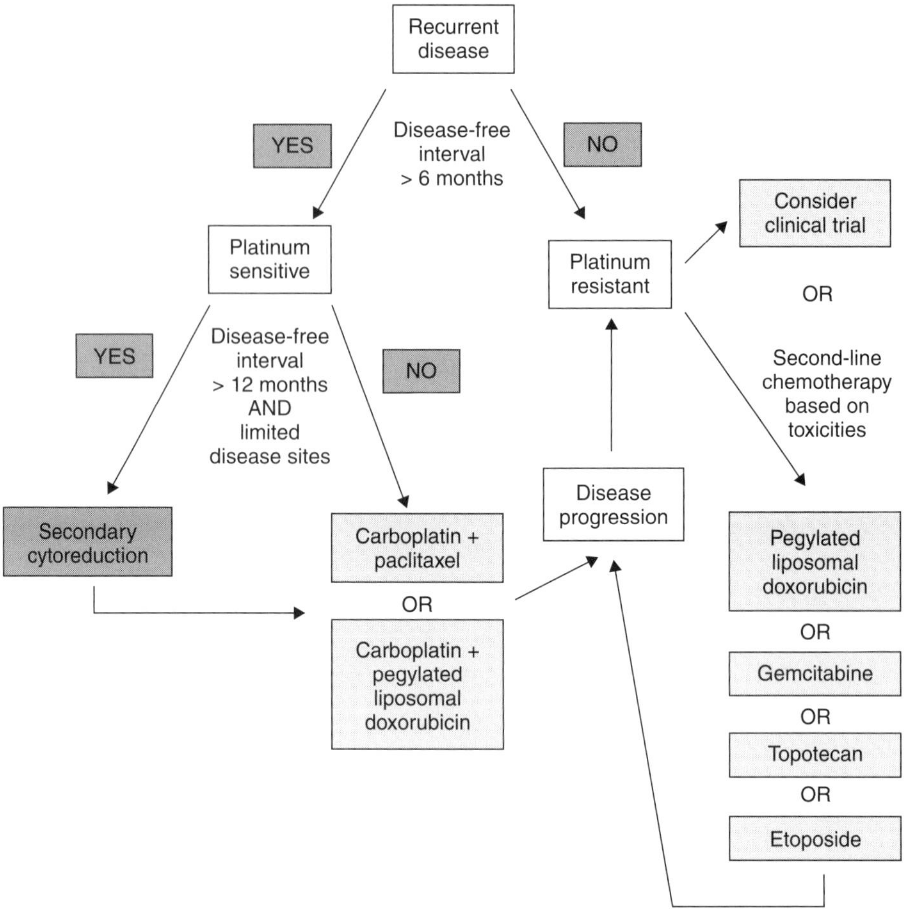

Figure 19.5

Decision analysis for recurrent epithelial ovarian cancer. Appropriate treatment of recurrent epithelial ovarian cancer is largely dependent on the disease-free interval. Once patients develop platinum-resistant disease, there are a number of second-line chemotherapies that have shown similar efficacy. An increasing number of clinical trials exist, and enrollment should be considered for any patient with recurrent disease.

cancer. However, the objective response rates to hormonal agents are relatively low, 10% to 20%, and patients generally demonstrate stable disease rather than a partial or complete response. Given the low side-effect profile and the fact that some patients can have prolonged stable disease on the agents, hormonal therapy should be considered in any patient with recurrent disease. Most commonly, these agents are used in asymptomatic patients desiring therapy.

Once a patient recurs with platinum-resistant disease there are still many chemotherapeutic options to consider (Figure 19.5). Studies have demonstrated multiple regimens with equivalent efficacy in this setting; response rates are typically low (15–30%) and the duration of response is often short. Because of the relative lack of efficacy of approved agents in platinum-resistant disease, clinical trials of novel agents should be considered for this patient population. When choosing among possible chemotherapeutic agents, given no clear survival advantage of a given regimen, chemotherapy choice should be driven by the side-effect profile of the specific agents as they apply to the individual patient. The use of multiagent chemotherapeutic regimens is not recommended. Although doublet regimens can improve response rates and progression-free survival, they have significant increased toxicity, and no phase III trial to date has demonstrated an improvement in overall survival rates with doublet therapy. Doublets can be considered when a rapid disease response is necessary. Due to the nature of epithelial ovarian cancer with multiple recurrences, most patients ultimately receive all of these potential "second-line" agents. Specific agents that have been shown to be effective include pegylated liposomal doxorubicin, gemcitabine, topotecan, and etoposide.

ACKNOWLEDGMENTS

We thank Dr. Jonathan Dillman in Radiology at the University of Michigan for his assistance with the images for Figures 19.2 and 19.4.

REFERENCES

1. Domchek SM, Friebel TM, Singer CF, et al. Association of risk-reducing surgery in BRCA1 or BRCA2 mutation carriers with cancer risk and mortality. *JAMA*. 2010;304(9):967–975.
2. Goff BA, Mandel LS, Melancon CH, et al. Frequency of symptoms of ovarian cancer in women presenting to primary care clinics. *JAMA*. 2004;291(22):2705–2712.
3. Young RC, Walton LA, Ellenberg SS, et al. Adjuvant therapy in stage I and stage II epithelial ovarian cancer. Results of two prospective randomized trials. *N Engl J Med*. 1990;322(15):1021–1027.

4. Trimbos JB, Parmar M, Vergote I, et al. International Collaborative Ovarian Neoplasm trial 1 and Adjuvant ChemoTherapy In Ovarian Neoplasm trial: two parallel randomized phase III trials of adjuvant chemotherapy in patients with early-stage ovarian carcinoma. *J Natl Cancer Inst.* 2003;95(2):105–112.
5. Bell J, Brady MF, Young RC, et al. Randomized phase III trial of three versus six cycles of adjuvant carboplatin and paclitaxel in early stage epithelial ovarian carcinoma: a Gynecologic Oncology Group study. *Gynecol Oncol.* 2006;102(3):432–439.
6. Chan JK, Tian C, Fleming GF, et al. The potential benefit of 6 vs. 3 cycles of chemotherapy in subsets of women with early-stage high-risk epithelial ovarian cancer: an exploratory analysis of a Gynecologic Oncology Group study. *Gynecol Oncol.* 2010;116(3):301–306.
7. Armstrong DK, Bundy B, Wenzel L, et al. Intraperitoneal cisplatin and paclitaxel in ovarian cancer. *N Engl J Med.* 2006;354(1): 34–43.
8. Bristow RE, Eisenhauer EL, Santillan A, and Chi DS. Delaying the primary surgical effort for advanced ovarian cancer: a systematic review of neoadjuvant chemotherapy and interval cytoreduction. *Gynecol Oncol.* 2007;104(2):480–490.
9. Berry E, Matthews KS, Singh DK, et al. An outpatient intraperitoneal chemotherapy regimen for advanced ovarian cancer. *Gynecol Oncol.* 2009;113(1):63–67.
10. Katsumata N, Yasuda M, Takahashi F, et al. Dose-dense paclitaxel once a week in combination with carboplatin every 3 weeks for advanced ovarian cancer: a phase 3, open-label, randomised controlled trial. *Lancet.* 2009;374(9698):1331–1338.
11. Parmar MK, Ledermann JA, Colombo N, et al. Paclitaxel plus platinum-based chemotherapy versus conventional platinum-based chemotherapy in women with relapsed ovarian cancer: the ICON4/AGO-OVAR-2.2 trial. *Lancet.* 2003;361(9375):2099–2106.
12. Meyer T and Rustin GJ. Role of tumour markers in monitoring epithelial ovarian cancer. *Br J Cancer.* 2000;82(9):1535–1538.
13. Rustin GJ, van der Burg ME, Griffin CL, et al. Early versus delayed treatment of relapsed ovarian cancer (MRC OV05/EORTC 55955): a randomised trial. *Lancet.* 2010;376(9747):1155–1163.
14. Chi DS, McCaughty K, Diaz JP, et al. Guidelines and selection criteria for secondary cytoreductive surgery in patients with recurrent, platinum-sensitive epithelial ovarian carcinoma. *Cancer.* 2006;106(9):1933–1939.
15. Pujade-Lauraine E, Wagner U, Aarall-Lundqvist E, et al. Pegylated liposomal Doxorubicin and Carboplatin compared with Paclitaxel and Carboplatin for patients with platinum-sensitive ovarian cancer in late relapse. *J Clin Oncol.* 2010;28(20):3323–3329.

20

Melanoma

KEVIN MCDONNELL AND CHRISTOPHER D. LAO

EPIDEMIOLOGY, RISK FACTORS, NATURAL HISTORY, AND PATHOLOGY

In 2010, there were approximately 68,130 new cases of melanoma and 8700 deaths secondary to this disease (1). The median age at diagnosis of melanoma is 60 years, but it is the most common malignancy diagnosed in women between the ages of 25 and 29. The incidence of melanoma is highest among Caucasians, with a rate of approximately 25 per 100,000 persons, with a 1.5:1 male to female predominance (2).

Melanoma is a malignancy originating from the neural crest-derived melanocyte. Thus, it can develop in sites to where these neural crest cells migrate, including the skin, mucosal membranes of the aerodigestive system, and uveal tissues of the eye. An association between sun exposure and melanoma exists; however, it appears more strongly associated with intermittent exposure resulting in sunburn. Recognized risk factors for the occurrence of melanoma include a previous personal or family history of melanoma, history of multiple (>100 nevi) benign and atypical nevi, a history of intermittent severe sunburns during adolescence, increased sensitivity to the sun, and an inherited susceptibility.

The most common histological subtype of melanoma is superficial spreading melanoma, representing up to three quarters of all diagnoses of the disease. This subtype often occurs in sun-exposed areas and appears as the classic irregular pigmented macule. Nodular melanomas represent the second most frequent histologic subtype, accounting for between 20% and 30% of melanoma cases. Nodular melanomas usually appear as rapidly growing, homogenous darkly pigmented nodules; microscopically, it may be either spindled or epithelioid. The third most frequent subtype is lentigo maligna, which most often originates in chronically solar-damaged skin, typically in older patients on skin of the head and neck. Acral lentiginous melanoma is a less frequent histological subtype in Caucasians, representing less than 10% of cases. However, among patients of Asian and African descent acral lentiginous melanomas occur more frequently than other subtypes. Acral lentiginous melanomas most typically occur on the palms, soles, and subungually. This subtype is not clearly related to sun exposure.

Less frequently occurring subtypes of melanoma include desmoplastic, mucosal, and uveal melanomas. Desmoplastic melanoma is a rare variant that is aggressive and deeply invasive. The desmoplastic melanoma is often amelanotic and therefore is often not initially appreciated as pathologic. It often occurs on areas of sun-exposed skin. Melanomas may also arise in nonsolar-exposed tissues such as the mucosal surfaces of the nose, esophagus, oral cavity, genitourinary tract, anus, and rectum. Melanomas uncommonly arise from the uvea of the eye. Uveal melanomas may manifest as pain or as a change in visual acuity and are often diagnosed without a biopsy. Metastasis from uveal melanoma is exclusively hematogenous, with a characteristic predilection for liver involvement.

The recognition of unique genetic events in certain subtypes of melanoma will likely result in the future molecular or genetic characterization of melanoma instead of histologic subtyping. Activating mutations of *BRAF* or *NRAS* have been found to be altered in 50% and 15%, respectively, of melanomas arising in nonchronically solar-damaged skin (3). In subsets of melanomas that are associated with chronic sun-damaged skin and minimal ultraviolet exposure history, such as mucosal and acral melanomas, the predominant foundational mutation may be an activating mutation in *KIT* rather than *BRAF* or *NRAS* (4). This may be clinically important, as targeted therapies have been developed against melanomas with known mutations. An inherited genetic susceptibility is present in approximately 5% to 10% of patients with melanoma. Such melanoma families can harbor alterations in the tumor suppressor gene *CDKN2A* that encodes for p16INK4A and p19ARF. *GNAQ* or *GNA11* mutations have recently been recognized to occur in nearly 50% of uveal melanomas, and genotyping that can distinguish high-risk uveal melanoma is already available for clinical risk stratification.

STAGING

Melanoma Pathologic Staging, Summarized From *AJCC TNM Staging, 7th Edition*

Stage	Definition
0	Primary tumor is confined to epidermis without lymph node or distant metastatic disease
IA	Primary tumor ≤1.00-mm thick, without ulceration and mitosis <1/mm² without lymph node or distant metastatic disease
IB	Primary tumor ≤1.00-mm thick, with ulceration or mitoses ≥1/mm² *or* 1.01–2.00-mm thick without ulceration without lymph node or distant metastatic disease
IIA	Primary tumor 1.01–2.00-mm thick with ulceration *or* 2.01–to 4.00-mm thick without ulceration without lymph node or distant metastatic disease
IIB	Primary tumor 2.01–4.00-mm thick with ulceration *or* 4.00-mm thick without ulceration without lymph node or distant metastatic disease
IIC	Primary tumor >4.00-mm thick with ulceration without lymph node or distant metastatic disease
IIIA	Primary tumor ≤1.00-mm thick and mitosis <1/mm² *or* >1.00-mm thick without ulceration, with 1 to 3 micrometastatic-positive lymph nodes and no distant metastatic disease
IIIB	Any tumor with 1 to 3 micro- or macrometastatic lymph nodes or in-transit metastases/satellites with no distant metastatic disease
IIIC	Any tumor with ulceration or mitoses ≥1/mm² with 1 to 3 macrometastatic-positive lymph nodes or in-transit metastases/satellites without distant metastatic disease *or* any tumor with >4 metastatic lymph nodes, matted nodes, or in-transit metastases/satellites with metastatic nodes without distant metastatic disease.
IV	Primary tumor of any size without or without lymph node disease, with distant metastases.

CASE SUMMARIES

Early-Stage Melanoma (Stage II/III)

S.K. is a 36-year-old previously healthy man who noted an enlarging, pigmented lesion on his right upper back. He reported a long history of a nevus that began to increase in size and bleed over the preceding few months. He subsequently sought care from his primary care physician. The patient had no significant past medical history and no family history of melanoma or other cancers. He reported a past history of nonblistering sunburns, with occasional tanning bed use and a history of smoking approximately 1 pack per day for 15 years. Physical examination was remarkable only for an approximately 8-mm raised, pigmented lesion on the right upper back. There were fewer than ten clinically atypical nevi, none meeting criteria for removal. He subsequently underwent an excisional biopsy of the index lesion which demonstrated a superficial spreading type melanoma, Breslow depth 5.6 mm, with ulceration, a focus of angiolymphatic invasion, and satellitosis (Figure 20.1). The patient subsequently underwent a radical excision of the melanoma with 2-cm margins and sentinel node mapping. The wide excision margins were negative, but a 0.9-mm tumor nodule was also noted in the resection specimen. One sentinel lymph node was identified in the right axilla and was positive for melanoma. No extracapsular extension was seen. The patient then underwent complete right axillary lymph node dissection, which demonstrated 1/12 lymph nodes to be positive for melanoma. A CT scan of the chest, abdomen, and pelvis and an MRI of the brain were obtained for staging and were negative for distant metastatic disease.

Evidence-Based Case Discussion

Prognostic Variables and Surgical Management

S.K. has a thick melanoma (≥4 mm), a focus of satellitosis, and a total of two lymph nodes positive for micrometastatic disease. He had no evidence of distant metastatic disease on staging workup. Overall this patient is presenting with stage IIIC melanoma that has been completely resected.

Several prognostic variables associated with primary cutaneous melanoma have been identified, which include lymph node positivity, Breslow depth (tumor thickness), microscopic ulceration, and mitotic rate for thin primary melanomas (<1-mm thick). Clark level is no longer considered an independent prognostic variable, unless the lesion is thin and mitotic rate is not available (5).

If no lymph nodes are involved, then the primary treatment modality is surgery with adequate margins. The extent of the resection is dependent on the initial tumor thickness, and several clinical trials have been performed to determine the most appropriate surgical margins. For melanoma in situ, standard recommendations are for surgical margins of 0.5 cm; for a tumor between 0.5 and 1 mm, the surgical margin should be 1.0 cm; for lesions greater than 1 mm and up to 2 mm, surgical margins should be 1 to 2 cm; and for all tumors > 2 mm a surgical margin of 2.0 cm should be obtained (Table 20.1).

Sentinel lymph node biopsy or mapping has proven to be an informative prognostic procedure for lesions ≥1 mm

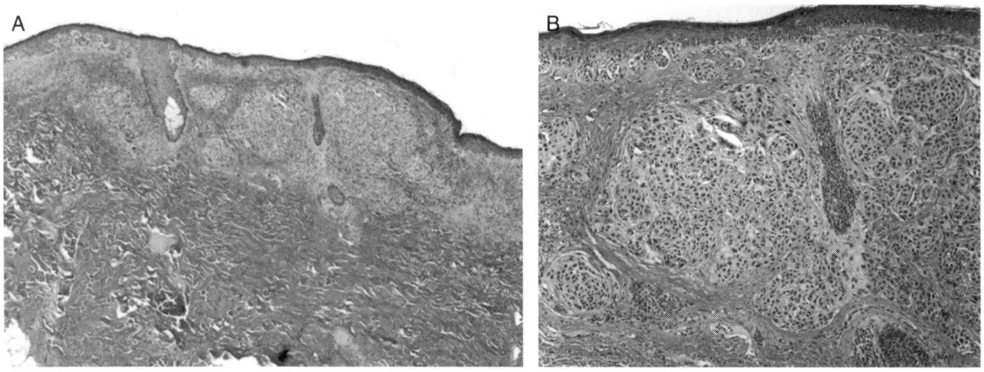

Figure 20.1

A. Invasive superficial spreading type melanoma (low power view, hematoxylin and eosin stain). Nodular areas of dense accumulations of malignant cells noted in the dermis. B. Magnified view (10×) of same melanoma. Aggregates of uniformly, large, atypical melanocytes with abundant cytoplasm evident. Scant melanin pigment dispersed throughout the lesion. (see color insert)

Table 20.1 Standard Workup, Evaluation, and Management of Cutaneous Melanoma

Melanoma	Surgical Margins	Sentinel Lymph Node	Radiologic Imaging	Labs
In situ	0.5 cm	No	No	No
<0.75 mm	1 cm	No	No	No
0.75 to 1 mm	1 cm	Consider	No	No
1 to 2 mm	1–2 cm	Yes	If LN positive	No
>2 mm	2 cm	Yes	If LN positive	No
In-transit disease	Negative margin	Consider	Consider	Consider LDH
Stage IV	N/A	N/A	Yes	LDH

LN: lymph node; N/A: not applicable; LDH: lactate dehydrogenase.

in Breslow depth. On the basis of the most recent update from the Multicenter Selective Lymphadenectomy Trial-1 (MSLT-1), in which patients with primary lesions between 1- and 4-mm thick were randomized to sentinel lymph node mapping or observation, there is a 5-year disease-free survival advantage to sentinel lymph node mapping, but no overall survival advantage (6). Documentation of lymph node involvement identifies patients at higher risk for recurrence; therefore, adjuvant therapy, including enrollment in clinical trials, can be considered for such patients. For lesions between 0.75 and 1 mm, sentinel lymph mapping can also be considered if additional higher-risk features are identified, including young age, positive deep margins, lymphovascular invasion, or a mitotic rate $\geq 1/mm^2$ (Table 20.1). When positive nodes are identified on sentinel lymph node mapping, a complete lymphadenectomy remains the standard of care. The importance of a subsequent completion node dissection following sentinel node biopsy is being evaluated in an ongoing randomized clinical trial (MSLT-2), in which patients are randomized to completion node dissection or surveillance. In the present clinical case, the Breslow depth of 5.6 mm was an indication for sentinel node lymph node biopsy.

Satellitosis can be defined as at least one separate focus of melanoma adjacent to the primary lesion. The presence of satellitosis increases the risk of recurrence. When disease is clinically detected in between the expected draining nodal basin and the primary lesion, but not immediately adjacent to the primary melanoma, it is considered in-transit metastasis. In-transit disease is typically managed with complete surgical excision if possible. Sentinel lymph biopsy for in-transit disease is controversial, as the lymphatics may be altered and unreliable.

Adjuvant Therapy

Lymph node involvement defines stage III disease. The 5-year survival rate is approximately 80%, 60%, and 40% for stages IIIA, IIIB, and IIIC, respectively (5). Following surgical management of the primary lesion, adjuvant therapy can be considered and includes enrollment on a clinical trial if available, high-dose interferon alpha-2b, or observation. There is evidence from one randomized clinical trial performed by an intergroup (Australia and New Zealand Melanoma Trials Group [ANZMTG] and Trans-Tasman Radiation Oncology Group [TROG]) that adjuvant radiation when compared to observation can improve disease-free survival, but not overall survival. Thus, in instances where regional control is required, radiotherapy can be considered.

The only FDA approved adjuvant therapy is high-dose interferon alpha-2b. Multiple randomized interferon trials have been performed comparing interferon to placebo or vaccine, but three U.S. cooperative group trials (Eastern Cooperative Group [ECOG] 1684, ECOG 1690, and ECOG 1694) have been performed with the high-dose regimen (20 million units/m^2 IV daily Monday-Friday for 4 weeks followed by 10 million units/m^2 subcutaneously three times a week for 48 weeks). ECOG 1684 was a randomized trial of high-dose interferon alpha-2b versus observation for patient with stages ≥IIB (T4) and III disease. A statistically significant difference in overall and disease-free survival was observed at 5 years (7). This trial was the primary reason for its FDA approval in 1995. However, results from a meta-analysis of the interferon trials and in a pooled analysis of high-dose regimens in which patients were followed for a median of 12.6 years showed that an overall survival advantage was no longer significant, although a relapse-free survival advantage remained significant (8,9). Interferon therapy is associated with a number of adverse effects that must be kept in mind when considering this therapy. In addition to generalized symptoms, such as anorexia, fatigue, malaise, headaches, nausea, vomiting, fever, chills, myalgias, and rash, interferon therapy may also induce liver dysfunction, myelosuppression, and depression. The latter is of concern particularly when contemplating this therapy for patients with a pre-existing psychiatric condition. Given the toxicities of treatment and the controversy surrounding the benefit of adjuvant interferon, observation has more recently been considered an appropriate option, including acceptance of observation as the control arm of clinical trials.

In the current case, after undergoing a lymph node dissection, the patient opted to proceed with clinical observation. Standard follow-up after surgical excision in the absence of additional adjuvant therapy includes a history and physical examination every 3 to 4 months for the first 2 years, every 6 months for the next 3 years, and then annually as clinically appropriate thereafter. No standard recommendation exists for imaging studies. Chest x-ray, CT, or PET scan as well as a brain MRI can be obtained at the discretion of the treating physician, but there is no evidence of a survival advantage to aggressive radiologic surveillance at this time. An LDH is the only laboratory study with prognostic significance, and thus can be checked periodically during follow-up as well. After 5 years, interval laboratory testing and imaging are performed as clinically indicated.

Locoregional and Metastatic (Stage IV) Melanoma

M.M. is a 70-year-old woman with a past history of coronary artery disease, hypertension, and a stage IB melanoma on her left lower leg (superficial spreading type, Breslow depth 0.6 mm, no ulceration, and mitotic rate of 2/mm^2). The lesion was treated with wide excision and no sentinel lymph node biopsy was performed due to the thin nature of the melanoma. The patient proceeded with follow-up physical examinations every 6 months with dermatology. Three years after her original diagnosis, the patient discovered a mass in the left groin. Physical examination confirmed a palpable mass, without other nodules or masses concerning for melanoma at that time. She underwent fine-needle aspiration of this mass, which confirmed malignant melanoma. Staging workup including a PET-CT demonstrated an FDG avid mass in the groin but failed to reveal any evidence of distant metastatic disease. Her regional recurrence was treated with left superficial inguinal lymph node dissection. This revealed one lymph node completely replaced with tumor. Following surgery she chose to continue with observation alone. Approximately, 1 year after surgery, the patient noticed multiple nodules in her leg developing over several weeks (Figure 20.2). Excision of one of these nodules confirmed recurrent melanoma. Repeat PET-CT again failed to reveal distant metastases, but multiple subcutaneous nodules were identified. She was not considered a candidate for isolated limb perfusion due to the proximal nature of her disease. She was being evaluated for participation in a clinical trial, but during the screening period she had repeat imaging studies that revealed findings concerning for metastatic disease in her lungs, mediastinum, and liver. Brain MRI was negative. CT guided biopsy of her liver confirmed metastatic disease. Measurement of the LDH was performed and was elevated to a level of 300 IU/L.

Evidence-Based Discussion

This is a patient initially diagnosed with low-risk stage Ib disease who presents with a palpable lymph node 3 years after her original diagnosis. She was being considered for management of her apparent unresectable regional disease, but developed biopsy proven distant metastatic (stage IV) disease in a short follow-up interval.

Locoregional Melanoma

Interval follow-ups are performed to detect recurrent disease, which if discovered within the locoregional area, defined as disease confined to the area of the primary lesion and the primary nodal basin, is still potentially

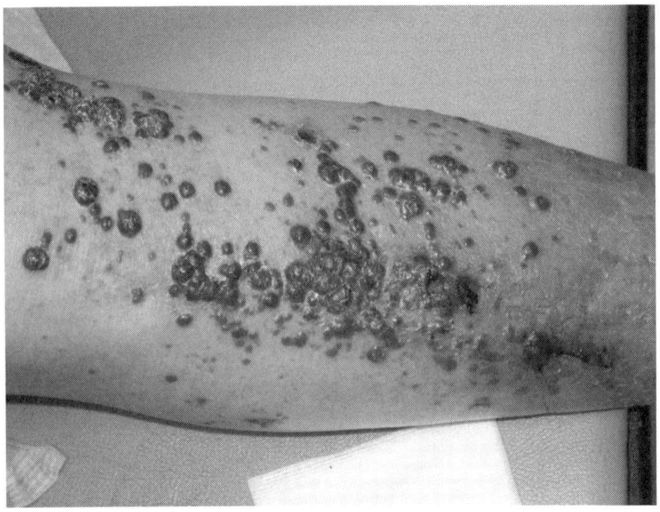

Figure 20.2

Representative photograph of multiple cutaneous and subcutaneous nodules of melanoma on an extremity of a patient. (see color insert)

curable with surgery. Recurrence can occur as either local recurrence at the primary tumor site, in-transit disease, nodal involvement, or distant metastatic disease. Imaging is at the discretion of the treating physician, but CT scans are standard and can pick up small volume disease. Melanoma tends to be FDG avid, and thus PET-CT is also an acceptable test, particularly when the extremities are involved. Brain MRI is a preferred test for ruling out brain involvement, as the sensitivity is higher for detecting metastasis, and melanoma can have a distinct resonance on MRI.

If recurrence occurs in the regional lymph node basin, complete surgical resection of the node should be performed, which may be incorporated in a complete lymph node dissection if not previously performed. For lymph node disease in the groin, consideration should be given to iliac or obturator node dissection, particularly if CT imaging documents pelvic disease, Cloquet's node is involved, or ≥3 lymph nodes are involved.

If the recurrence is considered unresectable, then hyperthermic isolated limb perfusion (ILP) or infusion (ILI) with melphalan (if isolated to an extremity), clinical trial participation, local ablation therapy, radiotherapy, systemic therapy, or topical imiquinod can be considered. These options are dependent on the location of the disease (whether previous treatment to the area was given, e.g., radiotherapy), characteristics of the disease (e.g., epidermotropic metastases), and comorbidities of the patient. In a large, randomized, phase III clinical trial, ILP did not demonstrate an improvement in overall survival in the adjuvant setting. The response rate to ILP, however, is between 50% and 90%, with a large proportion being complete responses. Therefore, this approach can be useful to control unresectable disease in appropriately selected patients. The use of surgery and/or radiation for regional recurrence in the setting of metastatic disease is based on whether a significant amount of morbidity would be expected from disease that could potentially grow uncontrolled. The current patient was not a candidate for ILP due to the proximal nature of the disease in her extremity. Also, given the pace of her metastatic disease, systemic therapy was indicated and locoregional treatment was deferred.

Stage IV Melanoma

Systemic therapy options for unresectable stage III and stage IV melanoma are similar. Stage IV disease is further classified based on the location of the disease and whether the LDH is elevated, as they are independent predictors of survival (5). Stage IV, M1a disease is defined as distant skin, subcutaneous, or nodal metastatic disease with a normal LDH. M1b disease includes lung metastases with a normal LDH, and M1c includes visceral metastases or any distant metastases with an elevated LDH value. The 5-year survival rates for stage IV patients with normal and elevated LDH values are 30% and 10%, respectively. Survival rates at 5 years for patients with M1a, M1b, and M1c disease are approximately 30%, 20%, and 10%, respectively.

The initial management decision in patients presenting with stage IV melanoma is whether the metastatic disease can be completely resected (see Figure 20.3 for workup and management algorithm). If the patient is surgically rendered free of disease from stage IV melanoma, the standard of care following surgery is observation or enrollment in a clinical trial. Survival in this cohort of patients is significantly better than in patients whose disease could not be resected, as demonstrated in at least two clinical trials.

In the case of disseminated, unresectable disease, several therapeutic options exist. Prior to 2011, there were only two FDA approved agents for Stage IV melanoma: dacarbazine and high-dose interleukin-2 (IL-2). Both agents were approved for the treatment of Stage IV melanoma based on clinical activity, some durability of responses for IL-2, and lack of other effective therapies at the time despite a lack of randomized phase III clinical trial evidence of a survival advantage. High-dose interleukin-2 is a specialized treatment for appropriately selected patients. The toxicities are significant with this therapy and include signs and symptoms mimicking sepsis. Treatment requires hospitalization for administration. For patients who are candidates for IL-2 therapy (younger age, patients over 50 years of age with normal cardiac function, no brain involvement, and normal organ function) there is potential for long term control, although the likelihood is on the order of 5% (10). In 2011, two

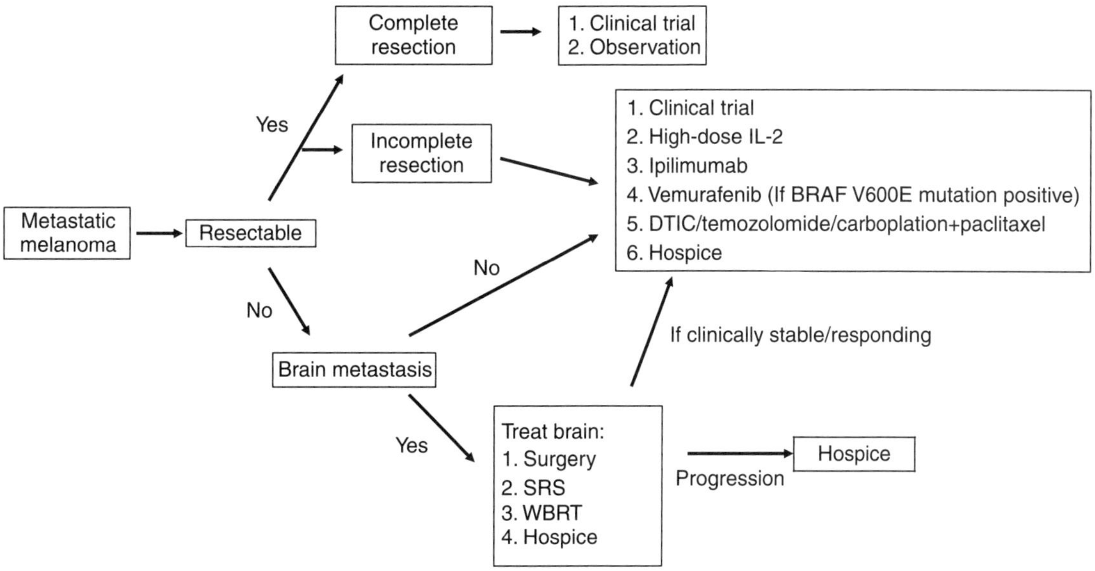

Figure 20.3

Workup and management algorithm for patients with metastatic (stage IV) melanoma.SRS, Stereotactic radiosurgery; WBRT, whole brain radiotherapy Note: All patients with unresectable or Stage IV melanoma should have BRAF mutational analysis

new agents, ipilimumab and vemurafenib, were approved by the US FDA based on statistically significant overall survival advantages in large randomized clinical trials. Ipilimumab, an antibody against CTLA-4, demonstrated a 4-month improvement in median overall survival (6.4 months for the nonipilimumab group compared with 10.1 months for ipilimumab), but more importantly, a subset of patients had disease control for greater than 2 years (11). Thus, for some patients this therapy may result in long-term control of the disease. As a result of these positive findings, ipilimumab was approved by the FDA early in 2011. *BRAF* mutations have been recognized to occur in approximately 50% of melanomas and therapeutic agents targeting *BRAF* V600E have now demonstrated response rates approaching 80% and improvements in survival. In a recently published phase III trial, 675 patients with previously untreated metastatic melanoma expressing *BRAF* V600E mutations were randomized to treatment with either an oral *BRAF* kinase inhibitor vemurafenib or with dacarbazine. In an interim analysis of overall survival and a final analysis of progression-free survival, vemurafenib therapy was associated with a 63% reduction in the risk of death and a 74% reduction in the risk of either death or cancer progression as compared to dacarbazine therapy ($P < .001$ for both comparisons)(12).

Other agents and regimens (e.g., temozolomide and carboplatin/paclitaxel) have demonstrated activity in clinical trials. The response rates range from 0% to 30% without an associated survival advantage. Biochemotherapy (cisplatin, vinblastine, dacarbazine, interferon, and IL-2) and other multidrug combinations (e.g., the Dartmouth regimen) correspond to the highest response rates, but no overall survival advantage has been demonstrated even when compared to dacarbazine alone (13). These regimens are now often reserved for disease that requires a response for palliation or if surgery might be possible with some shrinkage of a tumor that was previously considered unresectable. Currently, enrollment on a clinical trial remains a primary option for patients with stage IV melanoma.

A common complicating factor limiting treatment options is brain involvement. This is often associated with poorer survival. Clinical trials often require exclusion of brain metastases or documented disease control over time for consideration of enrollment. A brain MRI is thus often required in staging and periodically in follow-up, even if there was no brain involvement initially. If the brain is involved then resection, stereotactic radiosurgery, or whole brain radiotherapy are considered for palliative management.

The patient in this case was not considered to be a candidate for high-dose IL-2 due to her advanced age, comorbidities, and the risks associated with treatment. Ipilimumab was still only available on a clinical trial and no trial was available to her at the time. She was BRAF V600E negative. She was screened for first-line protocol therapy testing combinatorial targeted agents, and at first follow-up had a partial response by RECIST criteria. She continued on protocol therapy.

REFERENCES

1. Jemal A, Siegel R, Xu J, Ward E. Cancer statistics, 2010. *CA Cancer J Clin.* 2010;60:277–300.
2. ACS. Cancer Facts & Figures. 2009 [cited; Available from: http://www.cancer.org]
3. Davies H, Bignell GR, Cox C, et al. Mutations of the BRAF gene in human cancer. *Nature.* 2002;417:949–954.
4. Curtin JA, Busam K, Pinkel D, et al. Somatic activation of KIT in distinct subtypes of melanoma. *J Clin Oncol.* 2006;24: 4340–4346.
5. Balch CM, Gershenwald JE, Soong SJ, et al. Final version of 2009 AJCC melanoma staging and classification. *J Clin Oncol.* 2009;27:6199–6206.
6. Morton DL, Thompson JF, Cochran AJ, et al. Sentinel-node biopsy or nodal observation in melanoma. *N Engl J Med.* 2006;355:1307–1317.
7. Kirkwood JM, Strawderman MH, Ernstoff MS, et al. Interferon alfa-2b adjuvant therapy of high-risk resected cutaneous melanoma: the Eastern Cooperative Oncology Group Trial EST 1684. *J Clin Oncol.* 1996;14:7–17.
8. Kirkwood JM, Manola J, Ibrahim J, et al. A pooled analysis of Eastern Cooperative Oncology Group and intergroup trials of adjuvant high-dose interferon for melanoma. *Clin Cancer Res.* 2004;10:1670–1677.
9. Wheatley K, Ives N, Hancock B, et al. Does adjuvant interferon-alpha for high-risk melanoma provide a worthwhile benefit? A meta-analysis of the randomised trials. *Cancer Treat Rev.* 2003;29:241–252.
10. Atkins MB, Lotze MT, Dutcher JP, et al. High-dose recombinant interleukin 2 therapy for patients with metastatic melanoma: analysis of 270 patients treated between 1985 and 1993. *J Clin Oncol.* 1999;17:2105–2116.
11. Hodi FS, O'Day SJ, McDermott DF, et al. Improved survival with ipilimumab in patients with metastatic melanoma. *N Engl J Med.* 363:711–723.
12. Chapman PB, Hauschild A, Haanen JB, et al. Improved survival with vemurafenib in melanoma with *BRAF* V600E mutation. *N Engl J Med.* 2011;364:2507–2516.
13. Chapman PB, Einhorn LH, Meyers ML, et al. Phase III multicenter randomized trial of the Dartmouth regimen versus dacarbazine in patients with metastatic melanoma. *J Clin Oncol.* 1999;17:2745–2751.

21

Bone Sarcoma

VERA MARANCI AND SCOTT M. SCHUETZE

OSTEOSARCOMA

Epidemiology, Risk Factors, Natural History, and Pathology

Osteosarcoma is the most common nonhematopoietic bone tumor but accounts for fewer than 1000 cases per year. There is a bimodal age distribution most frequently arising during the second and sixth decades of life. In older patients, osteosarcoma is often secondary to Paget's disease, radiation, or enchondroma. Other risk factors for development of osteosarcoma include genetic syndromes such as familial retinoblastoma and Li-Fraumeni syndrome (germline *p53* mutation). Osteosarcoma is more common in males than in females.

Patients typically present with pain and a hardened mass. The most common site of disease are the intramedullary metaphyses of the long bones, typically the distal femur, proximal tibia, and proximal humerus. Osteosarcoma arising in the axial skeleton is more common in adults than in teenagers. Extraosseous osteosarcoma arises in the soft tissue, does not primarily involve bone, and is usually treated as a soft tissue sarcoma.

Osteosarcoma is typically composed of malignant spindle cells, osteoblasts, and bone matrix (osteoid). The common histologic subtypes of osteosarcoma include osteoblastic, chondroblastic, and fibroblastic variants. Osteosarcoma can arise on the surface of the bone or within the intramedullary canal, and it can be high or low grade. Grading is based on several components including mitotic count, pleomorphism, and cellular atypia. Intramedullary tumors are usually high grade, whereas low-grade tumors are found along the bone surface. Grade is more informative than histologic type because it affects prognosis and treatment decisions.

Osteosarcoma spreads hematogenously, with lung followed by bone being the most common sites of metastasis. At diagnosis, 10% to 20% of patients present with metastatic disease. Skip metastases within the medullary canal can occur. Lymph node or bone marrow involvement is very rare.

Staging

2006 AJCC Staging System for Osteosarcoma (1)

Stage	Definition
IA	Low grade, intracompartmental, ≤ 8 cm
IB	Low grade, extracompartmental, > 8 cm
IIA	High grade, intracompartmental, ≤ 8 cm
IIB	High grade, extracompartmental, > 8 cm
III	Any grade, bone skip metastases present
IVA	Any grade, lung metastases only
IVB	Any grade, nodal involvement, nonlung metastases

Case Summaries

Early-Stage Osteosarcoma

J.R. is a 19-year-old male college freshman who had been competing in cross-country and track developed pain in his left distal thigh when squatting during weight training 6 months prior to presentation. He was able to perform other weight training and to run without pain. One month prior to presentation he developed pain in his left distal thigh after running, and he began walking with a limp 1 week prior to medical evaluation. He was using ibuprofen occasionally for relief of pain after running, and fluticasone propionate and fexofenadine for treatment of seasonal rhinitis. He had no constitutional symptoms. His medical history included acute mononucleosis at age 4. Family medical history was notable only for tobacco-related lung cancer in a paternal grandmother in old age. On examination by his primary care provider, he had no point tenderness or effusion, and normal range of motion and stability in the left knee. He was prescribed naproxen and referred for orthopedic consultation.

During the orthopedic consultation, x-ray films of the left knee detected a mass in the distal femur. An MRI of the knee was performed and showed a 6.0 × 2.9 × 3.0 cm intraosseous mass in the distal femur invading the metaphysis and causing elevation of the medial periosteum and disruption of bone cortex (see Figure 21.1). Serum alkaline phosphatase and lactate dehydrogenase (LDH) were within normal range. A CT-guided core needle biopsy was diagnostic for high-grade osteoblastic osteosarcoma. Staging MRI of the left femur showed no skip metastasis in the bone. Chest CT was normal. Bone scan showed increased technetium uptake in the left distal femoral metaphysis but no other foci to suggest metastatic disease. Baseline audiology testing and echocardiogram were normal.

Evidence-Based Case Discussion

This is an otherwise healthy young adult presenting with a stage IIA (localized, intracompartmental, high-grade) osteoblastic osteosarcoma of the distal femur. Baseline studies showed normal levels of serum alkaline phosphatase and LDH, portending a favorable prognosis. There was also normal cardiac function, renal function, and hearing; if abnormal, these issues could impact the choice of chemotherapy. There were no skip metastases or distant disease noted. The presence of either of these factors would increase stage of disease and change sarcoma management.

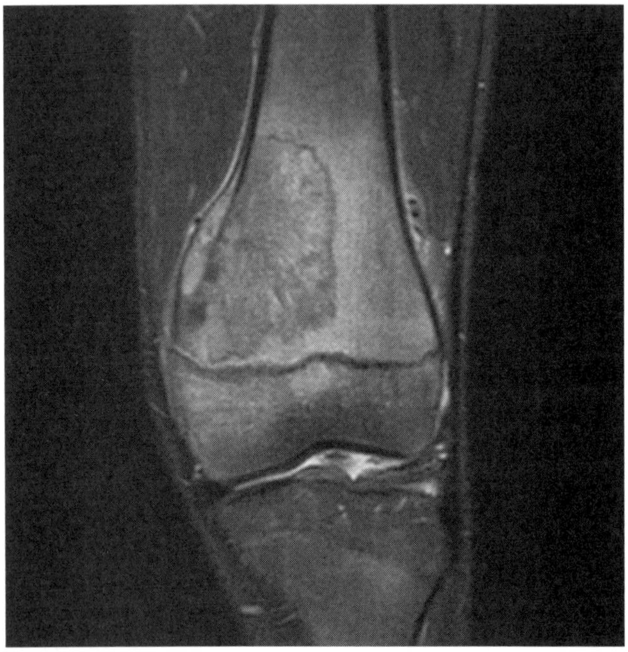

Figure 21.1

MRI (T2, STIR sequence; coronal image) of knee demonstrating intraosseous mass in distal femur.

With localized disease, the treatment paradigm is dependent on grade (see Figure 21.2). Low-grade lesions are treated with surgery alone, and high-grade lesions are treated with chemotherapy and surgery.

Osteosarcoma tends to be radiation resistant, and radiation has not been shown to be beneficial in the adjuvant setting. Radiation may be useful when the primary is unresectable or for palliation. The role of radiation in management of low-grade lesions is not defined but may be considered for treatment of unresectable disease.

Doxorubicin-based combinations make up the current backbone of chemotherapy, which is part of the standard of care for localized osteosarcoma. In early studies, adjuvant chemotherapy with single-agent doxorubicin or methotrexate improved 5-year survival rates to about 50% from 20% following amputation alone (2). Investigators at Memorial Sloan Kettering Cancer Center developed a T10 protocol using methotrexate, doxorubicin, cyclophosphamide, dactinomycin, bleomycin, ± cisplatin started prior to surgical resection that has demonstrated a 76% disease-free survival at 5 years from diagnosis in young adults with extremity primary osteosarcoma. There was a correlation between lower disease-free survival rate and elevated serum LDH or alkaline phosphatase levels at diagnosis (3).

The T10 regimen was the standard treatment for osteosarcoma for much of the 1970s and 1980s. It was not until the pivotal randomized trial performed by the European Osteosarcoma Intergroup (EOI) that a new standard was determined in the 1990s (4). This study compared 18 weeks (6 cycles) of doxorubicin and cisplatin versus 44 weeks (20 cycles) of the T10 multidrug regimen in nearly 400 patients with high-grade osteosarcoma. Surgery occurred during weeks 9 and 7 for the doublet and the multidrug regimen, respectively, with the remainder of chemotherapy being initiated 2 weeks postoperatively. Not surprisingly, more patients were able to complete the doublet treatment (94%) compared to the multidrug regimen (51%). Both overall survival and progression-free survival was similar in the treatment groups, 55% and 44%, respectively, at 5 years.

High-dose methotrexate is routinely used in the pediatric population and in young adults with osteosarcoma. The use of methotrexate in adults over the age of 40 is problematic because of decreased renal clearance and significantly increased risk of severe toxicity. Another study by the EOI compared doxorubicin and cisplatin for six cycles versus doxorubicin, cisplatin, and methotrexate for four cycles (5). Approximately 200 patients younger than age 40 were randomized between the two treatments. Twice as many patients in the methotrexate arm were unable to complete treatment compared to the

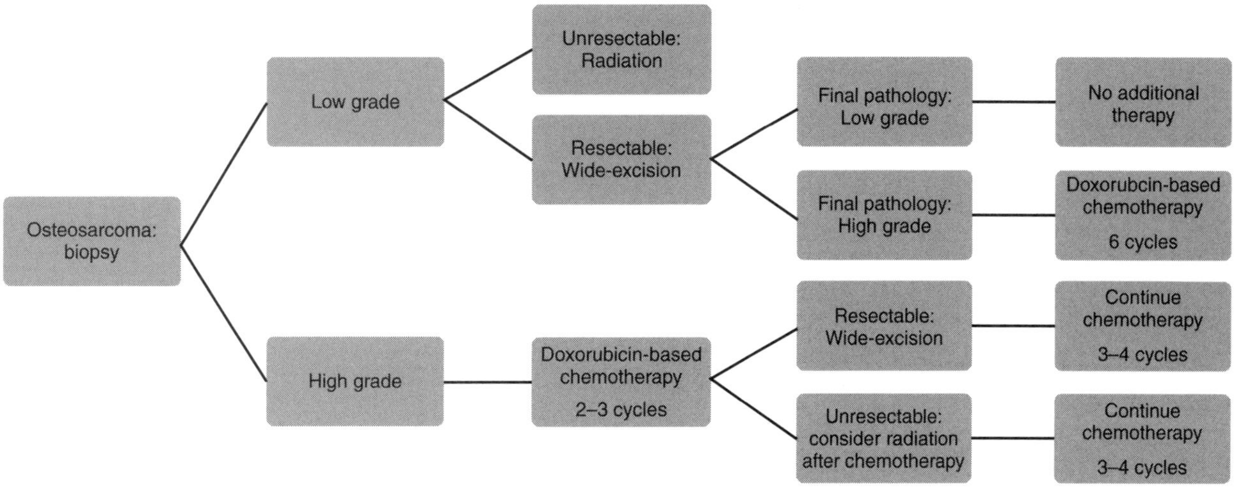

Figure 21.2

Treatment algorithm for localized osteosarcoma.

study arm. Overall survival was the same in both groups, and disease-free survival was better in the group without methotrexate. These results garnered criticism since the methotrexate arm received lower total doses of doxorubicin and cisplatin, which may have compromised the results. Two randomized studies comparing moderate-dose methotrexate to high-dose methotrexate in a doxorubicin-based regimen failed to demonstrate a difference in survival (6,7). Based on the available evidence, patients presenting with resectable, high-grade osteosarcoma should be offered chemotherapy using six cycles of doxorubicin and cisplatin as side effects permit. The addition of methotrexate to the chemotherapy may be considered in patients less than 40 years of age with two kidneys and normal renal function. Carboplatin is active in osteosarcoma and may be substituted for cisplatin in specific patients, for example, those with hearing impairments or neuropathy. However, a noninferiority comparison of carboplatin to cisplatin has not been performed in osteosarcoma.

The timing of chemotherapy does not seem to be critical with respect to survival. A randomized clinical study performed by the Pediatric Oncology Group compared surgery prior to the start of chemotherapy versus after 10 weeks of chemotherapy, which demonstrated equivalent 5-year event-free survival rates of 60% to 65% (8). Neoadjuvant chemotherapy is practically appealing because it allows time for careful surgical planning, manufacture of custom prosthetics, and collection of allograft bone used in limb-sparing surgical techniques. Tumor response to preoperative chemotherapy also provides prognostic and predictive information. Generally, in patients being considered for limb-sparing surgery, chemotherapy is given for about 10 weeks prior to surgery.

Other agents in the armamentarium to treat osteosarcoma include ifosfamide, with or without etoposide. Ifosfamide is an active agent in osteosarcoma, but its addition to standard chemotherapy does not improve survival in the front-line setting and results in more toxicity. A large international randomized trial is attempting to address whether the addition of ifosfamide and etoposide to postoperative chemotherapy for patients with a less than good histologic response to neoadjuvant chemotherapy will improve relapse-free and overall survival rates. Study enrollment is projected to reach maximum accrual in late 2010.

In summary, for localized, low-grade disease, surgical resection alone is the recommended treatment. For localized, high-grade disease, chemotherapy using six cycles of doxorubicin and cisplatin is recommended. Surgery may be performed prior to chemotherapy or after 2 to 3 cycles. The use of methotrexate and ifosfamide-etoposide doublet is more controversial. Most experts recommend that methotrexate be used in addition to cisplatin and doxorubicin for patients under the age of 40 with normal renal function and without pre-existing renal disease, administered under the supervision of physicians experienced in the management of methotrexate clearance and leucovorin rescue.

In the case of J.R. with stage IIA disease, consultation with orthopedic oncology confirmed that a limb-sparing resection with endoprosthetic reconstruction could be performed with acceptable morbidity and long-term functional outcome. The recommended therapy in this situation would be neoadjuvant doxorubicin, cisplatin, and methotrexate for 10 to 12 weeks, osteosarcoma resection, and completion of chemotherapy postoperatively. Radiation therapy would not be recommended.

Advanced Stage Osteosarcoma

T.R. is a 74-year-old retired dentist followed for Paget's disease involving the pelvis was noted to have a significant rise in serum alkaline phosphatase from 234 to 907 IU/L over a 2-year period. Bone scan detected abnormal uptake of technetium only in the left ilium. He had no pain in the pelvis or left leg and no constitutional symptoms. He biked and golfed regularly without difficulty. His medical history was notable for Paget's disease, hypertension, macular degeneration and a traumatic fracture of his left femur. Regular medications were aspirin, amlodipine, retinavites, glucosamine, and chondroitin sulfate. There were no cases of malignancy in his family history.

An MRI of the pelvis detected a 4.5 × 3.1 × 3.5 cm enhancing area involving the left ilium adjacent to the left sacroiliac joint. A CT-guided needle biopsy showed bone containing remodeling changes consistent with Paget's bone disease. An open biopsy was performed that detected high-grade, osteoblastic osteosarcoma arising in Paget's. Chest CT detected one subcentimeter, indeterminate, noncalcified nodule in the right upper lobe of the lung measuring 3mm. Cardiac, renal, and audiology evaluations were normal.

He was treated with three cycles of doxorubicin and cisplatin. Monitoring of cardiac function and hearing detected no significant change from baseline. Serum alkaline phosphatase level fell to 232 IU/L after the second cycle and was within the normal range after the third cycle of chemotherapy. The ilium mass appeared unchanged after the chemotherapy and the lung nodule was unchanged at 3 mm. He underwent a left internal hemipelvectomy to excise the residual osteosarcoma. Surgical margins were negative and there was no viable residual osteosarcoma. He completed an additional three cycles of doxorubicin and cisplatin postoperatively. Because the solitary lung nodule had nonspecific characteristics and did not change in size or appearance during chemotherapy the decision was made to follow the nodule by serial imaging.

Two years later he experienced a rise in serum alkaline phosphatase level. MRI and CT of the pelvis showed no local recurrence of osteosarcoma. Chest CT demonstrated the 3-mm noncalcified nodule in the right upper lobe that was unchanged in size and characteristics, but two new calcified nodules measuring approximately 1 cm were present in the left lung. A technetium bone scan showed photopenia in the left pelvis related to the hemipelvectomy, abnormal uptake in the two left lung nodules but no abnormal uptake in bone.

Evidence-Based Case Discussion

Here we have an older patient with osteosarcoma. An elevated serum alkaline phosphatase at presentation portends a poorer prognosis, but this is offset somewhat by small volume disease in the pelvis amenable to resection and confounded by the presence of Paget's bone disease that can cause an elevation in alkaline phosphatase. This case reminds us of the bimodal incidence of osteosarcoma. Older patients typically do not present with de novo disease. They instead present with osteosarcoma secondary to some other cause such as Paget's disease.

At initial presentation, it is unclear whether the subcentimeter pulmonary nodule is malignant, but since he had at worst limited pulmonary-only metastasis, following the treatment paradigm for localized osteosarcoma is appropriate (see Figure 21.2). Since the nodule remained stable following chemotherapy, proceeding with resection of the primary cancer alone was reasonable. His disease relapsed 2 years following diagnosis with metastases to the lung.

Pulmonary metastases are the most common site of metastasis. If lung is the only site of disease, surgical resection should be considered when feasible since this is the only potentially curative therapy in the metastatic setting. Retrospective series have demonstrated prolonged disease-free survival in 7% to 30% of patients who were able to undergo complete resection of osteosarcoma metastases (9). Those patients in whom osteosarcoma relapsed greater than two years from diagnosis and had only 1 to 2 metastatic nodules were shown to have the greatest event-free survival rate following metastasectomy. There are limited data from nonrandomized, retrospective series regarding additional benefit from postmetastasectomy chemotherapy giving conflicting results, but ifosfamide with or without etoposide and methotrexate can be considered.

In patients who at presentation have a high-grade lesion with a limited number of resectable pulmonary metastases, the treatment approach should follow that of early-stage disease (i.e., neoadjuvant chemotherapy, surgery with resection of primary and metastases, and adjuvant chemotherapy).

In those patients who are unable to undergo complete resection, chemotherapy, and radiation therapy are given with palliative intent. No standard approach has been established in the metastatic setting, but it is reasonable to attempt treatment with a doxorubicin-based regimen, if not used previously. If a patient was treated with doxorubicin initially, ifosfamide with or without etoposide would be an acceptable approach at the time of relapse. Ifosfamide and etoposide used in the relapsed setting has shown response rates of 50% to 60% (10,11).

Amputation should be considered for management of local relapse without distant disease as a potentially curative treatment. Radical surgery in the setting of distant metastasis may be considered for palliation of severe sequelae of local tumor progression.

In summary, in metastatic osteosarcoma, the treatment approach is determined by resectability. Preoperative treatment may be given for high-grade tumors, preferably using drugs not previously administered to improve the likelihood of resection of osteosarcoma with clear surgical margins. Preoperative chemotherapy also allows for detection of rapidly progressing, chemotherapy-resistant disease in which aggressive resection may not be advised. Metastatic low-grade tumors should be managed by surgery, if possible.

In the case of T.R. with relapsed disease, there was only limited involvement of the lung, making metastasectomy an appropriate choice. Given the long interval to relapse, benefit from chemotherapy postresection would probably be modest and the potential toxicity in an older patient must be considered. If chemotherapy is pursued, ifosfamide or ifosfamide and etoposide would be recommended. Methotrexate is not recommended in this case because of the patient's age.

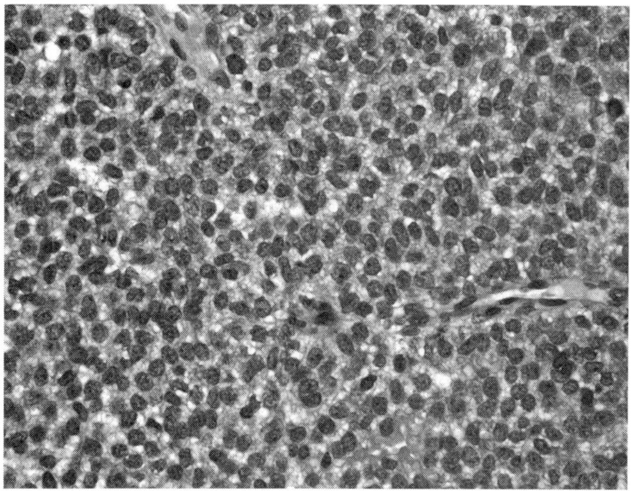

Figure 21.3

Photomicrograph of hematoxylin and eosin stained Ewing's showing finely granular chromatin and cytoplasmic vacuolization caused by glycogen accumulation (400×). (see color insert)

EWING'S SARCOMA

Epidemiology, Risk Factors, Natural History, and Pathology

Ewing's sarcoma makes up about 10% of bone sarcomas but is the second most common bone tumor in children and accounts for 350 cases per year in the United States. Both Ewing's sarcoma and primitive neuroectodermal tumor (PNET) are thought to arise from ectodermal tissue and not mesoderm. Older literature treats these two entities, along with Askin's tumor, as distinct diseases, but now all three fall into the Ewing's sarcoma family of tumors (ESFT) grouping based on common molecular characteristics. The majority of patients with Ewing's sarcoma are less than 18 years of age, and the peak incidence is 10 to 15 years of age. Males are more commonly affected than females. Caucasians are the most common race affected. There are no known risk factors.

Patients typically present with pain and can complain of fever, weight loss, or fatigue. These "B-type" symptoms correlate with a higher chance of developing metastatic disease. Tumors arise in the diaphysis of the long or flat bones, most commonly in the femur or pelvis (20% each) followed by the fibula, tibia, or humerus (10% each). Distal bone involvement is more favorable than proximal bone involvement and pelvic involvement carries the worst prognosis, presumably because tumor volume is often greater at the time of diagnosis when disease arises in the pelvis.

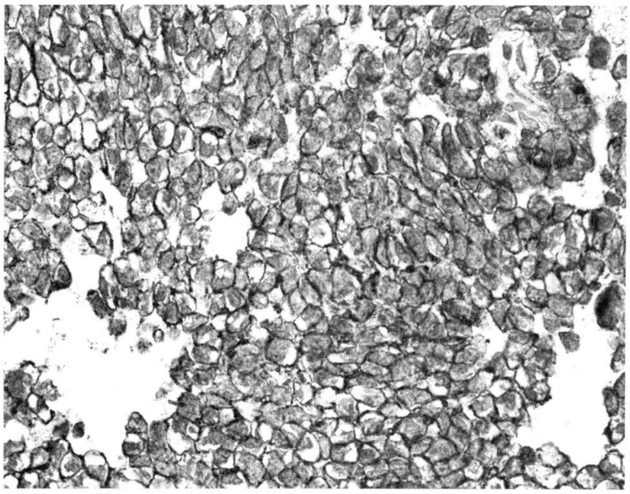

Figure 21.4

Photomicrograph of CD99 immunohistochemical stained Ewing's sarcoma showing intense cytoplasmic membrane staining (immunoperoxidase, 400×). (see color insert)

Ewing's sarcoma is classically described as highly cellular, uniform, round to ovoid, small blue cells separated by fibrous tissue (see Figure 21.3). Ewing's sarcoma can be characterized by the fusion of the *EWS* gene on chromosome 22 with *ETS* family members. More than 90% of Ewing's tumors will have either a t(11;22) or t(21;22) translocation involving *FLI-1* or *ERG*, respectively, and will be CD99 positive in a membranous staining pattern on immunohistochemistry (see Figure 21.4). Fluorescence in-situ hybridization (FISH) and polymerase chain reaction (PCR) techniques have been developed to detect the translocation.

Like osteosarcoma, there is a high rate of hematogeneous spread, with lung followed by bone being the most commonly affected by metastasis. Ewing's sarcoma may occasionally metastasize to lymph nodes and bone marrow. About one third of patients present with gross metastatic disease at presentation. Like osteosarcoma and other small blue cell cancers, micrometastatic disease at presentation should be assumed since there is a high relapse rate following local treatment alone. Diagnosis at a younger age and tumors less than 8 cm are better in terms of prognosis.

Staging

Staging for Ewing's sarcoma is not uniform. The AJCC staging schema may be adapted to Ewing's, but staging is more typically divided into two categories: localized and metastatic disease.

Case Summaries

Early-Stage (Localized) Ewing's Sarcoma

F.W. is a 49-year-old Caucasian corrections facility officer who developed pain in the right buttock approximately 6 months prior to diagnosis. He was treated for degenerative joint disease using nonsteroidal anti-inflammatory analgesics. The pain progressed and he began limping 3 months later. One month prior to diagnosis he developed weakness and severe pain in the right leg and could no longer ambulate independently. At the time of diagnosis he had no significant pain in the buttock/leg at rest but experienced severe pain with movement of or bearing weight on the right leg. He was using hydrocodone-acetaminophen for pain relief and a wheelchair for transportation.

He reported fatigue from the pain but no constitutional symptoms. His medications included synthroid for hypothyroidism and a daily multivitamin supplement. His mother and sister had hypothyroidism, and his father had prostate cancer at age 65. Family medical history was otherwise unremarkable. On examination he had a firm mass involving the right ilium that was not tender to palpation. He had reduced strength in the right hip flexors but the remainder of the examination was normal.

An MRI scan of the lower spine was performed that showed an expansile mass in the right ilium with ill-defined cortical margin and expansion of a soft tissue mass into the posterior aspect of the iliopsoas muscle. A CT-guided core needle biopsy was performed. Pathology showed a small, round, blue cell tumor. By immunohistochemistry, the tumor cells stained for CD99 in a membranous pattern, and vimentin, pancytokeratin, CD45, CD56, TdT, CD43, and CD79a were absent. FISH detected a translocation between chromosomes 11 and 22. Serum LDH, other chemistry values and complete blood counts were within normal ranges. CT scan of the chest, abdomen, and pelvis reidentified an approximately 8.0 × 5.5 cm mass in the right posterior iliac crest causing lysis of bone and extending anteriorly into the soft tissues, with no evidence of metastatic disease. FDG-PET imaging performed in lieu of a technetium bone scan showed enhanced uptake in the pelvic mass with a maximum standard uptake value of 66 but no evidence of metastasis. A bone marrow aspirate and biopsy from the left posterior iliac crest showed normal cellular marrow and no evidence of bone marrow metastasis. Baseline cardiac evaluation was normal.

Evidence-Based Case Discussion

This is an older patient with localized, pelvic, Ewing's sarcoma. Diagnosis was confirmed with cytogenetic analysis. Adverse features include his age, the location of the tumor, and the size of the tumor.

All Ewing's sarcomas are considered high grade and early-stage localized disease receives a standard approach to treatment (see Figure 21.5). Unlike osteosarcoma or other bone sarcomas, Ewing's sarcoma is radiation sensitive.

An initial treatment decision is whether to proceed with surgical resection or definitive radiation for local treatment. Choosing the primary modality of treatment depends on several practical factors. If the tumor is in an

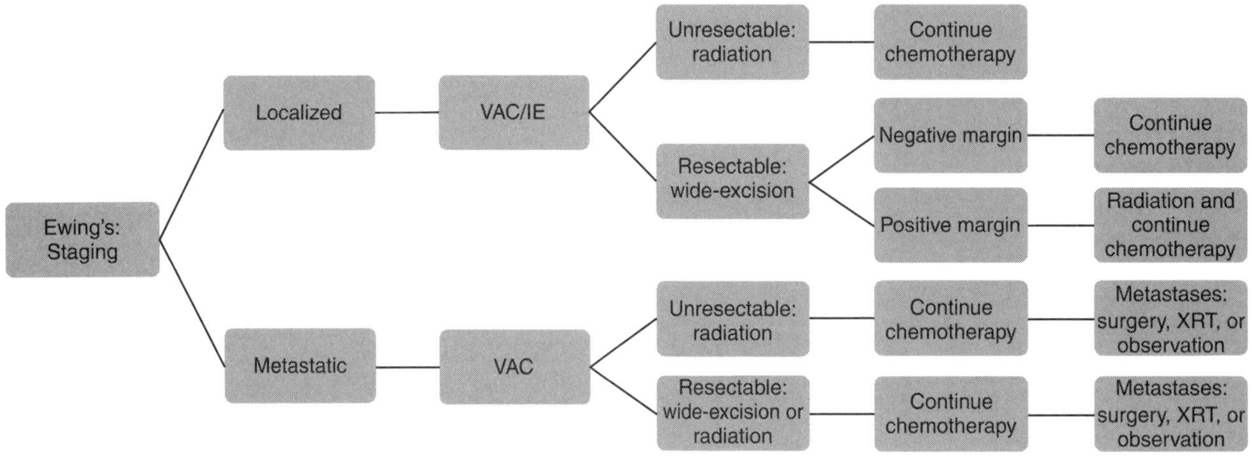

Figure 21.5

Treatment algorithm for Ewing's sarcoma. (VAC: vincristine, doxorubicin, and cyclophosphamide; IE: ifosfamide and etoposide; XRT: radiation therapy).

easily resectable location that would also allow reconstruction to occur, then surgery is preferred. If the location is not amenable to surgery, or if surgery is not able to be performed for other reasons, primary radiation therapy is recommended. Furthermore, adjuvant radiation therapy is recommended for incomplete surgical resection or positive surgical margin (tumor present at the inked surface of the specimen). Careful consideration should be given to the long-term effects of radiation therapy in growing children; radiation-induced sarcomas are the most common second malignancy in children with Ewing's sarcoma. In addition, the available evidence suggests that local failure rates are higher using radiation versus complete resection to control the primary tumor.

Regardless of the selected local treatment, the cure rate from local control measures alone is no better than 15% because of the high rate of distant disease recurrence. The inclusion of chemotherapy therefore becomes an important facet in the treatment of Ewing's sarcoma and like osteosarcoma, a combination of neoadjuvant and adjuvant treatment is preferred.

Current treatment for Ewing's sarcoma developed from the Intergroup Ewing's Sarcoma Studies (IESS) performed in the late 1970s and early 1980s. Nonrandomized trials had suggested a benefit to adjuvant chemotherapy. The first intergroup study, IESS-I, enrolled 342 children and adults with localized Ewing's sarcoma. The primary tumor was in place in the majority of patients; patients treated with surgical amputation were ineligible. Patients were randomized to vincristine, actinomycin-D, and cyclophosphamide, with or without doxorubicin. All patients received radiation therapy to the primary lesion. A separate randomization was to prophylactic bilateral whole lung radiation versus no lung radiation in those not receiving doxorubicin. Patients receiving doxorubicin along with vincristine, actinomycin-D, and cyclophosphamide had improved 5-year relapse-free (60% vs. 24%) and overall (72% vs. 36%) survival rates (12). The addition of prophylactic bilateral whole lung radiation was not as beneficial as the addition of doxorubicin to the backbone of vincristine, actinomycin-D, and cyclophosphamide.

The addition of ifosfamide and etoposide was evaluated by the Pediatric Oncology Group-Children's Cancer Group (POG-CCG). Patients less than 30 years of age with any stage of Ewing's were randomized to receive vincristine, actinomycin-D, cylophosphamide, and doxorubicin, with or without ifosfamide and etoposide given in alternating cycles every 3 weeks for 17 treatments. The 5-year event-free (69% vs. 54%) and overall survival (72% vs. 61%) rates favored the six-drug regimen in the nonmetastatic patients. The addition of ifosfamide and etoposide made no significant survival difference in those with metastatic disease (13). A follow-up study used the same six-drug regimen with G-CSF growth factor support for dose-dense scheduling every 2 weeks compared to every 3 weeks. A preliminary analysis suggested that the 3-year event-free survival rate was improved in the group receiving chemotherapy every 2 weeks (76% vs. 65%) (14).

Different regimens have been developed from these six core drugs, but the most commonly used regimen continues to be the POG-CCG treatment. Despite most of these studies being done in children or young adults, the same treatment is recommended for older adults if feasible.

In summary, four to eight courses of chemotherapy are recommended for nonmetastatic disease followed by local treatment that includes surgical resection alone, radiation therapy alone, or a combination of the two depending on the clinical situation. On recovery from surgery, the remainder of the chemotherapy is administered to provide a total of about 14 cycles. Cyclophosphamide, doxorubicin, and vincristine are administered together in cycles alternating with ifosfamide and etoposide. Actinomycin-D is substituted for doxorubicin after administering approximately 450 mg/m^2 body surface area of doxorubicin or if reduction in cardiac function occurs.

In the case of F.W. with localized disease, the recommendation would be to proceed with neoadjuvant chemotherapy using vincristine, cyclophosphamide, doxorubicin, ifosfamide, and etoposide. After 4 to 8 courses, local therapy with radiation would be considered given the location of the mass. Doxorubicin would be omitted during radiation, and the remainder of chemotherapy would be administered following completion of radiation.

Advanced Stage (Metastatic) Ewing's Sarcoma

M.S. is an 18-year-old Caucasian high-school senior who noted pain and swelling in her left arm that she attributed to a muscle pull sustained during conditioning exercises for lacrosse 3 months prior to diagnosis. The pain subsided but the swelling persisted. She detected a firm mass in the distal arm near the elbow 2 months later. She reported low-grade fevers and night sweats. She was prescribed a course of antibiotics for treatment of presumptive cellulitis that did not improve the pain, swelling, or constitutional symptoms. She was using hydrocodone-acetaminophen for management of arm pain. Her past medical and family histories were noncontributory.

On examination M.S. had a firm, tender, fixed mass in the left distal arm. There was normal strength and sensation in the arm. There were no palpable lymph nodes. Examination was otherwise normal. Serum LDH was elevated at 290 IU/L. Total white blood cell count was elevated at 11,200/mm^3 but the differential was normal. Other serum chemistries were within normal ranges.

An x-ray of the left elbow was performed and detected an ill-defined soft tissue mass posterior to the distal humerus without appreciable internal calcification. The mass appeared to arise from the distal humerus and there was a Codman's triangle-type periosteal reaction along with mild remodeling of the adjacent cortex. An MRI scan was performed and demonstrated a 9.4 × 7.5 × 8.2 cm heterogenous solid mass involving the distal humeral diaphysis and metaphysis with a large soft tissue component (see Figure 21.6). The soft tissue component extended circumferentially around the distal humerus, exerting mass effect upon the anterior and posterior muscle compartments. There was periosteal elevation at the superior aspect of the mass and abnormal signal intensity within the medial cortex of the distal humeral metaphysis.

A core needle biopsy was performed in the clinic. Pathology revealed the presence of a small, round, blue cell tumor. Immunohistochemical staining detected *CD99* in a membranous pattern, and *CD20*, *CD3*, and *TdT* were negative. PCR detected translocation involving *EWS* (on chromosome 22) and FLI-1 (on chromosome 11). A staging chest CT demonstrated multiple soft tissue nodules/masses in all lobes of both lungs with the largest in the left lower lobe measuring 2.5 × 1.3 cm. A technetium bone scan detected heterogeneous uptake centered in the left distal humerus but no suspicious focal uptake in the remainder of the skeleton. Bilateral bone marrow biopsies showed normal cellular marrow and no evidence of metastasis. Needle biopsy of a peripheral lung mass confirmed metastatic Ewing's sarcoma.

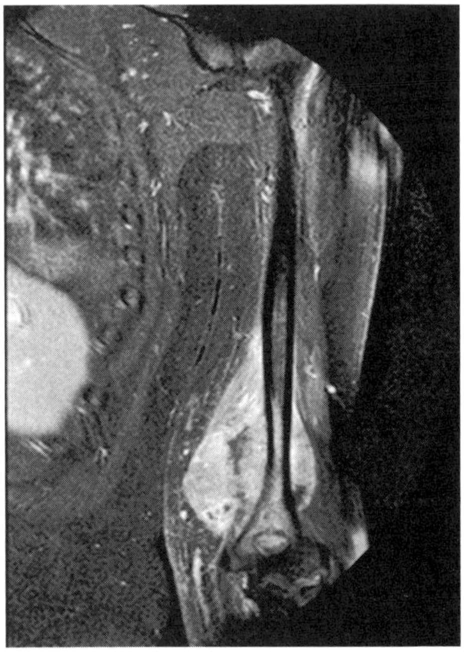

Figure 21.6

MRI (T1, postcontrast sequence, coronal image) of left arm demonstrating mass involving distal humeral diaphysis and metaphysis with cortical bone breach and involvement of surrounding soft tissue.

Evidence-Based Case Discussion

This is a young adult with pulmonary-only metastatic disease. Given the widespread involvement of the lungs, the Ewing's metastases may be considered unresectable. However, the treatment approach should be with curative intent because approximately 20% of patients presenting with metastatic Ewing's may be long-term survivors of the disease. Preoperated chemotherapy should be administered as described above in the localized Ewing's section for patients presenting de novo with metastatic Ewing's. Thereafter, surgical resection or definitive radiation of both the primary and metastatic lesions should be performed if feasible (see Figure 21.5).

A significant number of patients who were initially treated for localized Ewing's experience local and distant recurrence. Several characteristics influence the prognosis following relapse. A long interval to relapse after treatment of primary disease and lung-only disease are more favorable than their counterparts. When doxorubicin was administered as part of the initial therapy for localized disease, it is not given for relapsed disease due to the potential for cardiotoxicity to develop. Ifosfamide and etoposide may be used to treat relapsed Ewing's. When the primary disease treatment did not use these drugs, studies of the combination in relapsed Ewing's demonstrated response rates of 50% and 1- and 2-year overall survivals of 49% and 28%, respectively, in children and young adults (15).

Studies have also been done using topoisomerase I inhibitors. A study of 55 patients with participants aged 3 through 50 years, who were in first or second relapse, used cyclophosphamide with topotecan. The treatment provided an overall objective response rate (complete plus partial response) of 44%, with 25.9% of patients maintaining response after 23 months (16). A smaller study has evaluated the combination of irinotecan and temozolomide in patients with advanced Ewing's (17).

Docetaxel and gemcitabine have been evaluated in metastatic Ewing's. A small study of 22 patients with bone sarcomas showed a 29% overall objective response rate with this regimen; however, the median duration of response was short, at just under 5 months (18).

In summary, in advanced Ewing's sarcoma, the recommended treatment is chemotherapy followed by local therapy using radiation and/or surgery for residual disease, when feasible. For treatment of widely metastatic relapsed Ewing's, palliative care using chemotherapy, radiation, and/or surgery may be considered. Participation in clinical trials should be encouraged for patients with relapsed disease.

In the case of M.S. with advanced disease, treatment should include chemotherapy using doxorubicin, vincristine, cyclophosphamide, and actinomycin-D. Ifosfamide and etoposide could also be incorporated but are more cumbersome to administer and are unlikely to improve survival. Longer-term control of the primary site of the disease in the distal humerus would benefit from radiation or surgery and in this case, radiation would be preferred because of lower morbidity. If there is residual disease in the lung following chemotherapy, resection versus radiation may be considered to eliminate residual gross tumor. Patients with lung-only Ewing's metastasis fare better than patients with bone metastasis. Patients with visceral metastasis or diffuse involvement in the bone marrow have the poorest long-term survival rates.

REFERENCES

1. Greene FL, Page DL, Fleming ID, et al. *American Joint Committee on Cancer.* Sixth Edition. New York, Philadelphia, PA: Springer Science+Business Media LLC, 2002:213–219.
2. Rosen G, Marcove RC, Huvos AG, et al. Primary osteogenic sarcoma: eight-year experience with adjuvant chemotherapy. *J Cancer Res Clin Oncol.* 1983;106(Suppl):55–67.
3. Meyers PA, Heller G, Healey J, et al. Chemotherapy for nonmetastatic osteogenic sarcoma: the Memorial Sloan-Kettering experience. *J Clin Oncol.* 1992;10(1): 5–15.
4. Souhami RL, Craft AW, Van der Eijken JW, et al. Randomised trial of two regimens of chemotherapy in operable osteosarcoma: a study of the European Osteosarcoma Intergroup. *Lancet.* 1997;350(9082): 911–917.
5. Bramwell VH, Burgers M, Sneath R, et al. A comparison of two short intensive adjuvant chemotherapy regimens in operable osteosarcoma of limbs in children and young adults: the first study of the European Osteosarcoma Intergroup. *J Clin Oncol.* 1992;10(10):1579 –1591.
6. Bacci G, Gherlinzoni F, Picci P, et al. Adriamycin-methotrexate high dose versus adriamycin-methotrexate moderate dose as adjuvant chemotherapy for osteosarcoma of the extremities: a randomized study. *Eur J Cancer Clin Oncol.* 1986;22(11):1337–1345.
7. Krailo M, Ertel I, Makley J, et al. A randomized study comparing high-dose methotrexate with moderate-dose methotrexate as components of adjuvant chemotherapy in childhood nonmetastatic osteosarcoma: a report from the Children's Cancer Study Group. *Med Pediatr Oncol.* 1987;15:69–75.
8. Goorin AM, Schwartzentruber DJ, Devidas M, et al. Presurgical chemotherapy compared with immediate surgery and adjuvant chemotherapy for nonmetastatic osteosarcoma: Pediatric Oncology Group Study POG-8651. *J Clin Oncol.* 2003;21(8): 1574–1580.
9. Kempf-Bielack B, Bielack SS, Jürgens H, et al. Osteosarcoma relapse after combined modality therapy: an analysis of unselected patients in the Cooperative Osteosarcoma Study Group (COSS). *J Clin Oncol.* 2005;23(3):559–568.
10. Goorin AM, Harris MB, Bernstein M, et al. Phase II/III trial of etoposide and high-dose ifosfamide in newly diagnosed metastatic osteosarcoma: a pediatric oncology group trial. *J Clin Oncol.* 2002;20(2):426–433.
11. Gentet JC, Brunat-Mentigny M, Demaille MC, et al. Ifosfamide and etoposide in childhood osteosarcoma. A phase II study of the French Society of Paediatric Oncology. *Eur J Cancer.* 1997;33(2):232–237.
12. Nesbit ME Jr, Gehan EA, Burgert EO Jr, et al. Multimodal therapy for management of primary, nonmetastatic Ewing's sarcoma of the bone: a long-term follow-up of the First Intergroup study. *J Clin Oncol.* 1990;8(10):1664–1674.
13. Grier HE, Krailo MD, Tarbell NJ, et al. Addition of ifosfamide and etoposide to standard chemotherapy for Ewing's sarcoma and primitive neuroectodermal tumor of bone. *N Engl J Med.* 2003;348(8): 694–701.
14. Womer RB, West DC, Krailo MD, et al. Randomized comparison of every-two-week versus every-three-week chemotherapy in Ewing sarcoma family tumors (ESFT). *J Clin Oncol.* 2008;26:abstract 10504.
15. Miser JS, Kinsella TJ, Triche TJ, et al. Ifosfamide with mesna uroprotection and etoposide: an effective regimen in the treatment of recurrent sarcomas and other tumors of children and young adults. *J Clin Oncol.* 1987;5(8): 1191–1198.
16. Hunold A, Weddeling N, Paulussen M, et al. Topotecan and cyclophosphamide in patients with refractory or relapsed Ewing tumors. *Pediatr Blood Cancer.* 2006;47:795–800.
17. Wagner LM, McAllister N, Goldsby RE, et al. Temozolomide and intravenous irinotecan for treatment of advanced Ewing sarcoma. *Pediatr Blood Cancer.* 2007;48:132–139.
18. Navid F, Willert JR, McCarville MB, et al. Combination of gemcitabine and docetaxel in the treatment of children and young adults with refractory bone sarcoma. *Cancer.* 2008;113(2): 419–425.

22

Soft Tissue Sarcoma

DAWIT AREGAWI AND RASHMI CHUGH

EPIDEMIOLOGY, RISK FACTORS, NATURAL HISTORY, AND PATHOLOGY

Soft tissue sarcomas (STS) are rare malignancies that arise from mesenchymal tissue occurring in any site within the body. Sarcomas comprise less than 1% of all adult cancer, and approximately 10,660 cases are diagnosed annually in the United States (1). The majority of STS are sporadic, with no clearly defined cause. However, there are some established risk factors, including radiation, chemical exposure, chronic lymphedema, and certain genetic disorders such as Li Fraumeni syndrome, neurofibromatosis 1, and Gardner's syndrome. Traditionally, STS are classified based on morphology and tissue resemblance. However, the cell of origin is unclear in numerous sarcomas. Specific chromosomal translocations have been identified in approximately one third of all sarcomas (Table 22.1) (2). The resultant fusion protein, which often encodes for an aberrant transcription factor, has been shown in some cases to be directly related to pathogenesis of the tumor and is an appropriate target for therapy. These genetic abnormalities are now identified by fluorescence in-situ hybridization (FISH) and reverse transcriptase polymerase chain reaction (rt-PCR), which aid in the diagnosis of these challenging tumors.

STS can occur anywhere in the body. A multicenter cohort study of 4508 adults showed the anatomical distribution of STS to be thigh, buttock, and groin in 46%, while the torso, upper extremity, retroperitoneum, and head and neck accounted for 18%, 13%, 13%, and 9% of cases, respectively (3). It frequently presents as a painless mass. Suspicious extremity or trunk lesions, defined as masses that are deep, enlarging, or over 5 cm in diameter, should be imaged with magnetic resonance imaging (MRI). Visceral lesions are often visualized initially using CT. If imaging confirms a mass in which sarcoma is in the differential diagnosis, referral to the appropriate orthopedic or surgical oncologist is recommended for a properly performed biopsy that can be encompassed within the eventual surgical resection. Core needle biopsies guided by imaging, or physical examination in the case of palpable lesions, are often sufficient to make a diagnosis. Occasionally an incisional biopsy is required.

For the majority of STS, the spread of disease is hematogenous. The most common area of metastasis is the lung. A baseline chest CT should be included as part of the initial evaluation. Specific histologic subtypes may have different patterns of spread, including nodal disease with rhabdomyosarcomas, liver metastases with gastrointestinal stromal tumors, and abdominal and bony spread in myxoid liposarcomas. Thus, staging evaluation may need to be adjusted based on specific histologic subtype and site of origin.

With over 50 histologic subtypes and a continuously evolving classification nomenclature, accurate pathologic diagnosis of STS is challenging. Table 22.2 lists some of the most common histologies of STS and presumed cell of origin. Confirmation of the diagnosis of STS by a pathologist with sarcoma expertise is imperative. Access to molecular diagnostics to identify molecular abnormalities associated with STS is also instrumental in the diagnosis and treatment.

STAGING

The American Joint Committee on Cancer (AJCC) staging is based on the major prognostic factors of tumor size, grade, depth in relation to investing fascia, and the presence of metastatic disease (4); see table on the next page.

Staging System for STS, Adapted from the AJCC, 7th edition

Stage	Definition
Stage IA	Small tumor (≤5 cm), low grade; superficial or deep to muscular fascia
Stage IB	Large tumor (>5 cm), low grade; superficial or deep to muscular fascia
Stage IIA	Small tumor (≤5 cm), moderate or high grade; superficial or deep to muscular fascia
Stage IIB	Large tumor (>5 cm), moderate or high grade; superficial or deep to muscular fascia
Stage III	Large tumor (>5 cm), high grade; superficial or deep to muscular fascia; or any size or grade with regional nodal involvement
Stage IV	Any size or grade with distant metastasis

Table 22.1 Selected Sarcomas Associated With Chromosomal Translocations

	Genes	Translocation
Ewing's sarcoma	*EWSR1-FLI1*	t(11;22)(q24;q12)
Clear cell sarcoma	*EWSR1-ATF1*	t(12;22)(q13;q12)
Desmoplastic small round cell tumor	*EWSR1-WT1*	t(11;22)(p13;q12)
Myxoid chondrosarcoma	*EWSR1-NR4A3*	t(9;22)(q22–31;q11–12)
Alveolar rhabdomyosarcoma	*PAX3-FOXO1A*	t(2;13)(q35;q14)
Synovial sarcoma	*SYT-SSX*	t(X;18)(p11;q11)
Dermatofibrosarcoma protuberans	*COL1A1-PDGFB*	t(17;22)(q22;q23)
Alveolar soft-part sarcoma	*ASPL-TFE3*	t(X;17)(p11.2;q25)
Myxoid liposarcoma	*FUS-DDIT3*	t(2;16)(q13;p11)

Table 22.2 Common Subtypes of STS in Adults

Subtype	Presumed Tissue of Origin
Malignant fibrous histiocytoma	Unknown
Liposarcoma	Adipose tissue
Fibrosarcoma	Fibrous connective tissue
Synoviosarcoma	Unknown
Rhabdomyosarcoma	Striated muscle
Leiomyosarcoma	Smooth muscle
Neurofibrosarcoma, Schwannoma	Neural Sheath
Angiosarcoma	Blood or lymphatic vessels

CASE SUMMARIES

Locally Advanced STS

F.P. is a 58-year-old man who first presented to an outside physician in late 2006 with a painless left medial thigh mass. An MRI showed a 3.8-cm enhancing mass.

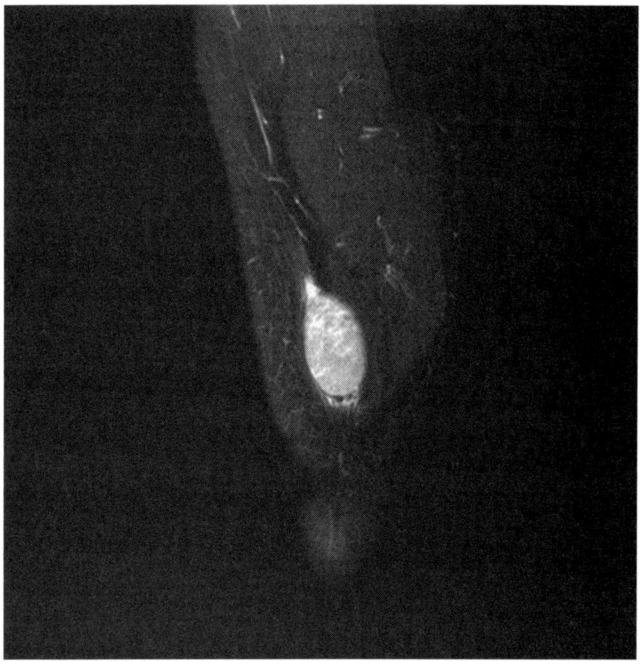

Figure 22.1

MRI of lower extremity leiomyosarcoma.

Observation was recommended, with a plan to repeat imaging in 1 year. The patient reported subjective enlargement that was confirmed on follow-up MRI in December 2007, showing a 5.4-cm mass. He denied any constitutional symptoms. The patient was referred for orthopedic consultation. Repeat MRI of the left thigh with gadolinium contrast (Figure 22.1) showed an enhancing mass measuring 6.1 cm arising between the sartorius and gracilis muscles. Core needle biopsy revealed a high-grade leiomyosarcoma. A chest CT was unremarkable. He received four cycles of neoadjuvant doxorubicin and ifosfamide with MESNA and filgrastim support. A subsequent wide local resection removed a superficial 6.7-cm mass contained in a pseudocapsule, with negative margins. He also received postoperative adjuvant radiation to a total dose of 63 gray. He is currently on observation, with no evidence of recurrent disease.

Evidence-Based Case Discussion

This is a relatively healthy patient presenting with stage III, high-grade STS of the left thigh. Imaging using tumor protocol MRI with gadolinium contrast was performed to define the extent of local disease and to evaluate for neurovascular involvement for eventual surgical resection. The tumor's high grade as well as large size (greater than 5 cm) confers a higher risk of eventual tumor recurrence. However, the determination of superficial tumor location is favorable as compared to a location deep to the fascia. Routine staging with chest CT showed no evidence of pulmonary nodules.

In general, management of newly diagnosed STS is complicated. Since centralization of treatment at a regional cancer center with access to multidisciplinary teams improves local control in all and survival in some (5), patients suspected of having STS should be referred to a center with expertise in sarcoma. Although many histologic subtypes of sarcoma are treated similarly when localized, certain subtypes have their own characteristic behavior and response to therapy. For instance, some subtypes of large, high-grade STS such as alveolar soft-part sarcoma and malignant hemangiopericytoma are known to be relatively chemoresistant, and thus standard chemotherapy in the adjuvant or neoadjuvant setting is not recommended. These nuances in therapy must be considered on an individual basis.

Figure 22.2 shows a generalized treatment algorithm for STS. Current treatment modalities of surgery and radiation for extremity STS yield excellent local control, but distant failure is common and almost universally fatal in high-risk STS. The sequencing of therapy, including surgery, chemotherapy, and radiation, is best considered in the multidisciplinary setting based on histologic subtype, tumor location, and patient-specific factors.

For patients with high-risk STS, which includes large (greater than 5 cm) and moderate- to high-grade tumors, the prognosis is generally poor, with approximately 50% of patients developing metastatic disease. For this reason, neoadjuvant or adjuvant chemotherapy is used in many centers for this population, even though its role remains controversial due to the lack of properly controlled and conducted clinical trials. Most published trials of adjuvant chemotherapy were inadequately powered, included a heterogeneous collection of sarcomas, and did not use full doses of the most effective cytotoxic agents, now known to be doxorubicin and ifosfamide. Because of this, some studies show benefit to adjuvant chemotherapy, whereas others show no benefit or are inconclusive. In 1997, the Sarcoma Meta-Analysis Collaboration published a meta-analysis of 14 trials of doxorubicin-based adjuvant chemotherapy consisting of 1568 patients. This revealed a longer local, distant, and overall recurrence-free survival with adjuvant chemotherapy (hazard ratios [HR] of 0.73, 0.70, 0.75; $P = .016$, $P = .0001$, $P = .0001$, respectively). There was no difference in overall survival, although there was a trend in favor of adjuvant chemotherapy (HR = 0.89, $P = .12$). Patients with extremity sarcomas did have a survival benefit on subgroup analysis, with a 7% absolute survival benefit at 10 years ($P = .029$) (6). Although a statistically significant survival benefit was not seen in all groups, only one study included in the meta-analysis used ifosfamide in addition to doxorubicin. As with any meta-analysis, the heterogeneous patient population, tumor inclusion criteria, and drug dosing make these data difficult to interpret. However, in the correctly selected patient with a high-risk extremity sarcoma, adjuvant chemotherapy with the most effective agents known (combination of doxorubicin and ifosfamide) may yield some benefit.

Although most studies performed have evaluated the role of adjuvant chemotherapy, many centers prefer the use of neoadjuvant treatment when possible. Response to neoadjuvant chemotherapy may improve surgical resection options, such as allowing a limb salvage operation, when otherwise not possible. The use of neoadjuvant chemotherapy may also allow identification of a subgroup of patients likely to benefit from additional adjuvant chemotherapy or those who should be considered for second-line or experimental treatments.

Given our patient's high-risk features of a large, high-grade STS and his otherwise good health, he received

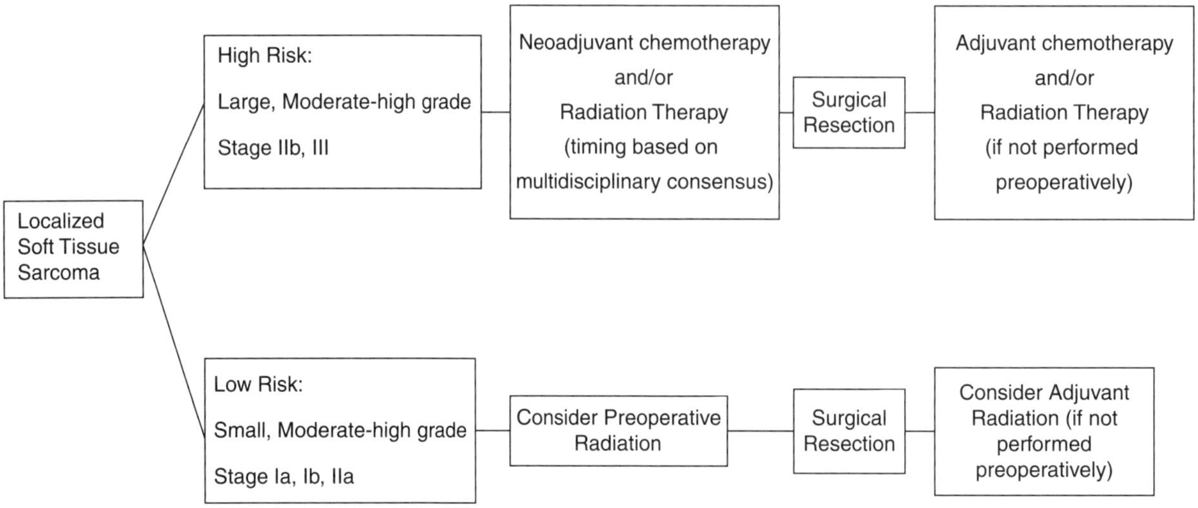

Figure 22.2

Treatment algorithm of localized soft tissue sarcoma.

neoadjuvant doxorubicin and ifosfamide. After two cycles of chemotherapy, repeat imaging showed stable disease, and he went on to complete the planned four cycles of therapy. If there was evidence of progressive disease, the patient would have proceeded directly to surgical resection after two cycles of treatment. Three weeks following completion of his chemotherapy, he underwent a wide resection that removed a superficial 6.7-cm high-grade leiomyosarcoma.

The patient is currently on observation and has been free of local or distant recurrence for more than 2 years after undergoing multimodality therapy.

Advances in reconstructive surgical techniques, institution of multimodality therapy, and improved selection of patients for neoadjuvant and adjuvant therapy have significantly increased the role of limb-sparing surgery with adequate local control of disease. Rosenberg et al. (7) published the first prospective randomized trial comparing limb-sparing surgery plus radiation compared to amputation in 43 adult patients with STS of the extremity. This demonstrated an increased limb salvage rate with the use of radiation following surgery, with no differences in disease-free survival and overall survival rates between the treatment groups. This and other randomized controlled trials have demonstrated low local recurrence rates (7–15%) with no detriment in overall survival when patients with extremity STS are treated with limb-sparing surgery and radiation as compared to amputation (7,8). Thus, limb-sparing surgery with or without adjuvant radiation therapy is an effective treatment option for extremity STS. Amputation, which was once considered standard, should be reserved only for cases of very large tumors involving a neurovascular bundle or where resection or re-resection with adequate margins cannot be performed without sacrificing functional outcome.

Several trials have shown the benefit of radiation in local control of STS combined with resection. In a prospective randomized trial from MSKCC, 5-year local control rates in high-risk lesions were 89% with brachytherapy and 66% without (9), whereas Yang et al. (10) randomized 91 patients with high-risk extremity sarcomas to receive postoperative chemotherapy and radiation or chemotherapy alone. With a median follow-up of 9.6 years, no patients in the radiation arm had local recurrence, whereas 19% in the chemotherapy-alone arm had local recurrence. On the basis of these randomized trials and several other single-institution retrospective studies, the addition of radiation, whether delivered preoperatively, postoperatively, or as brachytherapy, has become the standard of care for large, high-risk sarcoma.

The sequencing of radiation therapy in relation to surgery is a subject of debate, each with advantages and disadvantages but similar local control and progression-free survival rates. Preoperative radiation has an increased rate of acute wound complications, but can allow a smaller resection. When deciding between preoperative versus postoperative radiation therapy, one should consider the type of surgical procedure, extent of operative bed, likelihood of obtaining negative margins, factors of wound closure and tension, and grade of the sarcoma.

For the first 2 years after completion of treatment, serial tumor bed imaging with MRI is recommended every 6 months. Chest imaging and physical examinations are performed every 3 months. After 2 years, follow-up evaluations are spaced to every 4 to 6 months, for a minimum of 5 years of total follow-up. As late recurrences have been commonly reported, follow-up evaluations are often continued beyond the 5-year mark.

Advanced Metastatic Sarcoma

C.A. is a 63-year-old man who was found to have a palpable lower abdominal mass during a preoperative evaluation for a bariatric procedure in the fall of 2006. A CT showed a 15 × 15 cm pelvic mass. CT-guided biopsy revealed a high-grade pleomorphic sarcoma. He underwent a radical resection of the abdominal mass along with left nephrectomy, splenectomy, partial colectomy, and partial cystectomy, followed by adjuvant radiation. Following completion of radiotherapy, he was followed with serial imaging. Two years later, he was found to have 2.3-cm right middle and lower lobe pulmonary nodules and a retrocaval soft tissue mass measuring 3.6 cm. Symptoms at the time included a dry cough, but no shortness of breath or hemoptysis. A CT-guided core needle biopsy confirmed metastatic high-grade sarcoma.

Following the diagnosis, he was started on combination chemotherapy with gemcitabine and docetaxel. Follow-up chest CT after two cycles showed interval progression of disease. His treatment was switched to single-agent doxorubicin after a baseline echo showed an ejection fraction of 53%. He completed eight cycles, with an objective response, before commencing a chemotherapy holiday. After 6 months of serial imaging showing disease stability, he eventually developed progressive pulmonary disease. He was then enrolled in a clinical trial with cyclophosphamide and sirolimus.

Evidence-Based Case Discussion

Our patient is a 63-year-old man with a high-grade pleomorphic sarcoma who was on observation until he was found to have metastatic pulmonary and extrapulmonary lesions. Pulmonary metastases are the most common and usual first site of STS spread. Approximately 50% of patients with STS develop distant metastases and eventually die of disseminated disease, with a median survival of approximately 12 months from diagnosis of metastases (11,12).

For appropriately selected patients with isolated, limited pulmonary metastases from STS, surgical resection is often the treatment of choice and has been shown to be curative, with long-term disease-free survival rates of approximately 25% in retrospective studies (13–15). Figure 22.3 shows a treatment algorithm for patients with metastatic disease. Commonly used criteria for selecting patients include no extrathoracic disease, pleural effusion, or mediastinal/hilar adenopathy; good performance status of patient for thoracotomy and pulmonary resection; and technical feasibility of complete resection (16). Stereotactic radiosurgery is increasingly being used in some situations for small pulmonary metastases, but its true role is unclear.

Systemic chemotherapy is a therapeutic option for patients presenting with metastatic disease not amenable to complete surgical resection. For the majority of these patients, cytotoxic chemotherapy is regarded as palliative, although a small subset of patients achieve a long-term survival advantage (11). Active agents in metastatic STS with a 10% or greater response rate include single-agent doxorubicin, ifosfamide, gemcitabine, and dacarbazine. Doxorubicin, which was identified as an active drug in the 1970s, continues to be the most commonly used single agent. The response rate with doxorubicin averages approximately 10% to 25%, depending on the era and response criteria used. It has been shown to have a dose-response relationship in sarcoma, but its use is limited by the risk of cardiotoxicity after high cumulative doses.

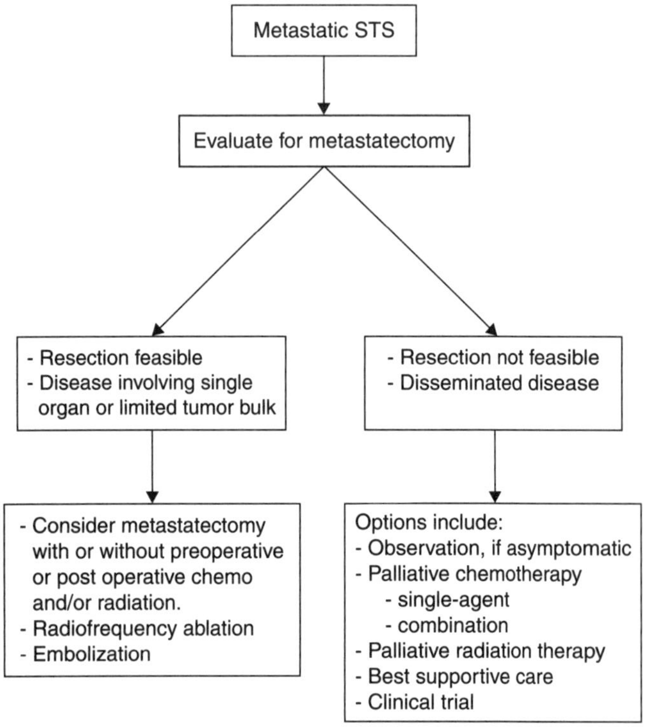

Figure 22.3

Treatment algorithm of metastatic soft tissue sarcoma.

Ifosfamide is the first drug to demonstrate significant efficacy in doxorubicin-refractory disease. Ifosfamide does have unique potential toxicities, including hemorrhagic cystitis, renal tubular acidosis, and neurotoxicity. Ifosfamide-induced hemorrhagic cystitis can be avoided by prophylactic use of 2-mercapto-ethane sulfonate sodium (mesna).

Combination chemotherapy for metastatic STS can yield higher response rates than single-agent chemotherapy, but may be more toxic. In 2003, the Sarcoma Disease Site Group published a meta-analysis including 2281 patients from eight randomized controlled trials comparing single-agent doxorubicin versus doxorubicin-based combination chemotherapy. No significant differences were seen in overall survival, although increased response rates as well as increased toxicities were seen with combination therapy (17). Doxorubicin-based combinations, including AIM (doxorubicin, ifosfamide, mesna), MAID (doxorubicin, ifosfamide, mesna, dacarbazine), and doxorubicin/dacarbazine, are still routinely used in clinical practice. However, they should be reserved for patients who may benefit from tumor shrinkage and can tolerate the potential increased toxicities of combination chemotherapy.

Combination chemotherapy with gemcitabine and docetaxel has recently emerged as a standard therapy for patients with metastatic STS. A study performed by the Sarcoma Alliance for Research through Collaboration adaptively randomized 122 patients with metastatic STS to either single-agent fixed dose rate gemcitabine or combination gemcitabine-docetaxel. There was an improvement in response rate (16% vs. 8%), median progression-free survival (6.2 months vs. 3.0 months), and overall survival (17.9 months vs. 11.5 months), with the combination as compared to the single agent, respectively (18). Other studies have confirmed this combination is active and have established it as an important regimen in the care of STS patients. Based on some observations, patients with the subtypes of leiomyosarcoma and high-grade undifferentiated sarcoma (also referred to as malignant fibrous histiocytoma) may have a higher chance of benefitting from gemcitabine-docetaxel.

Since our patient has an extrapulmonary metastatic lesion, he was not a candidate for metastatectomy and was started on combination chemotherapy. After initial progression on gemcitabine-docetaxel, the patient achieved a partial response to single-agent doxorubicin therapy. Given his history of nephrectomy with his primary tumor resection and his borderline renal function, he was not a candidate for ifosfamide-based chemotherapy. After eventual progression, he was treated on a clinical trial. As limited active agents exist for the treatment of metastatic STS, participation in clinical trials is an important part of patient care as well as in understanding the disease.

GASTROINTESTINAL STROMAL TUMOR

Epidemiology, Risk Factors, Natural History, and Pathology

Gastrointestinal stromal tumor (GIST) represents a unique subtype of STS derived from the interstitial cells of Cajal, the pacemaker cells of the gastrointestinal tract (GI). Approximately 4500 to 6000 adults are diagnosed annually in the United States. GISTs occur in equal frequency in men and women, with a median age of 60.

GISTs can occur anywhere along the GI tract, but mainly are found in the stomach (60%) and small intestine (jejunum and ileum, 30%) (19). Patients with GIST often present with symptoms, including early satiety, abdominal discomfort, palpable mass, or GI bleeding. Image-guided or endoscopic core biopsy or FNA is usually sufficient to make the diagnosis.

Approximately 85% of tumors possess mutations in the *c-kit* gene that result in constitutive activation of the KIT tyrosine kinase, which is felt to be the pathogenic event. Additional mutations within the PDGFR alpha gene have also been identified. Ten percent of GISTs are wild type and have no identifiable mutations.

Staging

Staging consists of a CT of the abdomen and pelvis, since peritoneal and hepatic spread occur most commonly. GISTs are also highly FDG avid, so PET scans are occasionally used for staging or assessing response to treatment.

The staging system for GIST is different from that for other STS and is shown in the following tables (according to the *AJCC, 7th Edition*):

Stage Grouping for GIST With a Primary Site in the Stomach or the Omentum

Stage IA	Tumor is ≤ 5 cm (T1 or T2), has not spread to regional lymph nodes (N0) or distant sites (M0), low mitotic rate.*
Stage IB	Tumor is > 5 cm but < 10 cm (T3), has not spread to regional lymph nodes (N0) or distant sites (M0), low mitotic rate.
Stage II	Tumor is ≤ 5 cm (T1 or T2), has not spread to regional lymph nodes (N0) or distant sites (M0), high mitotic rate* *or* tumor is > 10 cm (T4), has not spread to regional lymph nodes (N0) or distant sites (M0), low mitotic rate.
Stage IIIA	Tumor is > 5 cm but ≤ 10 cm (T3), has not spread to regional lymph nodes (N0) or distant sites (M0), high mitotic rate.
Stage IIIB	Tumor is > 10 cm (T4), has not spread to regional lymph nodes (N0) or distant sites (M0), high mitotic rate.
Stage IV	Tumor of any size (any T) that has spread to regional lymph nodes (N1) with no metastases (M0) *or* any tumor with distant metastasis (M1), any mitotic rate.

*Mitotic rate: (low ≤5 mitoses/50 high-powered field (HPF), high > 5 mitoses/50 HPF).

Stage Grouping for GIST of the Small Intestine, Esophagus, Colon, Rectum, and Peritoneum

Stage I	Tumor is ≤ 5 cm (T1 or T2), has not spread to regional lymph nodes (N0) or distant sites (M0), low mitotic rate.*
Stage II	Tumor is >5 cm but < 10 cm (T3), has not spread to regional lymph nodes (N0) or distant sites (M0), low mitotic rate.
Stage IIIA	Tumor is ≤ 2 cm (T1), has not spread to regional lymph nodes (N0) or distant sites (M0), high mitotic rate* *or* tumor is > 10 cm (T4), has not spread to regional lymph nodes (N0) or distant sites (M0), low mitotic rate.
Stage IIIB	Tumor is > 2 cm (T2 to T4), has not spread to regional lymph nodes (N0) or distant sites (M0), high mitotic rate.
Stage IV	Tumor of any size (any T) that has spread to regional lymph nodes (N1) with no metastases (M0) *or* any tumor with distant metastasis (M1), any mitotic rate.

*Mitotic rate: (low ≤ 5 mitoses/50 HPF, high> 5 mitoses/50 HPF).

In clinical practice, the staging system is not used frequently, since the patient's treatment course and decisions are usually based on whether the patient has localized or metastatic disease. If the patient does have localized disease, the determination of prognosis as well as consideration for adjuvant therapy is often based on whether the tumor confers a low-, intermediate-, or high-risk metastatic potential based on tumor and pathologic characteristics. Of note, the site of origin of the tumor (gastric vs. nongastric), size, as well as the mitotic rate (≤5 mitoses/50 HPF vs. >5 mitoses/50 HPF) are important variables affecting stage and prognosis.

Case Summary

Metastatic Gastrointestinal Stromal Tumor

M.Z. is a 69-year-old woman with a history of erosive esophagitis who presented with a new onset of lower abdominal pain, fatigue, and a 10-pound weight loss over 2 months. Abdominopelvic CT showed multiple intra-abdominal masses. The largest in the left upper quadrant measured 12 × 7.4 cm and was compressing the stomach, with at least six additional masses seen throughout the peritoneal cavity and pelvis, measuring from 3 to 12 cm. CT-guided biopsy demonstrated a spindle cell neoplasm that stained strongly positive for *c-kit*, consistent with GIST. Mutational analysis of *c-kit* revealed an exon 11 mutation.

Given the multiplicity of her lesions, the patient was felt not to be a surgical candidate and was started on imatinib 400-mg daily for her new diagnosis of metastatic GIST. Within 4 weeks of therapy she had improvement in her abdominal pain, with only minor complaints of bilateral periorbital edema. Imaging after 8 weeks showed a decrease in size of her tumor masses by approximately 20% (see Figure 22.4).

Evidence-Based Case Discussion

This patient has a biopsy proven metastatic GIST originating within the stomach, possessing the most common mutation in *c-kit*, exon 11.

GIST presents either as a localized/resectable or unresectable and/or metastatic disease. For localized or resectable GIST, surgical resection is the mainstay of treatment. However, the overall outcome of surgery is poor in certain patients due to the high risk of recurrence, and conventional chemotherapy and radiation are of limited benefit. Patients with GISTs possessing high-risk features (tumor size >10 cm or mitotic rate >10 per 50 HPF) have a more than 50% risk of recurrence within 2 years (20). The high rates of local and distant recurrence highlight the need for effective adjuvant treatment following the complete resection of GIST.

Imatinib, an oral inhibitor of the KIT, PDGFR alpha, and ABL tyrosine kinases has been shown to induce durable tumor responses in metastatic disease. These encouraging results led to the rationale of initiating trials in the adjuvant setting. To date, several trials have examined the role of adjuvant imatinib. In ACOSOG Z9001, 359 patients were randomized to 1 year of imatinib 400-mg daily and 354 patients received placebo following complete resection of a localized KIT positive GIST measuring at least 3 cm (21). With a median follow-up of 19.7 months, the estimated 1-year RFS was 98% (95% CI 0.96–1.00) in the imatinib arm compared to 83% (95% CI 0.78–0.88) in the placebo arm, with a corresponding 65% risk reduction of disease recurrence (HR 0.35; 95% CI 0.22–0.53; $P < .0001$). There was no statistical difference in overall survival.

This study led to the FDA approval of imatinib for adjuvant treatment of GIST over 3 cm in size. However, the true role of imatinib in the adjuvant setting is yet to be determined. As ACOSOG Z9001 was terminated early at a planned interim analysis based on the predetermined endpoint of relapse-free survival, it is unclear whether there is an overall survival benefit to adjuvant imatinib with continued follow-up. It is possible that GIST patients may have the same outcome if started on therapy in the adjuvant setting or at the first sign of metastasis. It is also unclear which patient population is most likely to benefit from adjuvant therapy, as many patients with low mitotic rate tumors are cured of disease surgically. The optimal length of therapy is also debated, as many patients treated with 1 year of therapy relapsed after imatinib discontinuation. Ongoing studies in the United States and Europe are evaluating the answers to these questions. Currently, adjuvant imatinib should be considered in the context of a clinical trial or reserved for the tumors with high-risk features.

Our patient presented with metastatic peritoneal disease, which is one of the two most common sites of metastases, the other being liver metastases. Figure 22.5 shows a treatment algorithm for patients with metastatic GIST. Imatinib has been approved as first-line therapy in advanced, inoperable, or metastatic GIST since 2002. Many studies have illustrated the role of imatinib in metastatic GIST. A multicenter trial of 147 patients with advanced GIST randomized patients to treatment with imatinib 400 or 600 mg once daily and

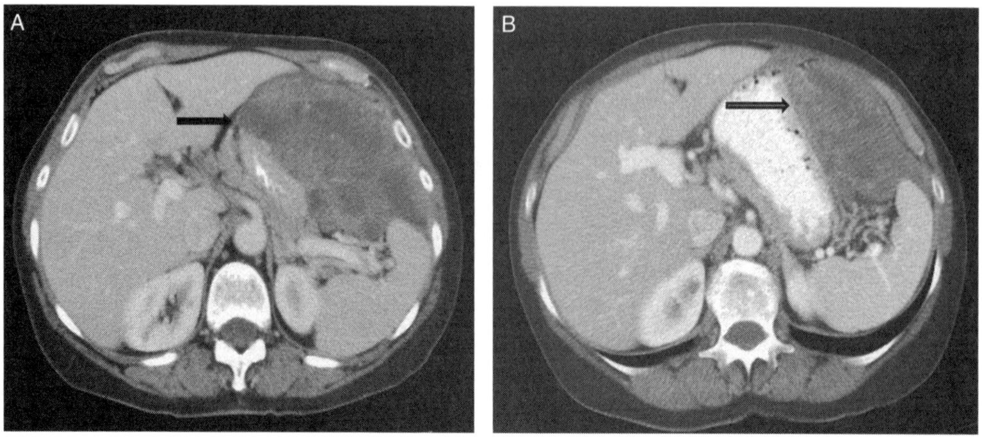

Figure 22.4

Metastatic GIST, prior to (A) and after (B) 8 weeks of imatinib therapy.

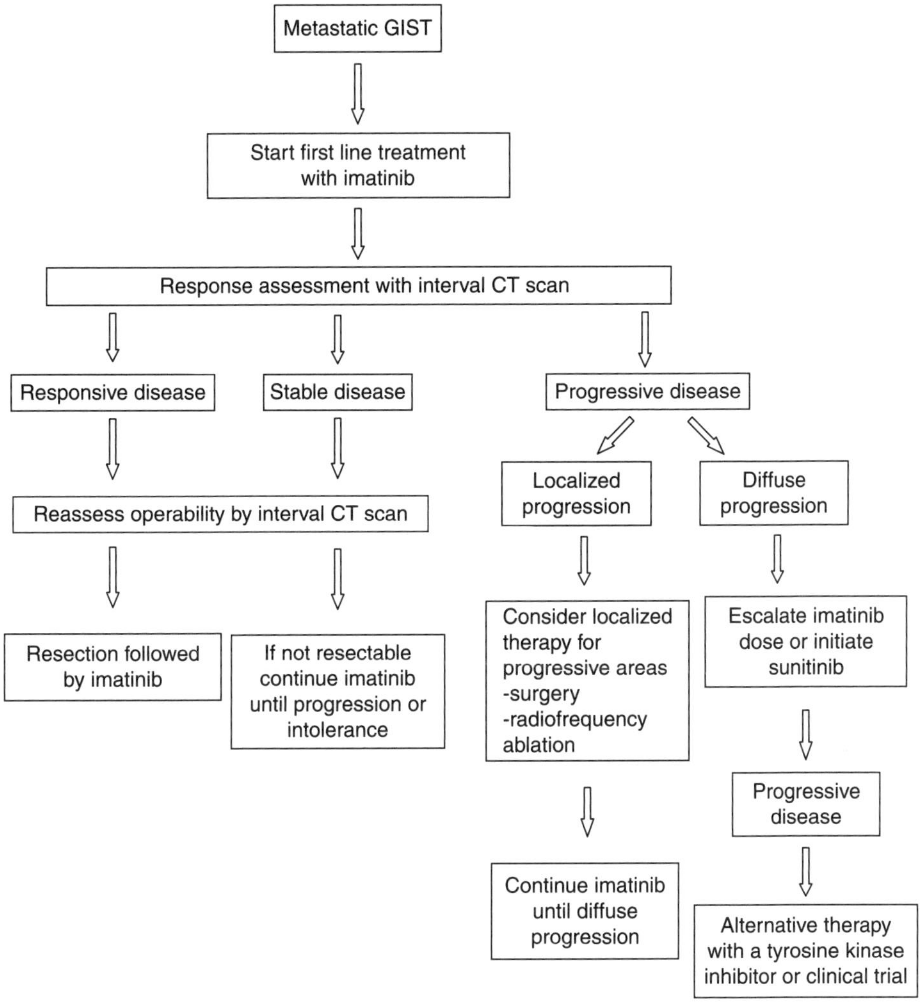

Figure 22.5

Treatment algorithm of metastatic GIST.

showed 53.7% partial response and 27.9% stable disease, with similar outcomes at both doses (22). EORTC 62005 and SWOG 0033 also evaluated the benefit of imatinib in this same population. In both of these phase III studies, patients were randomized to receive 400 or 800 mg/day imatinib and had equivalent response rates and overall survival with either dose, although more toxicity was seen at the higher dose (23,24). In a later meta-analysis, patients with GISTs with an exon 9 mutation were the only subset that demonstrated a progression-free survival benefit from the higher dose of imatinib, presumably because that mutation confers a higher MIC_{50} to imatinib.

Drug response also correlates with the location of the mutation within the *c-kit* exon. A phase II clinical trial demonstrated that GIST patients with an exon 11 mutation in *c-kit* had an 83.5% response rate to imatinib, compared with a 47.8% response rate in those with an exon 9 mutation (25). Based on these data, imatinib at 400-mg daily is recommended as first-line treatment for patients with metastatic GIST, although a higher dose of 800-mg daily can be considered for patients with a known exon 9 mutation. Imaging for response should be performed every 3 to 6 months, and the drug should be continued until progression or intolerable toxicity.

Unfortunately, the majority of patients treated with imatinib will eventually develop clinical resistance and progression of disease, primarily attributed to development of secondary mutations that confer resistance to imatinib. If progressing disease is localized or unifocal, surgery or local approaches such as radiofrequency ablation should be considered to address the resistant area, and effective systemic therapy for other areas of tumor involvement can be continued. Alternatively, sunitinib is a multitargeted tyrosine kinase inhibitor of KIT, VEGF, and PDGF that is approved by the FDA for GIST patients with imatinib resistance or intolerance. A randomized placebo-controlled trial of sunitinib in patients with imatinib-resistant GIST demonstrated a median time to tumor progression of 27.3 weeks compared with 6.4 weeks in the placebo arm (26).

Some patients with localized unresectable or metastatic GIST may be candidates for surgery after response to imatinib treatment or a period of disease stabilization, so there should be periodic reassessment for potential operability. Gronchi et al. (27) showed that advanced and/or metastatic GIST patients responsive to imatinib who underwent surgery had a postsurgery 2-year disease-specific survival rate of 100% compared with a 2-year disease-specific survival rate of 60% in patients with progressive disease. Furthermore, all patients with bulky primary GIST who received cytoreductive treatment were alive and without evidence of disease at a median follow-up of 21 months.

KAPOSI'S SARCOMA

Epidemiology, Risk Factors, Natural History, and Pathology

Kaposi's sarcoma (KS) is another entity that falls under the category of STS based on its malignant mesenchymal origin, despite fairly unique causative factors and epidemiology. KS is a multifocal indolent vascular tumor involving skin, mucosa, and viscera due to Kaposi sarcoma-associated herpesvirus (KSHV/HHV8) infection. On the basis of the clinical setting in which it occurs, KS is classified as classic (primarily affecting elderly men of Ashkenazi Jewish and/or Mediterranean descent), endemic (in Africa), iatrogenic (in patients with immune disorders, including following organ transplantation), and epidemic or AIDS-related. Yet, histologically, all four are indistinguishable.

In the Western world, AIDS-KS predominantly affects HIV-infected homosexual men, and patients tend to be younger. Even though no organ is consistently spared from involvement by AIDS-KS, the face and lower extremities, the oral cavity, and the GI and respiratory tracts are commonly involved.

Classic KS has a peak incidence of about 40 to 70 years with a wide range, affecting primarily people of Mediterranean or Central/Eastern European ancestry. The lesions usually occur on the distal extremities, particularly the lower legs and feet. Extracutaneous involvement is unusual and rarely is the presenting symptom. In general, oral mucosa and GI tract involvement is less common than with AIDS-KS, affecting less than 10% of patients.

Unlike classic KS, which has an indolent course and rarely accounts for mortality, AIDS-KS can present as an aggressive, life-threatening disease.

Factors associated with the risk of developing AIDS-KS include the presence of HIV infection and its detrimental effect on the immune system, the proangiogenic effect of HIV-1 transcriptional trans-activator (Tat) protein, as well as KSHV viremia, increasing anti-KSHV antibody titers, and lack of neutralizing antibodies.

The introduction and widespread use of highly active antiretroviral therapy (HAART) has led to a marked decline in the incidence of AIDS-KS.

Staging

There is no widely accepted staging system accepted for KS. A staging system for patients with classic KS was proposed based on observation of subjective criteria in 300 patients with classic KS, but has not yet been validated and is not routinely used in clinical practice (28). Subjective evaluation of patient tumors results in tumor classification of maculonodular (stage 1), infiltrative (stage 2), florid (stage 3), and disseminated (stage 4).

There is also no officially accepted AIDS-related KS staging system, but when needed most physicians use the AIDS Clinical Trials Group (ACTG) system that divides patients into good- or poor-prognosis disease groups according to the extent of the tumor (T), immune status (I), and severity (S) of systemic illness (Table 22.3) (29).

Case Summary

Metastatic Kaposi's Sarcoma

D.C. is a 35-year-old homosexual man who presented with an enlarging lesion in his hard palate of 4-weeks' duration, resulting in progressive dysphagia and a speech impediment. He was evaluated by an oral surgeon and

Table 22.3 AIDS Clinical Trial Group Staging of HIV Kaposi's Sarcoma

Disease Stage	Tumor State	Immune Status	Systemic Illness
Good prognosis (T0 I0 S0)	Tumor limited to skin and/or lymph node and/or minimal oral diagnosis	CD4 count ≥200 cells/mm^3	No history of opportunistic infections or thrush KPS ≥ 70 No B symptoms
Poor prognosis (T1 I1 S1)	Tumor associated edema/ ulceration, extensive oral KS, gastrointestinal KS, and visceral KS	CD4 count <200 cells/mm^3	History of opportunistic infections or thrush KPS <70 B symptoms Other HIV-related illness (e.g., neurological disease, lymphoma)

underwent a biopsy. Pathology showed Kaposi's sarcoma. Laboratory evaluation revealed a positive HIV test with a viral load of 164,000 and a CD4 count of 87. A diagnosis of AIDS-related KS was made. He was initiated on HAART with efavirenz/emtricitabine/tenofovir disoproxil fumarate and trimethoprim/sulfa for PCP prophylaxis.

Shortly after starting HAART, he noted erythematous to violaceous macular and patchy skin lesions involving his face, neck, and right groin. He also developed a dry cough without associated fever or dyspnea. A CT of the chest, abdomen, and pelvis showed ill-defined bilateral pulmonary nodules as well as multiple slightly enlarged mediastinal, axillary, retroperitoneal, mesenteric, and pelvic lymph nodes.

He was referred to the Oncology Clinic for further evaluation and management. His examination was remarkable for an extensive violaceous fungating mass within the upper palate and scattered purplish cutaneous macular lesions over the face, back, extremities, and right groin, with associated right lower extremity pitting edema. Over 35 cutaneous lesions were appreciated in total.

The patient was initiated on liposomal doxorubicin at a dose of 20 mg/m^2 every 3 weeks. He experienced tolerable side effects of mild nausea and fatigue on days 2 to 4 of each cycle. The oral/hard palate lesions steadily decreased in size, and the cutaneous lesions faded with each treatment cycle. After 6 months of therapy the patient had resolution of his oropharyngeal disease, dramatic improvement in his cutaneous lesions, and resolution of his lower extremity edema.

Evidence-Based Case Discussion

Our patient illustrates progressive AIDS-related KS with possible visceral (pulmonary), lymph node, oral, and extensive cutaneous involvement. There was worsening in the setting of HAART, suggesting immune reconstitution inflammatory syndrome. Even though the incidence of KS has decreased substantially after the introduction of HAART, it continues to be the most common neoplasm in patients with AIDS. AIDS-related KS can range from relatively indolent in behavior to fulminant spread. These highly vascular lesions most commonly manifest in the skin, although pulmonary and GI tract involvement is common. Upon pathologic diagnosis, screening for visceral involvement with stool guaiac and chest x-ray is recommended, but additional evaluations with CT scanning of the chest/abdomen/pelvis, endoscopy, and bronchoscopy are done as clinically indicated. Although there is no cure for AIDS-related KS, there are multiple effective therapies that are given with the goal of symptom palliation. Figure 22.6 is a treatment algorithm for patients with AIDS-related KS. HAART is used as front-line therapy and has decreased the incidence and mortality of AIDS-related KS. It can be effective as the sole modality of

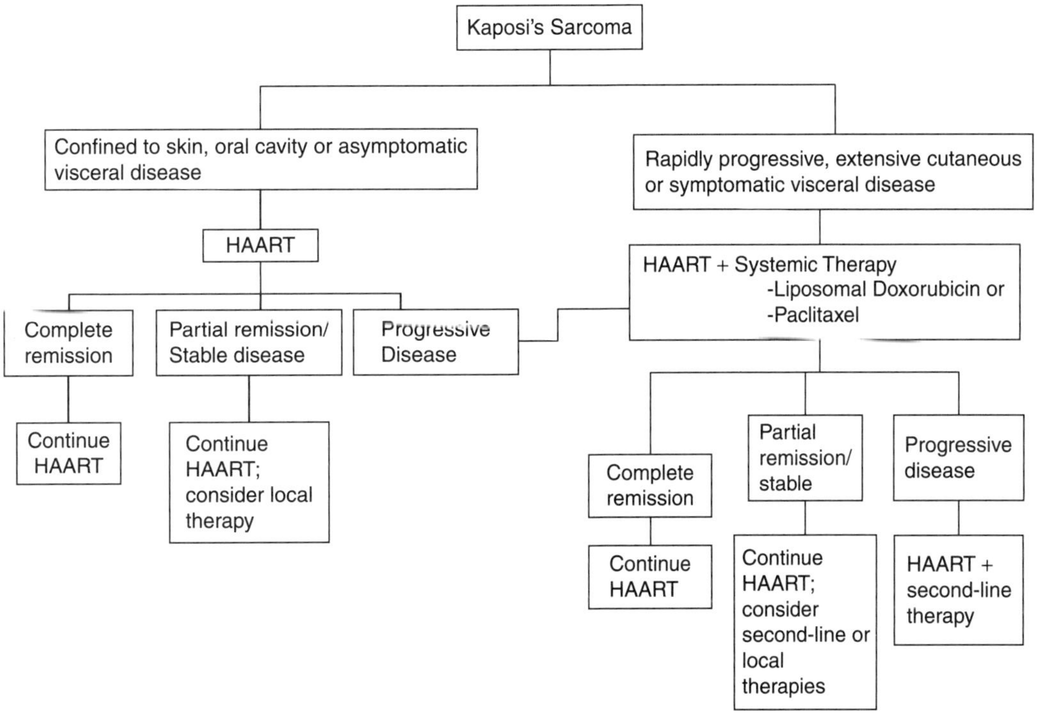

Figure 22.6

Treatment algorithm of metastatic Kaposi's sarcoma.

treatment for this disease. However, patients with visceral involvement, extensive cutaneous involvement (more than 25 skin lesions), rapidly progressive disease, or immune reconstitution inflammatory syndrome (worsening disease in the setting of HAART) require the use of systemic chemotherapy.

Liposomal doxorubicin is often used as front-line therapy, with response rates in the 30% to 60% range. A randomized trial of 73 patients with AIDS related KS showed that liposomal doxorubicin has a response rate of 46%, median PFS of 12.2 months, and 2-year survival of 78% (30). The effective dose of liposomal doxorubicin is 20 mg/m^2 every 3 weeks, which is substantially lower than the dose used for other malignancies. Treatment is typically well tolerated, although continuous assessment for overlapping toxicities with concomitant HAART, antibiotic, and antiemetic therapies is recommended.

Paclitaxel also induces tumor regression with acceptable toxicity and is associated with significant improvement in quality of life. It should be considered as a second-line therapy in patients with advanced KS who progress on liposomal doxorubicin (31). However, paclitaxel requires the use of dexamethasone in this already immunocompromised population and can have interactions with HAART based on its metabolism through the CYP450 system. Other potentially effective systemic therapies include vinorelbine, etoposide, and interferon alpha. For patients with symptomatic localized involvement, effective local strategies include radiation therapy and intralesional chemotherapy.

REFERENCES

1. Jemal A, Siegel R, Xu J, et al. Cancer statistics, 2010. *CA Cancer J Clin.* 2010;60(5):277–300.
2. Helman LJ, and Meltzer, P. Mechanisms of sarcoma development. *Nat Rev Cancer.* 2003;3(9): 685–694.
3. Lawrence WJr., Donegan WL, Natarajan N, et al. Adult soft tissue sarcomas. A pattern of care survey of the American College of Surgeons. *Ann Surg.* 1987;205(4):349–359.
4. Edge SB, Byrd DR, Compton CC, et al. *AJCC Cancer Staging Manual.* Seventh Edition. New York: Springer, 2010:175–180, 291–298.
5. Bhangu AA, B.J., Grimer RJ. Should soft tissue sarcomas be treated at a specialist center? *Sarcoma.* 2004:1–6.
6. Sarcoma Metaanalysis Collaboration. Adjuvant chemotherapy for localised resectable soft-tissue sarcoma of adults: meta-analysis of individual data. *Lancet.* 1997;350(9092):1647–1654.
7. Rosenberg SA, Tepper J, Glatstein E, et al. The treatment of soft-tissue sarcomas of the extremities: prospective randomized evaluations of (1) limb-sparing surgery plus radiation therapy compared with amputation and (2) the role of adjuvant chemotherapy. *Ann Surg.* 1982;196(3):305–315.
8. Baldini EH, Goldberg J, Jenner C, et al. Long-term outcomes after function-sparing surgery without radiotherapy for soft tissue sarcoma of the extremities and trunk. *J Clin Oncol.* 1999;17(10): 3252–3259.
9. Pisters PW, Harrison LB, Leung DH, et al. Long-term results of a prospective randomized trial of adjuvant brachytherapy in soft tissue sarcoma. *J Clin Oncol.* 1996;14(3):859–868.
10. Yang JC, Chang AE, Baker AR, et al. Randomized prospective study of the benefit of adjuvant radiation therapy in the treatment of soft tissue sarcomas of the extremity. *J Clin Oncol.* 1998;16(1):197–203.
11. Blay JY, van Glabbeke M, Verweij J, et al. Advanced soft-tissue sarcoma: a disease that is potentially curable for a subset of patients treated with chemotherapy. *Eur J Cancer.* 2003;39(1): 64–69.
12. Van Glabbeke M, van Oosterom AT, Oosterhuis JW, et al. Prognostic factors for the outcome of chemotherapy in advanced soft tissue sarcoma: an analysis of 2,185 patients treated with anthracycline-containing first-line regimens—a European Organization for Research and Treatment of Cancer Soft Tissue and Bone Sarcoma Group Study. *J Clin Oncol.* 1999;17(1):150–157.
13. Casson AG, Putnam JB, Natarajan G, et al. Five-year survival after pulmonary metastasectomy for adult soft tissue sarcoma. *Cancer.* 1992;69(3):662–668.
14. Putnam JB Jr, Roth JA, Wesley MN, et al. Analysis of prognostic factors in patients undergoing resection of pulmonary metastases from soft tissue sarcomas. *J Thorac Cardiovasc Surg.* 1984;87(2):260–268.
15. Jablons D, Steinberg SM, Roth J, et al. Metastasectomy for soft tissue sarcoma. Further evidence for efficacy and prognostic indicators. *J Thorac Cardiovasc Surg,* 1989;97(5):695–705.
16. McCormack, P. Surgical resection of pulmonary metastases. *Semin Surg Oncol.* 1990;6(5):297–302.
17. Bramwell VH, Anderson D, Charette ML. Doxorubicin-based chemotherapy for the palliative treatment of adult patients with locally advanced or metastatic soft tissue sarcoma. *Cochrane Database Syst Rev.* 2003;(3):CD003293.
18. Maki RG, Wathen JK, Patel SR, et al. Randomized phase II study of gemcitabine and docetaxel compared with gemcitabine alone in patients with metastatic soft tissue sarcomas: results of sarcoma alliance for research through collaboration study 002 [corrected]. *J Clin Oncol.* 2007;25(19):2755–2763.
19. Miettinen M, Lasota J. Gastrointestinal stromal tumors: review on morphology, molecular pathology, prognosis, and differential diagnosis. *Arch Pathol Lab Med.* 2006;130(10):1466–1478.
20. Rutkowski P, Nowecki ZI, Michej W, et al. Risk criteria and prognostic factors for predicting recurrences after resection of primary gastrointestinal stromal tumor. *Ann Surg Oncol.* 2007;14(7):2018–2027.
21. Dematteo RP, Ballman KV, Antonescu CR, et al. Adjuvant imatinib mesylate after resection of localised, primary gastrointestinal stromal tumour: a randomised, double-blind, placebo-controlled trial. *Lancet.* 2009;373(9669):1097–1104.
22. Demetri GD, von Mehren M, Blanke CD, et al. Efficacy and safety of imatinib mesylate in advanced gastrointestinal stromal tumors. *N Engl J Med.* 2002;347(7):472–480.
23. Verweij J, Casali PG, Zalcberg J, et al. Progression-free survival in gastrointestinal stromal tumours with high-dose imatinib: randomised trial. *Lancet.* 2004;364(9440):1127–1134.
24. Blanke CD, Rankin C, Demetri GD, et al. Phase III randomized, intergroup trial assessing imatinib mesylate at two dose levels in patients with unresectable or metastatic gastrointestinal stromal tumors expressing the kit receptor tyrosine kinase: S0033. *J Clin Oncol.* 2008;26(4):626–632.
25. Heinrich MC, Corless CL, Demetri GD, et al. Kinase mutations and imatinib response in patients with metastatic gastrointestinal stromal tumor. *J Clin Oncol.* 2003;21(23):4342–4349.
26. Demetri GD, van Oosterom AT, Garrett CR, et al. Efficacy and safety of sunitinib in patients with advanced gastrointestinal stromal tumour after failure of imatinib: a randomised controlled trial. *Lancet.* 2006;368(9544):1329–1338.

27. Gronchi A, Fiore M, Miselli F, et al. Surgery of residual disease following molecular-targeted therapy with imatinib mesylate in advanced/metastatic GIST. *Ann Surg.* 2007;245(3): 341–346.
28. Brambilla L, Boneschi V, Taglioni M, et al. Staging of classic Kaposi's sarcoma: a useful tool for therapeutic choices. *Eur J Dermatol.* 2003;13(1):83–86.
29. Krown SE, Metroka C, Wernz JC. Kaposi's sarcoma in the acquired immune deficiency syndrome: a proposal for uniform evaluation, response, and staging criteria. AIDS Clinical Trials Group Oncology Committee. *J Clin Oncol.* 1989;7(9): 1201–1207.
30. Cianfrocca M, Lee S, Von Roenn J, et al. Randomized trial of paclitaxel versus pegylated liposomal doxorubicin for advanced human immunodeficiency virus-associated Kaposi sarcoma: evidence of symptom palliation from chemotherapy. *Cancer.* 2010;116(16):3969–3977.
31. Tulpule A, Groopman J, Saville MW, et al. Multicenter trial of low-dose paclitaxel in patients with advanced AIDS-related Kaposi sarcoma. *Cancer.* 2002; 95(1):147–154.

23

Primary Brain Tumors

JANET WANG AND PAMELA NEW

EPIDEMIOLOGY, RISK FACTORS, NATURAL HISTORY, AND PATHOLOGY

Brain tumors account for 1.4% of all cancers and 2.3% of cancer-related deaths. The impact of mortality, disability, effect on family and caregivers, as well as the health care system, is significant. The worldwide incidence rate of malignant primary central nervous system (CNS) tumors is 3.7 per 100,000 person-years in males and 2.6 per 100,000 person-years in females. The incidence rates are higher in more developed countries than in less developed countries. The incidence of all primary nonmalignant and malignant CNS tumors in the United States is 18.71 cases per 100,000 person-years. Approximately, 22,000 new cases of malignant primary brain tumors are diagnosed in the United States annually (2009), representing 1.49% of all primary malignant cancers. The annual incidence of malignant primary brain tumors is 6.4 cases per 100,000 people. Gliomas comprise 32% of all primary brain tumors and 80% of all malignant brain tumors. Incidence of primary brain tumors increases with age, beginning at 20 years. The incidence for all brain and CNS tumors is highest in the 75- to 84-year-old range (65.5 per 100,000). The incidence rate of gliomas is higher in males (7.10 per 100,000 person-years) than in females (5.01 per 100,000 person-years); the frequency is doubled in whites compared to blacks.

There is no definite etiology for primary brain tumors. However, several genetic, environmental, and therapeutic factors have been implicated as risk factors. Previous exposure to ionizing radiation is an established risk factor. Studies have verified an increased risk of gliomas associated with various doses of radiation used to treat tinea capitis, adenoid hypertrophy, childhood leukemia, and other cancers. Low-dose radiation has been linked more often to the incidence of meningioma and nerve sheath tumors. Whether exposure to electromagnetic fields and cell-phone usage are risk factors is a source of continued controversy, but as yet no direct link has yet been established. Occupational studies of airline employees with exposure to cosmic radiation, and atomic energy employees remain equivocal. A recent cohort of U.S. nuclear workers has been examined and an increased risk of developing a primary brain tumor was found to be 15%. An increase in nervous system tumors was also found in survivors of the atomic bomb in Nagasaki and Hiroshima. Exposure to low doses of diagnostic radiation does not seem to play a role, except for a slight risk of meningioma from exposure to dental x-rays. Diet and smoking have also not been associated with increase in risk, nor has occupational exposure to chemicals. Exposure to various tumor-inducing viruses remains plausible and studies continue.

Familial aggregation of brain tumors occurs in 5%, and likely reflects the result of environmental exposures to heritable genetic mutability. Certain familial syndromes (tuberous sclerosis, neurofibromatosis, Turcot's, Li-Fraumeni) may predispose to gliomas in children or young adults. These account for approximately 5% to 10% of all brain tumors. Inherited mutations in the *TP53* gene in some families with Li-Fraumeni syndrome have an increased incidence of many cancers including breast, soft tissues, bone, leukemia, and brain tumors, including glioma and medulloblastoma. Patients with *p53* mutations are more likely to have a first-degree relative affected with cancer (58% vs. 42%), or a previously diagnosed cancer (17% vs. 8%).

Gliomas, occurring in the support tissues of the brain, are the most common primary brain tumor, accounting for more than 40% of primary CNS neoplasms. Subtypes include astrocytomas, oligodendrogliomas, and ependymomas. Gliomas display a broad spectrum of histologic features, and variation in their behavior most likely reflects the genes involved in their transformation. Astrocytomas are the most commonly occurring primary brain tumor in all ages. Oligodendrogliomas, arising from oligodendrocytes in the brain, account for less than 10% of intracranial tumors, and are less aggressive than astrocytomas. Nevertheless, they can invade and disseminate via the cerebrospinal fluid (CSF), causing swelling of the ventricles or hydrocephalus. Typically they are located in the supratentorial hemispheres and are potentially resectable. Ependymomas arise from the ependymal cells lining the brain ventricles. Their growth can block the flow of CSF causing enlargement of the ventricles or hydrocephalus. They tend not to infiltrate the brain and therefore may be amenable to surgical treatment. When not completely resectable, radiotherapy (XRT) is delivered. Chemotherapy has not been found to be effective in this tumor. Meningiomas arise from the dural sheathes surrounding the brain. Most occur near the surface of the brain and are surgically removable. Malignant variants are less frequent (25–30% of meningiomas). They are associated with deletions of loci on chromosome 1, 6p, 9q, and 17p. Medulloblastomas are primitive neuroectodermal tumors that arise in the cerebellum, replicate quickly and disseminate in the CSF. They occur most commonly in children. Chromosome 17p is a frequent site of deletion. Radiotherapy is the mainstay of treatment and usually includes the entire craniospinal compartment. Gangliogliomas are low-grade tumors containing both neurons and glial cells. They have a high rate of cure with surgery alone or surgery combined with radiotherapy. Schwannomas (neurolemomas) arise from Schwann cells that surround cranial and other nerves. These are most often benign tumors and occur near the cerebellum and around the eighth cranial nerve; they are responsible for hearing and balance.

Primary CNS lymphoma (PCNSL) is a diffuse large B-cell lymphoma (DLBCL) presenting in the brain or spinal cord in the absence of systemic lymphoma. About 1000 cases are diagnosed in the United States each year. The incidence of this tumor has been increasing steadily in the immunocompetent population since the 1970s. A reason for this may be improved methods of detection and diagnosis, rather than a true increase in the incidence of the tumor. Nevertheless, the number of patients diagnosed with PCNSL over the next decade is likely to continue to increase, particularly within the elderly population.

PCNSL most commonly presents as a contrast enhancing lesion in the deep brain parenchyma, but may also present as a multifocal or diffuse tumor, often with involvement of the leptomeningeal space. Regardless of initial presentation, the entire cranial-spinal axis is at risk for involvement because of the tendency for PCNSL cells to spread throughout the CSF pathways. Therapy targeted to the tumor site alone is never curative for this reason. It is not common for these lesions to spread outside of the CNS—although reports of relapse in patients systemically have increased (as high as 20% in some reports). This occurs despite the importance of standard screening procedures for systemic disease at the time of diagnosis. The eye is an important site for tumor spread with intraorbital involvement occurring in approximately 5% of patients at presentation. About 15% to 20% are at risk for relapse at this site since most systemically administered chemotherapeutic agents do not achieve cytotoxic concentrations within the eye, and standard radiation fields do not involve the orbits. PCNSL is also exquisitely sensitive to glucocorticoids, a factor that can obscure the initial diagnosis or limit interpretation of treatment. Approaches to treatment must also take into account the fact that these tumors reside in the normal tissues of the brain, spinal cord, and eye, protected by the microanatomical architecture of the blood-brain barrier. Therefore, inefficient drug delivery and neurotoxicity are also constant issues.

The approach to treatment for PCNSL involves biopsy only, as opposed to gross total or near total resection as in the case of other primary brain tumors. In the 1970s it was found that survival with surgical resection versus biopsy alone was not different (1–3 months), and therefore the standard surgical approach is biopsy alone. Because of the issues mentioned above, evaluation of the patient with PCNSL should include MRI of the entire neuraxis, CSF for cytology, and slit lamp examination of the eyes by an ophthalmologist. Evaluation for systemic disease may involve PET-CT of the entire body or CT scans of the chest, abdomen, and pelvis. A bone marrow aspirate is also recommended. Treatment with radiotherapy is controversial. The tumor is radiosensitive and will respond briskly, but unlike systemic B-cell lymphoma, the response is not durable. Also, taking into account the fact that the majority of these patients are the elderly, risk for radiation-induced leukoencephalopathy is high. There has been a growing trend of treating patients with chemotherapy to include high-dose methotrexate, the mainstay of treatment for this tumor, and reserving radiotherapy for recurrence. The use of rituxumab has also been found to be effective. The standard dose of radiation, when recommended, is 4500 cGy delivered to the whole brain to include the ventricular system.

STAGING

Grading System for Primary Brain Tumors and Prognosis

There is no formal staging system such as the TNM classification for primary brain tumors. Primary brain tumors are typically locally invasive and do not spread to lymph nodes or distant organs, therefore a TNM classification for these tumors is not relevant.

The pathological grading of primary brain tumors, however, is very important for treatment and prognosis.

The international classification of tumors published by the World Health Organization (WHO) was initiated in 1956 and has been updated for the fourth time in 2007. Its objective has been to create a classification and grading system of human tumors that can be accepted worldwide thus facilitating the international collection of epidemiologic data and clinical trials (1,2). This classification system is extremely important particularly for primary brain tumors since it directs prognosis and therapy. The 2007 WHO classification is focused on genetic data features that define tumor subsets, such as the 1p/19q codeletion in oligodendroglioma. Nevertheless, morphology is still the gold standard for the WHO classification. Astrocytomas that are well differentiated and low grade are classified as grade I (pilocytic)/grade II (diffuse) and comprise 15% to 20 % of all gliomas (Table 23.1). They are characterized by slow growth but can progress to anaplastic astrocytoma or glioblastoma. Anaplastic astrocytomas are classified as grade III and account for 30% to 35% of gliomas. They are characterized by increased cellularity and proliferative activity. Glioblastomas are classified as grade IV and comprise up to 40% to 50% of gliomas. Anaplastic astrocytomas and glioblastomas are frequently referred to as high-grade gliomas.

Low-grade gliomas have a median survival of 5 to 10 years with eventual risk of transformation to high-grade tumors. Prognosis worsens with increasing grade and age. Patients > 40 years of age with low-grade glioma may have a much more aggressive disease with a median survival of < 5 years. Even with standard treatment (surgical resection, radiotherapy, or chemotherapy), median survival for anaplastic astrocytomas is 3 years and only 1 year for glioblastoma.

Features of malignant gliomas that distinguish these tumors from other cancers and pose unique problems for treatment include the blood-brain barrier, which excludes many drugs that may have otherwise been effective; angiogenic edema, which increases tumor interstitial pressure that can reduce the penetration of drugs that do cross the blood-brain barrier; capacity of glioma cells to diffuse widely through the brain making local therapy difficult, including radiotherapy and surgery; heterogeneity of tumor microenvironments that may allow "tumor stem cells" to develop resistance to radiation and chemotherapy; genetic heterogeneity between tumors of different patients as well as within a specific tumor that limits the effectiveness of targeted therapies; and finally, the "immune sanctuary" provided by the brain that aids in tumor evasion of immune surveillance. The development of tumor immunotherapies has therefore been difficult.

Table 23.1 Astrocytoma

Grade	Tumor Type	Glioma %	Median Survival
I/II	Low-grade astrocytoma	15–20	5 years
III	Anaplastic astrocytoma	30–35	3 years
IV	Glioblastoma	40–50	1 year

Oligodendrogliomas are divided into two grades: grade II (well-differentiated oligodendrogliomas) and grade III (anaplastic oligodendrogliomas) (Table 23.2). Oligodendrogliomas account for 2.5% of all primary brain tumors and 5% of gliomas. These percentages, however, are increasing because of new diagnostic criteria, such as the specific molecular deletion of chromosomes 1p and 19q. This tumor has long been of interest to neuropathologists because of its distinctive appearance under the microscope, including small round nuclei with perinuclear halos (conveniently termed the "fried egg appearance"), a fine intricate vascular pattern (described as "chicken wire"), and microscopic calcification. Some tumors may also contain neoplastic astrocytes, resulting in the classification of oligoastrocytoma or mixed glioma. Grading of oligodendrogliomas is based on cellularity, mitotic rate, nuclear atypia, and the presence or absence of vascular proliferation or necrosis. Nevertheless, there was often lack of agreement among neuropathologists on the histologic diagnosis of this tumor, until molecular markers were discovered.

Patients with brain tumors typically present with headache, seizures, nonspecific cognitive or personality changes, or focal neurological deficits. The precise clinical features will depend on the location, histology, and rate of growth of the tumor.

CASE SUMMARIES

High-Grade Astrocytoma/ Glioblastoma Multiforme

J.B. is a 55-year-old woman with no past medical history, who presented to the emergency room with altered mental status, progressive difficulty in walking, and imbalance, slowly worsening over the prior 2 months. A CT scan performed in the emergency room revealed a left temporal-parietal mass with edema and midline shift. The patient was admitted to the hospital. An MRI of the brain with contrast was obtained and showed a 3.8 × 4.5 × 3.8 cm subcortical mass in the left posterior/superior temporal lobe/parietal region with surrounding vasogenic edema

Table 23.2 Oligodendroglioma

Grade	Tumor Type	Median Survival
II	Oligodendroglioma	4–10 years
III	Anaplastic Oligodendroglioma	3–4 years

resulting in marked effacement of the left cerebral sulci and 8-mm left to right midline shift with subfalcine herniation (Figure 23.1). Her neurological examination was remarkable for mild expressive aphasia and right hemiparesis. She was placed on dexamethasone 4 mg every 6 hours, which resulted in improvement in memory and balance. The patient underwent resection of the left temporal parietal mass. Pathology was consistent with Grade IV Glioblastoma Multiforme (GBM). She did very well postoperatively and began concurrent radiotherapy/temozolomide, totaling 6000 cGy of radiation delivered in 180 cGy fractions daily 5 times over 6 weeks. Temzolomide 75 mg/M^2 was prescribed daily for 7 days per week during this time, along with Bactrim 200 mg three times per week as prophylaxis for *Pneumocystis carinii* during this 6-week period. Two weeks after completion of radiotherapy J.B. began adjuvant temozolomide. The first dose was prescribed at 150 mg/M^2 for 5 days, and follow-up complete blood count (CBC) 3 weeks after beginning chemotherapy revealed a normal hemoglobin, platelet count, and WBC count and differential. The second and all following doses of temozolomide were prescribed as 200 mg/M^2 for 5 days every 28 days. J.B. tolerated 18 cycles of temozolomide. Speech and mobility returned to normal, and she continued to perform all activities of daily living and chores. MRI scans of the brain performed every 2 months continued to reveal no recurrence of tumor. CBC with platelet count and differential were checked 3 weeks after day 1 of each round of temozolomide. Several times during the 18-month period, J.B.'s absolute neutrophil count would decrease below 1500/μL, warranting a delay in starting the next dose of temozolomide. A delay of 1 week would allow her to recover and continue treatment.

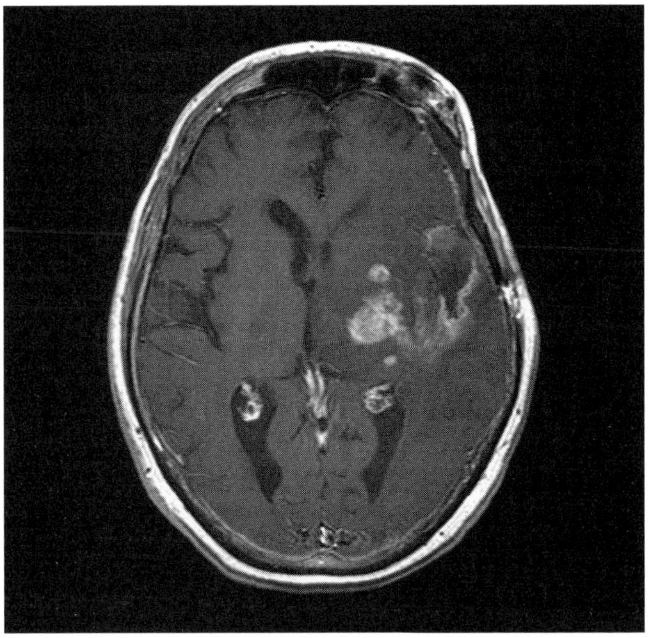

Figure 23.1

T-1 axial contrast-enhanced MRI scan of the brain revealing a large contrast enhancing mass involving the left temporal-parietal lobes as well as the basal ganglia, with edema and midline shift.

After completion of the 18 cycles of temozolomide, MRI scans of the brain were obtained every 4 to 6 months for surveillance. These remained free of disease until 46 months after diagnosis, when an MRI scan revealed a 5-mm contrast enhancing nodule in the posterior aspect of the resection cavity in the left temporal lobe. A follow-up MRI 4 weeks later revealed an increase in size of the lesion to 9 mm. During this time, J.B. remained asymptomatic, without speech problems, headaches, or seizures. She was referred to radiation oncology for consultation as to the possibility of receiving a boost of treatment to this nodule that was in the port of previous radiation. It was decided that she could safely receive 3000 cGy in five fractions over 12 days to this 9-mm lesion. The patient tolerated this treatment well, with the only complaint of fatigue at the end of the day.

A follow-up MRI scan 4 weeks after completion of radiotherapy revealed a much larger area of contrast enhancement with edema and necrotic areas. The patient continued to be asymptomatic at this time. The differential diagnosis for this mass included radiation effect, since this was the site of the previous nodule and stereotactic boost versus rapid tumor regrowth of a radio-resistant lesion. A repeat MRI scan of the brain was planned in 4 weeks, but J.B. presented earlier to the emergency room for evaluation of a seizure. A CT scan of the brain revealed a marked increase in size of the lesion, which now measured 4 cm with surrounding edema. For several days prior to the seizure, J.B.'s husband noted mild right-sided weakness and difficulty with expressive speech. She was admitted to the hospital and a PET scan was obtained. There was marked fludeoxyglucose (FDG) uptake in the region of abnormality on CT. Dexamethasone was prescribed and the patient improved in right limb strength and speech. A neurosurgical consultation was obtained, and J.B. underwent craniotomy with resection of tumor. Pathology was consistent with glioblastoma and treatment-related changes.

Postoperatively the patient did well, with residual weakness in her right extremities on neurological examination and expressive speech difficulties. She underwent rehabilitation and gained the ability to transfer from bed to chair with assistance, and speech therapy was provided. Treatment options at this time were reviewed with the patient, and treatment once again with temozolomide was included, either the previously tolerated 5-day schedule, or dose intense schedule (3 weeks at 75 mg/M^2 and 1 week off treatment in a 28-day cycle), or 150 mg/M^2 for 7 days on and 7 days off. J.B. was also eligible for enrollment in a research trial of temozolomide plus an angiogenesis inhibitor. After discussion of these options with the patient and family, their decision was to proceed with the investigational protocol. Consent was obtained and the patient enrolled in the study. She began treatment with temozolomide at 75 mg/M^2 daily for 21 days, and the experimental agent every morning. After one 4-week cycle, an MRI scan was performed since the patient seemed to be declining further in mobility and speech. The MRI scan of the brain revealed progression of disease in the left temporal lobe, as well as new involvement of the thalamus and brainstem. At this point J.B., was taken off study and bevacizumab 10 mg/M^2 plus BCNU 200 mg/M^2 was administered 4 weeks after study discontinuation. After one course of both agents, neurological function continued to deteriorate and hospice care was offered. The patient expired 4 months after the surgical resection of her recurrent glioblastoma.

Evidence-Based Case Discussion

J.B.'s case is a very typical clinical presentation of a high-grade glioma (GBM). The patient received standard of care treatment that included gross total resection. Pathology was consistent with glioblastoma multiforme. J.B. received postoperative radiotherapy concurrently with temozolomide followed by adjuvant temozolomide that has been shown to improve overall survival compared to radiotherapy alone (see below). J.B. responded very well to standard treatment but relapsed 4 years after her initial diagnosis.

High-grade gliomas represent the largest percentage of primary brain tumors and unfortunately, median survival for high-grade gliomas continues to be very poor. Elderly patients with GBM have an especially poor prognosis, with a median survival of 4 to 6 months. Malignant gliomas have high recurrence rates due to the infiltrative nature of the tumor. Most glioblastomas recur within 18 months of original diagnosis. Recurrent tumors often respond poorly to treatment and survival is often less than 6 months. Most recurrences are local, occurring within 2 cm of the original lesion (3).

Maximal total resection continues to be the overall goal. Resection of >98% of tumor volume has been shown to prolong overall survival in GBM and high-grade astrocytomas (13 months vs. 8.8 months) (4). More recent studies have shown that even 89% reduction of tumor burden can have a positive impact on survival.

External brain radiotherapy is standard of care postoperatively. Alternative dose fractionation schedules have been employed but without additional benefit in malignant gliomas. Other techniques for dose intensification such as hyperfractionation, brachytherapy, and stereotactic radiation boosts have been evaluated but are not superior to external beam XRT (5). There is a small benefit in median survival of 29.1 weeks compared to supportive care alone, 16.9 weeks (*P* = .002) (6).

Early trials in high-grade gliomas employing concurrent chemotherapy/radiotherapy were disappointing. Walker et al. (7) randomized patients to radiotherapy in combination with nitrosurea compared with radiotherapy alone. There was a slight improvement in overall survival; however, this was not statistically significant. In 2001, the largest adjuvant chemotherapy randomized controlled trial was conducted by the Medical Research Council (MRC) for high-grade astrocytomas. Six hundred and seventy four patients were assigned to radiotherapy plus PCV (procarbazine, CCNU, and vincristine) chemotherapy versus radiotherapy alone. Unfortunately, no survival benefit was seen even with the addition of PCV (*P* = .50; HR = 0.95) nor was there improvement in progression-free survival (*P* = 0.46, HR = 0.93) (8).

The European Organization for Research and Treatment of Cancer (EORTC) and National Cancer Institute of Canada (NCIC) then conducted a phase III randomized controlled trial comparing radiotherapy alone (60 Gy over 6 weeks) versus radiotherapy/temozolomide followed by adjuvant temozolomide in 573 newly diagnosed GBM patients. Side effects were well tolerated. Median survival was increased from 12.1 months to 14.6 months, *P* <.0001. Survival rate at 2 years was also improved from 10.4% to 26.5% (9). Temozolomide concurrent with XRT followed by adjuvant temozolomide became the new standard treatment of GBM postoperatively (10).

Post hoc subgroup analysis of these patients showed that patients with O^6-methylguanine-DNA methyltransferase (*MGMT*) gene promoter methylation had significantly improved median survival compared with patients whose tumors had unmethylated *MGMT* promoters (23.4 vs. 15.3 months). The cytotoxic effects of temozolomide were found to be mediated mainly through the methylation of the O6 position of guanine. Epigenetic silencing of *MGMT* via methylation prevented DNA damage caused by temozolomide from being rapidly repaired, which improved efficacy of the medication (9).

Carmustine or BCNU impregnated wafers (prolifspan) have also been found to provide benefit in the treatment of malignant gliomas. A phase III randomized, placebo-controlled trial evaluated 240 patients by implanting biodegradable polymers (either containing carmustine or placebo) into the tumor bed after resection followed by radiotherapy (11). These wafers contained 3.85% carmustine and were designed to release the drug slowly over a 2- to 3-week period after implantation. Median survival was improved from 11.6 to 13.9 months (*P* = .03). Adverse effects were comparable between the two groups, with a higher incidence of intracranial hypertension noted in the prolifspan group.

As shown in Figure 23.2 (algorithm for the initial management of glioblastoma), temozolomide remains the first-line chemotherapy in patients with malignant gliomas. Unfortunately, chemotherapy is not curative and despite treatment, all malignant gliomas eventually

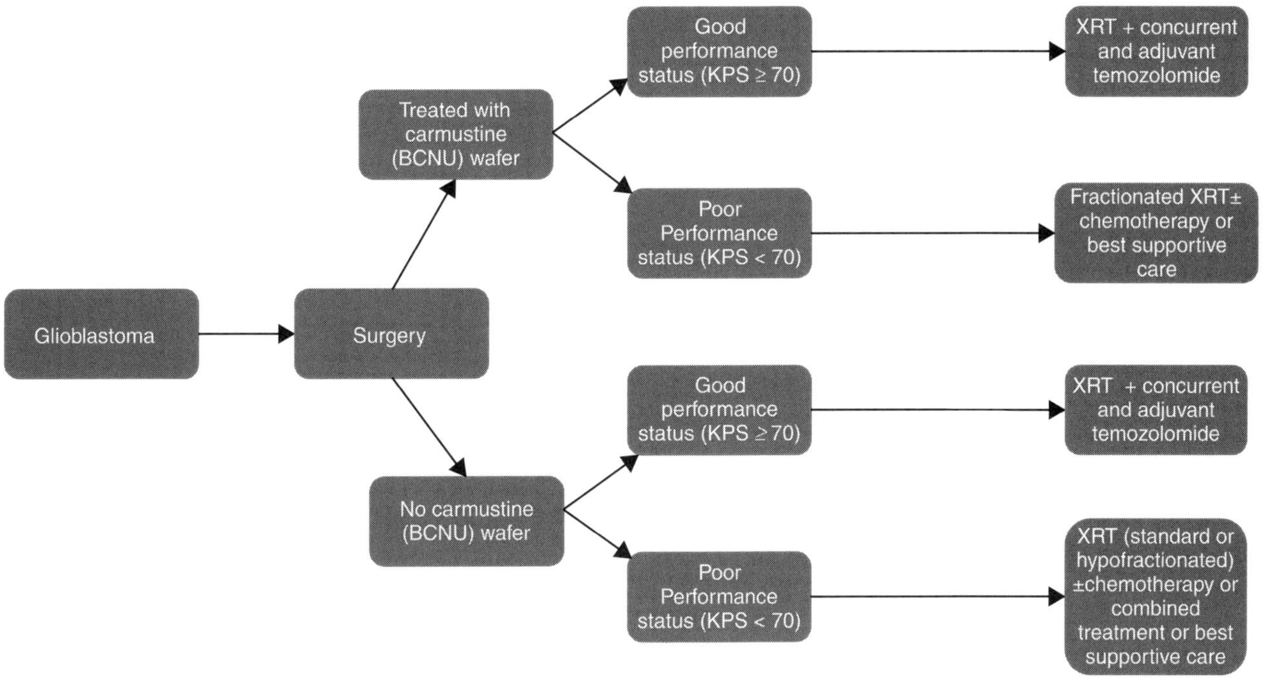

Figure 23.2

Algorithm for the initial management of glioblastomas.

recur. Patients may benefit from evaluation for re-resection. National Comprehensive Cancer Network (NCCN) guidelines recommend BCNU wafer, bevacizumab, systemic chemotherapy, clinical trials, or supportive care as reasonable options for recurrent high-grade gliomas that are not surgically resectable.

Data for second-line chemotherapy using systemic agents such as irinotecan, cisplatin, and etoposide agents have been disappointing with low response rates. There is growing popularity for the use of targeted agents in recurrent GBM (12).

A high percentage of GBM tumors have been found to express vascular endothelial growth factor (VEGF), which stimulates tumor angiogenesis and is associated with a poor prognosis. Bevacizumab is a humanized immunoglobulin IgG1 monoclonal antibody that inhibits the activity of VEGF. An initial phase II study (13) enrolled 35 patients who had experienced disease progression after radiotherapy/concurrent temozolomide to receive bevacizumab/irinotecan. Six-month progression-free survival was 46% with a median progression-free survival of 24 weeks. Six-month overall survival was 77% and median overall survival was 42 weeks. Out of the 35 patients, 20 (i.e., 57%) had at least a partial response, whereas 11 patients had to discontinue therapy due to toxicity. Only one patient developed CNS hemorrhage (in the tenth cycle) whereas four patients had thromboembolic events (13). In 2010, the Food and Drug Administration (FDA) approved the use of bevacizumab in patients with recurrent GBM.

Another recently approved therapy for recurrent glioblastoma is the NovoTTF-100Af, which received approval by the FDA on April 15, 2011. The treatment will be available during the fourth quarter of 2011. This device is a novel, noninvasive alternative to chemotherapy that has been shown in clinical trials to be safe and effective. It is a portable, wearable device that delivers low intensity, intermediate frequency electric fields (tumor treatment fields or ttf), which inhibit the replication of tumor cells. Nonproliferating cells and tissues are not affected. These electrical treatment fields disrupt the normal polymerization-depolymerization process of microtubules during mitosis. A 237 patient randomized pivotal trial demonstrated that patients who failed standard radiation and chemotherapy had a comparable median overall survival with fewer side effects and improved quality-of-life scores (14). The rate of progression-free survival at 6 months was 21% in the NovoTTF group and 15% in the chemotherapy group. The device, which weighs 6 pounds, is worn throughout the day by the patient.

Enrollment in clinical trials is also an option for patients with newly diagnosed glioblastoma or recurrent tumor. The roles of targeted therapy and immunotherapy are being explored in this venue.

Anaplastic Astrocytoma

M.F. is a 47-year-old man who had been noting increasing occurrence of left-sided headaches over a 4-month period of time. They gradually worsened in severity to the point of not responding to over-the-counter medications. The patient's family noted that he had difficulty with speech and word finding. His memory had also declined. The patient presented to the emergency room where an MRI scan of the brain revealed a left temporal lobe mass (Figure 23.3). The patient had no past medical history and was taking no medications at the time of diagnosis. He did not smoke or use alcohol. Family history was negative for brain tumors, but positive for an uncle with prostate cancer. Review of systems was entirely negative. He was admitted to the hospital and treatment with dexamethasone 4 mg every 6 hours was begun. M.F. was then noted to have improvement in speech and memory. The patient underwent craniotomy and resection of tumor. Pathology revealed an anaplastic (grade III) astrocytoma. The patient recovered fluent speech and mentation improved postoperatively.

Two weeks after surgery M.F. began intensity modulated radiotherapy (IMRT), to the tumor bed. He also began chemotherapy with temozolomide daily at a dose of 75 mg/M^2. These treatments were completed in 42 days, and a total of 6000 cGy was delivered. Two weeks following completion of radiation, M.F. began treatment with temozolomide on the fifth day of every 28-day regimen. He tolerated treatment very well, with minimal nausea, and no myelosuppression. MRI scans of the brain with and without gadolinium were obtained 4 weeks after the completion of radiotherapy and every 2 months thereafter. Subtle changes were noted approximately 6 months postoperatively that were worrisome for tumor progression. A perfusion sequence was added to his MRI study and this revealed no increase in blood volume in the region. Meanwhile M.F. continued to feel well, his speech returned to normal, and he continued to work full time. After 18 months of temozolomide treatments, and continued stable MRI scans, chemotherapy was stopped. Surveillance MRI scans then were scheduled for every 3 to 4 months and ultimately every 6 months. The patient continues to work full time and has a normal neurological examination 5 years after the original diagnosis.

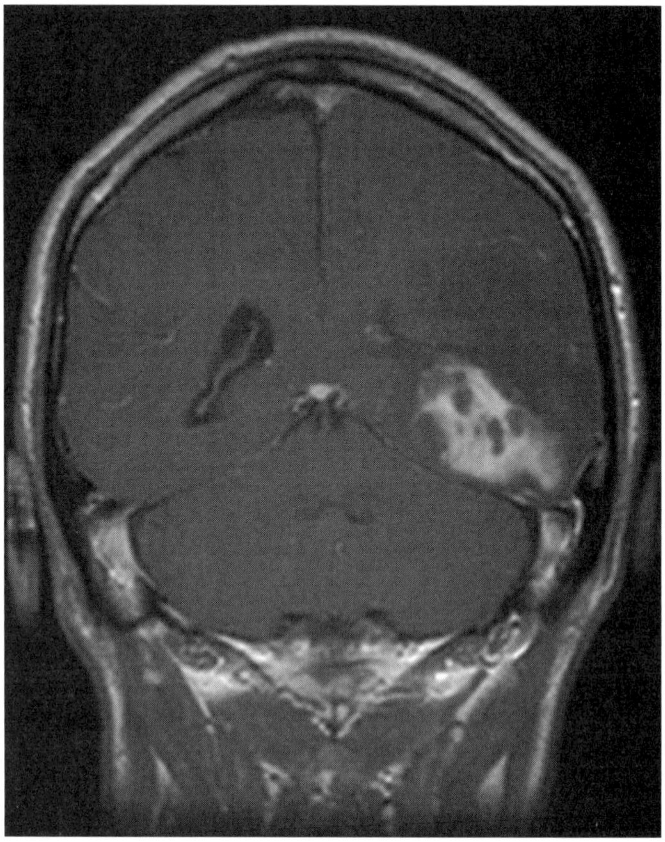

Figure 23.3

T-1 coronal enhanced MRI scan of the brain depicting a left temporal lobe cystic enhancing mass with surrounding edema.

Evidence-Based Case Discussion

M.F. presents as a typical case of dominant hemisphere tumor involvement with deterioration in expressive language on a background of several months of increasing headache. Anaplastic astrocytoma constitutes 8.3% of all CNS gliomas. The 5-year survival rate is poor at 28%. The mean age at the time of diagnosis is 41 years with a slight male predominance of 1.8 to 1.0 females. MRI is the diagnostic imaging tool of choice and usually presents a T-1 hypointense and T-2 hyperintense mass. Partial or heterogeneous enhancement may occur, lacking the ring enhancement/necrotic pattern seen often in glioblastoma. Anaplastic astrocytoma is characterized by increased cellularity, nuclear atypia, and increased mitotic activity.

M.F. received standard of care surgery with maximal resection as could safely be performed in the left temporal lobe. Maximal surgical resection is important, when possible, for bulk reduction of tumor mass and improvement in neurological function, adequate tissue sampling for pathological assessment, and cytoreduction to improve outcome. Intraoperative ultrasonography and image guided systems have influenced the safety with which maximal tumor volume can be resected without damaging important brain structures. Awake craniotomies and cortical mapping with somatosensory-evoked potentials are also useful tools for aggressive removal of tumor involving eloquent brain tissue. This technique highlights the area of cerebral cortex involved in speech, and the entire speech pathway can be outlined to aid the surgeon in his resection. Maximal surgical resection is important also for histological grading, since these tumors may present low-grade features in one portion and high-grade features in another portion of the same mass, therefore risking an inaccurate diagnosis with biopsy alone.

After surgery, M.F. went on to receive radiotherapy. In the history of treatment for high-grade gliomas, external beam radiation has been a cornerstone. Randomized trials in the 1970s and 1980s using whole brain radiation revealed an increase in survival from 5 months to 9 months (7). Involved field radiotherapy involving the T-2 weighted imaging abnormality and an additional 1- to 2-cm margin has replaced whole brain radiotherapy because it carries equivalent efficacy and less neurotoxicity. Conformal radiation fields have been estimated to reduce the dose of radiation to normal brain by 50%. Standard practice is to deliver 58 to 60 Gy in 1.8 to 2.0 Gy fractions administered 5 days per week for 30 to 35 fractions (5). Trials of radiosensitizers, such as hydroxyurea, misonidazole, carboplatin, and etoposide have added no benefit to survival. Brachytherapy (the implantation of radioactive sources, such as I-125, iridium-192, and gold-198) and stereotactic radiotherapy are other options for patients with recurrent anaplastic astrocytoma. However, there have been no randomized controlled trials to evaluate these techniques. A small trial of patients with recurrent anaplastic astrocytoma found that with stereotactic radiosurgery, time to progression averaged 4 to 7 months and median survival was 31 months. Other complications of both of these procedures include corticosteroid dependence and risk of symptomatic radiation-induced necrosis requiring further surgery. The risk of radiation-induced necrosis for recurrent malignant gliomas is reported as 6% to 14%, and following brachytherapy it is as high as 26% to 64% (15).

The first study to address the effect of chemotherapy in anaplastic astrocytoma was reported in 1978 and included 222 subjects in a four-arm randomized trial. Patients received radiation at doses of 50 to 60 Gy. The arms of the study consisted of best supportive care, radiotherapy alone, BCNU alone, and the combination of BCNU plus radiation. In each arm, patients received maximal surgical debulking. The combined group had an overall survival of 34.5 weeks, whereas the radiation-alone group had an overall survival of 35 weeks with less toxicity. From then on, radiation alone has been the standard treatment for anaplastic astrocytoma (16). Nevertheless, chemotherapy continued to be evaluated, and a phase III trial reported by Levin et al., in 1980, randomized patients with anaplastic astrocytoma and glioblastoma to receive either procarbazine, CCNU, and vincristine (PCV) or BCNU after standard radiotherapy. Overall survival was improved in both groups, but statistically so in the anaplastic astrocytoma cohort treated with PCV; 82 weeks versus 57 weeks in the BCNU arm (17). PCV then became the standard therapy for anaplastic astrocytoma.

Other investigators have explored the potential benefit of concomitant radiosensitizers such as BUdR (bromodeoxyuridine) an analogue of thymidine, or hydroxyurea in the treatment of newly diagnosed anaplastic astrocytomas. Radiation Therapy Oncology Group (RTOG) 94–04 was a randomized phase III study published in 1999, comparing radiation therapy with or without BUdR followed by adjuvant PCV (18). There was no added benefit in overall survival with the addition of BUdR to radiation therapy. Another RTOG trial (RTOG 98–13) randomized patients to radiotherapy (59.4 Gy in 33 fractions) concurrently with BCNU or CCNU versus temozolomide. The trial did not meet accrual goals and closed early (19).

Given the conflicting results of individual clinical trials, the impact of chemotherapy on outcomes in anaplastic astrocytoma has been evaluated in several meta-analyses. One such meta-analysis retrospectively reviewed 432 patients who had been treated on four RTOG protocols comparing BCNU versus PCV as adjuvant chemotherapy (20). There was no added benefit to overall survival, again questioning the results of the earlier phase III trial (18). Another meta-analysis reviewed 16 randomized control studies and revealed an estimated overall survival increase of 10% at 1 year and 9% at 2 years (21). For these reasons, the addition of adjuvant chemotherapy in the treatment of anaplastic astrocytoma remains controversial.

Temozolomide has been evaluated in the setting of recurrent anaplastic astrocytoma and in fact the drug was first approved by the FDA for this indication. A multicenter phase II trial enrolled 162 patients, of whom 111 were eligible. The primary endpoint for this trial, progression-free survival at 6 months, was 46%. Median progression-free survival was 5.4 months and median overall survival was 13.6 months (22). Because of a favorable toxicity profile as compared to PCV, temozolomide became the standard of care for recurrent anaplastic astrocytoma. Over the years following this study, trials in glioblastoma began to report the efficacy of temozolomide, and neuro-oncologists became familiar with the side-effect profile. Because of the toxicity of the PCV regimen, temozolomide became a more attractive alternative for use in *newly* diagnosed anaplastic astrocytoma. See Figure 23.4 for an algorithm for the management of patients with anaplastic astrocytoma.

A current ongoing trial, RTOG 0834, has been designed to shed light on these important issues. This study will determine whether concurrent and adjuvant temozolomide improves the outcome of patients with intact 1p,19q anaplastic gliomas. Patients are randomized to radiotherapy, radiotherapy with concomitant temozolomide, radiotherapy followed by adjuvant temozolomide, and radiotherapy with concurrent temozolomide followed by adjuvant temozolomide. Patients will be stratified for MGMT status as well. The primary objectives of this trial are to determine whether concomitant daily temozolomide with radiotherapy improves progression-free survival in this tumor compared to radiotherapy alone and to determine whether adjuvant temozolomide improves overall survival as compared to radiotherapy alone. Secondary objectives will assess whether the addition of temozolomide prolongs progression-free survival in patients with intact 1p, 19q anaplastic astrocytoma, as well as assess

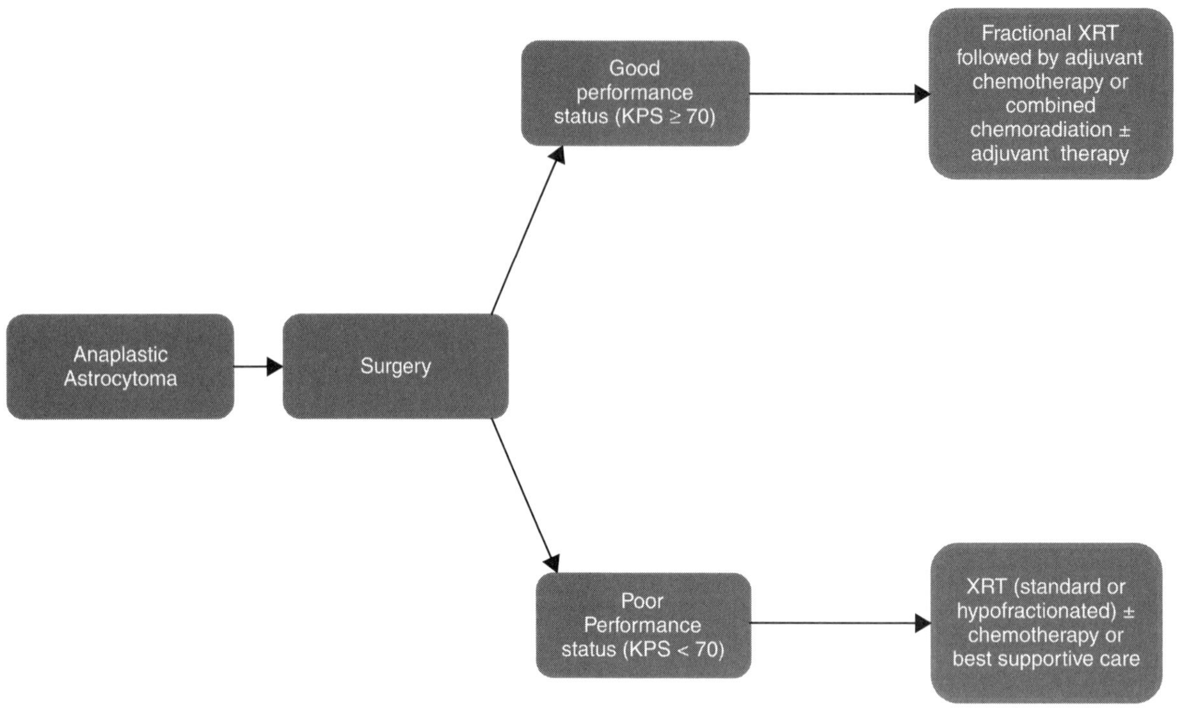

Figure 23.4

Algorithm for the management of anaplastic astrocytomas.

safety including long-term effects on cognition as well as quality of life.

Oligodendroglioma

N.H. is a 34-year-old woman who presented with a sensation of transient numbness in the left toe, which gradually progressed over 2 months to involve her left foot and entire left leg. These symptoms developed during her exercise routine in the sport of kickboxing and would then dissipate. At first, she felt that it was a pinched nerve. Finally the spells occurred while cleaning at home and involved shaking of her left leg. The patient presented to the emergency room where a CT scan was performed and revealed a right posterior parietal mass. An MRI scan with contrast revealed the mass to be nonenhancing (Figure 23.5). With initiation of the anticonvulsant, levetiracetam, the spells of lower extremity numbness resolved. Because of the location of the mass, the patient underwent biopsy, which revealed a low-grade oligodendroglioma. The genetic test for 1p, 19q heterozygocity was performed on the sample and codeletion was reported.

N.H. had a negative past medical history. Her social history was negative for tobacco or alcohol use. Her family history was significant for a maternal grandfather and several uncles who were diagnosed with prostate cancer. Her physical examination was entirely normal as was the neurological examination. The patient had normal speech and language, full strength, normal coordination, and sensory exam.

N.H. went on to treatment with temozolomide at 200 mg/M^2 daily for 5 days every 28 days. She completed a total of 18 courses of treatment. Treatment was well tolerated with an occasional delay of 1 week for myelosuppression. MRI scans performed every 3 months revealed stable disease. N.H. is working full time and has no neurological symptoms or signs, at 3.5 years postdiagnosis. She has had several sensory symptoms reminiscent of her original presentation over the years when engaged in vigorous workout. She remains on an anticonvulsant. Neurologic evaluation remains normal and Karnofsky performance status (KPS) is 100%.

Evidence-Based Case Discussion

N.H.'s case is a very typical clinical presentation of a low-grade oligodendroglioma, presenting with focal seizures, which were sensory in nature. Because of the location of the tumor, the surgeon chose to biopsy only. Surgical excision is the first line of therapy when this can be done without causing neurological deficit. The decision to proceed with radiotherapy versus chemotherapy may depend on the size of the tumor and the patient's performance status.

Radiotherapy was the mainstay of treatment for this tumor until the late 1980s, when investigators noted that

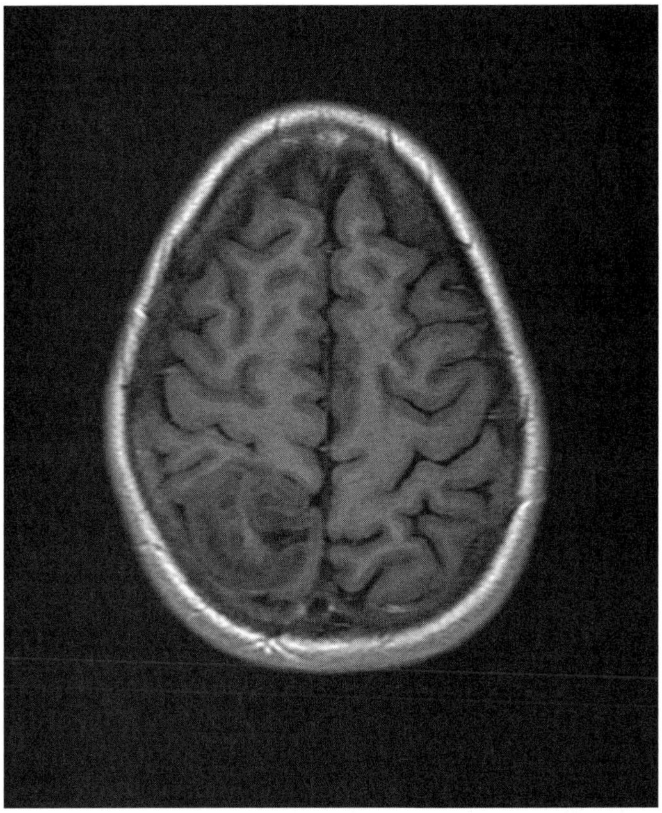

Figure 23.5

T-1 axial contrast-enhanced MRI scan revealing a large right posterior parietal nonenhancing mass with mild associated edema.

patients with anaplastic oligodendrogliomas responded to the multidrug regimen PCV (procarbazine, lomustine or CCNU, and vincristine). During the next decade, researchers acquired data on survival time when this drug regimen was added to radiotherapy. Interest peaked again when certain molecular subtypes were discovered, with different natural histories and responses to treatment. Durable responses to PCV and longer overall survival were found to correlate with simultaneous loss of the entire short arm of chromosome 1 (1p) and the entire long arm of chromosome 19 (19q) (23). In the initial study, all patients with the codeletion responded to PCV, and of those with intact 1p, 19q alleles, only 25% responded. Patients with intact alleles had a 5.7 times greater risk of recurrence or death after PCV. This codeletion of 1p, 19q is not often seen in other gliomas or cancers and is the earliest known molecular alteration in oligodendrogliomas, a molecular signature for these tumors. Up to 70% of oligodendrogliomas in adults have the codeletion. This tumor is rare in children and codeletion of 1p, 19q is uncommon when the tumor does occur in the pediatric population. In the mixed oligoastrocytic variant, the detection of 1p, 19q codeletion is less frequent. Other genetic alterations in low-grade oligodendrogliomas include overexpression of platelet-derived growth factor or receptor, epidermal growth factor receptor, or VEGF. Anaplastic tumors may have CDK4 or *MYC* amplification. These alterations occur in astrocytomas as well. A strong correlation has been observed between 1p, 19q codeletion and O^6 methylguanine-DNA methyltransferase (*MGMT*) gene silencing by promoter methylation (24). Whereas radiotherapy has demonstrated benefit in improving local control and survival (25), because of the chemosensitivity of these tumors, delay in radiotherapy has become a common practice, especially in patients with a good performance status. The original correlation of 1p, 19q LOH with treatment response was observed in patients treated with PCV. Further studies have shown that this susceptibility also includes temozolomide (81% response rate) that carries less toxicity than PCV (26). The NCCN recommends that in completely resected low-grade oligodendrogliomas, postoperative radiotherapy can be administered upfront or delayed. The use of front-line chemotherapy is still not definitive in oligodendrogliomas. Chemotherapy is recommended as a NCCN Category 2B recommendation in patients with stable controlled symptoms and good performance status.

Accordingly, the management of newly diagnosed low-grade oligodendroglioma, with codeletion of 1p, 19q, following gross total resection, would involve observation versus treatment with temozolomide for one year (Figure 23.6). If partially resected, treatment with temozolomide versus radiotherapy is acceptable. In the recurrent setting, resection is recommended if possible, followed by chemotherapy (temozolomide or PCV) or radiotherapy if not previously delivered. In patients with intact 1p, 19q status, a gross total resection would again allow for observation or chemotherapy/radiation. If partially resected, chemotherapy or radiotherapy and close observation are warranted. As in all patients with malignant primary brain tumors, decisions for therapy will rely on patient's age, performance status, location of tumor, as well as the molecular characteristics.

The chemosensitivity of oligodendroglial tumors has made upfront chemotherapy strategies popular, with the rationale to defer radiotherapy with its known impact on cognitive skills. The molecular characteristic of 1p/19q codeletion and the mechanisms by which these tumors are sensitive to chemotherapy and radiotherapy is unknown. Nevertheless, molecular signature tends to be the most important prognostic factor for survival and will direct therapy and impact all future trials of this tumor.

In recurrent low-grade oligodendroglioma, the 1p, 19q status is usually retained. However, in the salvage setting, response to temozolomide falls to 10% to 20%, even in the group with 1p, 19q deletions (24). Twenty percent of low-grade oligodendroglioma tumors may recur as the anaplastic variant. In the setting of recurrent oligodendrogliomas, NCCN guidelines recommend surgery for possible resection. In unresectable lesions, radiotherapy

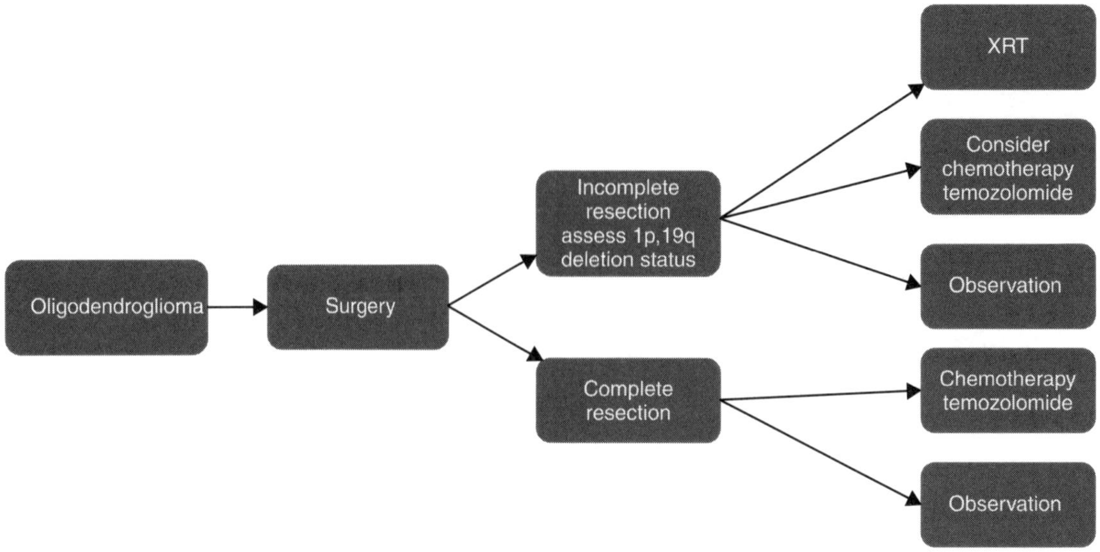

Figure 23.6

Algorithm for the management of oligodendrogliomas.

can be administered if none was administered previously. Chemotherapy would be a reasonable option if patients previously had radiotherapy alone (26). Options include temozolomide if not recently prescribed, PCV, carboplatin, and etoposide.

Patients with anaplastic (grade III) oligodendrogliomas with losses of chromosome 1p and 19q have also been found to be chemosensitive. In the 1990s, the RTOG and the EORTC conducted clinical trials of PCV plus radiotherapy versus radiotherapy alone for pure and mixed oligodendrogliomas (27,28). Both studies attempted to answer the question of whether the addition of PCV chemotherapy to radiotherapy could further impact survival in these patients. The results for both trials were identical. The addition of PCV to radiation at the time of diagnosis significantly prolonged progression-free survival, had no effect on overall survival, and was associated with greater toxicity than radiation alone. Both groups assessed the status of 1p, 19q LOH. Codeletion was noted in 46% of tumor samples in the RTOG study and 25% in the EORTC study. In both trials, codeletion was associated with longer progression-free and overall survival. However, survival was similar for those treated with PCV plus radiotherapy and radiotherapy alone regardless of deletion status in the EORTC trial. In the RTOG trial, longer progression-free survival was observed in those patients treated with combined modalities, but only in the subset of codeleted tumors. In both studies, patients who failed radiotherapy and then received PCV experienced a longer progression-free survival without longer overall survival. The conclusion of both trials was that the addition of early PCV to radiotherapy in oligodendroglioma is not superior to radiotherapy followed by chemotherapy at the time of recurrence. These results will shape future trials of oligodendroglioma and focus on the need for molecular stratification.

Options for these tumors in the recurrent setting would include reoperation, treatment with chemotherapy, such as temozolomide, if not previously delivered, PCV, or carboplatin/etoposide. Consultation to radiotherapy for a boost to the tumor bed is also an option.

REFERENCES

1. Louis D, Ohgaki H, Wiestler O, et al. The 2007 WHO classification of tumours of the central nervous system. *Acta Neuropathol.* 2007;(114):97–109.
2. Rousseau A, Mokhtari K, Duyckaerts C. The 2007 WHO classification of tumors of the central nervous system—what has changed? *Curr Opin Neurol.* 2008;21(6):720–727.
3. Clarke J, Butowski N, Chang S. Recent advances in therapy for glioblastoma. *Arch Neurol.* 2010;67(3):279–283.
4. Lacroix M, Abi-Said D, Fourney D, et al. A multivariate analysis of 416 patients with glioblastoma multiforme: prognosis, extent of resection, and survival. *J Neurosurg.* 2001;95:190–198.
5. Narayana A, Yamada J, Berry S, et al. Intensity-modulated radiotherapy in high-grade gliomas: clinical and dosimetric results. *Int J Radiat Oncol Biol Phys.* 2006;64(3):892–897.
6. Keime-Guibert F, Chinot O, et al. Radiotherapy for glioblastoma in the elderly. *NEJM* 2007;(356):1527–1535.
7. Walker M, Green S, Bayar D, et al. Randomized comparison of radiotherapy and nitrosureas for the treatment of malignant glioma after surgery. *NEJM.* 1980;(303):1323–1329.
8. Medical Research Council Brain Tumor Working Party. Randomized trial of procarbazine, lomustine, and vincristine in the adjuvant treatment of high-grade astrocytoma: a Medical Research Council Trial. *J Clin Oncol.* 2001;(19):509–518.
9. Stupp R, Hegi M, Mason W, et al. Effects of radiotherapy with comcomitant and adjuvant temozolomide versus radiotherapy alone on survival in glioblastoma in randomized phase III

study: 5-year analysis of the EORTC-NCIC trial. *Lancet Oncol.* 2009;10(5):459–466.
10. Stupp R, Mason W, Van den Bent M, et al. Radiotherapy plus comcomitant and adjuvant temozolomide for glioblastoma. *NEJM.* 2005;(352):987–996.
11. Westphal M, Hilt D, Bortey E, et al. A phase III trial of local chemotherapy with biodegradable carmustine (BCNU) wafers (Gliadel wafers) in patients with primary malignant glioma. *Neuro Oncol.* 2003;(5);79–88.
12. Wen P, Kesari S. Malignant gliomas in adults. *NEJM.* 2008;(359): 500–508.
13. Vredenburgh J, Desjardins A, Herndon J, et al. Bevacizumab plus irinotecan in recurrent glioblastoma multiforme. *J Clin Oncol.* 2007;(25):4722–4729.
14. Stupp R, Kanner A, Engelhard H, et al. A prospective, randomized, open-label, phase III clinical trial of NovoTTF-100A versus best standard of care chemotherapy in patients with recurrent glioblastoma [abstract]. Proc ASCO. *J Clin Oncol.* 2010;(28):LBA2007.
15. Laperriere N, Leung P, McKenzie S, et al. Randomized study of brachytherapy in the initial management of patients with malignant astrocytoma. *Int J Radiat Oncol Biol Phys.* 1998;(41): 1005–1011.
16. Walker M, Alexander E Jr., Hunt W, et al. Evaluation of BCNU and/or radiotherapy in the treatment of anaplastic gliomas. A cooperative clinical trial. *J Neurosurg.* 1978;(49):333–343.
17. Levin V, Silver P, Hanningan J, et al. Superiority of post-radiotherapy adjuvant chemotherapy with CCNU, procarbazine, and vincristine (PCV) over BCNU for anaplastic gliomas: NCOG 6G61 Final Report. *Int J Rad Oncol Bio Phys.* 1980;(8):321–332.
18. Prados M, Scott C, Sandler H, et al. A phase 3 randomized study of radiotherapy plus procarbazine, CCNU, vincristine (PCV) with or without BUdR for the treatment of anaplastic astrocytoma: A preliminary report of RTOG 9404. *Int J Radiat Oncol Biol Phys.*1999;(45):1109–1115.
19. Chang S, Cairncross G, Gilbert MR, et al. Radiation Therapy Oncology Group RTOG 98-13: A Phase III (Phase I Closed) randomized study of radiation therapy and temozolomide (IND#60,26) vs. radiation therapy and nitrosurea for anaplastic astrocytoma and mixed anaplastic oligoastrocytoma (astrocytoma dominant). ClinicalTrials.gov NCT00004259.
20. Prados M, Scott C, Curran W Jr., et al. Procarbazine, lomustine, and vincristine (PCV) chemotherapy for anaplastic astrocytoma: A retrospective review of radiation therapy oncology group protocols comparing survival with carmustine or PCV adjuvant chemotherapy. *J Clin Oncol.* 1999;(17):3389–3395.
21. Fine H, Dear K, Loeffler J, et al. Meta-analysis of radiation therapy with and without adjuvant chemotherapy for malignant gliomas in adults. *Cancer.* 1993;(71):2585–2597.
22. Yung W, Prados M, Yaya-Tur R, et al. Multicenter Phase II trial of temozolomide in patients with anaplastic astrocytoma or anaplastic oligoastrocytoma at first relapse. *J Clin Oncol.* 1999;(17)9:2762–2771.
23. Jenkins R, Curran W, Scott C, et al. Pilot evaluation of 1p and 19q deletions in anaplastic oligodendroglioma collected by a national cooperative cancer treatment group. *Am J Clin Oncol.* 2001;24(5):506–508.
24. Bromberg JE, Van den Bent MJ. Oligodendrogliomas: molecular biology and treatment. *Oncologist.* 2009;14:155–163.
25. Yeh S, Lee T, Chen H, et al. Treatment outcomes and prognostic factors of patients with supratentorial low-grade oligodendrogliomas. *Int J Radiat Oncol Biol Phys.* 2002;(54):1405–1409.
26. Kouwenhoven M, Kros J, French P, et al. 1p/19q loss within oligodendroglioma is predictive for response to first line temozolomide but not to salvage treatment. *Eur J Cancer.* 2006;(42): 2499–2503.
27. Cairncross G, Berkey B, Shaw E, et al. Phase III trial of chemotherapy plus radiotherapy compared with radiotherapy alone for pure and mixed anaplastic oligodendroglioma: Intergroup Radiation Therapy Oncology Group Trial 9402. *J Clin Oncol.* 2006;(24):2707–2714.
28. Van den Bent M, Carpentier A, Brandes A, et al. Adjuvant procarbazine, lomustine, and vincristine improves progression-free survival but not overall survival in newly diagnosed anaplastic astrocytomas and oligoastrocytomas: a randomized European Organization for Research and Treatment of Cancer Phase III trial. *J Clin Oncol.* 2006;24:2715–2722.

24

Cancer of Unknown Primary

YUVAL RAIZEN AND GERALD S. CYPRUS

EPIDEMIOLOGY, RISK FACTORS, NATURAL HISTORY, AND PATHOLOGY

The overall incidence of patients with cancer of unknown primary is difficult to accurately predict because of the variability in patient presentation as well as frequent classification of tumors as specific other diagnoses. On the basis of the statistics reported by the Surveillance, Epidemiology, and End Results (SEER) registries between 1973 and 1987, cancers of unknown primary account for about 2% of all cancer diagnoses. Jemal et al. report an incidence of 30,680 new cases of "other and unspecified primary sites" in the United States between 1995 and 2006. Similar to the data from the SEER registries, this accounts for 2% of all cancers diagnosed during this time period, with a very slight predominance in males. In this report, 7.7% of all cancer deaths were attributed to cancer of unknown primary (1). In other studies, the incidence was as high as 7%. This entity has been reported to be among the top ten most common cancer diagnoses worldwide. Based on pooled epidemiological data from various countries using a number of registries such as the SEER registry, the International Agency for Research into Cancer (IARC), as well as local registries from Australia, Netherlands, Germany, Russia, and Switzerland, Pavlidis et al. noted an overall frequency of 2.3% to 7.8%, as shown in Table 24.1 (2).

The median age at presentation is approximately 60 years. It is infrequently seen in children, accounting for less than 1% of cancer diagnoses, with those rare cases being mostly embryonal malignancies (such as small round blue cell tumors). There have not been any risk factors identified as an etiology for the development of cancer of unknown primary. The median overall survival in patients with carcinoma of unknown primary is reported to be between 4 and 9 months.

These tumors are often characterized by an aggressive nature and poor overall prognosis. Multiple metastatic sites are frequently observed due to early dissemination. As opposed to common metastatic patterns seen in known primary solid tumors, the pattern of metastasis is frequently unpredictable. An example of this difference is the frequency of bone metastases in patients with lung cancer presenting as cancer of unknown primary (CUP) (4%) compared with those presenting as a known lung cancer primary (30–50%) (2). Almost 30% of patients with CUP present with metastases in more than one location. Metastases are seen in liver in 24%, lung or pleura in 12%, lymph nodes in 11%, peritoneum in 9%, bone in 8%, brain in 2%, and other sites in 8%.

Evaluation of the tumor using light microscopy with hematoxylin and eosin (H&E) staining is often not sufficient to classify the histological subtype. Use of specialized pathological studies including immunohistochemical (IHC) markers, tumor markers, and specific cytogenetic alterations may assist in further classification. Various imaging modalities are also being used with increased frequency to narrow the differential diagnosis. According to a 1982 study by Neumann and Nystrom, the primary site may not be identified even in a postmortem examination in up to 20% to 50% of cases (3). In a more recent review of previously published autopsy studies (as well as studies using microarray technology) a primary site was identified in 73% of the cases. Among the sites identified, the reported relative frequencies by Pentheroudakis et al. were 27% lung, 19% pancreas, 11% bowel, 6% kidney/adrenals, 6% hepatobiliary, 5% gastric, 3% ovary/uterus, 2% prostate, and 21% "other," as seen in Figure 24.1 (4). Notably breast was noted to be the primary site with an incidence of <1%.

There is no clear evidence suggesting that cancers of unknown primary are distinct phenomena with unique

Table 24.1 Epidemiology of Cancer of Unknown Primary*

Geographical Area	Source	Frequency (%)	Period
USA	SEER	2.3	1973–1987
Australia	New South Wales Registry	4.2	1970–1990
Netherlands (Southeast)	Eindhoven Cancer Registry	4.0	1984–1992
Finland	IARC	2.5	—
Germany	—	7.8	1968–1984
Russia (Dniepropetrovsk region)	—	3.6	—
Switzerland (Vaud and Neuchâtel Cantons)	Local registries	2.3	1984–1993
Japan	IARC	3.0	—

SEER, Surveillance, Epidemiology, End Results; IARC, International Agency for Research Into Cancer

*Adapted with permission from Pavlidis et al. (2).

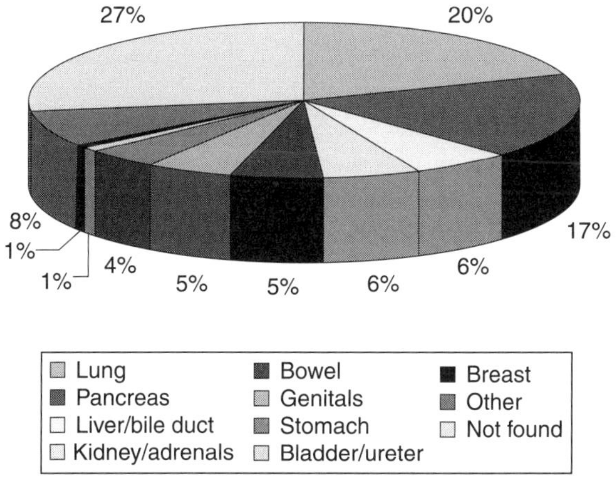

Figure 24.1

Distribution of sites of origin in cancer of unknown primary. Used with permission from Pentheroudakis et al. (4). (see color insert)

alterations in genetics and phenotypic expression. Thus far no consistent abnormalities have been identified that are common between different cancers of unknown primary. There is also no evidence that there are genetic differences between these tumors, which tend to have an atypical metastatic pattern, and those tumors with metastases from a known primary site. An area of interest is in the explanation of why the primary is not identifiable and several hypotheses have been proposed (5). These include involution or regression of the primary after the metastasis occurs. Some tumors may have arisen from fully differentiated embryonic epithelial cells that did not complete their migration in utero, thus presenting as a "metastatic" lesion. Alternatively, the primary neoplasm remains unrecognized because of its small size or location (obscured by surrounding tissue). A sequence of genetic events during carcinogenesis supports metastatic but not local growth (6). Finally, cancers of unknown primary may arise from yet undifferentiated pluripotent cells, which remain present in postnatal life, and display an ability to differentiate into multiple lineages (5).

STAGING

Whereas other tumors are customarily staged using systems such as the World Health Organization, cancers of unknown primary are by definition metastatic and are therefore not assigned a staging system. The challenge in assigning a staging system to cancers of unknown primary lies in the previously mentioned heterogeneity of the diseases with wide range of histopathology. For purposes of this chapter as well as clinical practice, cancers of unknown primary are considered metastatic by definition.

CASE SUMMARIES

Pathologic Evaluation and Role of Immunohistochemistry

J.H., a 52-year-old man with a history of hypertension, presented to his primary care physician with a 3-month history of vague abdominal pain associated with a 15-pound weight loss. Prior to this he had been healthy, only taking antihypertensive medication. He complained of early satiety with occasional nausea and nonbilious, nonbloody emesis, but normal bowel movements. He had an unremarkable colonoscopy at age 50. J.H.'s mother had breast cancer in her 60, but his family was otherwise healthy. He denied smoking or drug use, and drank alcohol socially. His lifestyle had been active and he worked as a restaurant manager. His physical examination revealed a soft but tender abdomen, mostly in the right upper quadrant, with palpable hepatomegaly of 17 cm. Laboratory studies showed a mild normocytic anemia, moderate hypoalbuminemia, and elevated AST and ALT. HIV and hepatitis tests were negative. A chest x-ray was unremarkable. Right upper quadrant ultrasound showed a number of masses in the liver with hepatomegaly. A CT of the chest, abdomen, and pelvis revealed six discrete masses in the enlarged liver, the largest measuring 3.3 cm. A number of enlarged retroperitoneal and perihepatic nodes were noted as well. Percutaneous CT-guided biopsy of one of the hepatic masses was performed, with pathology showing adenocarcinoma, with no further characterization or site of origin. Upper endoscopy and colonoscopy did not reveal any masses and were mostly unremarkable. An immunohistochemistry panel showed that the tumor was CK7-negative and CK20-positive, as well as CDX-2 positive. With this information, he was offered chemotherapy targeted at treating metastatic adenocarcinoma of colon origin.

Evidence-Based Case Discussion

Initial Pathologic Evaluation

The case of J.H. highlights the importance of the pathologic evaluation of unknown cancer, as well as the role of immunohistochemistry in determining the tissue site of origin. A stepwise approach, as described by Oien, can help direct this process (7).

Cancer of unknown primary is classified into a number of histological groups, with about 50% to 60% being classified as well- to moderately differentiated adenocarcinomas. Approximately 30% are classified as undifferentiated or poorly differentiated carcinoma, 5% to 15% as squamous cell carcinoma, 5% as undifferentiated neoplasm, and 1% as either well-differentiated or poorly differentiated neuroendocrine carcinoma (5,8). With evolving techniques pathologists have been able to more precisely identify not only the histology but the origin of the malignancy. A close collaboration between the pathologist and the medical oncologist is important in determining the management and optimal therapy of a cancer of unknown primary.

The initial pathological evaluation includes staining of the tissue with hematoxylin and eosin (H&E) with review under light microscopy, often to determine histological subtype. Light microscopy classifies 60% of cases as adenocarcinoma, 5% as squamous cell carcinoma, with the other 35% not clearly being classified, either as poorly differentiated adenocarcinoma, poorly differentiated carcinoma, or poorly differentiated neoplasm (9). Light microscopy alone infrequently identifies the site of origin in patients with cancer of unknown primary. After inspection by light microscopy, the tumor can then be subjected to immunohistochemical (IHC) investigation, using peroxidase-labeled antibodies against specific tumor antigens, performed on paraffin-embedded, formalin-fixed tissue. To rule out lymphoma, germ cell tumor, and melanoma, antibodies against epithelial antigens (pan-cytokeratins), lymphoid antigens (CD45, CD20, and CD3), melanotic antigens (PS100 and HMB45), and germ cell tumor antigens (αFP, βHCG, and PLAP) are employed (10). Notably none of the IHC tests is 100% specific and should thus be interpreted with caution, correlating the findings with the patient's clinical presentation.

Electron Microscopy

As IHC markers have been identified, the use of electron microscopy has fallen out of favor. It is disadvantageous in that it is expensive, not readily available, and time consuming. The use of electron microscopy has been essentially limited to situations in which patients are found to have poorly differentiated neoplasms with inconclusive immunoperoxidase staining.

Tumor Markers

Certain serum tumor markers may be helpful in ascertaining a primary tumor site, such as the prostate specific antigen (PSA), β-human chorionic gonadotropin (βHCG), and alpha fetoprotein (AFP). On the other hand, certain tumor markers commonly used as surrogate measures of response to therapy, such as carcinoembryonic antigen (CEA), CA125, CA19–9, and CA15–3, are not especially helpful in establishing the site of the primary cancer. This is due to the lack of specificity of these tests. Although their use in establishing the primary tumor is limited, these tumor markers play more of a prognostic role.

Cytogenetics

Conventional cytogenetics do not offer a significant advantage in narrowing a diagnosis, as few cytogenetic abnormalities specific to particular tumors have been found. One chromosomal alteration, isochrome 12p-i is seen in about 25% of patients with testicular carcinoma or other germ cell tumors. In addition to the predictive value of this cytogenetic abnormality, it is also prognostic in that patients with this abnormality have been noted to have a high sensitivity to chemotherapy for germ cell tumors. Other chromosomal abnormalities that have been found specific to particular tumors include t(11;22) in primitive neuroectodermal tumors (PNET), desmoplastic small round cell tumors, and Ewing's sarcoma. In some cases where the diagnosis of lymphoma is not initially evident, cytogenetics can be helpful, such as the presence of t(8;14)(q24;q32) in non-Hodgkin's lymphoma, t(14;18) in follicular lymphoma, and t(11;14) in mantle cell lymphoma.

Approaching the Diagnosis of Cancer of Unknown Primary

The initial approach once a biopsy is obtained is to determine that the abnormal cells are present within that biopsy specimen. Once that is confirmed, an assessment of whether those cells are malignant is made based on the presence of a "foreign" cell population, cytologic features, and abnormal architectural features, such as invasiveness. When a biopsy shows malignant cells, a decision must be made on their general classification as representing a carcinoma, germ cell tumor, melanoma, lymphoma, or sarcoma.

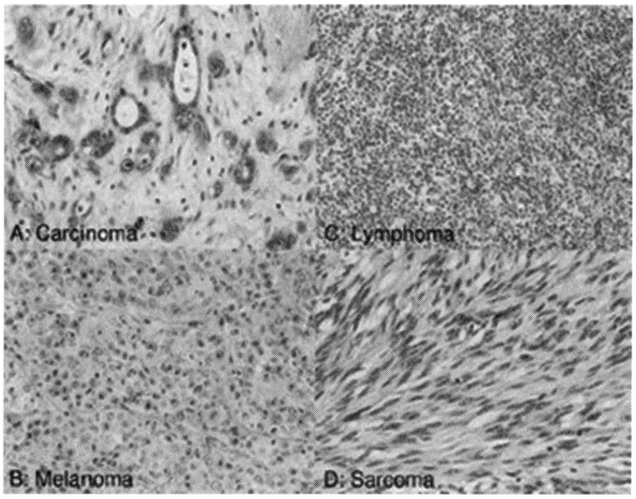

Figure 24.2

Microscopic appearance of cancer types.Carcinoma, as seen in (A), can be described as cohesive cells with a cuboidal or columnar shape, lying in tubules and glands. Melanoma, as seen in (B) with cohesive cells with large nuclei, prominent nucleoli and abundant brown melanin pigment. Lymphoma (C) has uniform small round lymphoid cells with little cytoplasm. Sarcoma (D) has cells with an elongated spindle shape, lying in sheets. The figures are used with permission from Oien (7). (see color insert)

This can often be distinguished based on morphology as seen by light microscopy (Figure 24.2). If a morphological evaluation is not sufficient to distinguish the general tumor type, a "first-line" immunohistochemistry (IHC) panel is performed. This panel typically includes an epithelial marker to evaluate for carcinomas, such as pancytokeratin. It would also include a melanocytic marker like S100 and a lymphoid marker like CLA. A second-line panel is then performed based on the positivity of the first-line markers. Additional melanocyte markers to evaluate for melanoma include Melan-A and HMB45, which are less sensitive than S100 but more specific. Positive IHC staining with these antibodies in the absence of staining with other first-line IHC markers is suggestive of melanoma. See Table 24.2 for a list of commonly used IHC markers. A number of additional markers that can be used in differentiating melanoma, lymphoma, and sarcoma, as well as further subclassification can be found in Figure 24.3.

Table 24.2 Immunohistochemical Markers Useful in the Diagnosis of Carcinoma of Unknown Primary*

Abbreviations	
CK	Cytokeratins KL_1, CK 5/6, CK7. CK19, CK 20, carcinoma markers
CD45	Leukocyte differentiation antigens
PS 100	Protein S100
CD20	B lymphocyte
CD3	T lymphocyte
EMA	Epithelial membrane antigen
CD30	Activation antigen
ALK	Anaplastic lymphoma kinase
HMB45, melan A	Melanic markers
SMA	Smooth muscle actin
SMD	Striated muscle desmin
CD31, CD34	Vascular "markers"
CD68	Histiocyte "marker"
CD99	Peripheral neuroectodermal tumor (PNET) "marker"
CD117	c-kit protein
VIM	Vimentin
Calretin, HBME1, WT1	Mesothelial markers
PLAP	Placental alkaline phosphatase
AFP	Alpha fetoprotein
βHCG	β-human chorionic gonadotropin
CGA	Chromogranin A
SYN	Synaptophysin
NSE	Neurone specific enolase
CEA	Carcinoembryonic antigen
Hep Par1	Hepatocellular antigen
PSA	Prostate specific antigen
TTF1	Thyroid transcription factor 1
GCDFP	Gross cystic disease fluid protein
ER	Estrogen receptor
PR	Progesterone receptor
GFAP	Glial fibrillary acidic protein
NF	Neurofilaments

*Adapted with permission from Bugat et al. (10).

Lymphoma

The use of common leukocyte antigen (CLA) is both very sensitive and specific for lymphoma, thus making the broad diagnosis of lymphoma much easier. Two lymphoid neoplasms, anaplastic large cell lymphoma (ALCL) and granulocytic sarcoma (chloroma of myeloid leukemia), are typically negative for CLA. To evaluate for these lymphoid malignancies, additional IHC markers are tested. ALCL is generally positive for either anaplastic lymphoma kinase protein (ALK1) or CD30. Granuclocytic sarcomas are typically positive for myeloid markers including CD15, CD43, CD68, and others. Once a diagnosis of lymphoma is made, additional markers can be used to further subtype, including B-cell markers CD20 and CD79a, T cell markers such as CD3, plasmacytic markers CD38 and CD138, CD30 positivity in Hodgkin lymphoma, as well as others.

Sarcoma

Sarcoma markers are typically not included in the initial IHC panel, since sarcomas are uncommon in CUP. If a general tumor type is not established with the first-line IHC panel, a second panel can be performed for evaluation of sarcoma. No single marker is used with high sensitivity for sarcoma. Vimentin is present in most sarcoma since it

Carcinoma

- Positive epithelial markers such as pancytokeratin
- Squamous cell carcinoma: CD 5/6, p63
- Solid organ carcinomas
  - Lung carcinoma: TTF-1, Napsin A
  - Gastrointestinal carcinomo: CDX-2
  - Breast carcinoma: ER, PR, HER2, GCDFP-15, MGB1
  - Hepatocellular carcinoma: Hepar-1; AFP; polyclonal CEA, CD10, or CD 13
  - Renal clear cell carcinoma: RCC, CD10, aquaporin-1, PAX-2
  - Papillary and follicular thyroid carcinoma: TTF1, Thyroglobulin
  - Gynecologic carcinomas: CA125, WT1, mesothelin
  - Medullary thyroid carcinoma: calcitonin
- Germ cell tumor: PLAP, OCT4 (embryonal carcinoma and seminoma), AFP (yolk sac tumor), HCG (choriocarcinoma)
- Neuorendocrine carcinoma: Chromogranin, synaptophysin, PGP9.5, CD56, TTF1 (small cell carcinomas), CDX2 (intestinal carcinoid tumors)
- Adrenocortical carcinoma: Alpha-inhibin, Melan-A

Melanoma

- Melanocyte markers
  - S100
  - HM645 and Melan-A (less sensitine, hot more specific than S100)

Sarcoma

- Vimentin, alpha smooth muscie actin, (SMA) despin, myoD1, myogenie, CD34, ckit (CD117), and CD99
- S100 melanocyte marker yositiee in nerve sheath tumors

Lymphoma

- Positive lymphoid markers such as CLA (CD45RB)
- B-cell markers: CD20, CD79a
- T-cell marker: CD3
- Anaplastic large cell lymphoma: ALK1 and CD30
- Granulocytic sarcoma: myeloid markers e.g. CD15, CD43, CD68, myeloperoxidase
- Hodgkin lyphoma: CD30
- Plasmacytic markers: CD38, CD138

Figure 24.3

Initial immunohistochemical panel for broad cancer types with additional panels for subtyping.

is present in most mesenchymal cells. It is also seen, however, in many carcinomas as well as 96% of melanomas. Other markers used in evaluating for sarcoma include smooth muscle actin (SMA), desmin, MyoD1, myogenin, S100, c-kit (CD117), CD34, and CD99.

Carcinoma

The most frequent general tumor types presenting as a cancer of unknown primary are carcinomas, which can be further subcategorized into adenocarcinomas; squamous cell carcinomas; carcinomas arising from liver, kidney, or endocrine glands; neuroendocrine tumors; and germ cell tumors. Aside from initial evaluation based on morphology, use of immunohistochemistry is valuable in further categorizing tumor types.

Adenocarcinomas

Adenocarcinomas make up at least 60% of cancers of unknown primary. The diagnosis of adenocarcinoma based on biopsy is suggested by the presence of glandular morphology. Occasionally the specific morphology of the adenocarcinoma can be suggestive of the primary site, with morphology able to correctly identify the primary site in about 25% of cases. Immunohistochemistry is used to further narrow the differential diagnosis, as was done in the case of J.H., ultimately determining that his cancer was most likely of colon origin. The most frequently used IHC markers are the cytokeratins (CK), which are cytoplasmic filaments that are specific to epithelial cells and are the key positive marker of carcinomas. Tumor sites of origin can be narrowed using monoclonal antibodies to specific subtypes of CK, most commonly two low-molecular-weight cytokeratins, CK7 and CK20. A general guideline for the interpretation of the CK7/CK20 phenotype is seen in Figure 24.4 (3). CK7 is normally expressed in simple glandular epithelium, and is seen in tumors of the lung, breast, pancreas, biliary tract, ovary, endometrium, and transitional eptithelium. Expression of CK7 is notably absent in lower gastrointestinal tract tumors. CK20 is expressed in gastrointestinal epithelium (especially colon), urothelium, and Merkel neuroendocrine cells of the skin. CK5 is expressed in the basal cells of squamous epithelium, as well as mesothelium. Analysis of the expression pattern of CK7 and CK20 can give the clinician a suggestion of the origin of the tumor, especially detailed subtyping of adenocarcinomas. A tumor that stains CK20–/CK7+ suggests that the tumor is most likely of lung (adenocarcinoma), breast, hepatobiliary, pancreatic, ovarian, endometrium, or transitional cell in origin. Up to 85% of carcinomas of lung origin stain positive for CK7, whereas only up to 15% stain positive for CK20. A tumor that stains CK20+/CK7– favors a lower gastrointestinal origin, such as colorectal or less likely, Merkel cell carcinoma. Positive staining for both CK7 and CK20 favors an upper gastrointestinal or urothelial-transitional cell carcinoma, whereas negative staining for both favors prostatic, renal, or liver carcinomas. Notably, expression of CK20 is mostly absent in lung adenocarcinoma, as well as carcinomas of the breast and prostate. A high false-positive and false-negative rate exists for these studies and care should be used when using these staining phenotypes alone in making a diagnosis of a primary site. A schematic approach to evaluating CK7 and CK20 phenotype can be found in Figure 24.4.

Other IHC markers used to distinguish cancers of unknown primary include thyroid transcription factor (TTF-1), thyroglobulin, gross cystic fibrous protein-15 (GCDFP-15), uroplakin III (UROIII), CDX-2, WT-1, and hep par 1. TTF-1 is a nuclear protein that is important in transcriptional activation during embryogenesis in the thyroid diencephalon and respiratory epithelium, and is thus positive frequently in carcinomas of the lung and thyroid. Thyroglobulin is a very specific marker for both papillary and follicular thyroid carcinoma. GCDFP-15 is a marker of apocrine differentiation, specifically seen with high frequency (62–72%) in patients with carcinoma of the breast. It is also found in the skin, salivary gland, bronchial gland, prostate, and seminal vesicle. UROIII positivity suggests urothelial origin, since the monoclonal antibody to UROIII is positive in up to 60% of primary urothelial cancers and 50% of metastatic urothelial cancers. This coexpressed with CK20, which is present in almost 50% of urothelial carcinomas, is strongly suggestive of urothelial origin. Caudal type homeobox transcription factor-2, that is, CDX-2, is normally found in the nucleus of intestinal epithelial cells from the proximal duodenum to the rectum. It is present in up to 90% of adenocarcinomas of the colon. A phenotype of CD7–/CD20+/CDX-2+ is highly suggestive of colon primary.

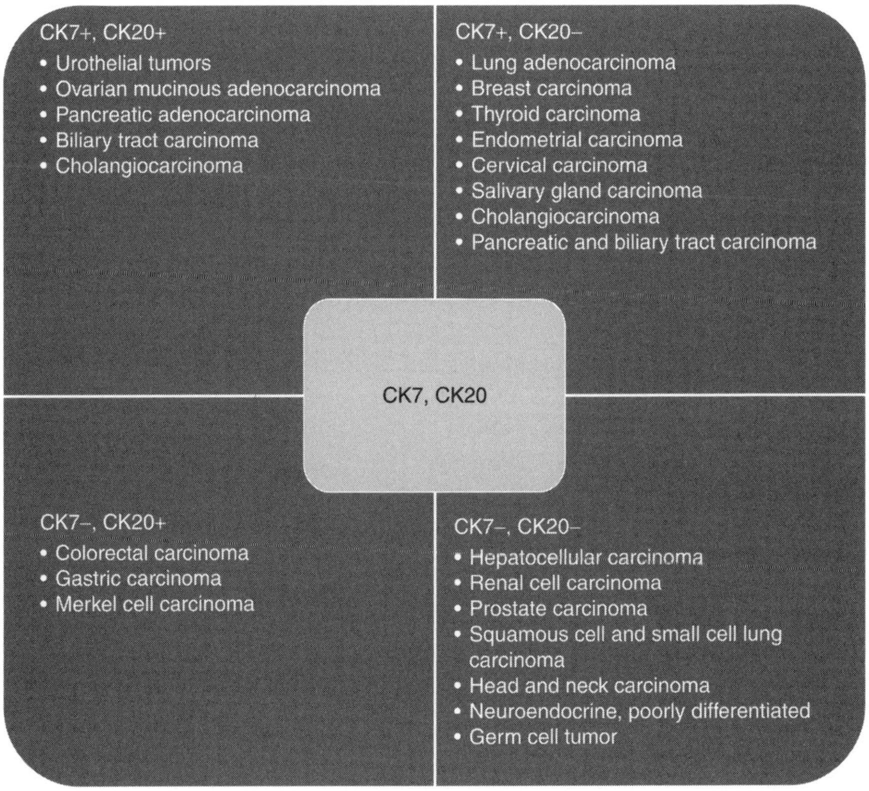

Figure 24.4

The use of cytokeratin markers. Adapted with permission from Varadhachary et al. (9).

It is also present in up to 30% of gastroesophageal adenocarcinomas, but rarely seen in pancreaticobiliary tumors. In addition to gastrointestinal tumors, all primary bladder adenocarcinomas express CDX-2, as do about 65% of ovarian mucinous adenocarcinomas. Wilm's tumor-1 (WT1) is a marker for epithelioid mesothelioma, it is also found to be positive in most cases of ovarian serous carcinoma. Hep par 1 expression is seen almost exclusively in hepatocytes, both benign and malignant. In patients presenting with liver-only metastases, diagnosis of hepatocellular carcinoma is supported by hep par 1 positivity, and cholangiocarcinoma is mostly excluded.

Lung is the most common primary site for adenocarcinomas, representing 27% of cancers of unknown primary. The majority of lung adenocarcinomas are CK7+/CK20–/TTF1+, though infrequently atypical expression is seen. For example, bronchoalveolar carcinomas are often CK20+ and mucinous carcinomas may be both CK20+ and TTF-1-negative. Of note, squamous cell carcinomas of the lung are typically TTF-1-negative and malignant mesotheliomas are always TTF-1-negative. Napsin A, a proteinase involved in surfactant B maturation, is an emerging marker thought to be more sensitive than TTF-1 for lung adenocarcinoma. It is expressed in up to 89% of cases.

Colorectal carcinomas are characterized by the phenotype CK7–/CK20+. This diagnosis can be further supported with CDX-2 staining, as described above. CDX-2, in contrast to many other markers that are either "positive" or "negative," is variably expressed. Most colorectal adenocarcinomas show strong and diffuse CDX-2 expression, as demonstrated in Figure 24.5, as do duodenal adenocarcinomas. Expression is low in gastroesophageal adenocarcinomas.

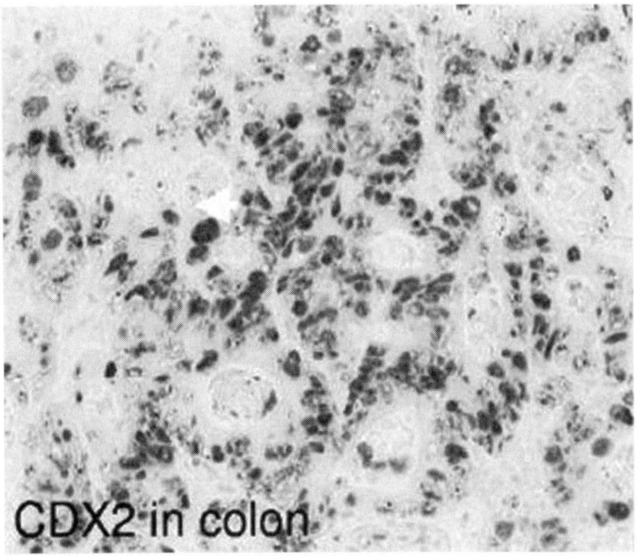

Figure 24.5

CDX-2 positivity in colon cancer. Used with permission from Oien (7). (see color insert)

Villin is another colonic marker, which is expressed in almost all adenocarcinomas of colorectal origin. However, it is also expressed in 90% of lung adenocarcinomas. Pancreaticobiliary and upper gastrointestinal tumors present a diagnostic dilemma. They account for a large percentage of cancers of unknown primary; however, a lack of sensitive and specific markers make their diagnosis challenging. CK and CDX-2 staining can be difficult to interpret since it relates to upper gastrointestinal tumors, and can be seen with any combination of phenotypes of CK7 and CK20, as well as any level of expression of CDX-2. Pancreaticobiliary cancers are CK7-positive in 96% of cases, with two thirds CK20-negative. CA19–9 is a tumor marker expressed in up to 90% of pancreaticobiliary tumors; however it lacks specificity. Another marker that lacks specificity, but can be helpful in differentiating pancreaticobiliary and upper gastrointestinal cancers from breast cancers is lysozyme, a secreted antibacterial enzyme.

Breast cancer infrequently presents as cancer of unknown primary, accounting for less than 1% of the cases. The majority of breast carcinomas are CK7+/CK20–. Other markers used in diagnosis of breast cancer as cancer of unknown primary are the estrogen receptor (ER) and GCDFP-15. ER expression is up to 85% specific to carcinomas of the breast and gynecologic tract, with 60% to 80% of breast cancers being ER-positive. As mentioned previously, GCDFP-15 is expressed frequently in breast cancers, often in ER-negative tumors, and is noted to have a specificity of up to 96% for breast cancer. Mammaglobin (MGB1) is a marker that is often expressed in otherwise diagnostically difficult breast cancers and can be useful in cases of suspected breast primary.

Gynecologic cancers, including ovarian and endometrial cancer, can often be easily differentiated from breast cancers since they are typically positive for other markers, such as CA125, WT1, and mesothelin. CA125, a membrane glycoprotein, is expressed in most gynecological malignancies, but infrequently in adenocarcinomas of other sites, with the exception of 50% to 60% of pancreaticobiliary carcinomas and 25% to 40% of lung adenocarcinomas. The use of CA125 in combination with ER-staining assists in differentiating gynecological primaries from breast primaries. Mesothelin is another membrane glycoprotein with a frequency of distribution similar to CA125. WT1 is frequently expressed in ovarian serous tumors, though negative in mucinous and endometrioid tumors. Positive staining for WT1 can be used to distinguish an ovarian primary from a pancreaticobiliary, gastrointestinal, and breast primary, since WT1 is typically negative in these tumor types. Absent WT1 staining can be useful as well in the setting of an ovarian mucinous or endometrioid cancer in combination with CEA to distinguish an ovarian primary from a gastrointestinal or pancreaticobiliary primary. They would all most likely be negative for WT1, but ovarian serous and endometrioid tumors do not express CEA.

Two percent of cancers of unknown primary are prostate adenocarcinomas. The typical cytokeratin phenotype is CK7–/CK20–. Use of PSA has an extremely high sensitivity and specificity for prostate adenocarcinoma in the setting of cancer of unknown primary, since PSA is expressed in 95% to 100% of these tumors and rarely in other sites. Other prostate markers include prostatic acid phosphatase (PAP), NKX3.1, and prostein (p501s).

Squamous Cell Carcinomas

Squamous cell carcinomas account for about 5% of all cases of cancer of unknown primary. Squamous histology can usually be assessed by light microscopy, but as with adenocarcinomas, immunohistochemistry can be used in cases where the histology is nondiagnostic. CK5 and p63 are the two markers most commonly used for squamous cell carcinoma. Unlike adenocarcinoma there are not any markers that consistently help to further narrow the primary to a specific site of origin. CK5 is expressed in up to 90% of squamous cell carcinomas as is p63, giving these tests a high sensitivity. Individually, CK5 and p63 have a lower specificity since expression is observed in a number of adenocarcinomas. Coexpression increases specificity of these tests for squamous cell carcinomas to 96%. Use of CK7 and CK20 can be useful in squamous cell carcinoma, which typically have a CK7–/CK20– phenotype, in contrast to adenocarcinomas that are mostly CK7-positive. Transitional cell carcinomas are typically positive for both CK7 and CK20, as well as uroplakin III, unlike squamous cell carcinomas.

Germ Cell Tumors

Germ cell tumors are typically very chemosensitive and potentially curable, making accurate diagnosis extremely important. These are classified as either seminomatous or nonseminomatous tumors. Nonseminomatous tumors are further classified into embryonal carcinoma, teratoma, yolk sac tumor, and choriocarcinoma. Immunohistochemistry is very helpful in confirming germ cell origin of a tumor. Placental-like alkaline phosphatase is very sensitive, but not completely specific for germ cell tumors. Nonseminomatous germ cell tumors stain with pancytokeratin whereas the seminomatous germ cell tumors do not. Octamer-binding transcription factor 4 (OCT4) is 100% specific for germ cell tumors since it is not expressed in any other tumor types. It is notably negative in yolk sac tumors and choriocarcinomas. Yolk sac tumors are positive for AFP and choriocarcinomas are positive for HCG.

Neuroendocrine Tumors

Neuroendocrine tumors are a heterogenous group accounting for 5% of cancers of unknown primary. Recognition of neuroendocrine tumors is prognostically important since they respond favorably to therapy. These are often easily recognized based on morphology alone; however, immunohistochemistry is very useful when this is not the case, given the existence of very sensitive and specific markers. Neuroendocrine markers include chromogranin A, synaptophysin, protein gene product 9.5 (PGP9.5), and CD56. The site of origin of carcinoid tumors (well-differentiated neuroendocrine tumors) can be determined using TTF1 and CDX-2. This is not the case with poorly differentiated tumors, although the site of origin is less important in neuroendocrine tumors than the degree of differentiation.

Solid Organ Carcinomas

Carcinomas arising in solid organs are occasionally considered in the realm of cancer of unknown primary in situations where primary tumors need to be distinguished from metastases—such as in liver or adrenal cancers, or in tumors that commonly present as metastatic disease, such as thyroid or kidney cancer. The morphology of carcinomas arising from solid organs is mostly distinctive and the tumors are generally well differentiated. Specific considerations include hepatocellular carcinoma, renal cell carcinoma, thyroid carcinoma, and adrenocortical carcinoma. The liver and biliary tract are the primary sites of origin in up to 10% of cancers of unknown primary. Hepatocellular carcinomas are mostly CK7+/CK20–. A number of other useful markers for hepatocellular carcinoma are Hepar-1, AFP, CD10, and CD13. Renal carcinomas account for 6% of cancer of unknown primary, 85% of which are renal clear cell carcinomas. Coexpression of vimentin and pan-cytokeratin is one characteristic of renal cell carcinoma; however, it is not absolutely specific. CD10 is often expressed in renal cell carcinomas, but CD10 has a low specificity. The antibody RCC, which reacts against a brush border protein of the proximal convoluted tubule in the kidney, appears to have a very high specificity for renal cell carcinoma. Aquaporin-1 and PAX-2 are additional markers that are frequently positive in renal cell carcinoma. Thyroid carcinomas, both follicular and papillary, are typically CK7+/CK20–, and use of TTF-1 and thyroglobulin yields high sensitivity. Medullary thyroid carcinoma can be distinguished by expression of calcitonin. Adrenocortical carcinomas are very uncommon as cancer of unknown primaries, though adrenal metastases are quite common. Alpha-inhibin and Melan-A are very sensitive and highly specific for adrenocortical carcinomas.

Prognostic Clinical Scenarios in Cancer of Unknown Primary

R.L., a 56-year-old man with a history of hypertension and dyslipidemia who presented to his primary care physician complaining of generalized fatigue and a 15-pound weight loss over 3 months. Prior to the onset of these symptoms he had been in good health, although he had not seen a doctor in many years. Other than the fatigue and weight loss, he had felt well but did notice a nontender lump on his neck that had developed over the same time period. He had a mild chronic cough, which he attributed to being a "smoker's cough." Notably, he had smoked one pack per day for 25 years. He drank a moderate amount of alcohol at least twice a week. His family history was significant: his father died of lung cancer at age 67 and his mother has breast cancer. His physical examination was remarkable for a 4-cm firm, nontender, nonmobile lymph node in the right anterior cervical chain with no overlying skin changes. Laboratory analysis did not show any abnormalities and a chest x-ray was also unremarkable. A fine-needle aspiration of the lymph node showed squamous cell carcinoma, negative for both CK7 and CK20. R.L. was referred to an otolaryngologist, who on extensive oropharyngeal examination and direct laryngoscopy, did not note any significant abnormalities. A CT of the neck revealed a 4.5 × 3.7 cm necrotic right cervical lymph node, with no other abnormalities. Panendoscopy did not show any visible lesions. Given the presentation and distribution of his adenopathy, R.L. was given therapy guided toward locally advanced squamous cell carcinoma of the head and neck: high-dose radiation therapy including the bilateral neck and the mucosa in the entire pharyngeal axis and larynx.

Evidence-Based Case Discussion

Prognostic Considerations in Cancer of Unknown Primary

The case of R.L. illustrates the importance of clinical scenarios in cancer of unknown primary. As can be seen with R.L., who was judged to have squamous cell carcinoma with a solitary cervical lymph node, certain presentations can dictate not only prognosis but also management. Clinical presentations in cancer of unknown primary can represent either a good or poor prognosis.

Because of the difficulty of determining the primary source of the metastatic malignancy, using specific disease-targeted therapy is often not possible. Many patients with cancer of unknown primary have tumors that are resistant to systemic treatments and chemotherapy, and the use of these therapies is often palliative. Median overall survival has been reported to range from 3 to 9 months depending on the study (NCCN and NCI), and the 5-year overall survival was less than 10%. Despite the overall poor prognosis, when considering this group as a whole, there are various factors that portend a better prognosis. A multivariate analysis by Abbruzzese et al. identified numerous variables with prognostic importance (6). A favorable prognosis was observed in patients with isolated neuroendocrine liver metastases and those with lymphadenopathy, excluding supraclavicular nodes. The presence of lymphadenopathy in and of itself was a favorable feature, although supraclavicular lymphadenopathy was associated with worse outcomes. The diagnoses of carcinoma, squamous cell carcinoma, and neuroendocrine carcinoma were all positive prognostic indicators. Male sex, identification of adenocarcinoma as the histological subtype, hepatic involvement, and greater number of involved organs were some of the variables associated with poorer outcomes. Specifically, metastatic involvement of the liver (non-neuroendocrine), lung, bone, pleura, or brain was associated with a poorer prognosis, as described by Greco et al. (11). Hainsworth et al. identified additional subsets of patients with desirable features, associated with specific clinical scenarios (12). These include women with isolated axillary lymph nodes, women with papillary serous peritoneal adenocarcinoma, young men with extragonadal germ cell syndrome, men with blastic bone metastases and elevated serum level PSA, and squamous cell carcinoma with either isolated cervical or inguinal lymph nodes. Tables 24.3 and 24.4 summarize the clinical scenarios with favorable and unfavorable prognoses.

Cancers of Unknown Primary With Favorable Prognostic Factors: Neuroendocrine Carcinoma

Neuroendocrine carcinomas uncommonly present as cancers of unknown primary, accounting for 5% of unknown primary diagnoses. Presenting as cancers of unknown primary, neuroendocrine carcinomas represent a group with a favorable prognosis, regardless of grade. Categorization of these tumors is based on pathologic grade and degree of differentiation, which can predict the clinical behavior and response to therapy.

Table 24.3 Favorable Prognostic Factors in Patients With Carcinoma of Unknown Primary

Poorly differentiated carcinoma with midline distribution
Women with papillary adenocarcinoma of the peritoneal cavity
Women with adenocarcinoma involving only axillary lymph nodes
Squamous cell carcinoma involving cervical lymph nodes
Isolated inguinal adenopathy with squamous histology
Poorly differentiated neuroendocrine carcinomas
Men with blastic bone metastases, adenocarcinoma, and elevated PSA
Patients with single, small, and potentially resectable tumor

Table 24.4 Unfavorable Prognostic Factors Patients With Carcinoma of Unknown Primary

Male gender
Adenocarcinoma with multiple metastases involving other organs (liver, lung, or bone)
Nonpapillary malignancy ascites (adenocarcinoma)
Multiple cerebral metastases (adenocarcinoma or squamous cell carcinoma)
Adenocarcinoma with multiple lung/pleural or multiple bone osseous metastases

Low-grade, well-differentiated neuroendocrine tumors appear similar to typical carcinoid tumors, islet cell tumors, paragangliomas, pheochromocytomas, and medullary thyroid carcinomas. When presenting as cancer of unknown primary, they typically present in the liver, bone, or lymph nodes. It is more uncommon for low-grade neuroendocrine tumors to present as cancers of unknown primary than for the higher-grade tumors, representing only 10% of neuroendocrine carcinomas of unknown primary. Typical primary sites for these tumors should be investigated, which include the stomach, small intestine, colon, rectum, pancreas, and bronchus. This should be done with imaging including CT scan, as well as invasive investigations including bronchoscopy, upper endoscopy, and colonoscopy. Other imaging modalities, such as octreotide scan, PET scan, and/or magnetic resonance imaging (MRI) can be implemented, which will be discussed in a later section (Imaging of Cancer of Unknown Primary and Future Directions). These tumors have an indolent behavior, with a median overall survival of 124 months. Management should be similar to that of metastatic typical carcinoid with either local therapy or therapy aimed at symptomatic control. Systemic chemotherapy does not play a significant role in treatment of low-grade neuroendocrine tumors since they tend to be relatively unresponsive. Local therapeutic options include resection, radiation, chemoembolization, or ablation. Octreotide, a somatostatin analogue, is often used as a monthly depot injection as first-line therapy in low-grade neuroendocrine tumors. It is well tolerated and has a significant impact on control of symptoms due to hormone excess.

The high-grade or anaplastic, poorly differentiated neuroendocrine tumors include atypical carcinoids, small cell carcinomas, and poorly differentiated large cell neuroendocrine tumors. Although still considered to have a "favorable prognosis" when presenting as cancer of unknown primary, high-grade neuroendocrine tumors are significantly more aggressive than low-grade tumors. The median overall survival is 10 months. Large cell carcinomas are the most common high-grade neuroendocrine tumors, accounting for 75% of neuroendocrine carcinomas of unknown primary. These have a very heterogeneous presentation, and can involve a variety of sites, often more than one. Small cell carcinomas represent 15% of neuroendocrine carcinomas of unknown primary. A number of more rare tumors are often mistaken for small cell carcinomas due to similar morphology, such as germ cell tumors with neuroendocrine differentiation, peripheral neuroectodermal tumors, Ewing's sarcoma, and desmoplastic small round cell tumors. Both small cell and large cell carcinomas are highly aggressive, though they tend to be sensitive to systemic chemotherapy. Treatment of large cell carcinoma of unknown primary mirrors that of small cell carcinoma of unknown primary. Surgical resection or radiation therapy is considered in cases where the disease is localized to a limited region. Systemic chemotherapy with a platinum-based combination regimen, most commonly cisplatin and etoposide, is the recommended treatment, following guidelines of therapy for treating small cell lung cancer. Addition of paclitaxel has not been shown to have advantage over two-drug platinum-based therapy, and carries additional toxicity. Compared to low-grade neuroendocrine tumors, overall response rates to chemotherapy are high, approaching 70% in some studies. This is in contrast to the very low overall response rates of less than 10% seen in the use of chemotherapy in low-grade neuroendocrine tumors (see Chapter 9, Neuroendocrine Tumors).

Women With Axillary Lymph Node Metastases

A woman who is found to have a cancer of unknown primary presenting as adenocarcinoma with isolated axillary lymph node metastases should raise a suspicion in the clinician for breast cancer. Imaging should be directed toward investigating a possible breast primary. If mammography is unrevealing, breast MRI should be obtained with consideration of PET scanning as well to look for an occult breast primary. IHC staining of the biopsy should include ER, PR, and HER2 testing—their presence is highly suggestive of breast cancer. Occasionally, despite this workup, no definitive breast primary can be identified. In that situation treatment should be initiated following guidelines for management of stage II breast cancer. This should include a surgical approach with either a modified radical mastectomy or an axillary lymph node dissection. If an axillary lymph node dissection is performed, it should be followed by radiation therapy and should not be done as stand-alone therapy. Mastectomy is often very effective in identifying the occult primary, with reports of up to 82% of primaries found on pathologic evaluation of the resected breast. Identified primaries are typically less than 2 cm, and occasionally only noninvasive tumor is discovered. Following surgical management, adjuvant therapy is indicated as administered to patients with node-positive breast cancer. As in known primary breast cancer, selection of adjuvant therapy depends on hormone receptor status, HER2 status, menopausal status, and the number of involved lymph nodes. Prognosis for these patients is similar to that of women with stage II breast cancer. Of note, men may present in this manner as well, although rarely, and should be managed in the same way.

In the setting of axillary lymph nodes identified as adenocarcinoma with metastases in a distribution typical of metastatic breast cancer, such as multiple bone metastases or pleural metastases, breast cancer should remain the primary consideration. These patients should be managed based on guidelines for metastatic breast cancer, with careful attention to ER, PR, and HER2 status.

Women With Peritoneal Carcinomatosis

Peritoneal carcinomatosis is often seen in women with carcinoma of the ovary, but it is also seen less commonly in the setting of gastrointestinal, lung, or breast cancer. It can also be seen in women with no clear intra-abdominal primary and normal ovaries, presenting as a cancer of unknown primary or in primary peritoneal carcinomatosis. This is a situation with a favorable prognosis given the effectiveness of chemotherapy directed against ovarian cancer. One clinical scenario in which this is seen is in women at high risk for ovarian cancer due to genetic predisposition (such as in BRCA1 families) who have undergone prophylactic oophorectomy. The histologic appearance of the malignant cells in the peritoneal fluid frequently resembles ovarian carcinoma, but can be variable and is occasionally poorly differentiated. Treatment of women with isolated peritoneal carcinomatosis should follow guidelines for the management of advanced ovarian cancer, including initial maximal surgical debulking, followed by combination chemotherapy. Chemotherapy should include taxane and a platinum agent, with the combination of cisplatin and paclitaxel being the most commonly used. The presence of minimal residual disease following debulking surgery has been associated with better outcomes, including increased frequency of complete response as well as prolonged overall survival. Up to 15% of patients receiving such therapy may experience prolonged survival.

Young Men With Features of Extragonadal Germ Cell Tumor

In young men with poorly differentiated carcinoma with midline distribution in either the mediastinum or retroperitoneum, a diagnosis of extragonadal germ cell tumor should be suspected. This diagnosis would be supported by elevation in either HCG or AFP, and can also be supported by cytogenetic evaluation with an isochrome 12p abnormality. If these tests are equivocal or there is limited availability of cytogenetic analysis, young men with poorly differentiated carcinoma in either of these locations should be treated based on guidelines for poor-prognosis germ cell tumor. This should include combination chemotherapy with a platinum-containing regimen, such as cisplatin, etoposide, and bleomycin. If after a partial response to four cycles of chemotherapy, residual tumor is noted on follow-up imaging, surgical resection should be considered.

The "extragonadal germ cell tumor syndrome" was described in 1979 in men younger than 50 years, with midline tumors (mediastinum or peritoneum) or multiple pulmonary nodules, short symptom interval with rapid tumor growth, elevated levels of serum AFP and/or HCG, and a good response to chemotherapy or radiation (5). Patients rarely are seen to have all of these clinical features, but the presence of any two suggest the possibility of a germ cell tumor.

Men With Adenocarcinoma and Osteoblastic Bone Metastases

Men with predominant bone metastases with adenocarcinoma should be suspected to have prostate cancer, especially if the bone metastases are osteoblastic. IHC staining of the biopsy should include PSA as well as PAP. Serum PSA levels should be measured for confirmation of the diagnosis and the patients should be treated based on guidelines for metastatic prostate cancer. In the presence of multiple osteoblastic bone metastases with unknown primary, androgen deprivation therapy should be given as a trial empirically, irrespective of PSA level. Response to androgen deprivation therapy has also been noted in men with PSA levels suggestive of prostate cancer but who have atypical metastatic patterns. These patients should thus also be managed using guidelines for metastatic prostate cancer.

Adenocarcinoma Presenting as a Single Metastatic Lesion

In some cases (such as R.L.'s) only one metastatic lesion can be identified. Additional metastatic lesions frequently become evident in a short period of time in those who present with a single metastatic lesion. Local treatment with radiation therapy or definitive resection, if feasible, should be considered in this subset of patients. Adjuvant radiation therapy after resection to improve chances of local control may be considered as well. A significant number of these patients have a prolonged disease-free survival with local therapy. The role of adjuvant chemotherapy in combination with local therapy has not been strictly defined. It is reasonable to offer a short course of adjuvant chemotherapy using an empiric chemotherapy regimen for cancer of unknown primary.

Squamous Carcinoma

Squamous cell carcinoma of unknown primary is an uncommon entity, representing about 5% of all patients with cancer of unknown primary. Effective therapies exist for certain clinical syndromes including squamous carcinoma of either cervical or inguinal lymph nodes.

Squamous Cell Carcinoma Involving Cervical Lymph Nodes

The cervical lymph nodes are the most common site for metastatic squamous cell carcinoma of unknown primary and the presence of these metastases is suggestive of a head and neck cancer, as is described in the case of R.L. This is especially true if the lymph nodes are in the middle or upper cervical lymph node region. Many of the patients with these isolated nodes have risk factors for head and neck cancer, such as smoking, alcohol use, and exposure to HPV. When this situation is identified, further investigation should be performed in search of the occult primary with panendoscopy. This should include examination of the head and neck by an experienced otolaryngologist, examining the oropharynx, nasopharynx, hypopharynx, larynx, and upper esophagus with direct endoscopy. Bronchoscopy should be included in this evaluation as well if chest imaging and examination of the head and neck are unrevealing. Biopsies should be taken of any suspicious areas. Tonsillectomy should be performed empirically in patients with subdigastric, submandibular, or midjugulocarotid adenopathy, since these patients have a high likelihood of having a tonsillar primary. Ipsilateral tonsillectomy can be performed in patients with a single node in this distribution. Bilateral tonsillectomy should be performed in those patients who present with bilateral adenopathy as described. Tonsillectomy can identify a primary site in about 25% of cases. Imaging in this scenario should include plain radiographs of the chest and CT of the neck. PET scanning is recommended since it identifies primary site in up to 25% of patients with this presentation. The biopsy sample should be evaluated for the presence of Epstein-Barr virus genome, the presence of which would be suggestive of a nasopharyngeal primary site. The tumor tissue should also be examined for the presence of HPV-16, which is specific for an oropharyngeal primary site, seen increasingly in nonsmokers and nondrinkers.

If no primary is located, treatment should follow guidelines for management of locally advanced squamous cell carcinoma of the head and neck. This should involve local therapy with high-dose radiation therapy, radical neck dissection, or a combination of these approaches. Responses to these treatments have been similar, with 30% to 60% of patients achieving long-term, disease-free survival. Surgery is typically not offered alone except in select patients, such as those with pN1 neck disease with no extracapsular extension. Radiation therapy should include the bilateral neck and the mucosa in the entire pharyngeal axis and larynx. This approach is superior to radiation to ipsilateral cervical lymph nodes alone. Although concurrent chemotherapy and radiation therapy is standard in locally advanced head and neck cancer, the role of chemotherapy in metastatic squamous cell carcinoma in cervical lymph nodes with unknown primary is controversial. Platinum-based chemotherapy given concurrently with radiation appears to be beneficial, especially in patients with N2 or N3 lymph node involvement.

Poorer prognosis is seen in patients with extensive lymphadenopathy or those with poorly differentiated tumors. Those patients with lower cervical or supraclavicular lymph nodes also do not do as well as those with higher cervical nodes. These patients are more likely to have an occult primary lung cancer. Despite the poorer prognosis, the recommended therapy is similar to that for patients with higher cervical nodes. They should receive aggressive local therapy and should be considered for concurrent chemotherapy.

Squamous Cell Carcinoma Involving Inguinal Lymph Nodes

Patients with inguinal lymphadenopathy with squamous histology should undergo thorough genitourinary examination, with careful attention paid to the penis, scrotum, vulva, vagina, and cervix. Any suspicious lesion should be biopsied. The anorectal area should be examined as well with digital rectal exam and anoscopy. If the primary cannot be identified, treatment should be offered with definitive local therapy, including inguinal lymph node dissection, with or without radiation therapy. Long-term survival can result from local therapy, especially in patients found to have squamous cell carcinoma of the anus, vulva, vagina, or cervix. Combined therapy with concurrent radiation and chemotherapy improves prognosis for a number of primary cancers originating in the inguinal region. Systemic therapy with concurrent platinum-based chemotherapy and radiation should be considered in patients without an identified primary site.

Cancer of Unknown Primary With Single Small Metastasis

Patients with a single small site of metastasis with an unidentified primary are a group with a favorable prognosis, often with a long-term disease-free survival, independent of the pathology. These patients should be offered aggressive local therapy with radiation, resection, or both.

Poorly Differentiated Carcinoma

Approximately 20% of patients with cancer of unknown primary site are identified to have poorly differentiated carcinoma. Despite the heterogeneity of this group there is a subset of these patients who have chemotherapy-sensitive tumors. Occasionally, specific diagnoses can be made using specialized pathologic studies, allowing for more disease-guided therapy. In cases of poorly differentiated carcinoma with unknown primary site, a trial of empiric combination chemotherapy should be offered. Use of platinum-based chemotherapy (with or without combination taxane chemotherapy) has produced relatively high response rates, with the substitution of carboplatin for cisplatin being equally effective with less toxicity.

Cancers of Unknown Primary With Unfavorable Prognostic Factors

While approximately 20% of patients with cancer of unknown primary are considered to have a favorable prognosis as detailed in the previous section, the majority of patients continue to have a poor prognosis. No chemotherapeutic regimen has been found to be convincingly effective in this subset of patients and treatment is empiric, with aim at palliation. The historical and current data for survival in patients with cancer of unknown primary is described by Greco et al. (11). In a retrospective review of an extensive series of almost 45,000 patients, the combined median overall survival was noted to be 4.5 months, with 20% 1-year survival, 4.7% 5-year or greater survival. Of note, the patients in this series with long-term survival were mostly those with favorable prognostic factors. When excluding 3871 of those patients who either had squamous or epidermoid carcinoma or well-differentiated neuroendocrine carcinoma, 1-year survival dropped to 12% in the remaining 40,828 patients. Initial chemotherapeutic trials throughout the 1970s involved mostly single-agent regimens with very low response rates and very rare long-term survival. Platinum-based combination chemotherapy was evaluated starting in the 1980s. A review of 38 phase II trials performed between 1964 and 1996 showed a response rate of about 20% and median overall survival of 6 months. Some of the larger trials showed longer survival and increased response; however, these trials included many patients with previously unrecognized favorable prognostic factors. It is important to note when discussing older data in cancer of unknown primary that all of the trials were small, with no large randomized phase III data. Long-term follow-up results were rarely published due to either patient death or rapid publishing of results.

In the last decade, with the development of new drugs with broad activity and new targeted agents, a number of larger prospective phase II trials have been conducted. Nine sequential studies were reported by the Minnie Pearl Cancer Research Network (MPCRN) since 1997, including 692 patients with cancer of unknown primary. These studies used various combinations of paclitaxel, docetaxel, cisplatin, carboplatin, gemictabine, irinotecan, capecitabine, oxaliplatin, bevacizumab, and erlotinib, either as front-line therapy or salvage therapy. Only those patients not identified to have favorable features were included in first-line therapy trials. Among the 396 patients included in the first five studies done by the MPCRN, there was an objective response rate of 30% with 24% partial response and 6% complete response. The median overall survival was 9.1 months with 38% 1-year, 10% 5-year, and 8% 10-year survival, as seen in Figure 24.6. There was a 5-month median progression-free survival with 17% 1-year, 4% 5-year, and 3% 10-year progression-free survival. In comparing the various regimens there was no significant difference in survival between the groups.

The use of targeted agents, which have been approved for use in advanced cancers of known primary such as colorectal, breast, and non-small cell lung cancer, has been studied in cancer of unknown primary. A phase II trial was conducted by the MPCRN combining bevacizumab (inhibitor of vascular endothelial growth factor) and erlotinib (inhibitor of epidermal growth factor receptor) in 51 patients with cancer of unknown primary. Most of the patients were previously untreated, with the untreated patients all having poor prognostic features. Twenty-nine of the patients (61%) had stable disease and 5 of the patients (10%) had a partial response, with the majority of patients receiving at least 8 weeks of therapy. The median overall survival was 7.4 months, with a 33% 1-year survival. In a retrospective comparison to second-line chemotherapeutic agents, these responses were superior. Based on the positive results with these targeted agents, a recent MPCRN phase II trial evaluated use of targeted agents in the front-line setting. Patients received paclitaxel/carboplatin/bevacizumab every 21 days with daily erlotinib for a total of four cycles, followed by up to 1 year of maintenance therapy with bevacizumab and erlotinib. Only the 56 patients who were not known to be in a favorable subset were included in the trial. An objective response rate of 38% was noted with 19 patients (34%) having stable disease. Median progression-free survival was 10.4 months, with median overall survival of 11.6 months, 1-year survival of 46.5%, and a tolerable toxicity profile. It appears that targeted agents may have a beneficial role in the management of cancer of unknown primary with unfavorable

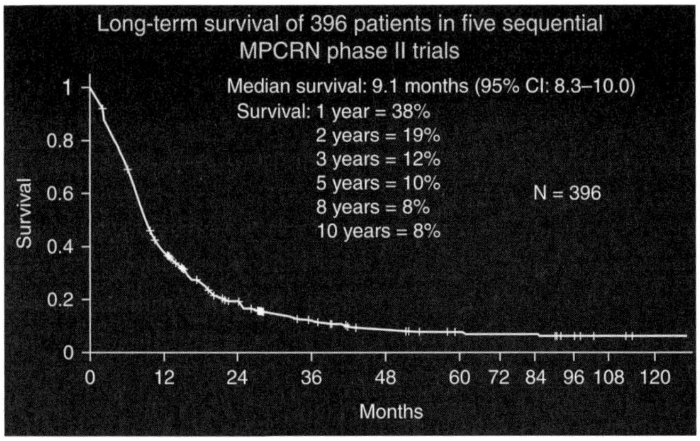

Figure 24.6

Survival curve for 396 patients treated on the first 5 sequential prospective phase ii trials by the Minnie Pearl Cancer Research Network (MPCRN). Used with permission from Greco and Pavlidis (11).

prognostic factors, though larger phase III trials need to be done.

The recently published phase III multicenter Sarah Cannon Oncology Research Consortium Trial randomized 198 patients to receive paclitaxel, carboplatin, and etoposide (PCE) versus gemcitabine and irinotecan first line, both followed by gefitinib (13). In this trial, which is one of the largest phase III trials in cancer of unknown primary to date, patients were given between four and six cycles of chemotherapy, after which those with no progression of disease were maintained on gefitinib until disease progression. Notably this trial was stopped early due to slow accrual. The trial, which did not meet the primary endpoint of showing a 10% difference in overall survival (increasing the 2-year overall survival to 30%), showed that the two regimens were not statistically different in median overall survival, median progression-free survival, and response rate. In comparing PCE with gemcitabine/irinotecan, median 2-year survival was 15% versus 18%, median overall survival was 7.4 months versus 8.5 months, median progression-free survival was 3.3 months versus 5.3 months, and response rate was 18% in both arms. The authors concluded that the gemcitabine/irinotecan combination is favorable due to its toxicity profile. The trial was not powered to detect a difference in efficacy with the addition of gefitinib, and its inclusion was intended to assess the possible activity of this agent. Based on the available data from this trial, gefitinib did not appear to have significant activity as a single-agent therapy in maintenance.

Analysis of all patients in the MPCRN showed that in patients with cancer of unknown primary with poor prognostic factors, there is no difference in survival for adenocarcinoma over poorly differentiated carcinomas. Men have a shorter survival than women in this category, as do patients with an Eastern Cooperative Oncology Group (ECOG) performance status of 2 or greater compared to those with and ECOG performance status of 0 or 1. Other identified poor prognostic variables included elevated lactate dehydrogenase level, low serum albumin, and the presence of liver metastases.

In addition to the MPCRN trials, 12 trials have reported long-term follow-up with 1-year survival data, and 8 of those 12 trials reported a 2-year survival data. These phase II trials used multiple regimens, mostly platinum-, paclitaxel-, docetaxel-, gemcitabine-, irinotecan-, or vinorelbine-based. Inclusive of the MPCRN trials, the mean 1-year survival was 34.6%, mean 2-year survival was 13%, mean 3-year survival was 12%, and median overall survival was 8.9 months, as can be seen in Table 24.5.

Despite the fact that no phase III studies have clearly shown a benefit of systemic chemotherapy over best supportive care in survival of patients with cancer of unknown primary with poor prognostic features, aggregate data of numerous phase II studies does appear to suggest such a benefit.

Imaging in Cancer of Unknown Primary and Future Directions

A.W., a healthy 41-year-old woman, presented to her primary care physician with a slowly growing nontender nodule in her right axilla that was noted during a self-breast examination at home. She had been up to date on her health maintenance and had her first mammogram the previous year, which was normal. Her only previous hospitalization was for a cesarian section, and she did not have any pertinent family history. She was previously a smoker with 14 pack-years, although she quit smoking 5 years earlier. Her physical examination showed a 3-cm firm, nontender, mobile nodule in the right axilla. Laboratory studies including a CBC, serum chemistries, and liver function tests which were normal, as was a chest x-ray. A bilateral mammogram did not reveal any abnormalities in the breast tissue, but a breast ultrasound showed a hypoechoic nodule in the right axilla measuring 3.4 × 2.7cm. A fine-needle aspiration showed adenocarcinoma, though tissue site of origin was indeterminate. An immunohistochemistry panel showed that the tumor was CK20 negative, CK7 positive, ER positive, PR negative, and HER2 negative. A CT scan of the chest, abdomen, and pelvis was otherwise unremarkable, as was a breast MRI and bone scan. An axillary lymph node dissection was performed, identifying only the one positive lymph node. Because of these findings, A.W. was treated as if she had node-positive breast cancer.

Evidence-Based Case Discussion

The Role of Imaging in Cancer of Unknown Primary

A.W.'s case provides another example in which the clinical scenario points to a good prognosis in cancer of unknown primary, as well as dictating therapy. It also shows the importance of imaging in the management of cancer of unknown primary.

Chest X-Ray and Computed Tomography

Routine radiographs of the chest are included as part of the initial evaluation in all patients with cancer of unknown primary. Autopsy studies suggest that chest x-ray alone is able to differentiate a primary and secondary malignancy in only one third of cases. The routine use of computed tomography (CT) of the chest is somewhat more debatable. An argument could be made to only obtain a CT of the chest in those patients with chest x-ray abnormalities. However, a chest CT is often included in the initial evaluation due to frequent involvement of the mediastinum in

Table 24.5 Long-Term Survival in Patients with Unknown Primary Carcinoma and Unfavorable Prognostic Factors. Used with permission from Greco and Pavlidis (11).

Greco and Pavlidis (11).	No. of patients	Regimen	Medlan Survival (mo)	1-Year survival (%)	2-Year survival (%)	3-Year survival (%)
Briasoulis et al, 2000	33	PCb	10	25	5	NR
Dowell et al, 2001	34	P5FUL (17)	8.3	26	NR	NR
		CbE (17)	6.4			
Balana et al, 2003	30	GCE	7.2	36	14	NR
Park et al, 2004	37	PC	11	38	11	NR
Piga et al, 2004	102	CbDoxE	9	35.3	18	11
Pouessel et al, 2004	35	GD	10	43	7	NR
El-Rayes et al, 2005	22	PCb	6.5	27	NR	NR
Pittman et al, 2006	51	GCb	7.8	26	12	NR
Palmeri et al, 2006	66	GPC (33)	9.6	30	NR	NR
		GVC (33)	13.6	52	NR	NR
Berry et al, 2007	42	PCb	8.5	33	17	NR
Briasoulis et al, 2007	47	Oxlr	9.5	40	NR	NR
Schneider et al, 2007	33	GCaCb	7.6	35.6	14.2	NR
MPCRN (5 trials) 1997–2008	396	Multiple regimens (see text)	9.1	38	19	12
Total	928		8.9*	34.6*	13*	12*

Abbreviations: G, gemcitabine; Ox, oxaliplatin; Ir, irinotecan; 5FUL, 5-fluorouracil/leucovorin; V, vinorelbine; C, cisplatin; Ca, capecitibine; Cb, carboplatin; P, paclitaxel; Dox, doxorubicin; E, etoposide; D, docetaxel; NR, not reported
* Mean survivals of all studies.
* Used with permission from Greco FA and Pavlidis N. Treatment for patients with unknown primary carcinoma and unfavorable prognostic factors. Seminars in Oncology 2009; 36(1): 65–74.

cancer of unknown primary. Another factor supporting the use of initial CT scanning of the chest is the frequency of identifying lung carcinoma as the primary tumor. If pathologic testing is suggestive of a lung primary, a CT of the chest should certainly be performed. CT of the abdomen and pelvis in patients with cancer of unknown primary has a well-studied benefit and detects a primary site in 30% to 35% of patients. This is routinely performed in the initial evaluation and is often useful in determining the extent of disease, as well as localizing the most favorable site for biopsy.

Mammography and Other Breast Imaging Tests

A mammogram should be routinely performed in all women who are found to have adenocarcinoma of unknown primary, regardless of the pathologic evaluation. This, along with a breast ultrasound, should especially be done in women with adenocarcinoma with positive supraclavicular, axillary, or mediastinal nodes. In cases where a breast primary is strongly suspected and mammography and ultrasound are noncontributory, bilateral MRI of the breast should be considered, as was done for A.W. MRI scanning is very sensitive for the detection of occult breast cancers in women with malignant axillary lymphadenopathy. Though not included in the routine initial evaluation, MRI of the breast should be used when mammography and ultrasound are inadequate in assessing the extent of the disease, particularly in women with dense breast tissue, malignant axillary adenopathy, and an occult primary breast tumor. It is also helpful in evaluation of the chest wall.

^{18}F-fluorodeoxyglucose Positron Emission Tomographic Scan (FDG-PET)

The use of PET scan in cancer of unknown primary is not yet a clearly proven diagnostic modality but it does have various indications for which it is very valuable. Most of the trials that have been performed using PET scans in the diagnostic evaluation of patients with cancer of unknown primary have involved patients with squamous cell carcinoma with cervical lymphadenopathy. A number of both prospective and retrospective studies have been performed in this subset, with mostly small sample sizes (no more than 50) (9). In these trials, a primary tumor was identified through the use of PET scanning in up to 30% of patients with metastatic cervical lymph nodes. In these patients, PET scan appears to have a clear benefit, allowing for guidance of biopsy, determining extent of disease, guiding therapy such as narrowing radiation fields to limit toxicity, and surveillance after treatment.

Aside from patients with cervical adenopathy on presentation, the use of PET is not recommended as part of a standard evaluation in patients with cancer of unknown primary. Small retrospective studies have suggested that PET studies are able to detect a primary tumor in about 20% of cancer cases of unknown primary in patients not presenting with neck adenopathy.

One limitation of PET studies is the absence of significant accumulation of the ^{18}F-fluorodeoxyglucose tracer in some neoplastic tissues, leading to limited accuracy of anatomic localization. Combination of PET with CT using intravenous contrast has become increasingly routine, improving localization. Combination PET-CT has been noted to identify primary tumors in 33% to 35% of patients with cancer of unknown primary, and up to 57% in smaller studies. To date, there have not been any large prospective trials comparing PET or PET-CT with conventional imaging modalities. Larger clinical studies with long-term follow-up need to be performed using PET scanning before it can be routinely recommended as a diagnostic tool in cancer of unknown primary. In addition to efficacy, cost-effectiveness should be evaluated as well given the expense of this imaging, which thus far has not been studied.

In addition to the evaluation of patients with cervical adenopathy, there are a number of situations where PET appears to be a valuable imaging modality. One example is the use of PET when there is a single site of metastasis, and therapy with curative intent is planned. This allows for the possible identification of disease beyond the single metastatic site, if it is present. Assessment of residual cancer in patients who are candidates for postsurgical adjuvant therapy can be achieved with PET. When surgical resection or radiation therapy is being considered for residual tumor following systemic therapy, PET can be useful in localization of the residual disease. Another situation in which PET scanning would be useful is in patients with an iodine dye allergy who would be unable to undergo conventional CT scanning.

Magnetic Resonance Imaging

The role of MRI in the diagnosis of cancer of unknown primary, outside of its use in the diagnosis of occult breast cancers, is unclear. Those patients who are unable to have CT scans due to contraindications may have MRI as an alternative. Otherwise, there have not been large studies comparing the accuracy of MRI versus CT scanning in the diagnostic evaluation of cancer of unknown primary. Used as an adjunct to CT scanning, it does not appear that MRI significantly alters the treatment plan in most cases. Also due to high costs, routine use of MRI in the initial evaluation of cancer of unknown primary is not recommended. As discussed above, MRI is accepted in patients with isolated axillary lymph node metastases and suspected occult breast cancer. A number of small studies suggest that a negative MRI is predictive of low yield of mastectomy in patients with suspected breast cancer. It is also beneficial in identifying and localizing the site of the primary tumor in up to 70% to 75% of women with isolated axillary lymphadenopathy and suspected occult breast cancer. This provides the advantage of improved surgical planning and the possibility of breast-conserving surgery.

Future Directions

Treatment of cancer of unknown primary often requires the use of empiric therapies. In the absence of a specific diagnosis or suggestive clinical scenario, this creates the possibility of choosing a suboptimal treatment for an individual patient. Current research is aimed at shifting from empiric therapy for all patients with management of cancer of unknown primary as a single entity to specifically tailored therapy using targeted agents and novel therapies. Improved diagnostic methods, with more accurate identification of the tissue of origin is needed to better tailor therapy. As seen in clinical practice in the treatment of breast cancer, one area of growth in the diagnostic arena of cancer of unknown primary is that of molecular profiling. This allows for a subcellular look at phenotypes of the tumor cells, expanding on the concept that the gene profile of particular tumors should be conserved when they metastasize (15). The expression profile of a primary tumor should be mostly the same as that of a metastasis. This allows for comparison of a pattern of gene expression of a cancer of unknown primary to known patterns of different tumor types (which can be very useful in identification of the primary site), or it allows for further classification. This pattern of gene expression can be identified using microarray or by reverse transcription polymerase chain reaction (RT-PCR).

Gene Expression Profiling: Microarray

Measurement of mRNA, and thereby measurement of gene expression, has been used to guide prognostication as well as therapeutics in known primary malignancies, most notably in breast cancer. The use of gene expression profiling in breast cancer creates a genomic taxonomy of the tumor, which stratifies patients according to the likelihood of recurrence. This allows the physician to assess the benefit of adding chemotherapy to the treatment regimen, which individually tailors therapy based on various characteristics of the tumor. The process of gene expression profiling involves extraction of mRNA from tissue, amplifying the mRNA, fluorescently labeling it, and hybridizing it to a microarray. The microarray contains a variety of DNA spots, which code for a unique sequence of a specific gene. After hybridization of the amplified mRNA to the microarray, the fluorescent signal is quantitated at a particular DNA spot. Microarray allows for measurement of thousands of genes simultaneously; however, as such, it is not highly sensitive and is often difficult to reproduce.

Real-Time Polymerase Chain Reaction

RT-PCR allows for quantitation of a specific desired amount of mRNA. RT-PCR is notably more sensitive than gene expression using microarray and unlike microarray allows for quantitative measurement of mRNA. However, unlike microarray, only tens to hundreds of genes can be measured simultaneously. It is also a more time-intensive and expensive test, which needs to be highly sensitive to be compatible with most tumor biopsies that are formalin-fixed, paraffin-embedded (FFPE).

Gene Expression Assays

A number of gene expression assays to determine primary tumor origin have been developed (14). Five of these are currently commercially available in the United States and Europe or are in development. Two of the assays are compatible with FFPE samples. These assays have been validated using mostly samples from primary tumors or known metastatic sites. Metastases from cancer of unknown primary represents a minority of those tested. A retrospective study by Varadhachary et al. evaluated a 10-gene RT-PCR assay performed in 104 FFPE biopsies from patients with cancer of unknown primary (15). This study was the first to evaluate RT-PCR molecular profiling in a large group of patients with cancer of unknown primary. This assay was designed to detect tumors originating from the lung, breast, colon, ovary, pancreas, or prostate. A specific diagnosis was identified in 63 (61%) of the tested specimens using this assay. Validation of such data in cancer of unknown primary is complicated because identification of the primary tumor is rare. Therefore, the authors used indirect variables, including clinicopathologic features, treatment response, and disease course, as measures of validation. This is illustrated in those patients in the aforementioned study who were found by assay to have a colon cancer profile. In the 23 patients with a profile consistent with a colon primary, a colonoscopy did not find the primary in 17 patients. A retrospective analysis revealed that only one of the seven patients treated with a standard empiric cancer of unknown primary regimen (taxane and platinum) had a response, with none of the three patients responding to gemcitabine and irinotecan. Nevertheless, all of the patients who were given a standard colon cancer regimen had a clinical response. Despite these promising results, large prospective studies using assay results to guide therapy need to be performed, and data on impact of these assays on survival are not available.

REFERENCES

1. Jemal A, Siegel R, Xu J, Ward E. Cancer statistics, 2010. *CA Cancer J Clin.* 2010; doi:10.3322/caac.20073
2. Pavlidis N, Briasoulis E, Hainsworth J, et al. Diagnostic and therapeutic management of cancer of an unknown primary. *Eur J Cancer.* 2003;39:1990–2005.
3. Neumann KH, Nystrom JS. Metastatic cancer of unknown origin: nonsquamous cell type. *Semin Oncol.* 1982;9(4):427–434.
4. Pentheroudakis G, Golfinopoulos V, Pavlidis N. Switching benchmarks in cancer of unknown primary; from autopsy to microarray. *Eur J Cancer.* 2007;43:2026–2036.
5. Greco GA, Hainsworth JD, et al. Cancer of unknown primary site. In: DeVita Jr. VT, Hellman S, Rosenberg SA, eds: *Cancer: Principles and Practice of Oncology*, Eighth Edition. Philadelphia, PA: Lippincott Williams & Wilkins. 2008:2363–2387.
6. Abbruzzese JL, Abbruzzese MC, Hess KR, et al. Unknown primary carcinoma: natural history and prognostic factors in 657 consecutive patients. *J Clin Oncol.* 1994;12(6):1272–1280.
7. Oien, Karin A. Pathologic evaluation of cancer of unknown primary. *Semin Oncol.* 2009;36(1):8–37.
8. Pavlidis N, Fizazi K. Carcinoma of unknown primary (CUP). *Crit Rev Oncol/Hematol.* 2009;69:271–278.
9. Varadhachary G, Abbruzzese J, Lenzi R. Diagnostic Strategies for Cancer of unknown primary. *Cancer.* 2004;100(9):1776–1785.
10. Bugat R, Bataillard A, Lesimple T et al. Summary of the Standards, Options, and Recommendations for the management of patients with carcinoma of unknown primary site (2002). *Br J Cancer.* 2003;89(suppl. 1):S59–S66.
11. Greco FA and Pavlidis N. Treatment for patients with unknown primary carcinoma and unfavorable prognostic factors. *Semin Oncol.* 2009;36(1): 65–74.
12. Hainsworth JD and Fizazi K. Treatment for patients with cancer of unknown primary and favorable prognostic factors. *Semin Oncol.* 2009;36(1):44–51.
13. Hainsworth JD, Spigel DR, Clark BL, et al. Paclitaxel/carboplatin/etoposide versus gemcitabine/irinotecan in the first-line treatment of patients with carcinoma of unknown primary site. *Cancer J.* 2010;16(1):70–75.
14. Bender RA and Erlander MG. Molecular classification of cancer of unknown primary. *Semin Oncol.* 2009;36(1):38–43.
15. Varadhachary GR, Talantov D, Raber M, et al. Molecular profiling of carcinoma of unknown primary and correlation with clinical evaluation. *JCO.* 2008;26(27):4442–4448.

25

Hodgkin Lymphoma

POLLY NIRAVATH AND CATHERINE M. BOLLARD

EPIDEMIOLOGY, RISK FACTORS, NATURAL HISTORY, AND PATHOLOGY

Hodgkin lymphoma (HL) is a lymphoid tumor that comprises about 10% of all lymphomas and 0.6% of all cancers diagnosed in the developed world each year. This amounts to approximately 7800 new cases and 1290 deaths annually in the United States. A hallmark feature of HL is its bimodal pattern of incidence, with one peak at 15 to 34 years of age, and a second peak at greater than 55 years old. There is also a slight male predominance, with a male:female ratio of 1.4:1 (1).

Interestingly, HL is classically associated with higher socioeconomic status. In developed countries, HL, particularly the nodular sclerosing subtype, is associated with factors that are linked to higher socioeconomic status such as single family homes, smaller family sizes, and higher level of maternal education. In contrast, mixed cellularity HL is inversely related to socioeconomic status. It is commonly postulated that delayed exposure to some environmental antigen may trigger development of HL, though this has never been proven. Of relevance, it has been observed that higher rates of certain childhood infections such as chicken pox, measles, mumps, rubella, and pertussis are negatively associated with development of HL (2).

The possible genetic predisposition of HL is incompletely understood, but first-degree relatives do have a higher risk of developing HL, including a two to five-fold increased risk for siblings. Among same sex siblings, the risk may be increased as much as nine-fold. There is also an increased risk among parent-child pairs, though not between spouses, again supporting a genetic predisposition (3).

In addition, there are environmental factors involved in the development of HL. Individuals with a history of infectious mononucleosis infection have two to three times increased risk of developing HL as compared to age-matched controls (4). Though this association has been known for many years, it was only in 1987 when Weiss et al. was actually able to demonstrate the Epstein-Barr virus in malignant Hodgkin and Reed-Sternberg (HRS) cells (4). Of note, the association with EBV seems to vary among populations. Approximately half of all HL cases in economically developed countries harbor EBV in the HRS cells, whereas up to 90% of patients in developing countries carry the virus in their HRS cells (3). One EBV protein in particular, known as latent membrane protein 1 (LMP1), is thought to be key in the oncogenic process, as it is known to elicit B lymphocyte transformation in vitro (4).

There is clearly a relationship between the development of HL and immune deficiency. Patients with HIV and common variable immune deficiency are at higher risk for getting HL, and it has also been noted clinically that HL patients have higher rates of bacterial, fungal, and viral infections even before starting chemotherapy and radiation treatment. HL patients also typically have T cell dysfunction, as evidenced by impaired delayed-type hypersensitivity reaction. Transfusion-related graft versus host disease has also been described in HL patients. In more advanced stages of the disease, $CD3^+$ T cells tend to be reduced in number, and lymphopenia is a common finding in HL patients of all stages. It remains unclear whether the underlying immune deficiency commonly seen in HL is primary, secondary, or both in some cases (5).

Although HL is included among the World Health Organization HIV-associated lymphomas, and there has been an increased incidence of HL in HIV patients since the introduction of highly active antiretroviral therapy (HAART), the exact nature of this association remains unclear. There is a ten-fold increased risk among HIV positive individuals to develop HL, and this risk seems to decline with lower CD4 counts. Interestingly, 80% to 100% of HIV-associated HL is associated with EBV infection. In particular, the above-mentioned EBV-encoded LMP1 is expressed in nearly all HIV-HL cases (6). Furthermore, EBV proliferation is typically kept under check in immunocompetent individuals by T cell immunity. Logically, it seems that the EBV-infected cells may proliferate more rapidly in HIV patients because of their impaired T cell activity. The sum of this data suggests that HIV-associated HL is most likely an EBV-related lymphoma that has developed in the setting of impaired EBV-specific T cell immunity (6).

HL is generally considered to be a slow-growing lymphoma. It is felt that some cases of HL may be preceded by a condition called "progressive transformation of the germinal center." The term refers to a type of follicular lymphoid hyperplasia containing many small B cells of mantle zone type. This pathologic entity is seen in about one fifth of lymph nodes in nodular lymphocyte predominant HL. However, there are many cases in which patients have this condition without ever developing HL. Thus, its significance is not totally clear. Another notable feature of HL is its tendency to spread to contiguous lymph nodes. Eventually, with more advanced disease, the lymphoma can invade blood vessels and spread to more distant organs (3).

In the past several decades, significant advances have been made in the treatment of HL, such that at least 80% of patients are now cured with chemotherapy and radiation. In fact, the overall 5-year survival rate for all patients with HL from 1999 to 2006 was 84.7%. Even for those with stage III and IV disease at diagnosis, 5-year overall survival is 82.3% (1). Clearly, recent treatment advances have dramatically changed the landscape of this disease.

Pathologically, HL is notable for its characteristic HRS cells in a background of inflammatory cells. Reed-Sternberg cells are clonal B cells of follicle center cell origin (3). The composition of the milieu in which the Reed-Sternberg cells reside determines the subtype of HL. The REAL/WHO classification identifies two main subtypes: classical Hodgkin lymphoma (classical HL) and lymphocyte predominant Hodgkin lymphoma (LPHL).

Classical HL accounts for 95% of cases and is characterized morphologically by typical Reed-Sternberg cells. Immunophenotypically, 70% to 85% of classical HL cases will express CD15; CD30 and fascin are positive in nearly all cases. CD20 may be positive in 30% to 40% of cases, more commonly in lymphocyte rich HL. The B cell marker CD79a may be expressed in 10% of classical HL. Finally, the inflammatory background cells in classical HL are T cells, except for the lymphocyte rich subtype of classical HL, which has a background similar to that of LPHL (3).

LPHL comprises the remaining 5% of all HL cases and typically contains lymphohistiocytic or "popcorn" cells. LPHL is more commonly CD15 and CD30 negative, with strong CD20 and CD45 positivity, thus distinguishing it from classical HL. Staining for CD3 may further support the diagnosis because T cells characteristically form rosettes around the lymphocyte predominant cells, characteristic of LPHL. The background cells in LPHL are usually CD20 and CD79a positive B cells (3).

STAGING

HL is staged using the Ann Arbor staging mechanism with subsets A and B used for the absence or presence of B symptoms, respectively.

Hodgkin Lymphoma Staging System

Stage	Definition
I	Involvement of a single lymph node region (I), or localized involvement of a single extralymphatic organ or site (I_E).
II	Involvement of two or more lymph node regions on the same side of the diaphragm (II), or localized involvement of a single associated extralymphatic organ or site and its regional lymph node(s), with or without involvement of other lymph node regions on the same side of the diaphragm (II_E)
III	Involvement of lymph node regions on both sides of the diaphragm (III), which may also be accompanied by localized involvement of an associated extralymphatic organ or site (III_E), by involvement of the spleen (III_S), or by both (III_{E+S}).
IV	Disseminated (multifocal) involvement of one or more extralymphatic organs, with or without associated lymph node involvement, or isolated extralymphatic organ involvement with distant (nonregional) nodal involvement.
Further Classification Applicable to Any Stage	
A	No systemic symptoms present
B	Unexplained fevers >38°C, drenching night sweats, or weight loss >10% of body weight
X	Bulky disease: mediastinal widening more than 1/3 the diameter of the chest, or nodal mass >10 cm
E	Involvement of a single extranodal site that is contiguous or proximal to the known nodal site

CASE SUMMARIES

Early-Stage Disease

N.P. is a 23-year-old Caucasian woman with no significant past medical history who presented to her primary care doctor with 4 months of a slowly enlarging right neck mass. She denied fevers, chills, night sweats, pruritis, and weight loss. Physical examination revealed no other lymphadenopathy, although CT scans showed right-sided cervical lymphadenopathy as well as mediastinal lymphadenopathy measuring 4 cm in greatest dimension. Laboratory results included normal CBC, albumin, and erythrocyte sedimentation rate (ESR). Urine pregnancy test was negative. Excisional biopsy of the right cervical lymph node revealed classic Reed-Sternberg cells, and immunohistochemistry showed CD15 and CD30 positivity, with CD20 negativity. Bone marrow biopsy was negative for lymphomatous involvement.

Evidence-Based Case Discussion

In summary, N.P. is a 23-year-old woman with stage IIB classical HL, nodular sclerosing subtype. She has favorable early-stage disease. Her age brings to light the issue of HL in pregnancy. Even though this particular patient was not pregnant, HL is the fourth most common malignancy among pregnant women (3). In staging a pregnant woman, MRI or ultrasound is usually chosen over CT scan in order to avoid any radiation exposure to the fetus. Likewise, PET scanning should also not be used because the radioactive tracer crosses the placenta and is associated with higher radiation exposure than CT scan. In terms of treatment, chemotherapy should not be given in the first trimester when the fetus is particularly susceptible to teratogenic effects from chemotherapy. Therapy for this slow-growing lymphoma can usually be delayed until the second or third trimester, when it has not been associated with higher rates of malformations, but has been linked to higher rates of intrauterine death, growth retardation, preterm delivery, and low birth weight. Generally, though, most pregnant women can be offered chemotherapy with adriamycin, bleomycin, vinblastine, and dacarbazine (ABVD) in the second or third trimester with little risk to the fetus, since several case series and case reports have shown little adverse effect on the fetus from this particular regimen. Radiation exposure, on the other hand, presents much more potential harm and should be avoided if at all possible. Radiation to the fetus results in significantly higher risk of developing leukemia or a solid malignancy in the first decade of life. Also, radiation to the chest in a pregnant or lactating woman confers a much higher risk of breast cancer in the future for the mother (7).

For N.P., with early-stage, favorable disease, treatment is based on prognostic features present at the time of diagnosis in order to optimize therapy while minimizing toxicity. Long-term toxicities of HL therapy typically include cardiac and pulmonary damage, infertility, and secondary malignancies. In fact, among patients with early-stage favorable HL, mortality from these other causes increases over time, eventually overtaking HL-related mortality after 12 to 15 years (8). In an attempt to achieve high cure rates while decreasing side effects, many early studies asked whether radiation alone is sufficient for early-stage favorable disease, or whether both chemotherapy and radiation are necessary. The SWOG 9133/CALGB 9391 trial enrolled 348 patients with stage IA and IIA disease, excluding patients with adverse prognostic features such as bulky lymphadenopathy and/or B symptoms. Half of the patients were randomized to receive two cycles of chemotherapy (adriamycin and vinblastine) followed by subtotal lymphoid irradiation (STLI), and the other half received STLI only. The trial was closed early because of the clearly superior failure-free survival of 94% versus 81% in the combined modality therapy (CMT) arm versus the STLI-only arm, though there was no demonstrable difference in overall survival. However, hematologic toxicity was higher in the combined modality arm, with 37 patients experiencing grade 4 myelosuppression in the CMT arm, versus 4 patients in the STLI-only arm (9).

The German Hodgkin Study Group performed a similar study, HD7, which compared two cycles of ABVD chemotherapy followed by extended field radiotherapy (EFRT) versus EFRT alone. EFRT consisted of 30 Gy to the extended field and 10 Gy to the involved field. They enrolled 650 patients, excluding those with large mediastinal mass, extranodal disease, massive splenic involvement, or high ESR. The GHSG also demonstrated decreased relapses in the combined modality arm (3% vs. 22%), though this did not translate into an improvement in overall survival (10).

Finally, in the H8-F trial that enrolled stage I and II HL patients with favorable risk factors, the investigators found a significantly higher rate of complete remission and improved 10-year overall survival in patients who received three cycles of MOPP-ABV followed by involved field radiotherapy as compared to those who received only subtotal nodal irradiation alone (11).

Although it is apparent that sequential chemotherapy and radiation is superior to radiotherapy alone, the question of how much irradiation is actually necessary remained unanswered until relatively recently. In their HD8 study, the German Hodgkin Study Group asked the question of whether involved field radiotherapy could be used instead of extended field radiotherapy (12). They analyzed 1064 early-stage, unfavorable risk patients, randomized to four cycles of chemotherapy followed by either extended field radiotherapy (30 Gy in the extended field volume and 10 Gy to the initial bulky disease) or involved field radiotherapy (30 Gy in the involved field and 10 Gy to initial bulky disease). The chemotherapy in each arm consisted of two cycles of cyclophosphamide, vincristine, procarbazine, and prednisone (COPP) alternating with two cycles of ABVD. All patients had at least one adverse risk factor: large mediastinal mass (at least 1/3 of the thoracic diameter), extranodal disease, massive splenic involvement, elevated ESR, or more than two lymph node areas of involvement. Patients with stage IIIA disease with no risk factors were also included in the study. There was no difference between the two arms in terms of freedom from treatment failure or overall survival. However, the EFRT arm was more toxic, with significantly higher rates of nausea and vomiting, GI toxicity, leukopenia, and thrombocytopenia. With a median observation time of 55 months, there was a 4.6% rate of secondary malignancies in the EFRT arm versus 2.8% in the IFRT arm, although this was not statistically significant with a *P*-value of 0.191. The investigators concluded that four cycles of chemotherapy followed by involved field radiotherapy is effective and sufficient treatment for early-stage disease with unfavorable risk factors (12).

The next question to be asked was the number of chemotherapy cycles required and the amount of involved field radiation needed for effective treatment. The HD10 trial randomized patients with favorable stage I or II disease with no risk factors in a 2 × 2 design to four versus two cycles of ABVD and 30 Gy versus 20 Gy of IFRT. Both interim analysis at 2 years and updated 4-year follow-up data showed no difference in freedom from treatment failure or overall survival (13).

Finally, two major trials looked at chemotherapy alone for early-stage HL. The first trial, conducted in Memorial Sloan-Kettering Cancer Center, randomized 152 patients with stage IA, IB, IIA, IIB, or IIIA HL without bulky disease to either six cycles of ABVD alone or six cycles of ABVD and radiotherapy. Eleven patients in the ABVD plus radiotherapy arm received involved field radiotherapy, and the remaining patients received extended field. Although there was a trend for improved overall survival with ABVD + XRT versus ABVD alone (97% vs. 90% at 60 months), this was not statistically significant, with $P = .08$. Similarly, there was no significant difference in terms of CR duration or FFP between the two arms. Also of note, there were five secondary malignancies in the RT arm and three in the chemotherapy-alone arm, but the size of this study prevented detection of differences of <20% (14).

The other major trial investigating chemotherapy alone versus combined modality therapy was conducted by NCI Canada Clinical Trials Group and ECOG. They randomized 399 patients with nonbulky stage I to IIA disease to 4 to 6 cycles of ABVD chemotherapy alone versus combined modality therapy with ABVD and radiation. A significantly higher freedom from disease progression at 5 years was observed in the combined modality arm (93% vs. 87%, $P = .006$), but there was no significant difference in terms of event-free survival or overall survival. However, in subset analysis, the difference in freedom from disease progression did seem to come primarily from the unfavorable cohort rather than the favorable cohort of patients (15).

With the somewhat conflicting results of these two studies, the currently accepted recommendation is to treat

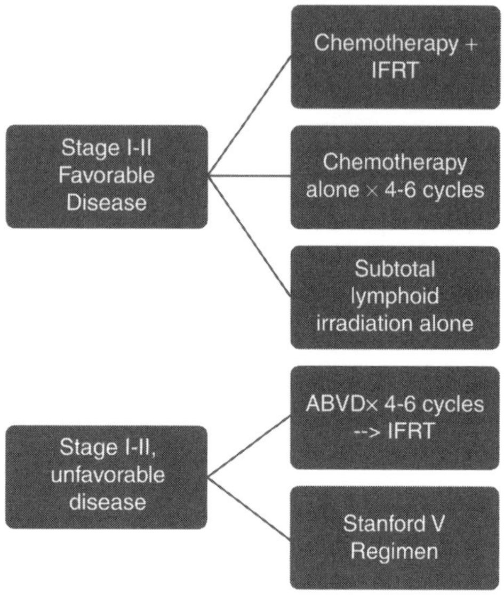

Figure 25.1

Treatment of early stage disease.

patients with favorable stage I and II disease with combined modality therapy, though this may be only two cycles of ABVD followed only by IFRT, as shown by the HD 10 trial. For select cases of favorable stage I and II disease with relative contraindications to radiation therapy, some patients may receive only 4 to 6 cycles of ABVD chemotherapy, particularly if they have a negative PET scan after two cycles of chemotherapy. However, those with unfavorable stage I and II disease should be treated with combination chemotherapy and involved field radiotherapy (see Figure 25.1).

Advanced Stage Disease

L.Z., a 46-year-old Hispanic woman with no past medical history, presented to the emergency room complaining of a left neck mass enlarging over the previous 6 months, fevers to 101 degrees, chills, sweats, and a 30-pound weight loss. Her physical examination revealed a 6-cm firm left neck mass, along with other palpable lymphadenopathy in the right cervical, left axillary, and bilateral inguinal regions. Laboratory values were significant for anemia with a hemoglobin of 10.5 g/dL, a platelet count of 125,000/µL, an albumin of 2.9 g/dL, and an ESR of 78 mm/hr. A CT scan revealed hepatosplenomegaly and diffuse bulky lymphadenopathy, including enlargement of mediastinal, bilateral cervical, left axillary, retroperitoneal, pelvic, and bilateral inguinal lymph nodes. Biopsy of the left cervical lymph node was positive for nodular sclerosing HL, and bone marrow biopsy was positive for HL involvement as well. She was treated with two cycles of ABVD chemotherapy, and subsequent PET scan showed partial response (Figure 25.2).

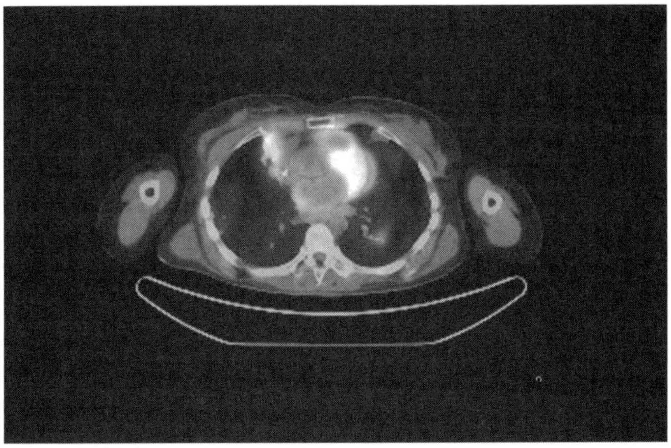

Figure 25.2

PET scan showing residual FDG-avid disease in the mediastinum. (see color insert)

Evidence-Based Case Discussion

L.Z. has stage IVB HL with several poor prognostic features, including B symptoms and bulky lymphadenopathy. Furthermore, the lack of complete response on PET scan following two cycles of ABVD is a very poor prognostic indicator. Studies have shown markedly improved 2-year progression-free survival with negative PET scan after two cycles of chemotherapy (95% vs. 12%). A retrospective study analyzed 165 patients with advanced HL who initially received two cycles of ABVD followed by PET scan. Those with negative PET scan were given four more cycles of ABVD and irradiation, and those with positive PET scan were given four cycles of dose-escalated bleomycin, etoposide, adriamycin, cyclophosphamide, vincristine, procarbazine, and prednisone (BEACOPP) followed by four cycles of standard dose BEACOPP and irradiation. The 2-year failure-free survival was 65% for the PET positive patients and 92% for the PET negative patients (P = .0004). When compared to historical controls who did not change treatment based on the PET scan results, the 2-year progression-free survival for PET positive patients was improved from 12% to 62% (16). Although these results do support a prognostic role for PET scan, randomized controlled trials are still ongoing to support the predictive role of PET in the management of HL.

For advanced stage HL, chemotherapy with mechlorethamine, vincristine, procarbazine, and prednisone (MOPP) was once the standard treatment; however, it was associated with development of acute leukemia, sterility, and severe myelosuppression. Thus, CALGB conducted a randomized, prospective trial of 361 patients with stage III or IV disease comparing 6 to 8 cycles of MOPP versus 6 to 8 cycles of ABVD versus 12 cycles of MOPP alternating with ABVD. Although the overall survival was not significantly different, the complete response rate was higher in the ABVD-containing regimens, and they were associated with fewer hematologic adverse events and fewer dose reductions (17).

Although ABVD has emerged as the accepted standard therapy for HL in many institutions, the Stanford V regimen is also widely used. By decreasing the total dose of alkylating agents, doxorubicin, and bleomycin while increasing the dose density and intensity of chemotherapy, the Stanford V regimen aims to decrease the risk of sterility, secondary leukemia, and cardiopulmonary toxicities. This regimen consists of doxorubicin, vinblastine, mechlorethamine, vincristine, bleomycin, etoposide, and prednisone, which is given only for a period of 12 weeks, followed by consolidative radiotherapy. The initial phase II trial included 126 patients with stage II bulky disease or stage III to IV disease and resulted in a 5-year freedom from progression of 89%, and the overall survival of 96% at 4.5 years (18).

The Stanford V regimen has been directly compared to ABVD in a randomized trial that included 520 patients with advanced stage disease, defined as stage III to IV disease, or B symptoms, or locally extensive disease within any stage. Seventy-three percent of the Stanford V patients received radiation therapy, compared to only 53% in the ABVD arm. Although the overall response rate and the overall survival were not significantly different between the two arms, there was a higher complete response rate with ABVD as compared to Stanford V (55% vs. 36%, $P < .001$). However, this came at the expense of more pulmonary toxicity with ABVD (10% vs. 2%) and higher probability of needing G-CSF (75% vs. 41%) (19).

In cases of advanced HL, even more aggressive regimens can be justified based on potentially higher cure rates, but with increased toxicity. Diehl et al. examined 1201 patients with newly diagnosed unfavorable stage II or stage III to IV HL. Patients were randomized to one of three arms: eight cycles of cyclophosphamide, vincristine, procarbazine, and prednisone alternating with doxorubicin, bleomycin, vinblastine, and dacarbazine (COPP-ABVD); bleomycin, etoposide, doxorubicin, cyclophosphamide, vincristine, procarbazine, and prednisone (BEACOPP); or increased-dose BEACOPP. When indicated, patients also received radiation therapy after chemotherapy. Even with the use of G-CSF, there was a stunning 98% incidence of grade 3 to 4 leukopenia, with 22% grade 3 to 4 infections in the dose-escalated BEACOPP arm. Similarly, 47% of patients experienced grade 4 thrombocytopenia. The rate of secondary acute leukemia 5 years after the diagnosis of Hodgkin's disease was 0.4% in the COPP-ABVD group, 0.6% in the BEACOPP group, and 2.5% in the increased-dose BEACOPP group (P = .03). However, the rate of complete remission was higher with dose-escalated BEACOPP (96% vs. 85% for COPP-ABVD and 88% for standard dose BEACOPP), and early progression was significantly lower in the dose-escalated BEACOPP arm as well, with only 2% early progressers, as compared to 10% in the

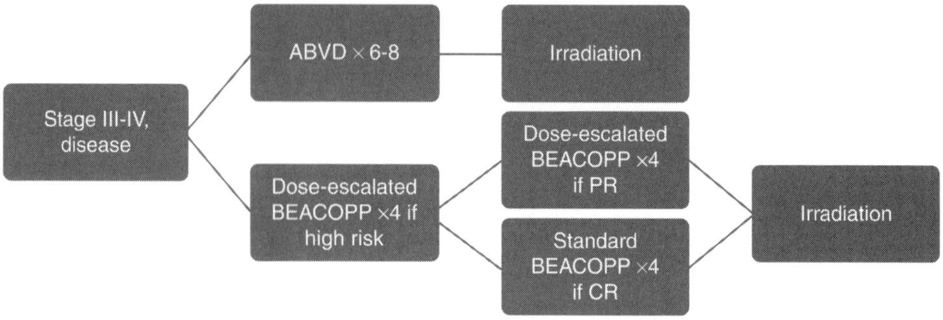

Figure 25.3

Treatment for advanced Hodgkin lymphoma.

COPP-ABVD arm and 8% in the standard BEACOPP arm. Finally, the 5-year overall survival was significantly improved in the patients who received dose-escalated BEACOPP (91% vs. 83% for COPP-ABVD) (20). In an updated report, the 10-year overall survival rate remained significantly higher with dose-escalated BEACOPP (86% vs. 80% for standard BEACOPP and 75% for COPP-ABVD) (20).

ABVD and BEACOPP were compared head-to-head in an Italian trial as front-line therapy for 307 patients with stages IIB, III, and IV HL. BEACOPP demonstrated improved progression free survival as compared to ABVD (81% vs. 69% at median of 41 months, with $P = .038$). However, this did not translate into a significantly higher overall survival rate, and patients in the BEACOPP arm experienced significantly higher rates of grade 3 to 4 neutropenia and severe infections (21).

Overall, these studies suggest that intensifying initial chemotherapy with dose-escalated BEACOPP is a double-edged sword improving disease control but with increased toxicity. Furthermore, a clear advantage in overall survival has not been demonstrated for dose-escalated BEACOPP versus standard ABVD chemotherapy.

Another major question for advanced HL is whether patients should receive stem cell transplant as first-line treatment. Several studies have addressed this question. In the first study, 163 adults with advanced stage disease and at least two adverse prognostic features received four courses of chemotherapy with ABVD, MOPP/ABVD, or MOPP/ABV. Patients who achieved complete response were then randomized to receive either four more courses of the same chemotherapy, or high-dose therapy followed by autologous stem cell transplant. There was no difference between the two arms in terms of complete response, 5-year failure-free survival rates, or 5-year overall survival (22). In a second study, patients with high-risk, advanced stage disease were randomized to receive either prednisolone, vinblastine, doxorubicin, chlorambucil, etoposide, bleomycin, vincristine, procarbazine (PVACE-BOP) for three cycles, followed by autologous stem cell transplant, or PVACE-BOP for five cycles. Only 65 patients accepted randomization, and there was no difference in terms of time to treatment failure or overall survival (23). Thus, patients who respond well to initial chemotherapy for advanced stage HL are unlikely to derive added benefit from early intensification with autologous stem cell rescue in the first-line setting.

A final question for the treatment of advanced stage HL is whether to irradiate radiologically eradicated disease since 80% of relapsed HL cases recur in sites of previous lymphadenopathy (3). In order to answer this question, 208 patients who had achieved complete remission after six cycles of nitrogen mustard, vincristine, prednisone, bleomycin, doxorubicin, and procarbazine (MOP-BAP) chemotherapy were randomized to either receive involved field radiotherapy (IFRT) to all initially involved sites or no further treatment. There was no significant difference between the two arms with respect to remission duration, relapse-free survival, or overall survival. However, the pattern of relapse was different in the two groups. Seventy-nine percent of the relapsed patients in the no further treatment arm had disease recurrence exclusively in previously involved sites, and only 47% of those who relapsed in the "radiotherapy" arm had disease in areas of previous involvement (24).

A similar study was conducted in India from 1993 through 1996 in which 179 patients with advanced stage HL who had achieved complete remission after six cycles of ABVD were randomized to receive either consolidation radiation therapy (most patients received IFRT) or no further treatment. The 8-year overall survival was 89% in the chemotherapy-alone group, versus 100% in the radiotherapy group ($P = .002$) (25). Whereas these findings seem to contradict the previous study, it should be noted that 70% of the patients had mixed cellularity (MC) histology, as compared to the majority of Americans who have nodular sclerosing (NS) histology. MC HL is known to be more sensitive to therapy with generally better outcomes than NS HL (3). Hence, it is not clear whether the two histologies would benefit differently from consolidation radiation therapy. In an attempt to resolve the issue of consolidation with radiation therapy, a large meta-analysis examined data on 1740 patients with all stages of disease across 14 trials. The trials were divided into two groups: those that evaluated chemotherapy alone versus the same chemotherapy plus radiation therapy (additional RT design), and those that tested whether radiotherapy as part of a combined modality treatment can be substituted by chemotherapy (parallel RT/CT design). The meta-analysis found that there were significantly more durable complete remissions at 10 years in the additional RT design trials for those patients who received radiotherapy ($P \leq .001$). However, in the parallel RT/CT design, continuous complete remission rates were statistically similar when either additional radiotherapy or additional chemotherapy was given. Interestingly, there was an 8% improvement in overall survival at 10 years in patients who received no radiotherapy in the parallel RT/CT design, which was due to a statistically significant increased rate of deaths unrelated to HL in the combined modality groups. In particular, the relative risk of dying from leukemia was 2.48 times greater in groups who received radiation versus those who did not (26). This meta-analysis seems to suggest that additional chemotherapy can substitute for radiation therapy, possibly with less long-term toxicity and increased overall survival. However, the trials that included an additional RT component used 6 to 8 cycles of MOPP or BCVPP (carmustine, cyclophosphamide, vinblastine, procarbazine, and prednisone), which are not as efficacious as newer, anthracycline-containing regimens such as ABVD. Thus, it is still debatable whether these results are truly applicable in the present day.

In summary, 6 to 8 cycles of chemotherapy with ABVD or the Stanford V regimen are effective treatments for advanced stage HL. Although dose-escalated BEACOPP may provide improved remission rates for high-risk patients, this is at the risk of higher toxicity (increased cytopenias, treatment-related mortality, infertility, and secondary cancers), and there is no increase in overall survival as compared to ABVD. There is no role for stem cell transplant in the first line setting. Patients who are not in complete remission after completing chemotherapy, or those with bulky mediastinal disease initially, should receive consolidative irradiation. For patients who achieve complete remission with chemotherapy alone, consolidative irradiation may be a consideration, though more studies are needed to clarify its role. See Figure 25.3 for a management algorithm. Further studies are also ongoing to evaluate whether PET scan after two cycles of chemotherapy can be used to determine subsequent chemotherapy.

Relapsed and Refractory Disease

M.M. is a 54-year-old Caucasian woman with stage IV HL as manifested by cervical, axillary, and bulky mediastinal lymphadenopathy as well as bone marrow involvement. She was treated with eight cycles of ABVD and mediastinal irradiation. A restaging PET scan performed 2 months after the completion of treatment still shows residual FDG-avid disease in the mediastinum that is biopsy-proven to be HL.

Evidence-Based Case Discussion

M.M. has highly aggressive, refractory HL. Although initial CR rates are quite high in HL, approximately 20% to 30% of patients relapse, presenting a complicated treatment decision. Some of the features associated with higher rates of relapse include advanced stage, B symptoms, and extranodal disease. At relapse, all patients should be re-biopsied because of the relatively high risk for secondary tumors. Once HL is confirmed, the type of relapse should be ascertained because of the marked difference in prognosis and response to treatment. Patients with primary progressive HL who never achieved a CR, or relapse within 3 months of completing treatment, have a markedly poorer prognosis than those patients who are early relapsers (within 3–12 months of treatment completion) or late relapsers (more than 12 months after treatment is completed). The projected 20-year overall survival for primary progressive HL is 0%, compared to 11% for early and 22% for late relapsers (3).

In a small percentage of patients with relapsed disease who have very limited areas of involvement in which radiotherapy was not used in first line, salvage radiotherapy may be very effective. However, for the majority of patients with relapsed or refractory disease, the favored treatment plan is salvage chemotherapy followed by autologous stem cell transplant (ASCT). Two randomized controlled trials have established the role of ASCT in relapsed HL; both of these trials have shown improved progression-free survival without difference in overall survival. The first trial enrolled 40 patients in which 20 received high-dose chemotherapy with BEAM (carmustine, etoposide, cytarabine, and melphalan) followed by ASCT, and the remaining 20 patients received mini-BEAM (the same drugs as BEAM, at lower doses, not requiring stem cell rescue) alone. The ASCT arm demonstrated improved 3-year event-free survival (53% vs. 10%, $P = .025$). At a median follow-up of 34 months, five patients in the BEAM arm had died, two from complications of ASCT, and three from disease progression, while nine patients died in the mini-BEAM group, all from disease progression. The overall survival difference was not statistically significant, and it is unclear whether an overall survival difference would have been demonstrated with a higher powered study (27). The second randomized trial treated 161 relapsed patients with two cycles of dexamethasone-BEAM. Those with CR or PR were randomized to two more cycles of dexa-BEAM versus high-dose BEAM followed by ASCT. Freedom from treatment failure at 3 years was significantly improved in the ASCT arm (55% vs. 34%, $P = .019$). However, overall survival was not significantly different between the two groups (28).

Allogeneic transplant has also been studied in relapsed and refractory HL; however, its toxicities generally seem to outweigh its benefits. One trial that examined 100 allogeneic transplants from HLA-identical siblings discovered a

35% incidence of acute graft versus host disease (GVHD) and 45% chronic GVHD. Three-year survival was dismal at only 21% (29). Similarly, another study retrospectively compared 45 allogeneic transplants with 45 matched autologous transplant controls from the European Bone Marrow Transplantation Registry, and they found a significantly improved 4-year survival with autologous transplant (64% vs. 30%, $P = .007$). Transplant related mortality (TRM) was felt to be the primary culprit for this difference, with 65% TRM after allogeneic transplant compared with only 12% after autologous transplant (30). At present, autologous bone marrow transplant remains the widely accepted standard of care for relapsed and refractory HL.

The choice of salvage regimen for relapsed or refractory HL is not entirely clear, as there are many available options and no randomized controlled trials to establish the superiority of any one regimen over the others.

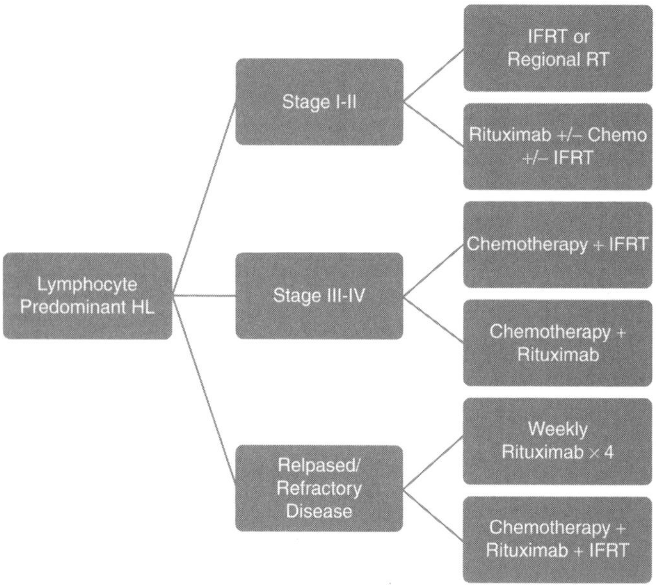

Figure 25.4

Treatment of lymphocyte predominant Hodgkin lymphoma.

Lymphocyte Predominant HL

R.T. is an otherwise healthy 35-year-old male who presented with a 6-month history of an enlarging right axillary mass. He denied fatigue, fevers, chills, sweats, and weight loss. On physical examination, he was noted to have bilateral axillary lymphadenopathy. Laboratory tests including CBC, electrolytes, and liver function tests were unremarkable. ESR was elevated at 56 mm/hour. A CT scan showed only bilateral axillary lymphadenopathy. Bone marrow biopsy shows LPHL, positive for CD20 and negative for CD15 and CD30.

Evidence-Based Case Discussion

This young man has stage II LPHL, which behaves quite differently from classical HL. LPHL generally is less aggressive, carries a better prognosis, and tends to be identified at earlier stages with 53% of patients diagnosed in stage I disease, and only 6% in stage IV (3). However, LPHL has a slightly higher rate of transformation to secondary non-HL and tends to relapse multiple times as compared to classical HL (3).

It is now widely held that LPHL should be treated differently from classical HL due to its unique behavior with frequent relapses and remissions, as well as its CD20 positivity (Figure 25.4). In a recent study of 113 patients with stage I or II LPHL, 82% were treated with radiation therapy alone, 12% with combined chemoradiotherapy, and 6% with chemotherapy alone. Interestingly, those who received chemotherapy alone had worse progression-free survival than those who received radiation alone, with six out of seven patients who received chemotherapy relapsing compared to only 20 of 106 patients who received radiation therapy. Furthermore, overall survival rates did not differ among patients who received extended field, regional field, or limited field radiotherapy (31). Another review examined 131 cases of stage IA LPHL in the German Hodgkin Study Group. They found no significant difference in complete remission or overall survival at 43 months for those patients who had radiation alone or combined chemoradiotherapy (32). These results indicate that involved field radiation therapy alone may be sufficient for early-stage LPHL, with little, if any, added benefit of chemotherapy.

There has also been much interest in using rituximab in LPHL, given its CD20 positivity and the relative tolerability of rituximab. The German Hodgkin Study group examined 15 patients with confirmed relapsed or refractory LPHL, of whom 40% had stage III or IV disease. Treating with four weekly doses of rituximab resulted in 94% overall response rate, with a 53% complete response. Median time to progression was 33 months, and median overall survival was not yet reached at 7 years (33).

In summary, evidence supports using radiation as a single treatment modality for early-stage LPHL, with the addition of chemotherapy +/– rituximab for the treatment of more advanced LPHL. For relapsed or refractory disease, four doses of single agent rituximab may be sufficient to stave off disease for a prolonged period of time, though the likelihood of eventual relapse is quite high.

REFERENCES

1. Altekruse SF, Kosary CL, Krapcho M, et al (eds). *SEER Cancer Statistics Review, 1975–2007*. Bethesda, MD: National Cancer Institute.

2. Montella M, Maso LD, Crispo A, et al. Do childhood diseases affect NHL and HL risk? A case control study from Northern and Southern Italy. *Leukemia Res.* 2006;30:917–922.
3. Diehl V, et al. Hodgkin lymphoma. In: DeVita VT, Lawrence TS, Rosenberg SA, eds. *Cancer: Principles and Practice of Oncology.* Philadelphia, PA : Lippincott Williams & Wilkins; 2008:2167–2220.
4. Weiss LM, Strickler JG, Warnke RA, et al. Epstein–Barr viral DNA in tissues of Hodgkin's disease. *Am J Path.* 1987;129:86–91.
5. Kennedy-Nasser A, Bollard C, Rooney C. Adoptive immunotherapy for Hodgkin lymphoma. *Int J Hem.* 2006;83:385–390.
6. Carbone A, Gloghini A, Serraino D, et al. HIV-associated Hodgkin lymphoma. *Curr Opin HIV AIDS.* 2009;4(1):3–10.
7. Pereg D, Koren G, Lishner M. The treatment of Hodgkin's and non-Hodgkin's lymphoma in pregnancy. *Haematologica.* 2007;92:1230–1237.
8. Ng AK, Bernardo MP, Weller E, et al. Long term survival and competing causes of death in patients with early stage Hodgkins disease treated at age 50 or younger. *J Clin Oncol.* 2002;20:2101–2108.
9. Press OW, LeBlanc M, Lichter AS, et al. Phase III randomized intergroup trial of subtotal lymphoid irradiation versus doxorubicin, vinblastine, and subtotal lymphoid irradiation for stage IA to IIA Hodgkin's disease. *J Clin Oncol.* 2001;19:4238–4244.
10. Engert A, Franklin J, Eich HT, et al. Two cycles of doxorubicin, bleomycin, vinblastine, and dacarbazine plus extended-field radiotherapy is superior to radiotherapy alone in early favorable Hodgkin's lymphoma: final results of the GHSG HD7 Trial. *N Eng J Med.* 2007;25:3495–3502.
11. Fermé C, Eghbali H, Meerwaldt JH, et al. Chemotherapy plus involved field radiation in early stage Hodgkin's disease. *N Eng J Med.* 2007;357:1916–1927.
12. Engert A, Schiller P, Josting A, et al. Involved-field radiotherapy is equally effective and less toxic compared with extended field radiotherapy after four cycles of chemotherapy in patients with early stage unfavorable Hodgkins lymphoma: results of the HD8 trial. *J Clin Oncol.* 2003;21:3601–3608.
13. Diehl V, Brilliant C, Engert A, et al. Investigating reduction of combined modality treatment intensity in early stage Hodgkin's lymphoma. *J Clin Oncol.* 2005;23(16S):6506.
14. Straus DJ, Portlock CS, Qin J, et al. Results of a prospective randomized clinical trial of doxorubicin, bleomycin, vinblastine, and dacarbazine (ABVD) followed by radiation therapy (RT) versus ABVD alone for stages I, II, and IIIA nonbulky Hodgkin disease. *Blood.* 2004;104:3483–3489.
15. Meyer RM, Gospodarowicz MK, Connors JM, et al. Randomized comparison of ABVD chemotherapy with a strategy that includes radiation therapy in patients with limited stage Hodgkin's lymphoma: NCI Canada Clinical Trials Group and the ECOG. *J Clin Oncol.* 2005;23:4634–4642.
16. Gallamini A, Patti C, Viviani S, et al. Early chemotherapy intensification with BEACOPP in advanced stage Hodgkin lymphoma patients with a interim PET positive after two ABVD courses. *Brit J Haem.* 2010 Dec 20. doi: 10.1111/j.1365-2141.2010.08485.x. [Epub ahead of print]
17. Canellos GP, Anderson JR, Propert KJ, et al. Chemotherapy of advanced Hodgkins disease with MOPP, ABVD, or MOPP alternating with ABVD. *N Eng J Med.* 1992;327:1478–1484.
18. Bartlett NL, Rosenberg SA, Hoppe RT, et al. Brief chemotherapy, Stanford V, and adjuvant radiotherapy for bulky or advanced stage Hodgkin's disease: a preliminary report. *J Clin Oncol.* 1995;13:1080–1088.
19. Hoskin PJ, Lowry L, Horwich A, et al. Randomized comparison of the Stanford V regimen and ABVD in the treatment of advanced Hodgkin's lymphoma: UK NCRI Lymphoma Group Study ISRCTN 64141244. *J Clin Oncol.* 2009;27:5390–5396.
20. Engert A, Diehl V, Franklin J, et al. Escalated dose BEACOPP in the treatment of patients with advanced stage Hodgkins lymphoma:10 years of follow up of the GHSG HD9 study. *J Clin Oncol.* 2009;27:4548–4554.
21. Federico M, Luminari S, Iannitto E, et al. ABVD compared with BEACOPP compared with CEC for the initial treatment of patients with advanced Hodgkin's lymphoma: results from the HD2000 Gruppo Italiano per lo Studio dei Linfomi Trial. *J Clin Oncol.* 2009;27:805–811.
22. Federico M, Bellei M, Brice P, et al. High-dose therapy and autologous stem-cell transplantation versus conventional therapy for patients with advanced Hodgkin's lymphoma responding to frontline therapy. *J Clin Oncol.* 2003;21:2320–2325.
23. Proctor SJ, Mackie M, Dawson A, et al. A population-based study of intensive multi-agent chemotherapy with or without autotransplant for the highest risk Hodgkin's disease patients identified by the Scotland and Newcastle Lymphoma Group (SNLG) prognostic index. A Scotland and Newcastle Lymphoma Group study (SNLG HD III). *Eur J Cancer.* 2002;38:795–806.
24. Fabian CJ, Mansfield CM, Dahlberg S, et al. Low-dose involved field radiation after chemotherapy in advanced Hodgkin disease. A Southwest Oncology Group randomized study. *Ann Int Med.* 1994;120:903–912.
25. Laskar S, Gupta T, Vimal S, et al. Consolidation radiation after complete remission in Hodgkin's Disease following six cycles of doxorubicin, bleomycin, vinblastine, and dacarbazine chemotherapy: Is there a need? *J Clin Oncol.* 2004;22:62–68.
26. Loeffler M, Brosteanu O, Hasenclever D, et al. Meta-analysis of chemotherapy versus combined modality treatment trials in Hodgkin's disease. International Database on Hodgkin's Disease Overview Study Group. *J Clin Oncol.* 1998;16:818–829.
27. Linch DC, Winfield D, Goldstone AH, et al. Dose intensification with autologous bone-marrow transplantation in relapsed and resistant Hodgkin's disease: results of a BNLI randomised trial. *Lancet.* 1993;341:1051–1054.
28. Schmitz N, Pfistner B, Sextro M, et al. Aggressive conventional chemotherapy compared with high-dose chemotherapy with autologous haemopoietic stem-cell transplantation for relapsed chemosensitive Hodgkins Disease: a randomized trial. *Lancet.* 2002;359:2065–2071.
29. Gajewski JL, Phillips GL, Sobocinski KA, Armitage JO, Gale RP, Champlin RE. Bone marrow transplants from HLA-identical siblings in advanced Hodgkins disease. *J Clin Oncol.* 1996;14:572–578.
30. Milpied N, Fielding AK, Pearce RM, et al. Allogeneic bone marrow transplant is not better than autologous transplant for patients with relapsed Hodgkins disease. *J Clin Oncol.* 1996;14: 1291–1296.
31. Chen RC, Chin MS, Ng AK, et al. Early-stage, lymphocyte-predominant Hodgkin's lymphoma: patient outcomes from a large, single-institution series with long follow-up. *J Clin Oncol.* 2010;28:136–141.
32. Nogová L, Reineke T, Eich HT, et al. Extended field radiotherapy, combined modality treatment or involved field radiotherapy for patients with stage IA lymphocyte-predominant Hodgkin's lymphoma: a retrospective analysis from the German Hodgkin Study Group (GHSG). *Ann Oncol.* 2005;16:1683–1687.
33. Schulz H, Rehwald U, Morschhauser F, et al. Rituximab in relapsed lymphocyte-predominant Hodgkin lymphoma: long-term results of a phase 2 trial by the German Hodgkin Lymphoma Study Group (GHSG). *Blood.* 2008;111:109–111.

26

Non-Hodgkin Lymphoma

MICHELINA CAIRO, A. EDWARD YEN, AND HELEN E. HESLOP

EPIDEMIOLOGY, RISK FACTORS, NATURAL HISTORY, AND PATHOLOGY

In 2010, approximately 65,540 individuals in the United States developed non-Hodgkin lymphoma (NHL) and 20,210 died from these disorders (SEER website, http://seer.cancer.gov/). NHL represents the sixth most common malignancy in U.S. among men and women with a median age of 67 at diagnosis.

Several viruses including HIV, hepatitis B and C, EBV, HTLV1, and HHV8 are implicated in the pathogenesis of NHL subtypes as are other infectious agents (Tables 26.1 and 26.2). Other risk factors for developing lymphoma include autoimmune disorders, immune deficiency and exposure to certain toxins.

Presentation can range from the incidental finding of an enlarged lymph node to a history of classic B symptoms (fevers, chills, night sweats, and weight loss) to symptomatic cytopenias or organ-specific dysfunction due to lymphoma involvement.

Non-Hodgkin lymphomas are a heterogeneous group of lymphoproliferative malignancies involving B, T, or NK lymphocytes, ranging from indolent to aggressive types and currently categorized by the World Health Organization (WHO) classification of lymphoma (Tables 26.1 and 26.2) (1). B-cell lymphoma cases far outweigh T-cell and NK-cell types.

Mechanisms of pathogenesis include aberrant somatic hypermutation or chromosome translocations that may reflect errors in antigen receptor gene rearrangements since many translocations involve the immunoglobulin or T-cell receptor gene loci. Determination of NHL type is extremely important as management can vary from watchful monitoring of disease for indolent types to aggressive chemotherapy and bone marrow transplant for highly aggressive types. NHLs are classified by morphology, histology, immunophenotype, extent of nodal involvement, and genetic aberrations. An excisional lymph node biopsy is preferred over a fine needle aspirate (FNA) to ensure there is sufficient material for an accurate diagnosis which includes immunophenotypic and cytogenetic analyses. End-organ evaluation may be indicated in tumors with predilection for certain organ systems, such as CSF analysis for Burkitt lymphoma. PET-CT is more sensitive and specific than CT and is currently recommended for high grade lymphomas which are more avid for FDG (2).

Genomic expression profiling (GEP) using microarrays in NHL has delineated the role of chromosomal translocations, aberrant signaling pathways, and dysregulation of molecules involved in abnormal proliferation and apoptosis in the pathogenesis of NHL and led to stratification based upon genetic differences (3–6). For example, diffuse large B-cell lymphoma (DLBCL) can be classified into "germinal center" or "activated" B-cell types with the former having better overall survival than the latter (3). GEP studies have also emphasized the importance of interactions between the tumor cells and the microenvironment including both stromal elements and infiltrating lymphocytes in lymphoma biology and prognosis (5,7). While GEP analysis is confined to clinical trials, surrogate immunohistochemistry markers such as BCL-6 and MUM-1 have been identified to differentiate germinal center and activated B-cell DLBCL.

STAGING

Patients with non-Hodgkin lymphoma are assigned an anatomic stage using the Ann Arbor system and are also evaluated using the International Prognostic Index (IPI), which assigns a risk category. The original IPI index remains the best prognostic assessment for patients with

Table 26.1 Mature B-Cell Neoplasms, Non-Hodgkin Type (WHO 2008) and Associated Risk Factors and Genetic Aberrations

Neoplasm	Associations
Chronic lymphocytic leukemia/ small lymphocytic lymphoma	Deletion 13q24, 11q23, 6q21, 17p13, trisomy 12, CD38, ZAP-70, IgVH mutation, CD5
B-cell prolymphocytic leukemia	
Splenic marginal zone lymphoma	
Hairy cell leukemia	
Splenic lymphoma/leukemia, unclassifiable	
*Splenic diffuse red pulp small B-cell lymphoma**	
*Hairy cell leukemia-variant**	
Lymphoplasmacytic lymphoma	
Waldenström macroglobulinemia	
Heavy chain diseases	
Alpha heavy chain disease	
Gamma heavy chain disease	
Mu heavy chain disease	
Plasma cell myeloma	
Solitary plasmacytoma of bone	
Extraosseous plasmacytoma	
Extranodal marginal zone B-cell lymphoma of mucosa-associated lymphoid tissue (MALT lymphoma)	t(1;14), BCL10, H.pylori, Chlamydia psitacci, C. jejuni, B. burgdorferi infections
Nodal marginal zone B-cell lymphoma (MZL)	CD11c, t(11;18), API2/MALT1
Pediatric type nodal MZL	
Follicular lymphoma	
Pediatric type follicular lymphoma	CD10, BCL2, t(14;18)
Primary cutaneous follicle center lymphoma	
Mantle cell lymphoma	CD5, Cyclin D1, FMC7, t(11;14)
Diffuse large B-cell lymphoma (DLBCL), not otherwise specified	BCL2, BCL6,
T cell/histiocyte rich large B-cell lymphoma	
DLBCL associated with chronic inflammation	
Epstein-Barr virus (EBV)+ DLBCL of the elderly	Epstein-Barr virus (EBV)+
Lymphomatoid granulomatosis	EBV
Primary mediastinal (thymic) large B-cell lymphoma	
Intravascular large B-cell lymphoma	
Primary cutaneous DLBCL, leg type	
ALK+ large B-cell lymphoma	t(2;5)(p23;q35), CD30
Plasmablastic lymphoma	
Primary effusion lymphoma	HHV-8
Large B-cell lymphoma arising in HHV8-associated multicentric Castleman disease	HHV-8
Burkitt lymphoma	t(8,14), t(2,8), t(8,22), CMYC, Epstein-Barr virus (EBV)
B-cell lymphoma, unclassifiable, with features intermediate between diffuse large B-cell lymphoma and Burkitt lymphoma	
B-cell lymphoma, unclassifiable, with features intermediate between diffuse large B-cell lymphoma and classical Hodgkin lymphoma	

*These represent provisional entities or provisional subtypes of other neoplasms. Diseases shown in italics are newly included in the 2008 WHO classification.

Table 26.2 Mature T-Cell and NK-cell Neoplasms (WHO 2008), and Associated Risk Factors and Genetic Aberrations

Neoplasm	Associations
T-cell prolymphocytic leukemia	
T-cell large granular lymphocytic leukemia	
Chronic lymphoproliferative disorder of NK-cells*	
Aggressive NK cell leukemia	
Systemic EBV+ T-cell lymphoproliferative disease of childhood(associated with chronic active EBV infection)	EBV
Hydroa vacciniforme-like lymphoma	EBV
Adult T-cell leukemia/ lymphoma	
Extranodal NK/T-cell lymphoma, nasal type	EBV
Enteropathy-associated T-cell lymphoma	
Hepatosplenic T-cell lymphoma	Chromosome 7 abnormalities
Subcutaneous panniculitis-like T-cell lymphoma	
Mycosis fungoides	
Sézary syndrome	
Primary cutaneous CD30+ T-cell lymphoproliferative disorder	
Lymphomatoid papulosis	
Primary cutaneous anaplastic large-cell lymphoma	
*Primary cutaneous aggressive epidermotropic CD8+ cytotoxic T-cell lymphoma**	
Primary cutaneous gamma-delta T-cell lymphoma	
*Primary cutaneous small/medium CD4+ T-cell lymphoma**	
Peripheral T-cell lymphoma, not otherwise specified	
Angioimmunoblastic T-cell lymphoma	EBV, HHV6
Anaplastic large cell lymphoma (ALCL), ALK+	Anaplastic lymphoma kinase
*Anaplastic large cell lymphoma (ALCL), ALK–**	

*These represent provisional entities or provisional subtypes of other neoplasms. Diseases shown in italics are newly included in the 2008 WHO classification.

diffuse large B-cell lymphoma, but modifications (outlined in the pertinent sections) have proved more predictive for patients with mantle cell lymphoma (MCL) or follicular lymphoma (8,9).

Ann Arbor Classification of Non-Hodgkin Lymphoma

Stage	Description
I	Involvement of a single lymph node region or lymphoid structure (e.g., spleen, thymus, Waldeyer's ring)
II	Involvement of two or more lymph node regions on the same side of the diaphragm
III	Involvement of lymph regions or structures on both sides of the diaphragm
IV	Involvement of extranodal site(s) beyond that designated E
For all stages	
A	No symptoms
B	Fever (>38°C), drenching sweats, weight loss (10% body weight over 6 months)
For stages I to III	
E	Involvement of a single, extranodal site contiguous or proximal to known nodal site

International Prognostic Index—for Non-Hodgkin Lymphoma

Prognostic Factors	
Age	>60 years
Performance status	>1
Lactate dehydrogenase	>1 × normal
Extranodal sites	>1
Stage	III or IV
Risk Category	**Number of Factors**
Low	0 or 1
Low-intermediate	2
High-intermediate	3
High	4 or 5

CASE SUMMARIES

Advanced Diffuse Large B-Cell Lymphoma

B.B., a 68-year-old white man, was in good health until he noticed difficulty in swallowing solids. Physical exam showed he had cervical, axillary and supraclavicular lymphadenopathy and a CT scan revealed a posterior pharyngeal mass. He denied any history of fever, night sweats or weight loss. Biopsy of the posterior pharyngeal mass revealed large, transformed B-cells with prominent nucleoli. Immunohistochemical stains were positive for MUM1 and BCL6. Ki-67 was 80%. Flow cytometry showed the cells to be CD19+, CD20+, CD22+, and surface IgM+. A PET-CT scan revealed diffuse disease, involving the tonsillar lymph nodes, bilateral cervical lymph nodes, submental, supraclavicular, inguinal lymph nodes and an intra-abdominal mesenteric mass. Basic laboratory studies were within normal range except the LDH, which was elevated. Hepatitis B, C and HIV were negative. Cardiac evaluation with MUGA demonstrated that the patient had a normal ejection fraction. A bone marrow biopsy showed no evidence of lymphoma.

Evidence-Based Case Discussion

This patient with DLBCL was classified as Ann Arbor stage IIIA because PET-CT scan showed lymphadenopathy on both sides of the diaphragm. A lumbar puncture was not performed as part of the staging since the patient did not present with CNS symptoms or testicular, marrow, or sinus involvement. Currently, gene expression profiling is not routinely used in the diagnosis of diffuse large B-cell lymphoma, but immunohistochemistry showed positivity for the markers MUM1 and BCL6 (see Figure 26.1) suggesting that he did not fall into the better prognosis "germinal center" type (3). Patients may also be stratified into prognosis groups with the International Prognosis Index (IPI). Applying the age-adjusted IPI, this patient's stage III disease, elevated LDH, and age >60 together indicate high-intermediate risk. The prognosis for 2-year survival is 48% and for 5-year survival is 37%. Favorable features include his performance status of 1 and the absence of extranodal disease. Since anthracyclines have been associated with cardiac dysfunction, it is important to verify the ejection fraction prior to using an anthracycline-containing regimen. It is also important to ascertain his hepatitis status since hepatitis B viral reactivation has been reported with the use of rituximab in combination with chemotherapy. HIV testing is essential as DLBCL occurs in HIV+ patients with a higher frequency compared to the general population and is associated with a higher risk of disease in the CNS.

The paradigm-shifting GELA study of DLBCL in the elderly comparing CHOP (cyclophosphamide, doxorubicin, vincristine, prednisone) with CHOP + rituximab (R-CHOP) showed a highly significant advantage in response rate, failure-free survival, and overall survival in the rituximab-containing arm (10). Several other studies confirmed these results and R-CHOP has become the standard of care for this disease in all age groups. Repeat imaging may be performed after 4 cycles with the intention of assessing response and treating 2 cycles past complete response for a total of 6 to 8 cycles. If complete response has not been achieved by 6 cycles, alternative therapy may be considered. Several other first-line approaches with increased dose density or alternative dose schedules have been the focus of clinical studies. For example R-EPOCH

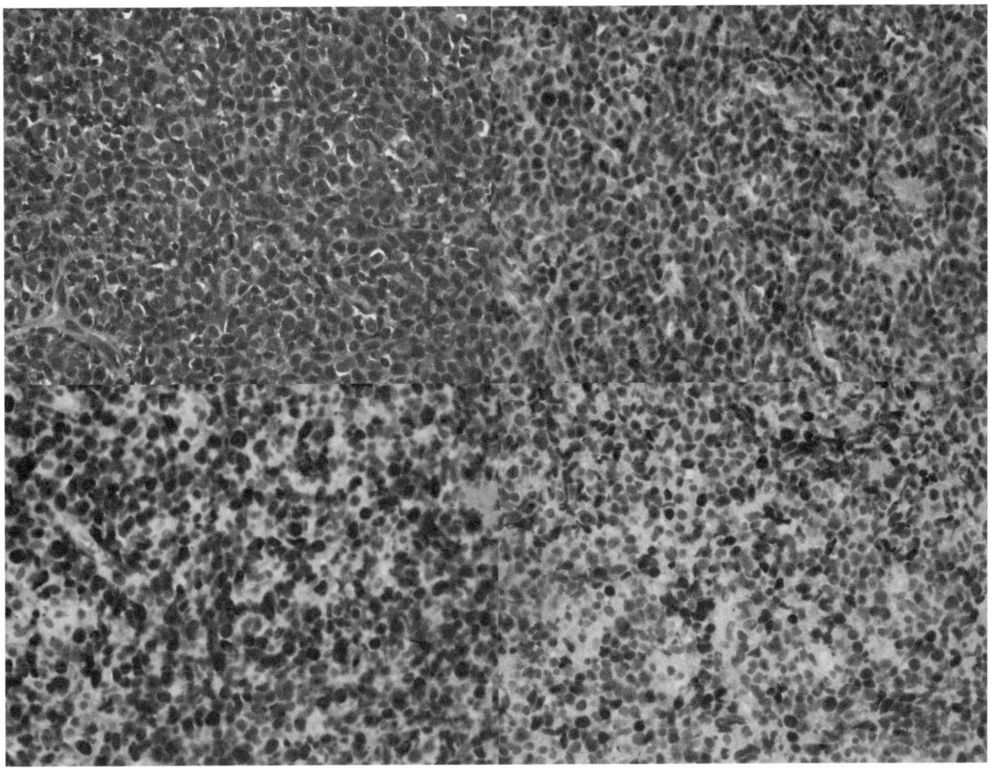

Figure 26.1

Diffuse large B-cell lymphoma. Upper left—H&E, 200 × magnification; upper right—bcl-6 positive, 200 × magnification; bottom left—MIB1 80% positive, 200 × magnificaton; bottom right—MUM1 positive, 200 × magnification. (see color insert)

(rituximab, etoposide, prednisone, vincristine, cyclophosphamide and doxorubucin) is an alternative regimen that has similar activity for carefully selected younger patients. If there is a very bulky (>10 cm) mass at any site, radiotherapy may be considered. Figure 26.2 represents a management algorithm for the treatment of patients with diffuse large B-cell lymphoma.

B.B. received 8 cycles of R-CHOP-21 since restaging after 4 cycles revealed a partial response. After chemotherapy was completed, a PET-CT scan was repeated to assess response and to provide a new baseline for comparison should he show signs of relapse. When PET-CT scanning is used it is advisable to wait 6 to 8 weeks postchemotherapy to avoid a false positive result. This patient's PET-CT showed no evidence of disease 8 weeks after treatment and he entered surveillance.

Advanced DLBCL in Relapse

Eight months after diagnosis and 4 months after completing therapy, B.B. noted a 1-cm node in the left posterior auricular area. Three months later, the posterior auricular lymph node, which had been quiescent, doubled in size over a few days. A biopsy revealed diffuse large B-cell lymphoma with Ki-67 >90%. Restaging PET-CT scan revealed disease in the neck and posterior auricular area.

Evidence-Based Case Discussion

Relapse is common in diffuse large B-cell lymphoma, especially within the first 2 to 3 years when more than 30% of patients treated with rituximab-containing regimens will relapse. Careful assessment of new symptoms and repeat biopsy of suspicious lesions are indicated. Because autologous stem cell transplant provides significant survival benefit in relapsed patients, it is important to establish that the tumor is sensitive to chemotherapy (11). Thus, a salvage regimen is usually administered. An ideal salvage regimen should have a high response rate, low hematologic and non-hematologic toxicity, and no impaired mobilization of stem cells. Platinum-containing regimens such as ESHAP (etoposide, methylprednisolone, cytarabine, and cisplatin) or ICE (infosfamide, mesna, carboplatin, and etoposide) with rituximab are frequently used although comparative trials are not available. B.B. was treated with rituximab-ESHAP with a very good partial response after two cycles. He underwent stem cell mobilization with GCSF after his third cycle followed by autologous hematopoietic stem cell transplant complicated only by neutropenic fever. He remains in remission 1 year posttransplant.

Burkitt Lymphoma

A.Y. is a 52-year-old Hispanic man with a 20-year history of HIV infection on HAART therapy, a recent CD4 count of 300, and an undetectable viral load. He presented to the clinic with complaints of difficulty in swallowing, numbness and tingling in his hands and feet, blurry vision, headache, and neck pain. Physical exam confirmed the presence of a large pharyngeal mass and right neck swelling. His gaze was mildly disconjugate. A biopsy of the right tonsillar mass demonstrated a high-grade B-cell

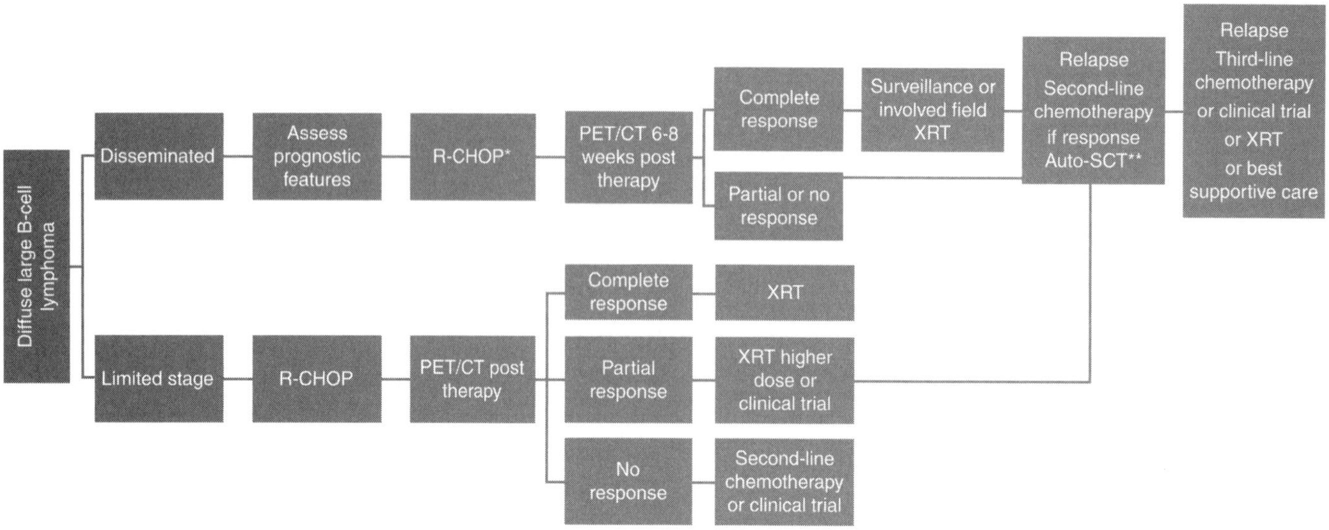

*R-CHOP refers to rituximab, cyclophosphamide, doxorubicin, vincristine, and prednisone. Those patients with depressed cardiac function should receive an alternative to doxorubicin. Those patients with adverse prognostic features may consider clinical trial.

**Second-line chemotherapy options include R-ICE, R-ESHAP, R-DHAP among others. Avoid severely myelotoxic chemotherapy for transplant-eligible patients. Those unfit to proceed to autologous stem cell transplant (Auto-SCT) may be treated according to their fitness and physician preference. Carefully selected patients may be eligible for allogeneic stem cell transplant.

Figure 26.2

Suggested algorithm for the treatment of diffuse large B-cell lymphoma.

lymphoma with Ki67 >99% and a "starry-sky" pattern consistent with Burkitt lymphoma. Immunophenotyping showed the cells to be positive for CD19, CD20, CD22, CD10 and HLA-DR and negative for EBV-encoded RNA (EBER), CD5 and Bcl-2. Cytogenetic testing confirmed a t(8;14) translocation. On a staging CT, masses were found in both orbits surrounding the optic nerve, the left maxillary antrum and the right tonsil. There were no parenchymal brain abnormalities. A large mass of lymph nodes encased the celiac axis and there was a large abdominal soft tissue mass and a soft tissue mass anterior to the sacrum. A bone marrow biopsy was negative for lymphomatous involvement. A lumbar puncture was performed as part of the staging and no malignant cells were found in the CSF.

Evidence-Based Case Discussion

Burkitt lymphoma is a highly aggressive B-cell malignancy characterized by a high proliferation index and translocations of the c-myc oncogene on chromosome 8 to the Ig heavy chain gene on chromosome 14 (t(8;14)), the kappa light chain gene on chromosome 2 (t(2;8)) or the lambda light chain gene on chromosome 22 (t(8;22)). In this patient, the Ki-67 index was greater than 99%, and the most common translocation between c-myc and immunoglobulin heavy chain was present. The characteristic "starry sky" appearance under the microscope was also noted (Figure 26.3). Up to 5% of patients lack c-myc rearrangements. Despite this, a diagnosis may be made if there is a high proliferation index and if morphology and immunophenotyping are consistent with Burkitt lymphoma. Burkitt lymphoma has both an endemic form, seen in Africa, and a sporadic form which is more commonly seen in children and adolescents and also in subjects with immunodeficiency. If an adult Burkitt lymphoma patient is not known to be HIV positive, then HIV should be tested. Type 1 latency EBV infection can be detected in tumor cells in almost all endemic BL and in 30% to 40% of sporadic and immunodeficiency-associated cases.

The staging evaluation for Burkitt lymphoma includes imaging from brain to pelvis, bone marrow biopsy, and lumbar puncture as described above. PET scanning is not used since it does not provide additional information that would influence management. Despite neurological symptoms, this patient's CSF sample did not show lymphoma cells by cytology. Nevertheless, CNS involvement is so common in Burkitt lymphoma that intrathecal chemotherapy should be given with or without symptoms or signs of CNS involvement. Additional laboratory studies include chemistries, renal function tests, lactate dehydrogenase and uric acid levels. This tumor is very sensitive to chemotherapy and highly intensive combination chemotherapy regimens with central nervous system prophylaxis are employed including hyper-CVAD (which includes cyclophosphamide, vincristine, doxorubincin, dexamethasone, methotrexate and cytarabine), EPOCH (etoposide, vincristine, doxorubicin, cyclophosphamide, and prednisone), CODOX-M (cyclophosphamide, vincristine, doxorubicin, and cytarabine), and CALGB 9251 (which includes cyclophosphamide, ifosfamide, methotrexate, vincristine,

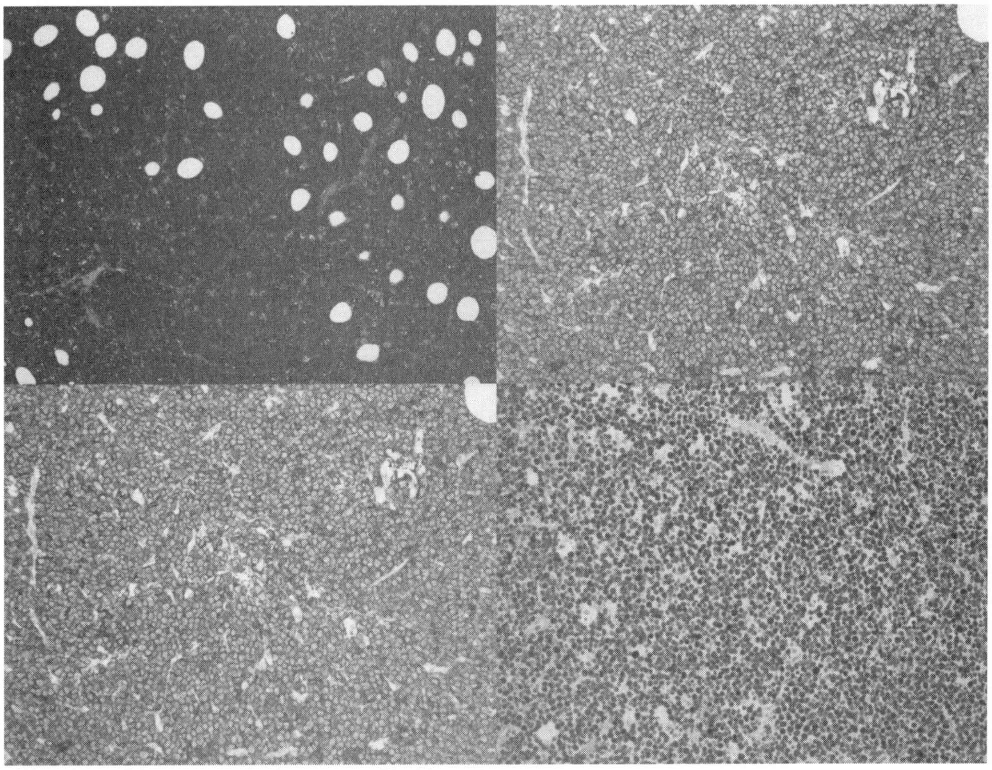

Figure 26.3

Burkitt lymphoma. Upper left—H&E, 40 × magnification; upper right—CD20, 100 × magnification; bottom left—CD10, 100 × magnification; bottom right—MIB1 with >95% positivity, 100 × magnification. (see color insert)

doxorubicin, cytarabine, and etoposide). Overall, intensive multidrug chemotherapy results in remission rates of 65% to 100% and long-term survival of 40% to 80%. Recent studies suggest the incorporation of Rituximab is beneficial. Regardless of which chemotherapy regimen is chosen, a brisk tumoricidal response is expected placing the patients at high risk of developing tumor lysis syndrome. Aggressive prophylaxis for this complication is required and at a minimum, allopurinol and IV hydration should be instituted. In cases where uric acid is already elevated or the tumor burden is particularly substantial, uric acid blocking drugs such as rasburicase may be used. Although there is concern in HIV-positive patients that chemotherapy may exacerbate immunodeficiency, patients who remain on highly active antiretroviral therapy (HAART), as well as patients without HIV infection, generally tolerate these chemotherapy regimens. Figure 26.4 shows a suggested algorithm for the management of patients with Burkitt lymphoma.

Hyper-CVAD with rituximab was chosen for A.Y. He tolerated his full first course of the chemotherapy with very limited side effects including nausea, decreased appetite, and shaking chills on day 1, which resolved. He received intensive hydration and allopurinol and his uric acid, which was in the normal range prior to initiation of chemotherapy, remained stable. He received intrathecal chemotherapy with methotrexate and cytarabine. During the admission for the first cycle of chemotherapy, the patient's chest mass and neck mass both decreased in size and his vision improved. His first cycle and several subsequent cycles of chemotherapy were complicated by neutropenic fever that resolved along with his neutrophil count. Despite concern that rituximab might worsen his immunodeficiency, he did not develop any opportunistic infections. Restaging at the completion of chemotherapy confirmed complete remission. Five years later, the patient remains in remission with no recurrence of Burkitt lymphoma and remains on HAART therapy.

Posttransplant Lymphoproliferative Disorder

C.M. is a 30-year-old African American woman who received a cadaveric kidney transplant for end-stage renal disease 3 months ago. Her transplant course was complicated by multiple urinary tract infections and a rejection episode requiring additional immunosuppression. She presented to her transplant physician complaining of daily fever to 102°F and suprapubic pain and fullness. As part of her evaluation for fever of unknown origin, a CT revealed a suspicious $4 \times 5 \times 5$ cm^3 mass inferior to the transplanted kidney. A PET/CT showed the mass had an SUV of 18. A biopsy showed diffuse large cell lymphoma that tested positive for EBV-encoded RNA (EBER) and latent membrane protein 1 (LMP1). Her peripheral EBV viral load was elevated at 1202 (normal <200). A bone marrow aspirate and biopsy were negative for lymphoma.

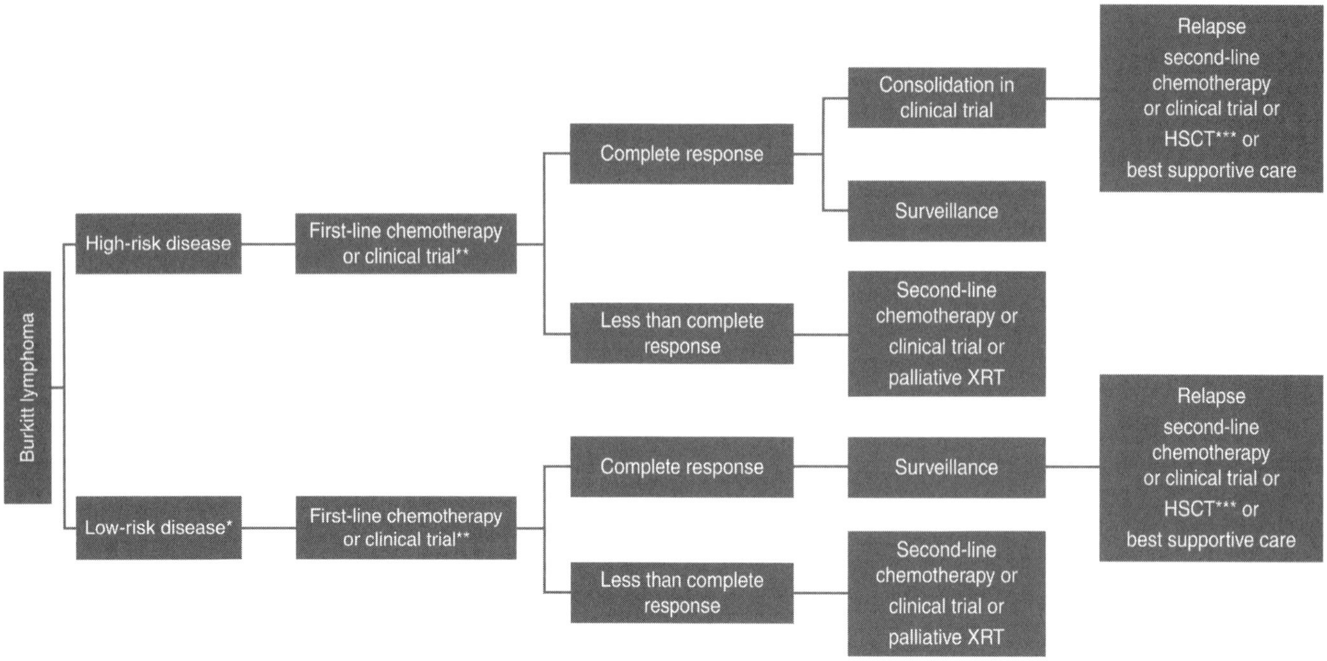

*Low risk disease is marked by low LDH and excised abdominal mass less than 10 cm.

**First line chemotherapy may be hyper-CVAD, CODOX-M, or other regimens as discussed in the text with CNS prophylaxis or treatment as appropriate.

***HSCT refers to hematopoietic stem cell transplant

Figure 26.4

Suggested algorithm for the treatment of Burkitt lymphoma.

Evidence-Based Case Discussion

EBV is a latent herpes virus that infects nearly 90% of the world's population. After primary infection, reactivation in latently infected B cells is controlled by a strong EBV specific T-cell response, but in severely immunocompromised hosts, such as patients on immunosuppression after solid organ transplant (where T-cell immunity is impaired), B-cell proliferation can occur (12). Risk factors for posttransplant lymphoproliferative disease (PTLD) include the degree of immunosuppression, with this complication most commonly occurring within 6 months of solid organ or hemopoietic stem cell transplant (HSCT). A rise in serum EBV viral load can predict the development of PTLD, and regular surveillance has been recommended by European consensus guidelines in high-risk HSCT recipients (13). While this assay is sensitive, it is not specific, and less than 50% of solid organ transplant recipients with an elevated EBV DNA will develop PTLD. Consequently, the decision of when to intervene depends on the clinical scenario. When a patient is symptomatic with fever and a mass as in the case of C.M., the decision is clear. The evaluation includes biopsy and full-body imaging.

Treatment options for PTLD include restoring immunity to EBV or directly targeting the B-cells. Reducing the immunosuppression, in consultation with the transplant team, is often the first step, and in some patients with early disease will result in sufficient immune recovery to obtain disease control. Second line therapy involves direct targeting of the B-cells with monoclonal antibodies such as rituximab or cytotoxic chemotherapy. Rituximab is often used as monotherapy with reported response rates of 44% to 100% (12). Chemotherapy with regimens such as CHOP can be reserved for patients who fail to respond or who have more extensive or progressive disease. Radiation therapy and surgical resection may have a role in limited disease or in organ-threatening disease. Clinical trials are exploring means of reconstituting the EBV specific response with antigen specific T cells. For PTLD occurring post-HSCT, infusion of donor lymphocytes is an option when the donor is EBV seropositive although this therapy carries the risk of GVHD. Figure 26.5 is a suggested management algorithm for PTLD.

C.M. initially had a trial of reduction of immunosuppression, but had persistent disease so received 4 doses of rituximab. Her mass regressed and serum EBV DNA fell to zero; she is currently being monitored for recurrence.

Mantle Cell Lymphoma

H.R. is a 66-year-old woman who was noted to be anemic at a routine office exam. Her physical exam

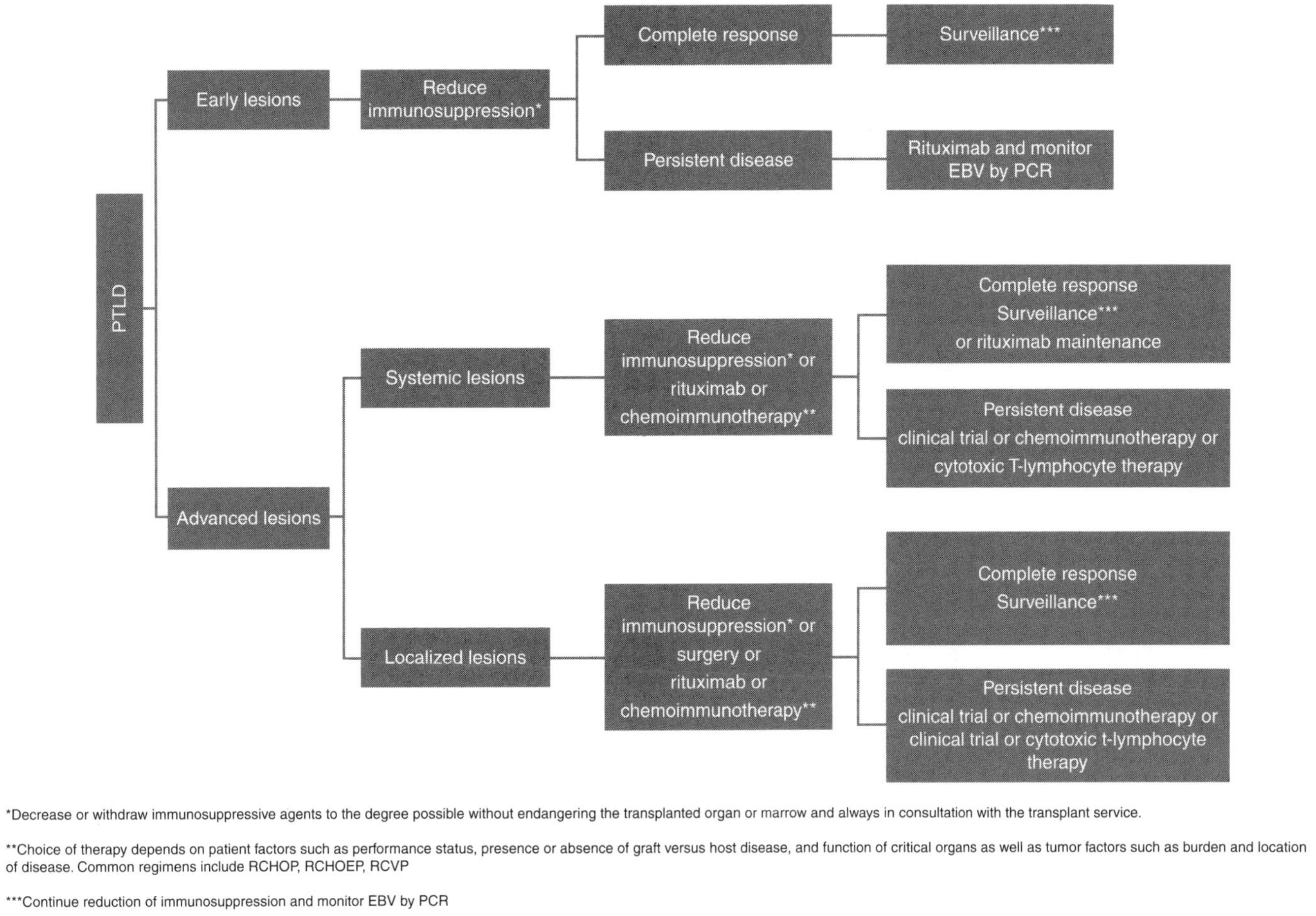

Figure 26.5

Suggested algorithm for the treatment of posttransplant lymphoproliferative disorder.

revealed scattered small cervical lymph nodes, 4 × 5 cm^2 left axillary lymphadenopathy, and two 1 cm inguinal lymph nodes. She reported fatigue and feeling hungry, but weight loss over the previous three months. She also reported night sweats over the previous two months. Fecal occult blood test was positive and colonoscopy was normal. An EGD revealed several solid nodules in the stomach and small intestine. Pathologic exam of these nodules demonstrated medium sized lymphoid cells with notched nuclei consistent with. Immunohistochemistry was positive for CD20, BCL-2, CD43, IgGM immunoglobulin, CD5 and cyclin D1 and negative for CD10. The t(11;14) translocation was detected by fluorescence in situ hybridization (FISH). Proliferation was assessed by MIB stain and was intermediate. Bone marrow biopsy and aspirate were positive for disease with 3% MCL cells on flow cytometry. A staging PET/CT showed metabolically active nodes on both sides of the diaphragm. A hepatitis panel was negative and her LDH and β-2 microglobulin were both elevated. Her ECOG performance status was 0.

Evidence-Based Case Discussion

Many patients with MCL present with advanced disease and frequently have extranodal involvement in the spleen, liver or gastrointestinal tract where lymphomatous lesions may be asymptomatic at presentation. The typical immunophenotypes are surface IgM+ and IgD+, CD5+, CD20+, CD43+, CD23–/+, cyclin D1+, and CD10–/+ (Figure 26.6). Most MCLs contain t(11;14), which involves translocation of the immunoglobulin heavy chain promoter and the proto-oncogene CCND1 that encodes cyclin D1. FISH may be required to detect the translocation (14).

Some MCLs have a Ki-67 index <10% and may have an indolent course, but the majority behave as an aggressive lymphoma. Four independent prognostic factors (age, performance status, lactic dehydrogenase, and leukocyte count) can be used to stratify patients into risk groups (8). The high risk group has overall survival of 2 years, intermediate risk group has an overall survival of 4 years and the low risk group has an overall survival of 6 years.

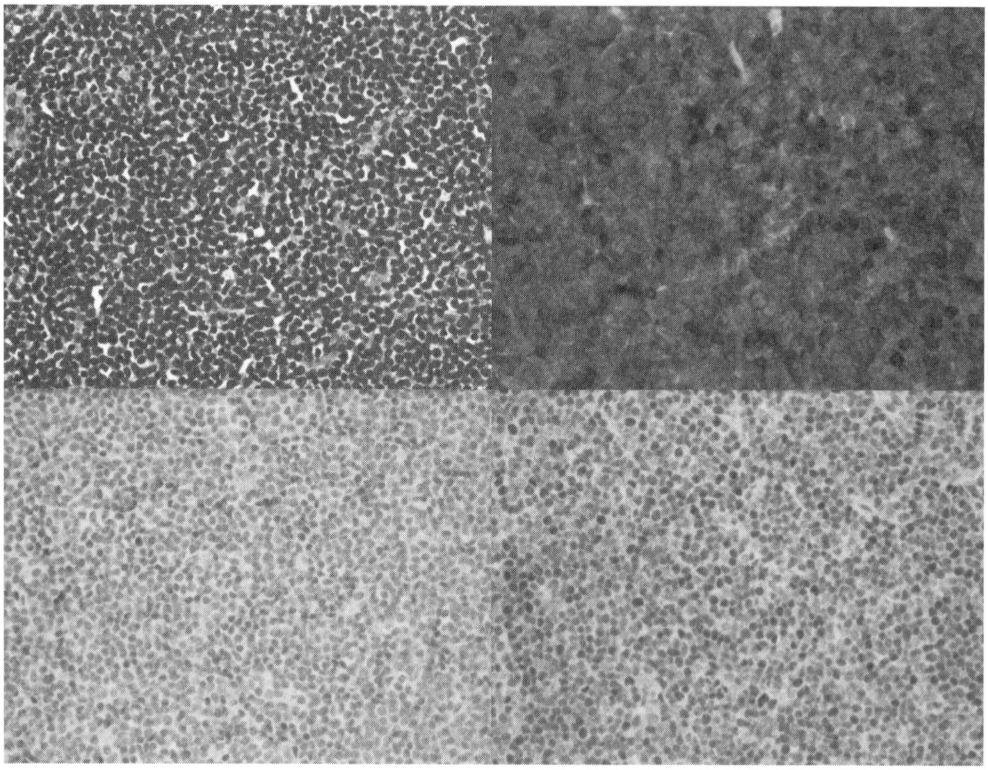

Figure 26.6

Mantle cell lymphoma. Top left—H&E, 100 × magnification; top right—CD5, 100 × magnification; bottom left—CD10, 100 × magnification; bottom right—Cyclin D1, 100 × magnification. (see color insert)

Standard staging procedures include CT of the chest, abdomen, and pelvis. A PET/CT may be used, but is not required. MCL often presents with extranodal disease in the gastrointestinal tract, and endoscopy is included in staging if it will change stage and management. MCL is frequently present at stage III or IV, and chemotherapy is indicated unless patient performance status dictates otherwise. There are no randomized prospective clinical trials comparing induction chemotherapy regimens for MCL, but the two most common treatment approaches are CHOP-rituximab or more aggressive regimens developed to introduce cytarabine or methotrexate early in treatment such as Hyper-CVAD and the Nordic regimen or the CALGB 59909 regimen. The combination of rituximab + Hyper-CVAD alternating with methotrexate and cytarabine was studied in a phase II randomized single-institution clinical trial of 97 patients and resulted in 3-year overall failure-free survival of 73% (15). An alternative regimen is the Nordic regimen using maxi-CHOP alternating with cytarabine followed by autologous stem cell transplant (ASCT) in first complete remission. The six-year progression free survival was 66% with this approach (16). The CALGB 59909 regimen used R-CHOP plus methotrexate followed by intensification with high doses of cytarabine and etoposide then autologous transplant after conditioning with carmustine, etoposide, and cyclophosphamide. This regime resulted in a 2-year PFS of 76% (17). For elderly patients, less aggressive alternatives such as RCHOP, R-CVP (cyclophosphamide, vincristine, and prednisone), bendamustine + rituximab, or dose-adjusted EPOCH may be considered.

Although most patients will achieve remission with intensive therapy, the majority will subsequently relapse. If the patient has a good performance status at the first relapse, aggressive salvage regimens can be used with the goal of proceeding to allogeneic stem cell transplant if the disease is chemosensitive. However, many patients with relapsed MCL will not be transplant candidates. Alternative options include standard lymphoma salvage regimens or monotherapy if the goal is palliative. Maintenance therapy with rituximab prolongs the duration of response to salvage therapy (18). For palliative therapy, both bortezomib and lenalidomide have activity as single agents, and the combination of bendamustine and rituximab has also produced good response rates (19). Figure 26.7 shows a suggested management algorithm for patients with MCL.

H.R. had renal dysfunction at baseline. This abnormality combined with her age led her physicians to give a more moderate regimen and she received 6 cycles of a modified Nordic regimen (R-CHOP alternating with cytarabine). Hyper-CVAD was not given because methotrexate could further compromise her renal function. She gained weight after the first cycle and maintained her baseline renal function throughout therapy. A PET/CT scan performed 8 weeks after completion of chemotherapy revealed a complete response. The patient was referred for consideration of autologous stem cell transplant in first remission, but the potential benefit was not judged to be

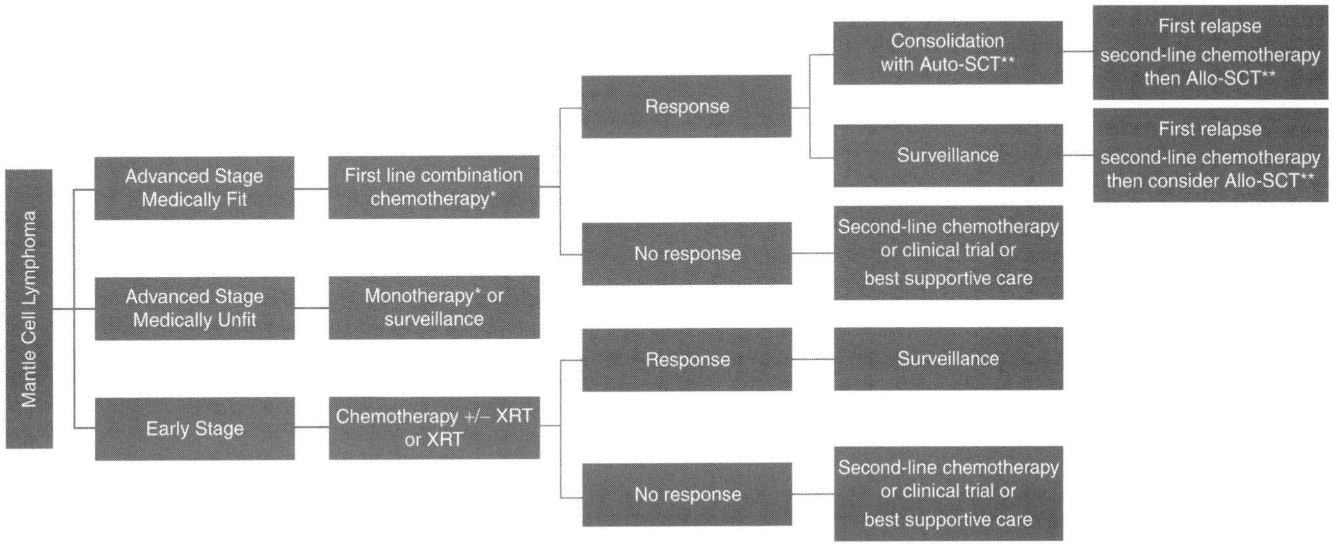

*First line combination chemotherapy, monotherapy, second line chemotherapy options and indications for autologous stem cell transplant are discussed in greater detail in the evidence-based case discussion.

**Patients appropriate for Auto-SCT (autologous stem cell transplant) and Allo-SCT (allogeneic stem cell transplant) must be carefully selected.

Figure 26.7

Suggested algorithm for the treatment of mantle cell lymphoma.

positive enough given her age and renal comorbidities. The patient was placed on rituximab maintenance every 6 months and remains recurrence-free 7 months after achieving remission.

Follicular Lymphoma

S.S. is a 60-year-old Hispanic woman who presented with a right-sided neck mass. She reported no fevers, chills, or night sweats, her weight had been stable and she had good appetite and energy. Examination of her neck confirmed multiple 1 to 2 cm enlarged lymph nodes limiting her range of motion. CBC and chemistries including LDH were normal and HIV and hepatitis serologies were negative. A CT scan identified bilateral jugular, supraclavicular, hepatogastric and para-aortic lymph nodes. An excisional biopsy of a right cervical lymph node showed a nodular growth pattern with centrocytes mixed with centroblasts, 11 per high-powered field, consistent with lymphoma. Flow cytometry confirmed the diagnosis of lymphoma, showing a monoclonal B-cell population positive for CD19, CD20, CD22 HLA-DR, CD5 (partial dim), CD23 (partial), CD11c (partial), and negative for kappa, lambda, CD10, and CD25. Cytoplasmic staining for BCL-2 was strongly positive. A bone marrow biopsy showed no lymphomatous involvement.

Evidence-Based Case Discussion

S.S. has grade 2 follicular lymphoma (FL) stage IIIA based on the Ann Arbor system. In deciding treatment options it is important to determine the pathologic grade, which depends on the number of centroblasts in a high-power field.

Grade 1—0 to 5 centroblasts/hpf
Grade 2—6 to 15 centroblasts/hpf
Grade 3—More than 15 centroblasts/hpf

The distinction has clinical relevance since grade 1 and 2 FL is categorized and treated like indolent NHL, while, grade 3 FL is treated like large-cell lymphoma with more aggressive chemotherapy regimens.

The Follicular Lymphoma International Prognostic Index (FLIPI) score, comprised of the five features below, is a useful tool in predicting the survival of patients with FL (9).

- Age > 60 years
- Ann-Arbor stage III or IV
- 4 or more involved nodal sites
- Elevated LDH
- Serum hemoglobin less than 12

The FLIPI score subdivides FL into low (0–1 factors), intermediate (2 factors), or high (three or more factors) risk groups. The relative 10-year overall survival for each group is 70.7%, 50.9%, and 35.5%, respectively, with non-overlapping confidence intervals. S.S. falls into the intermediate risk category with 2 factors (Ann Arbor stage III and four involved nodal sites).

Follicular lymphoma is an indolent, heterogeneous disease that is generally responsive to treatment, but associated with high relapse rates. Eighty-five percent of patients with FL have t(14;18) which results in the overexpression of B-cell leukemia/lymphoma 2 (BCL-2) protein.

One of the hallmarks of the disease is transformation to an aggressive histology. Higher grade and more extensive disease not only carry a higher risk of relapse, but also a higher risk of transformation to large-cell lymphoma. Since follicular lymphoma typically affects an older population, the functional status and comorbidities of the patient may affect treatment decisions.

For low-grade FL, early stage disease can be treated with involved-field radiation alone or in some cases, a period of observation. For patients with more advanced disease (stage 3 or 4) a period of observation may be appropriate if the patient is asymptomatic, but most will eventually require rituximab-containing chemotherapy regimens. The addition of rituximab to cyclophosphamide, anthracycline and fludarabine-based regimens has improved response rates and response duration with time to progression and overall survival both significantly extended (20). A recent trial (published only in abstract form) randomized patients to first line R-CHOP versus R-bendamustine and demonstrated a higher CR rate, and longer PFS in the bendamustine arm. Single-agent rituximab may also be used in the frontline setting for patients who are unable to tolerate treatment with alkylating agents.

A meta-analysis of several small studies suggests that maintenance rituximab may improve progression-free survival rate for patients with relapsed disease, but the benefit is less clear after first line therapy. A prospective intergroup trial is evaluating the role of rituximab after first line therapy, the results are not yet published. The use of hematopoietic stem cell transplantation (HSCT) in FL is reserved for second line therapy (21). Allogeneic HSCT should be considered in younger patients with good performance status since a 5-year progression-free survival rate of 83% has been reported using a reduced intensity regimen of fludarabine, cyclophosphamide and rituximab (22). Figure 26.8 shows a suggested treatment algorithm for low-grade follicular lymphoma.

S.S. was treated with 6 cycles of R-CHOP with a complete response and remained in remission for two years when she developed recurrence of cervical lymphadenopathy. Biopsy confirmed recurrence of Grade II follicular lymphoma with no evidence of transformation. Since she has no other symptoms she is currently being observed.

Peripheral T-Cell Lymphoma

Y.A., a previously healthy 33-year-old man, was transferred to the emergency room by his primary care doctor for increasing somnolence, worsening appetite, and new visual hallucinations. He had lost 50 pounds over the last 10 months, and reported recurrent fevers and sweating at night. In the emergency room, Y.A. was found to be hyponatremic and pancytopenic with elevated liver function tests. His mental status acutely declined and he was transferred to the intensive care unit. On examination, he was noted to have a rash and inguinal lymphadenopathy. An MRI of his brain showed no masses, bleeding,

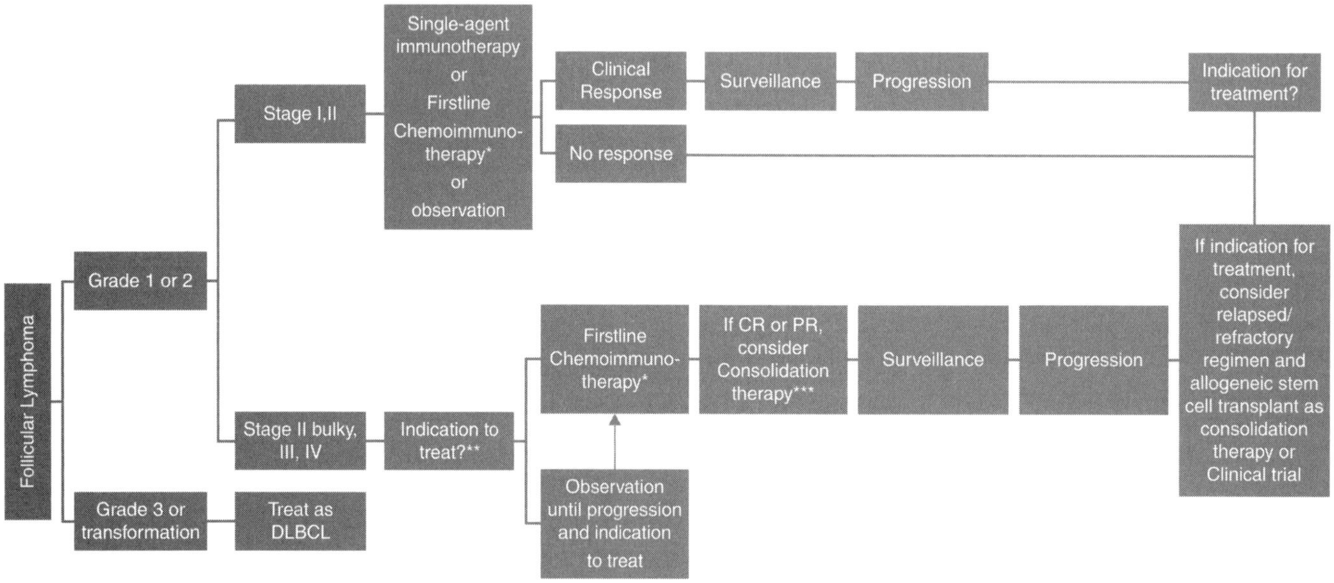

*Avoid severely myelotoxic chemotherapy for transplant-eligible patients. Firstline chemoimmunotherapy refers to fludarabine, cyclophosphamide, doxorubicin, or bendamustine based regimens with rituximab.

**Indications include clinical trial, end-organ dysfunction, cytopenias due to lymphoma, bulky disease, steady progression, or patient preference.

***Consolidation therapy refers to rituximab up to 2 years.

Figure 26.8

Suggested algorithm for the treatment of low-grade follicular lymphoma.

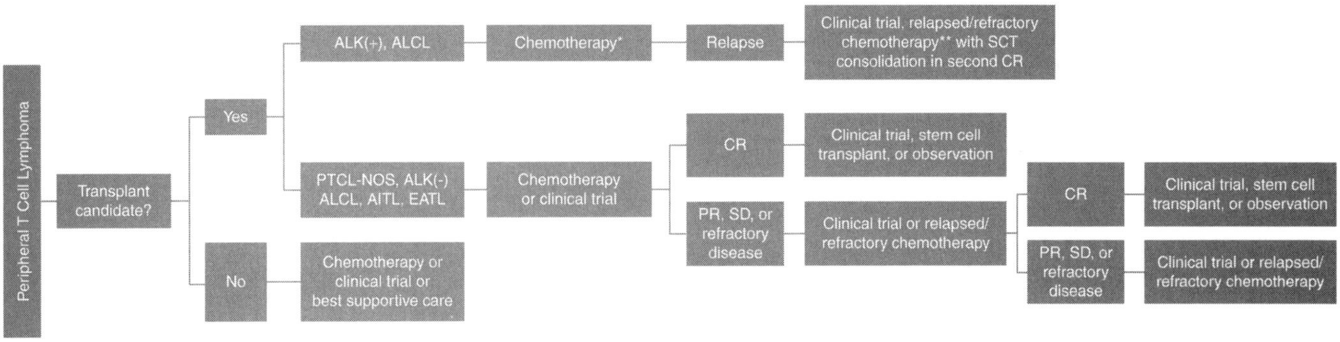

*Combination chemotherapy with CHOP in ALK+ ALCL has shown improved survival compared to other subtypes.

Figure 26.9

Suggested treatment algorithm for PTCL.

or demyelination. His sodium was carefully corrected and the confusion improved. Peripheral blood flow cytometry, FNA of the lymph node, and bone marrow biopsy were nondiagnostic. An excisional biopsy of the inguinal node was performed and showed a monoclonal population of large, atypical, pleomorphic lymphoid cells. Flow cytometry revealed a population of CD3 positive T cells with aberrant loss of CD2, CD5, CD7, CD4, and a high Ki-67 proliferation index of 80% to 90%. CD57, TdT, and CD34 were all negative as were ALK, pancytokeratin and EBV-LMP1. CSF cytology was negative for lymphoma. Serum uric acid and LDH were normal. A CT scan showed additional retroperitoneal lymphadenopathy and an enlarged spleen.

Evidence-Based Case Discussion

The immunophenotype of the monoclonal lymphocyte population is consistent with a peripheral T-cell lymphoma not otherwise specified (PTCL-NOS) (REAL-WHO classification (1)) since it does not meet criteria for other subtypes of T-cell lymphoma. Compared to B-cell lymphomas, peripheral T-cell lymphomas respond less well to chemotherapy and have a poorer survival. NCCN guidelines recommend participation in a clinical trial if one is available and intensive chemotherapy with a regimen such as CHOP if no trial is available (23). More intensive regimens such as HyperCVAD have been used, but they do not result in improved outcome (24). Because 3-year overall survival rates are only 40% to 50% for patients with ALK-negative disease, autologous transplant should be considered as consolidation in first remission (23). Figure 26.9 represents a treatment algorithm for peripheral T-cell lymphoma.

Y.A. was treated with CHOP, which he tolerated well. Since he is young with a high IPI score and ALK-negative disease, he has been referred for autologous stem cell transplant.

REFERENCES

1. Swerdlow SH, Campo E, Harris NL. *Classification of Tumours of Haematopoietic and Lymphoid Tissues.* 4th ed. Lyon, France: International Agency for Research on Cancer; 2008.
2. Seam P, Juweid ME, Cheson BD. The role of FDG-PET scans in patients with lymphoma. *Blood.* 2007;110(10):3507–3516.
3. Lenz G, Staudt LM. Aggressive lymphomas. *N Engl J Med.* 2010;362(15):1417–1429.
4. Dave SS, Fu K, Wright GW, et al. Molecular diagnosis of Burkitt's lymphoma. *N Engl J Med.* 2006;354(23):2431–2442.
5. Dave SS, Wright G, Tan B, et al. Prediction of survival in follicular lymphoma based on molecular features of tumor-infiltrating immune cells. *N Engl J Med.* 2004;351(21):2159–2169.
6. Dunleavy K, Pittaluga S, Czuczman MS, et al. Differential efficacy of bortezomib plus chemotherapy within molecular subtypes of diffuse large B-cell lymphoma. *Blood.* 2009;113(24):6069–6076.
7. Lenz G, Wright G, Dave SS, et al. Stromal gene signatures in large-B-cell lymphomas. *N Engl J Med.* 2008;359(22):2313–2323.
8. Hoster E, Dreyling M, Klapper W, et al. A new prognostic index (MIPI) for patients with advanced-stage mantle cell lymphoma. *Blood.* 2008;111(2):558–565.
9. Solal-Céligny P, Roy P, Colombat P, et al. Follicular lymphoma international prognostic index. *Blood.* 2004;104(5):1258–1265.
10. Coiffier B, Lepage E, Briere J, et al. CHOP chemotherapy plus rituximab compared with CHOP alone in elderly patients with diffuse large-B-cell lymphoma. *N Engl J Med.* 2002;346(4):235–242.
11. Oliansky DM, Czuczman M, Fisher RI, et al. The role of cytotoxic therapy with hematopoietic stem cell transplantation in the treatment of diffuse large B-cell lymphoma: Update of the 2001 evidence-based review. *Biol Blood Marrow Transplant,* 2011;17(1):20–47.
12. Heslop HE. How I treat EBV lymphoproliferation. *Blood.* 2009; 114(19):4002–4008.
13. Styczynski J, Reusser P, Einsele H, et al. Management of HSV, VZV and EBV infections in patients with hematological malignancies and after SCT: guidelines from the Second European Conference on Infections in Leukemia. *Bone Marrow Transplant.* 2009;43(10):757–770.
14. Pileri SA, Falini B. Mantle cell lymphoma. *Haematologica.* 2009;94(11):1488–1492.
15. Romaguera JE, Fayad L, Rodriguez MA, et al. High rate of durable remissions after treatment of newly diagnosed aggressive mantle-cell lymphoma with rituximab plus hyper-CVAD alternating with rituximab plus high-dose methotrexate and cytarabine. *J Clin Oncol.* 2005;23(28):7013–7023.

16. Geisler CH, Kolstad A, Laurell A, et al. Long-term progression-free survival of mantle cell lymphoma after intensive front-line immunochemotherapy with in vivo-purged stem cell rescue: a non-randomized phase 2 multicenter study by the Nordic Lymphoma Group. *Blood*. 2008;112(7):2687–2693.
17. DamonLE,JohnsonJL,NiedzwieckiD,etal.Immunochemotherapy and autologous stem-cell transplantation for untreated patients with mantle-cell lymphoma: CALGB 59909. *J Clin Oncol*. 2009;27(36):6101–6108.
18. Forstpointner R, Unterhalt M, Dreyling M, et al. Maintenance therapy with rituximab leads to a significant prolongation of response duration after salvage therapy with a combination of rituximab, fludarabine, cyclophosphamide, and mitoxantrone (R-FCM) in patients with recurring and refractory follicular and mantle cell lymphomas: Results of a prospective randomized study of the German Low Grade Lymphoma Study Group (GLSG). *Blood*. 2006;108(13):4003–4008.
19. Ghielmini M, Zucca E. How I treat mantle cell lymphoma. *Blood*. 2009;114(8):1469–1476.
20. Hiddemann W, Buske C, Dreyling M, et al. Treatment strategies in follicular lymphomas: current status and future perspectives. *J Clin Oncol*. 2005;23(26):6394–6399.
21. Oliansky DM, Gordon LI, King J, et al. The role of cytotoxic therapy with hematopoietic stem cell transplantation in the treatment of follicular lymphoma: an evidence-based review. *Biol Blood Marrow Transplant*. 2010;16(4):443–468.
22. Khouri IF, McLaughlin P, Saliba RM, et al. Eight-year experience with allogeneic stem cell transplantation for relapsed follicular lymphoma after nonmyeloablative conditioning with fludarabine, cyclophosphamide, and rituximab. *Blood*. 2008;111(12):5530–5536.
23. Zelenetz AD, Abramson JS, Advani RH, et al. NCCN Clinical Practice Guidelines in Oncology: non-Hodgkin's lymphomas. *J Natl Compr Canc Netw*. 2010;8(3):288–334.
24. Vose JM. Peripheral T-cell non-Hodgkin's lymphoma. *Hematol Oncol Clin North Am*. 2008;22(5):997–1005, x.

27

Multiple Myeloma

KEVIN MCDONNELL AND ANDRZEJ J. JAKUBOWIAK

EPIDEMIOLOGY, RISK FACTORS, NATURAL HISTORY, AND PATHOLOGY

There were an estimated 20,580 new cases of, and 10,580 deaths secondary to, multiple myeloma in 2009. Between 2003 and 2007, the median age at diagnosis was 70 years. There is an approximate 1.5:1 male to female predominance; the incidence is highest among patients of African descent with more than a twofold increased risk compared with Caucasians.

There exist few established risk factors associated with the development of multiple myeloma. Among the recognized risk factors are exposure to radiation, a family history of multiple myeloma, occupational exposures to petroleum products and agricultural pesticides, as well as obesity.

Multiple myeloma is a malignant hematological disorder characterized by the clonal proliferation of a terminally differentiated malignant plasma cell. Pathological expansion of the clone within the bone marrow compartment results in hematologic dysfunction including anemia and recurrent infection. Clonal B-cell immunoglobulin overproduction may result in renal compromise secondary to renal tubular light chain deposition. Furthermore, increased release of pro-osteoclastic mediators such as macrophage-inflammatory factor-1α and receptor activator of nuclear factors-κB ligand (RANKL) may lead to hypercalcemia and the development of lytic bone lesions.

Multiple myeloma evolves from the premalignant state of monoclonal gammopathy of undetermined significance (MGUS). Clinicians define MGUS as the presence of a serum monoclonal protein without significant bone marrow involvement or end-organ damage (see Table 27.1). The precise molecular and cellular evolution of MGUS has not yet been established; however, it has been proposed to originate with antigenic stimulation of the B cell accompanied by the activation of Toll-like receptors and augmented interleukin-6 expression. These events lead to B-cell proliferation and predispose to genetic mutations permitting progression of the disease.

An intermediate state of myeloma, termed asymptomatic or smoldering myeloma, may precede the symptomatic state and is defined as an increased serum monoclonal of ≥30 g/L and/or bone marrow clonal plasma cells ≥10%, with no related organ damage (Table 27.1). The final stage of multiple myeloma progression is symptomatic myeloma characterized by myeloma with end-organ dysfunction with either hyper*C*alcemia, *R*enal impairment, *A*nemia or *B*ony symptoms (the CRAB criteria; Table 27.1). The emergence of these clinical symptoms has become the key diagnostic criterion determining when to initiate treatment (1).

A monoclonal gammopathy that shares a common etiology with multiple myeloma is the solitary plasmacytoma that similarly derives from a single B-cell clone but distinguishes itself from multiple myeloma as a solitary lesion, most frequently in bone. In addition, with the solitary plasmacytoma there is noted to be a normal bone marrow without evidence of a B-cell clone, no bony disease apart from the plasmacytoma itself and no evidence of end-organ damage (Table 27.1).

Progression of multiple myeloma occurs secondary to intrinsic genetic mutations that accrue to the myeloma cell, per se, and additionally by virtue of alterations to the bone marrow microenvironment that result in increased angiogenesis and myelomagenesis.

There exists a variety of clinical, laboratory, and molecular variables associated with multiple myeloma that define the pathological state and prognosis of the disease. Historically, variables intrinsic to the patient have included the performance status, age, beta-2 microglobulin value, C-reactive protein level, LDH, serum

Table 27.1 Diagnostic Criteria for Monoclonal Gammopathies*

Monoclonal Gammopathy	Criteria
Monoclonal gammopathy of undetermined significance	(A) M protein in serum < 30g/L (B) Bone marrow clonal plasma cells <10% (C) No evidence of B-cell proliferation (D) No end-organ damage
Asymptomatic (smoldering) myeloma	(A) M protein in serum ≥ 30 g/L and /or bone marrow clonal plasma cells ≥10% (B) No end-organ damage
Multiple myeloma requiring treatment	(A) M protein in serum and/or urine (B) Clonal plasma cells in the bone marrow (C) End-organ damage including one of the following CRAB (creatinine, renal, anemia, bone) criteria: Calcium > 11.5 g/dL Renal Impairment with creatinine > 2 mg/dL Anemia with hemoglobin < 10 or 2 g < normal Bony disease
Solitary plasmacytoma	(A) Solitary lesion of bone or soft tissue as demonstrated by biopsy (B) Normal bone marrow without evidence of clonal plasma cells (C) Except for primary plasmacytoma, normal skeletal survey and MRI of spine and pelvis (D) Absence of end-organ damage

*Adapted from Durie et al. (1).

creatinine, and platelet count. Ancillary to these variables, molecular and cytogenetic assessments of the myeloma serve as additional diagnostic and prognostic criteria.

Gene expression profiling (GEP) has recently been demonstrated to be a valuable clinical, prognostic tool to identify patients with high-risk multiple myeloma (2). In addition to clarifying prognosis, GEP has also been used to define the complex molecular pathways involved with the role of the bone marrow microenvironment in multiple myeloma progression and the identification of fundamental molecular alterations, such as aberrant cyclin D expression, underlying the development of multiple myeloma (2).

Cytogenetic assessment of multiple myeloma can be achieved by employing either metaphase cytogenetic analysis or interphase fluorescent in-situ hybridization (FISH). Interphase FISH is the more frequently employed cytogenetic technique in multiple myeloma since relative to metaphase cytogenetics, interphase FISH is a more sensitive technique.

Cytogenetic characterization dichotomizes multiple myeloma into a favorable prognostic hyperdiploid class (defined as chromosome number between and including 48 and 74) and a poor prognostic nonhyperdiploid class (defined as a chromosome number less than 48 or greater than 74).

The hyperdiploid state constitutes approximately 50% of multiple myeloma cases and consists of cells with trisomies of chromosomes 3, 5, 7, 9, 11, 19, and 21. Nonhyperdiploid multiple myeloma represents the remaining 50% of cases and is typified by hypodiploid, pseudodiploid, and near tetraploid states accompanied by IgH translocations partnered with chromosome loci on chromosomes 11 (*cyclin D1* gene), chromosome 4 (*FGFR-3* gene), chromosome 6 (*cyclin D3* gene), chromosome 16 (*C-maf* gene), or chromosome 20 (*mafB* gene). Various of these mutations confer a better prognosis than others: a more favorable prognosis is associated with the t(11;14)(q13;q32) and t(6;14) translocations, whereas the del(17p), t(4;14)(p16;q32), and t(14;16) translocations are associated with a worse prognosis, although the significance of t(14;16) translocation has recently been questioned.

To these fundamental genetic defects may accrue secondary mutations that permit progression of the multiple myeloma resulting in a worsening prognosis. These secondary mutations include deletion of 17p13 (the p53 tumor suppressor gene locus), chromosome 1 abnormalities, activation of NF-κB, K-ras mutations, 12p deletions, methylation of p16, inactivation of p18, microRNA dysregulation and 16q defects, among others.

In addition to molecular characteristics of the myeloma, specific cellular phenotypes are also associated with differing prognosis. For example, the specific cellular immunophenotype CD138+, CD117–, CD28–, and CD19– is associated with a favorable prognosis, whereas the immature or plasmablastic cellular morphology demonstrates a poor prognosis. As well, an increased tumor grow rate, as indicated by the plasma cell labeling index (PCLI), has been associated with a worse prognosis.

STAGING

The most current staging system for multiple myeloma is the International Staging System (ISS) (3) and has largely replaced the older Durie-Salmon staging system. The ISS is summarized below. More recently, International Myeloma Working Group has categorized myeloma into two stages: asymptomatic and symptomatic myeloma. This distinction is based on the presence or absence of organ damage. Myeloma-related organ damage (i.e., hypercalcemia, renal insufficiency, anemia, or bone disease) identifies a subset of patients with symptomatic myeloma requiring treatment (Table 27.1) (1).

ISS for Multiple Myeloma

Stage	Definition
I	Serum beta-2 microglobulin < 3.5 mg/L Serum Albumin ≥ 3.5 g/dL
II	Not either stage I or stage III
III	Serum beta-2 microglobulin ≥ 5.5 mg/L

Response to treatment in multiple myeloma is described in reference to the International Uniform Response Criteria defined by the International Myeloma Working Group (1). These criteria distinguish among stringent complete response, complete response, very good partial response, partial response, progressive disease, clinical relapse, and relapse from complete response, and are summarized in Table 27.2. These categories are important for evaluating

Table 27.2 Response Criteria for Multiple Myeloma*

Response	Criteria
Complete response (CR)	Negative immunofixation on the serum and urine, disappearance of any soft tissue plasmacytomas and ≤5% plasma cells in the bone marrow.
Stringent complete response (sCR)	CR with a normal free light chain ratio and with an absence of clonal cells in the bone marrow by immunohistochemistry or immunofluorescence.
Very good partial response (VGPR)	Serum and urine M-protein detectable by immunofixation but not on electrophoresis or 90% or greater reduction in serum M-protein plus urine M-protein level <100 mg per 24 hours.
Partial response (PR)	≥50% reduction of serum M-protein and reduction in 24 hour urine M-protein ≥90% or to <200 mg per 24 hours. If the serum and urine M-protein are unmeasurable, a ≥50% decrease in the difference between involved and uninvolved FLC levels is required in place of the M-protein criteria. If the serum and urine M-protein are unmeasurable and serum free light assay is also unmeasurable, ≥50% reduction in plasma cells is required in place of M-protein, provided baseline bone marrow plasma cell percentage was ≥30%. In addition to the above listed criteria, if present at baseline, a ≥50% reduction in the size of soft tissue plasmacytomas is also required.
Stable disease (SD)	Not meeting the criteria for CR, VGPR, PR, or progressive disease
Progressive disease (PD)	Occurs when one or more of the following has occurred: increase of ≥25% from baseline in 1. Serum M-component and/or (the absolute increase must be ≥0.5 g/dL) 2. Urine M-component and/or (the absolute increase must be ≥200 mg/24 hours) 3. Only in patients without measurable serum and urine M-protein levels: the difference between involved and uninvolved FLC levels. The absolute increase must be >10mg/dL. 4. Bone marrow plasma cell percentage: the absolute % must be ≥10% 5. Definite development of new bone lesions or soft tissue plasmacytomas or definite increase in the size of existing bone lesions or soft tissue plasmacytomas 6. Development of hypercalcemia (corrected serum calcium >11.5 mg/dL or 2.65 mmol/L) that can be attributed solely to the plasma cell proliferative disorder
Clinical relapse	Requires one or more of: Direct indicators of increasing disease and/or end-organ dysfunction (CRAB features). It is not used in calculation of time to progression or progression-free survival but is listed here as something that can be reported optionally for use in clinical practice. 1. Development of new soft tissue plasmacytoma or bone lesions 2. Definite increase in the size of existing plasmacytomas or bone lesions. A definite increase is defined as a 50% (and at least 1 cm) increase as measured serially by the sum of the products of the cross-diameters of the measurable lesion 3. Hypercalcemia (>11.5 mg/dL) [2.65 mmol/L] 4. Decrease in hemoglobin of ≥ 2g/dL [1.25 mmol/L] 5. Rise in serum creatinine by 2 mg/dL or more [177 µmol/L or more]
Relapse from CR	Any one of the following: Reappearance of serum or urine M protein by immunofixation or electrophoresis. Development of ≥5% plasma cells in the bone marrow. Appearance of any other sign of progression (i.e., new plasmacytoma, lytic bone lesion, or hypercalcemia).

*From Durie et al. (1).

response to therapy, identifying disease progression, and guiding future treatment recommendations.

CASE SUMMARIES

Intermediate-Stage Multiple Myeloma Asymptomatic (Smoldering Myeloma)

A.B. is a 55-year-old man who on routine physical examination was noted to have an elevated serum protein level of 9.4 g/dL. This abnormal protein level then prompted an evaluation for multiple myeloma. The following laboratory results were obtained:

White blood count	6700/μL
Hemoglobin	14.2 g/dL
Platelet	218,000/μL
Calcium	9.4 mg/dL
Creatinine	1.0 mg/dL
Albumin	3.9 g/dL
LDH	149 IU/L
β2-microglobulin	2.2 mg/L

The urine protein electrophoresis and Bence-Jones protein quantitation demonstrated trace amounts of intact monoclonal IgG monoclonal protein. The serum protein electrophoresis and immunofixation demonstrated an elevated total protein of 8.9 g/dL and an IgA kappa monoclonal gammopathy of 2.6 g/dL. A serum free light chain assay was obtained and values were within normal limits with a kappa free light value of 0.78 mg/dL, a lambda free light chain value of 22.20 mg/dL, and kappa/lambda free light chain ratio of 0.04. Serum quantitative immunoglobulins were performed that demonstrated an elevated immunoglobulin A level of 2990, a normal immunoglobulin G level of 51, and a low immunoglobulin M level of 20. A skeletal survey revealed mild degenerative changes but otherwise no evidence of lytic lesions. The bone marrow biopsy demonstrated a normocellular marrow with 23% plasma cells; flow cytometry did not reveal any definite evidence of a monoclonal B-cell population. Cytogenetics and FISH were performed that revealed a normal male karyotype; the del(13q), del(17p), t(4;14), t(11;14), and t(14;16) mutations were absent.

Evidence-Based Case Discussion

The patient in the present case meets the diagnostic criteria for asymptomatic (smoldering) multiple myeloma (Table 27.1). Although the patient's monoclonal protein does not exceed 3.0 g/dL, we do note that his bone marrow plasma cells are greater than 10%. We also observe that his calcium, creatinine, and hemoglobin remain within normal limits, and his skeletal survey does not reveal any lytic lesions. Based on these parameters, the patient has asymptomatic or smoldering multiple myeloma (Table 27.1).

Clinically, asymptomatic myeloma is distinguished both from MGUS and symptomatic myeloma. Asymptomatic myeloma has an increased risk of progressing to symptomatic myeloma relative to MGUS, with the risk of progression 10% for each year during the initial 5 years, 3% per year during the next 5 years, and 1% each year for the last 10 years (4). NCCN guidelines (2011) recommend monitoring asymptomatic multiple myeloma at 3- to 6-month intervals with laboratory evaluation including a complete blood count, serum laboratories to assess creatinine, albumin, LDH, calcium, beta-2 microglobulin and quantitative immunoglobulins, serum protein electrophoresis, serum immunofixation electrophoresis, serum free light chain assay, urine protein electrophoresis, and urine immunofixation electrophoresis. A skeletal survey may be included annually in the assessment and a bone marrow biopsy may be considered as clinically indicated. In accordance with NCCN guidelines (2011)—provided the myeloma remains asymptomatic, that is, without evidence of organ damage—no treatment is recommended. However, once the patient meets the criteria for symptomatic myeloma (Table 27.1), treatment should be initiated. Currently, a number of trials are ongoing with thalidomide, lenalidomide, and dexamethasone to consider whether institution of these agents may retard progression from the asymptomatic to the symptomatic phase of multiple myeloma.

Symptomatic Myeloma in a Patient Eligible for Autologous Stem Cell Transplant

B.C. is a 43-year-old woman who reported the onset of increasing fatigue. As part of her workup, a complete blood cell count was performed that demonstrated a normochromic, normocytic anemia with a hemoglobin of 8.2 g/dL. A bone marrow biopsy was performed that revealed 30% clonal plasma cells. Additional laboratory values included the following:

White blood cell count	6000/μL
Hemoglobin	8.2 g/dL
Platelet	279,000/μL
Calcium	10.0 mg/dL
Creatinine	1.1 mg/dL
Albumin	4.4 g/dL
LDH	214 IU/L
β2-microglobulin	5.7 mg/L

A urine protein electrophoresis and urine immunofixation with quantitation (Bence-Jones quantitation) identified intact monoclonal IgG kappa protein with a monoclonal component of 15 mg/24 hours, but with no light chain (or Bence-Jones) protein component. A serum protein electrophoresis and immunofixation assay was performed that demonstrated an IgG kappa monoclonal gammopathy of 2.87 g/dL. A serum free light chain assay was obtained, which was normal with a kappa free light value of

1.04 mg/dL, lambda free light chain value of 1.10 mg/dL, and a kappa/lambda free light chain ratio of 0.95. Serum quantitative immunoglobulins revealed an elevated immunoglobulin G level of 3280 mg/dL, a normal immunoglobulin A level of 50 mg/dL and a decreased immunoglobulin M level of 245 mg/dL.

Cytogenetics and FISH were performed that revealed 1/30 abnormal clones with a 54 XX karyotype containing a combination of trisomies 3, 5, 7, 9, 11, 15, 19, and 21. A skeletal survey did not demonstrate any evidence of bony pathology.

Evidence-Based Case Discussion

This case represents a patient with newly diagnosed, ISS stage III multiple myeloma given her elevated serum beta-2 microglobulin level of 5.7. The patient also meets the criteria for symptomatic myeloma based on her anemia (Hgb 8.2).

The initial clinical consideration with regard to treatment of symptomatic multiple myeloma is whether the patient qualifies for stem cell transplantation as the treatment regimens that are employed for multiple myeloma can significantly impact the ability to achieve successful transplantation. In most cancer centers the criteria for an autologous stem cell transplant include age ≤ 65 years, normal organ system functioning, and an acceptable performance status (Karnofsky > 70%, ECOG < 3); however, in many centers in the United States there is no upper age limit to transplantation. In the present case, the patient is aged 43 with no major clinical barriers to stem cell transplantation.

Induction Regimens

Standard treatment for symptomatic multiple myeloma entails induction therapy with successive consolidative high-dose chemotherapy and autologous stem cell transplantation. Historically, alkylating agents such as melphalan, anthracyclines, vincristine, and high-dose steroids have constituted primary components of the induction regimens employed for the treatment of multiple myeloma; the use of alkylating agents, though, compromises the viability of stem cells, limiting the ability to harvest sufficient stem cells prior to autologous stem transplant. The recent discovery of alternative antimyeloma chemotherapeutic agents such as the immunomodulatory agents (IMiDs), thalidomide and lenalidomide, and the proteasome inhibitor, bortezomib, have allowed the implementation of effective induction regimens that do not employ stem cell harmful alkylating agents. For transplant-eligible candidates, the NCCN recognizes a number of Category 1 (based on randomized controlled trials) induction regimens that include

- bortezomib/dexamethasone, lenalidomide/dexamethasone,
- bortezomib/doxorubicin/dexamethasone (PAD and VDD regimens),
- cyclophosphamide/bortezomib/dexamethasone (CyBorD),
- bortezomib/thalidomide/dexamethasone (VDT), and bortezomib/lenalidomide/dexamethasone (RVD).

These novel regimens achieve response rates (≥PR) in 90% to 100% of patients and very good partial response (VGPR) in 50% to 60% of patients, compared to response rates of 60% to 70% and low rates of VGPR for traditional regimens, such as VAD. The superiority of a novel two-drug regimen (bortezomib/dexamethasone) versus traditional induction regimen with vincristine, doxorubicin, and dexamethasone (VAD), was demonstrated in a recently published randomized study (5).

In addition, there is emerging evidence that induction with a novel three-drug regimen is superior to induction with two-drug regimens (6) and that the achievement of at least 90% reduction of disease (VGPR) or CR prior to transplant predicts better outcome posttransplant (7,8).

With the recent, improved understanding of the genetics and identification of reliable prognostic variables for multiple myeloma, many clinicians have advocated for the use of risk-adapted approaches for the treatment of multiple myeloma. One such risk-adapted approach is the Mayo Stratification of Myeloma and Risk-Adapted Therapy (mSMART) (9). In the mSMART approach, using FISH, cytogenetic, and plasma cell labeling index (PCLI) parameters, patients who are transplant candidates are initially stratified into high-risk and standard-risk cohorts. High-risk characteristics include del(17p), t(4;14), t(14; 16) identified by FISH, cytogenetic deletion 13, hypoploidy or PCLI ≥ 3%; standard-risk features entail all other FISH, cytogenetic, and PCLI variables including hyperdiploid, t(11;14) and t(6;14) states.

With high-risk disease, specifically t(4;14) disease, it has been found that the use of bortezomib relative to thalidomide has resulted in the achievement of superior response rates, and thus within the mSMART risk-adapted approach, bortezomib-containing regimens are recommended for induction regimens with high-risk disease. In the case of standard-risk disease, either bortezomib- or IMiD-containing regimens are acceptable options for the induction regimen (Figure 27.1). Stem cells are subsequently collected after 4 to 6 cycles of induction therapy to permit stem cell transplantation.

In the present case, the patient demonstrated standard-risk disease and she underwent four cycles of bortezomib, lenalidomide, and dexamethasone followed by stem cell collection in anticipation of receiving an autologous stem cell transplant.

Consolidation Therapy

Following induction therapy, consolidation therapy may be considered. The standard approach to consolidation therapy in multiple myeloma has included administration of high-dose melphalan (HDM) accompanied by autologous

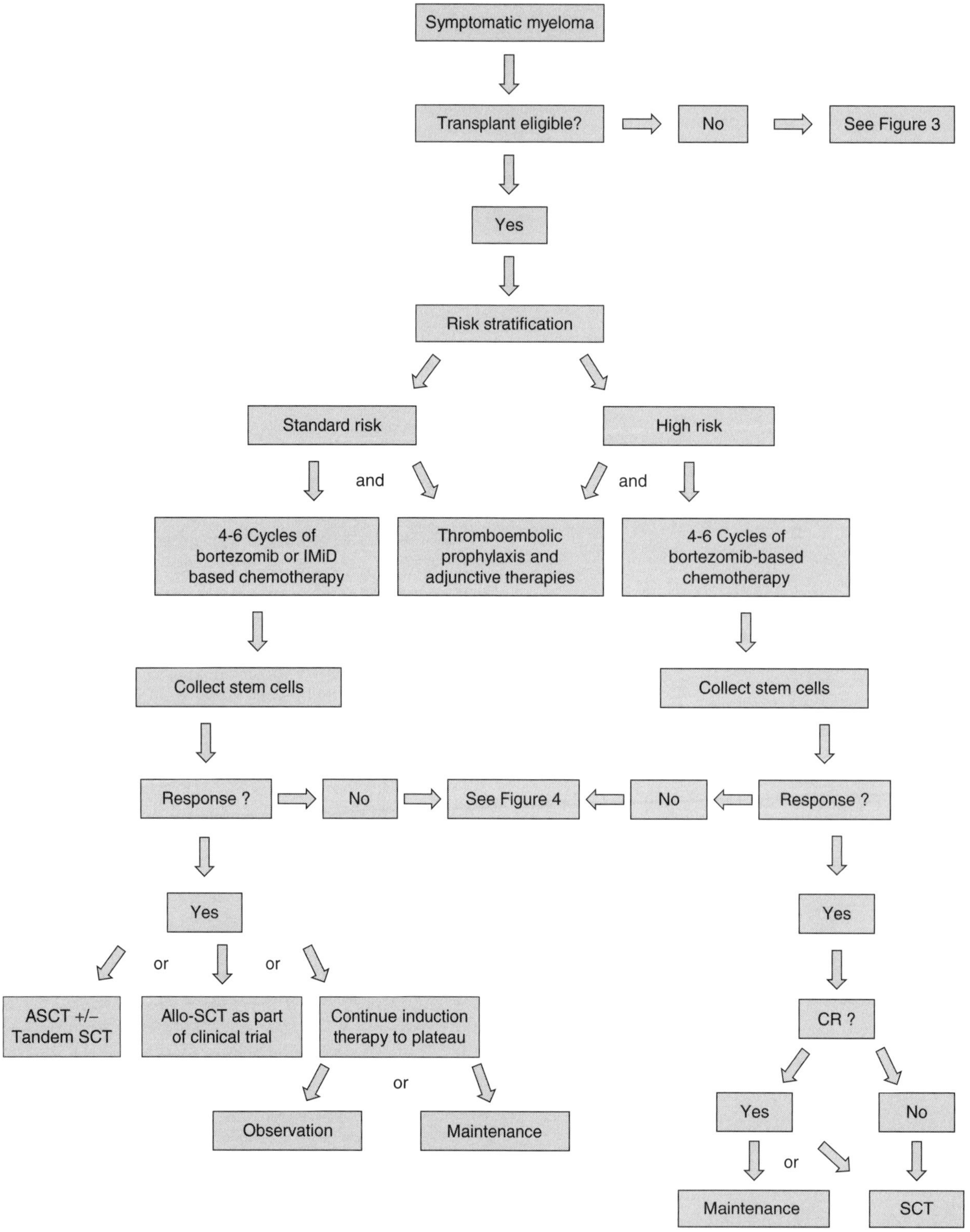

Figure 27.1

Treatment algorithm: symptomatic multiple myeloma in transplant-eligible candidate.

stem cell transplantion (ASCT) (10). However, the therapeutic successes achieved with the IMiDs and bortezomib have afforded new options with regard to consolidation therapy. Overall, high-dose melphalan with autologous stem cell transplantation following induction therapy does provide a small, though significant improved response rate (VGPR or better) relative to induction therapy alone. However, the excellent response rates achieved with the bortezomib- and IMiD-containing regimens allow for some flexibility regarding the timing of consolidative HDM/ASCT. Again, specific recommendations for consolidative therapy may be informed by risk stratification.

In the case of high-risk disease, the mSMART guidelines recommend proceeding with consideration of ASCT following induction therapy unless a CR has been achieved; in the case of high-risk CR, it is reasonable to maintain the initial response with continued bortezomib- or IMiD-containing regimens. More latitude with regard to ASCT can be given in the case of standard-risk disease in which case one can consider continued bortezomib/IMiD-based chemotherapy, provided a response has been achieved with induction therapy. Clinical investigations are currently underway to more fully clarify the role of high-dose induction chemotherapy, specifically whether RVD +/– autotransplantation followed by RVD consolidation and lenalidomide maintenance are comparable regimens.

Tandem ASCT

Tandem ASCT following an initial ASCT has been demonstrated to result in improved clinical outcomes relative to single ASCT. Patients receiving the tandem ASCT achieved an improved event-free and overall survival (11). Thus, tandem ASCT can be considered following the initial ASCT in either the high-risk or standard-risk cohorts.

Allogeneic Stem Cell Transplantation

Allogeneic stem cell transplants theoretically afford the additional therapeutic benefits of graft without contamination with myeloma cells and graft versus myeloma effect. However, the role of allogeneic transplant in management of myeloma has not been established. The results of studies provide conflicting results. ASCT followed by a reduced-intensity conditioning allogeneic stem cell transplantation has recently been demonstrated to provide improved progression-free survival rates, and therefore represents one therapeutic option for newly diagnosed patients with multiple myeloma, especially those with high-risk disease (12). However, at least two other studies did not show such benefit if compared to tandem autotransplant (13,14).

Maintenance Therapy

Following induction and consolidation, patients have been demonstrated to improve their survival and time to progression rates by the implementation of maintenance therapy. IMiD-based maintenance therapy using either thalidomide or lenalidomide is recommended both within the NCCN and mSMART guidelines.

In the present clinical case the patient opted to undergo a single ASCT; she, however, chose, after ASCT, to proceed with observation only, without maintenance therapy.

Supportive Care for Patients With Symptomatic Myeloma on Treatment

Once the patient demonstrates symptoms from their myeloma and begins treatment, consideration should be given for relief of these symptoms as well as preventing further complications from their treatment regimens.

Patients with multiple myeloma demonstrate an increased risk for thrombotic events and this risk is augmented in multiple myeloma patients undergoing IMiD-based therapeutic regimens. For this reason, the International Myeloma Working Group has advocated the initiation of thrombosis prophylaxis based on the presence of various risk factors including the specific myeloma therapy that the patient is receiving. These risk factors include obesity; previous history of thromboembolism; the presence of a central venous catheter; cardiac, renal, or diabetic disease; infection; immobilization; surgery; use of erythropoietin and hypercoagulability. If one of these risks factors is present then daily aspirin is recommended; if more than one risk factor is present then full anticoagulation with low molecular heparin or warfarin is advocated. If high-dose dexamethasone, doxorubicin, or multiagent chemotherapy is employed, full anticoagulation is also recommended.

Because of the unique pathophysiological nature of multiple myeloma and the associated unique clinical manifestations of the disease, NCCN guidelines endorse the implementation of a number of adjunctive therapies when treating a patient with multiple myeloma. The adjunctive therapies include institution of bisphosphonate therapy for patients with active bone disease, radiation therapy for palliation of bony disease, recognition and treatment of hypercalcemia, hyperviscosity and anemia, infection control including PCP, herpes, and antifungal prophylaxis, and careful monitoring and prevention of renal dysfunction.

Advanced Myeloma in a Patient Not Eligible for Autologous Stem Cell Transplant

C.D. is a 74-year-old woman with a previous history of IgA kappa MGUS. At the time of her diagnosis at age 65, her monoclonal protein was measured at 1.2 g/dL and there was a small amount of Bence-Jones protein noted in the urine; otherwise she was asymptomatic without any evidence of end-organ damage and her other laboratory values and radiographic studies were within normal limits. She had been followed at regular intervals, and over the past 24 months it had been noted that her monoclonal protein level had been rising, her hemoglobin had been decreasing, and her β2-microglobulin values were increasing; furthermore, she had developed increasing symptoms of fatigue and bony pain. Her most recent laboratory values revealed the following:

White blood count	5600 cells per μL
Hemoglobin	9.2 g/dL
Platelet	293,000 cells per μL
Calcium	10.6 mg/dL
Creatinine	0.8 mg/dL
Albumin	3.5 g/dL
LDH	102 IU/L
β2-Microglobulin	7.2 mg/L

A urine protein electrophoresis and Bence-Jones quantitation were performed that contained trace amounts of intact monoclonal IgA kappa protein. A serum protein electrophoresis and immunofixation assay demonstrated an IgA kappa monoclonal gammopathy of 3.5 g/dL. A serum free light chain assay was obtained that revealed a Kappa free light chain value of 2.18 mg/dL, Lambda free light chain value of 0.10 mg/dL and a Kappa/Lambda free light chain ratio of 21.80. Serum quantitative immunoglobulins identified a decreased immunoglobulin G level of 297 mg/dL, an elevated immunoglobulin A level of 3030 mg/dL, and a decreased immunoglobulin M level of 8 mg/dL. A skeletal survey demonstrated the development of numerous lytic lesions within the calvarium. A bone marrow biopsy revealed clonal plasma cells of ~ 20%. A flow cytometric analysis did not show any evidence of a monoclonal B-cell population. Cytogenetics and FISH documented a del(13q) and t(11;14).

Evidence-Based Case Discussion

C.D. describes a patient with a history of MGUS who progressed to ISS stage III multiple myeloma based on the elevation of her β2-microglobulin value to 7.2 mg/L, and meeting criteria for symptomatic myeloma based on anemia and bone disease.

Because of the patient's symptoms including the drop in her hemoglobin value and development of bony lesions, she was advised to initiate therapy; however, given her advanced age she was deemed not eligible for a stem cell transplant at the clinical center where she was receiving her care.

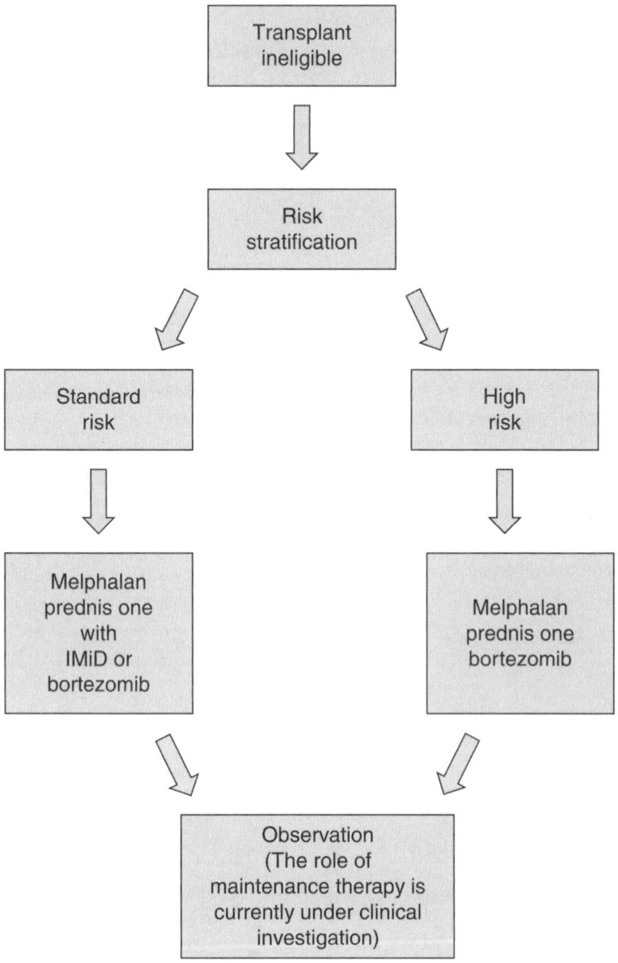

Figure 27.2

Treatment algorithm: symptomatic multiple myeloma in transplant-ineligible patient.

Induction Therapy for Transplant-Ineligible Patients

For patients who are ineligible for stem cell transplantation, the inclusion of alkylating agents such as melphalan, which is stem cell toxic, is not a concern. Traditionally, melphalan and prednisone have been employed as the foundation for induction therapy in this transplant-ineligible patient population.

The introduction and success of the IMiDs and bortezomib as effective agents for induction therapy has allowed investigators to improve induction response rates when using IMiDs and bortezomib in combination with the traditional melphalan/prednisone regimen for transplant-ineligible candidates. NCCN guidelines recognize melphalan/prednisone/bortezomib, melphalan/prednisone/thalidomide, and lenalidomide/low-dose dexamethasone as Category 1 therapeutic induction options for treatment of transplant-ineligible patients. The mSMART guidelines recommend melphalan/prednisone/bortezomib (Category 1–2) in high-risk patients, and melphalan/prednisone combined with either thalidomide or lenalidomide (Category 1–2) in standard-risk patients (Figure 27.2). Recently, several nonmelphalan-based regimens have been more commonly adopted in nontransplant candidates, including bortezomib/dexamethasone and RVD. Which MP-based regimen or other available regimen should be selected for nontransplant candidates is not established. A randomized Intergroupe Francophone du Myelome (IFM) study comparing Rev/Dex with MPT is expected to report its results soon.

Maintenance Therapy for Transplant-Ineligible Patients

Maintenance therapy following induction therapy in the transplant-ineligible patient has not been extensively investigated. NCCN guidelines are not explicit in this regard, but generally recommend observation or maintenance therapy with thalidomide following induction. mSMART guidelines endorse observation only following induction therapy. A recent study provided evidence that lenalidomide maintenance after induction with melphalan/prednisone/lenalidomide provides superior outcome than melphalan/prednisone or melphalan/prednisone/lenalidomide without maintenance (15).

Advanced Stage Myeloma—Relapsed Disease

This case involves the previously discussed patient, B.C., who was diagnosed with symptomatic, stage III multiple myeloma, underwent induction therapy with bortezomib, lenalidomide, and dexamethasone, followed by ASCT, and then decided to proceed with observation only rather than with maintenance therapy. For approximately 2 years, the patient sustained a complete response with no detection of a monoclonal protein. At 24 months posttransplantation the patient was noted to have a detectable IgG monoclonal protein of 0.4 g/dL, her β2-microglobulin was 1.7 mg/L and her hemoglobin was 11.9 g/dL. At 36 months posttransplantation, the patient presented for reassessment at which time her laboratory values were found to be the following:

White blood count	7300 cells per μL
Hemoglobin	9.3 g/dL
Platelet	268,000 cells per μL
Calcium	9.7 mg/dL
Creatinine	1.4 mg/dL
Albumin	4.0 g/dL
LDH	205 IU/L
β2-Microglobulin	6.3 mg/L

A urine protein electrophoresis and Bence-Jones quantitation was performed that contained intact monoclonal IgG kappa protein, 10.1 g/24 h. A serum protein electrophoresis and immunofixation assay demonstrated an IgG kappa monoclonal gammopathy of 2.6 g/dL.

A serum free light chain assay indicated a Kappa free light chain value of 4.04 mg/dL, Lambda free light chain value of 0.34 mg/dL, and a Kappa/Lambda free light chain ratio elevated at 11.88. Quantitative immunoglobulins indicated an elevated immunoglobulin G value of 3280 mg/dL, an immunoglobulin A value of 50 mg/dL, and decreased immunoglobulin M value of 24 mg/dL. A skeletal survey was normal with no evidence of any lytic lesions. A bone marrow biopsy revealed 20% plasma cells. Cytogenetics and FISH were performed on the bone marrow aspirate and demonstrated a hyperdiploid clone with trisomy 7, 11, 14, 9, and 15.

Evidence-Based Case Discussion

This case involves a patient who is status post-ASCT 36 months previously who decided against maintenance therapy and who now has symptomatic, relapsed disease. Her FISH and cytogenetic studies are consistent with standard-risk disease.

In the present clinical case the patient is demonstrating relapse following ASCT. A number of treatment options are available. NCCN guidelines endorse participation in a clinical trial or a repetition of the original induction regimen provided that the relapse has occurred greater than 6 months following the original induction regimen. Other Category 1 salvage treatment regimens recognized by the NCCN include bortezomib, bortezomib/liposomal doxorubicin, and lenalidomide/dexamethasone. One also has the option of repeating an ASCT if the patient remains SCT eligible. mSMART guidelines recommend these same treatment options for standard-risk disease. In the case of high-risk disease, the mSMART guidelines recommend repeating the bortezomib- or IMiD-based pretransplant induction regimen followed by a repeat ASCT with consideration of a tandem mini-AlloSCT or full-AlloSCT. In the case of relapse after initial IMiD-based therapy alone, mSMART guidelines recommend ASCT followed by thalidomide or lenalidomide maintenance or AlloSCT. If the patient is not eligible for SCT, the mSMART guidelines recommend initiation of a bortezomib-based regimen. In the situation of a relapse following a bortezomib-based-only initial therapy, ASCT is also recommended followed by thalidomide maintenance or AlloSCT. In patients not eligible for SCT, initiation of an IMiD-based regimen is recommended (Figure 27.3).

For subsequent relapses, other salvage regimens are available including NCCN Category 2A regimens such as lenalidomide, cyclophosphamide/vincristine/doxorubicin/dexamethasone (C-VAD), dexamethasone/thalidomide/cisplatin/doxorubicin/cyclophosphamide/etoposide (DT-PACE) and high-dose cyclophosphamide/dexamethasone.

Recently, a variety of novel therapeutic agents have been introduced for the treatment of multiple myeloma. Among these agents are new proteasome inhibitors including carfilzomib and NPI0052. More advanced investigation of carfilzomib showed promising clinical activity in relapsed and relapsed/refractory multiple myeloma (16). In addition, carfilzomib appears to be better tolerated without many of the off-target effects such as peripheral neuropathy that are associated with other proteasome inhibitors such as bortezomib. As well, carfilzomib, when employed in a combination with lenalidomide and dexamethasone, adds to the antimyeloma effects of these agents (17). Another promising agent is pomalidomide, a novel IMiD similar to thalidomide and lenalidomide. When used alone or in combination with dexamethasone, pomalidomide has demonstrated clinical efficacy in patients with multiple relapses of multiple myeloma (18). Encouraging results were also reported (2010 American Society of Hematology national meeting) for vorinostat and panobinostat, two new deacetylase inhibitors targeting histones. Finally, the implementation of novel antibody-based therapies, specifically elotuzamab, a humanized monoclonal antibody against CS-1 (an antigen expressed on the surface of myeloma cells) has produced promising clinical effects. Elotuzamab when given to patients with relapsed/refractory multiple myeloma appears to enhance the effect of bortezomib (19). Even more promising is the

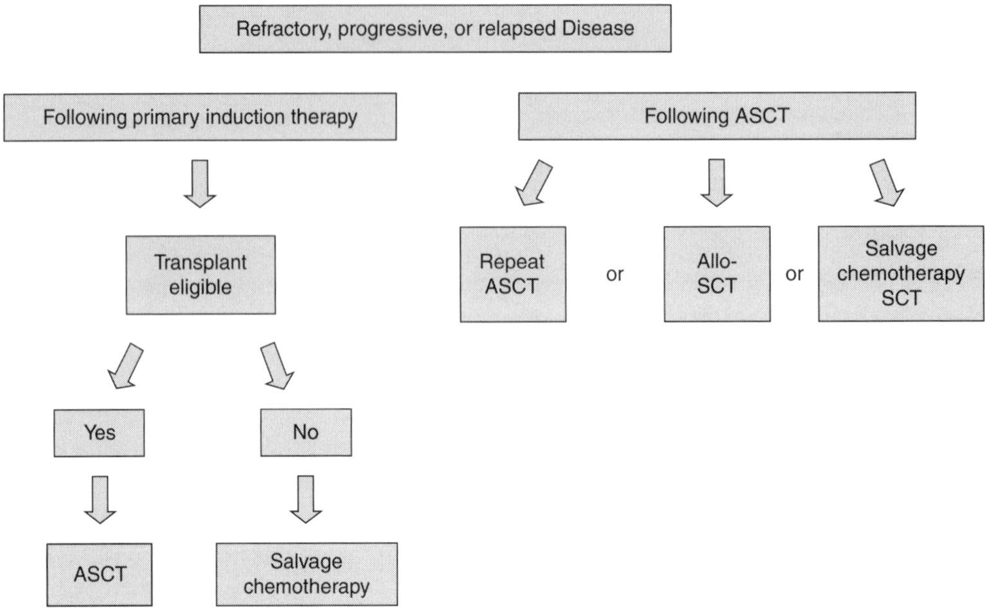

Figure 27.3

Treatment algorithm: refractory, progressive, or relapsed disease.

combination of elotuzamab with lenalidomide and dexamethasone, possibly the most therapeutically active regimen for relapsed multiple myeloma (20). In the present case, the patient opted to enroll in a clinical trial aimed at further clarifying the clinical efficacy of elotuzamab. Although none of these novel agents has yet been approved by FDA for the treatment of myeloma, it is envisioned that if approved they may substantially improve clinical outcomes.

REFERENCES

1. Durie BG, Harousseau JL, Miguel JS, et al. International uniform response criteria for multiple myeloma. *Leukemia*. 2006; 20(9):1467–1473.
2. Zhou Y, Barlogie B, Shaughnessy JD Jr. The molecular characterization and clinical management of multiple myeloma in the post-genome era. *Leukemia*. 2009;23(11):1941–1956.
3. Greipp PR, San Miguel J, Durie BG, et al. International staging system for multiple myeloma. *J Clin Oncol*. 2005;23(15): 3412–3420.
4. Kyle RA, Remstein ED, Therneau TM, et al. Clinical course and prognosis of smoldering (asymptomatic) multiple myeloma. *N Engl J Med*. 2007;356(25):2582–2590.
5. Harousseau JL, Attal M, Avet-Loiseau H, et al. Bortezomib plus dexamethasone is superior to vincristine plus doxorubicin plus dexamethasone as induction treatment prior to autologous stem-cell transplantation in newly diagnosed multiple myeloma: results of the IFM 2005–01 phase III trial. *J Clin Oncol*. 2010;28(30):4621–4629.
6. Cavo M, Tacchetti P, Patriarca F, et al. Bortezomib with thalidomide plus dexamethasone compared with thalidomide plus dexamethasone as induction therapy before, and consolidation therapy after, double autologous stem-cell transplantation in newly diagnosed multiple myeloma: a randomised phase 3 study. *Lancet*. 2010.
7. Jakubowiak AJ, Kendall T, Al-Zoubi A, et al. Phase II trial of combination therapy with bortezomib, pegylated liposomal doxorubicin, and dexamethasone in patients with newly diagnosed myeloma. *J Clin Oncol*. 2009;27(30):5015–5022.
8. Harousseau JL, Palumbo A, Richardson PG, et al. Superior outcomes associated with complete response in newly diagnosed multiple myeloma patients treated with nonintensive therapy: analysis of the phase 3 VISTA study of bortezomib plus melphalan-prednisone versus melphalan-prednisone. *Blood*. 2010;116(19):3743–3750.
9. Kumar SK, Mikhael JR, Buadi FK, et al. Management of newly diagnosed symptomatic multiple myeloma: updated Mayo Stratification of Myeloma and Risk-Adapted Therapy (mSMART) consensus guidelines. *Mayo Clin Proc*. 2009;84(12):1095–1110.
10. Attal M, Harousseau JL, Stoppa AM, et al. A prospective, randomized trial of autologous bone marrow transplantation and chemotherapy in multiple myeloma. Intergroupe Francais du Myelome. *N Engl J Med*. 1996;335(2):91–97.
11. Attal M, Harousseau JL, Facon T, et al. Single versus double autologous stem-cell transplantation for multiple myeloma. *N Engl J Med*. 2003;349(26):2495–2502.
12. Bruno B, Rotta M, Patriarca F, et al. A comparison of allografting with autografting for newly diagnosed myeloma. *N Engl J Med*. 2007;356(11):1110–1120.
13. Garban F, Attal M, Michallet M, et al. Prospective comparison of autologous stem cell transplantation followed by dose-reduced allograft (IFM99–03 trial) with tandem autologous stem cell transplantation (IFM99–04 trial) in high-risk de novo multiple myeloma. *Blood*. 2006;107(9):3474–3480.
14. Krishnan A, Pasquini MC, Ewell M, et al. Tandem autologous hematopoietic stem cell transplants (AuHCT) with or without maintenance therapy (auto-auto) versus single AuHCT followed by HLA matched sibling non-myeloablative allogeneic HCT (auto-allo) for patients with standard risk (SR) multiple myeloma (MM): results from the Blood and Marrow Transplant Clinical Trials Network (BMT CTN) 0102 Trial. *ASH Annual Meeting Abstracts*. 2010;116(21):41.
15. Palumbo A, Dimopoulos MA, Delforge M, et al. A phase III study to determine the efficacy and safety of lenalidomide in combination with melphalan and prednisone (MPR) in elderly patients

with newly diagnosed multiple myeloma. *ASH Annual Meeting Abstracts.* 2009;114(22):613–.

16. Siegel D, Martin T, Wang M, et al. Results of PX-171–003-A1, an open-label, single-arm, phase 2 (Ph 2) study of carfilzomib (CFZ) in patients (pts) with relapsed and refractory multiple myeloma (MM). *ASH Annual Meeting Abstracts.* 2010;116(21):985–.
17. Jakubowiak AJ, Dytfeld D, Jagannath S, et al. Carfilzomib, lenalidomide, and dexamethasone in newly diagnosed multiple myeloma: initial results of phase I/II MMRC trial. *ASH Annual Meeting Abstracts.* 2010;116(21):862–.
18. Richardson PG, Siegel D, Baz R, et al. A phase 1/2 multi-center, randomized, open label dose escalation study to determine the maximum tolerated dose, safety, and efficacy of pomalidomide alone or in combination with low-dose dexamethasone in patients with relapsed and refractory multiple myeloma who have received prior treatment that includes lenalidomide and bortezomib. *ASH Annual Meeting Abstracts.*2010;116(21):864–.
19. Jakubowiak AJ, Benson DM Jr., Bensinger W. *Elotuzumab in combination with bortezomib in patients with relapsed/refractory multiple myeloma: updated results of a phase 1 study. ASH Annual Meeting Abstracts.* 2010;116(21):3023–.
20. Richardson P, Weber D, Mitsiades CS, et al. A phase I study of vorinostat, lenalidomide, and dexamethasone in patients with relapsed or relapsed and refractory multiple myeloma: excellent tolerability and promising activity in a heavily pretreated population. *ASH Annual Meeting Abstracts.* 2010;116(21):1951–.

28

Acute Lymphoblastic Leukemia

NAVAL G. DAVER AND MARK M. UDDEN

EPIDEMIOLOGY, RISK FACTORS, NATURAL HISTORY, AND PATHOLOGY

Acute lymphoblastic leukemia (ALL) is a clonal disease arising from somatic mutations in a lymphoid progenitor cell that alter regulation of cellular proliferation, differentiation, and apoptosis. Rapid accumulation of precursor lymphoid cells usually occurs in the bone marrow displacing normal hematopoiesis resulting in neutropenia, thrombocytopenia, anemia, and dissemination of leukemic cells in the peripheral blood. ALL may arise in lymph nodes or the mediastinum and may not have bone marrow or peripheral blood involvement at presentation. Such patients are said to have lymphoblastic lymphoma that is usually treated as ALL. The central nervous system (CNS) is a significant site of involvement at presentation or relapse.

ALL accounts for 12% of all leukemias diagnosed in the United States. It is estimated that 5330 new cases of ALL were diagnosed in the United States in 2010 and approximately 1400 deaths were attributable to ALL per Surveillance, Epidemiology and End Result (SEER) registry data. ALL is the most common malignancy in patients younger than 15 years of age, accounting for 75% of all leukemia diagnosed in this age group. Twenty percent of acute leukemia in adults is ALL. There is a bimodal age incidence, characterized by a peak between the ages of 1 and 4, followed by a second peak in the elderly (>60 years of age). ALL tends to affect men more often than women although in infancy there is a slight female preponderance. ALL is more common in Caucasians than Blacks and in the United States there seems to be higher incidence among Hispanic populations.

Down syndrome and Ataxia-telangiectasia have been associated with a 30 to 70 times greater risk of developing B-cell and T-cell ALL, respectively (1,2). Increased incidence has also been noted in patients with Bloom syndrome and patients with auto-immune conditions such as Sjögren syndrome. It is unknown whether the chromosomal instability or immunosuppression caused by these diseases is the driving factor in leukemogenesis. Multiple environmental factors including nuclear, electromagnetic, and cosmic radiation and chemical agents such as insecticides, DDT, and vitamin K have been implicated as risk factors, but the data supporting these are inconclusive. Intrauterine exposure to radiation increases the risk of childhood leukemia.

Our understanding of the leukemogenic process has improved significantly as a result of recent progress in the field of genomic analysis. This is especially true in pediatric and young adult B- and T-cell ALL. Recent identification of novel gene fusion transcripts and altered gene expression has significantly enhanced our knowledge regarding the biology and etiopathogenesis of ALL. These markers seem to have prognostic, predictive, and possible therapeutic implications.

The best known genetic mutation in ALL involves *BCR-ABL* gene rearrangement resulting in the formation of the "Philadelphia chromosome"—named for the geographic location of its discovery. The Philadelphia chromosome is found in up to 20% of adult ALL cases (3). The resulting gene transcript in ALL patients is usually 190 kD compared to the 210 kD gene product expressed in patients with chronic myelogenous leukemia. Insight into the *BCR-ABL* transcript has permitted development of tyrosine kinase inhibitors (TKIs) for treatment of both CML and Ph+ALL (4). Other genetic changes associated with ALL are summarized in Table 28.1.

Recent genomewide studies in pediatric ALL have identified hitherto unrecognized gene mutations in high-risk groups. One such mutation is deletion of the *IKZF1* gene on chromosome 9 that encodes the IKAROS transcription

Table 28.1 Cytogenetic Classification and Prognosis in Adult/Childhood B-cell ALL

Karyotype	Incidence in Adults (%)	Incidence in Children (%)	Adults Achieving CR (%)	Adults Achieving 3-Year Survival (%)
Normal	30–40	15–20	82	50
t (9;22)	25–30	3	78	18
+8	10–12	2	87	17
t(4;11)	4–7	2	76	18
+21	0–3	20–25	84	30
Abnormal 9p	6–30	7–10	89	43
Abnormal 12p	4–6	7–10	82	82
t(14q11)			100	78
t(1;19)	2–3	3–11	5–6	
t(12;21)	5	25–30	90	90
Hyperdiploidy	4–5	23–26	90	70–80

factor. A second mutation is in the Janus kinase 2 (*JAK2*) gene. Mutation of the *JAK2* gene, resulting in replacement of valine by phenylalanine at position 617 (V617F), is well recognized in myeloproliferative diseases including polycythemia vera and myelofibrosis. However, in pediatric ALL, a group of mutations at R683 was observed in 10% to 15% of patients with high-risk disease. This mutation is also frequently found in Down syndrome-related ALL and is uniformly associated with overexpression of CRLF2 (cytokine receptor-like factor 2) due to gene rearrangement. It appears that *CRLF2* overexpression in combination with mutation of *JAK1* or *JAK2* genes and deletion or mutation of *IKZF* promotes leukemogenesis. The genetic signature in these cases overlaps significantly with the *BCR-ABL* signature (5). Ultimately these newly identified mutations may serve as therapeutic targets in ALL.

Gene expression profiling studies also enable classification of T-cell ALL into at least four distinct prognostic subtypes. The *TLX1* and *TLX3* subgroups are characterized by rearrangements solely of the *TLX1* or *TLX3* genes; whereas the *TAL/LMO* and *HOXA* groups are characterized by various rearrangements that affect functionally equivalent oncogenes. These genetic subgroups are associated with expression of specific immunophenotypic markers that reflect arrest at specific stages of T-cell development. In addition to these mutually exclusive "driver" mutations, other mutations have been found in more than one genetic subgroup. These additional mutations affect various cellular processes and include *NOTCH1* activating mutations (seen in 56% of children with ALL) and *FBXWZ* inactivating mutations that are associated with favorable outcomes (6). These additional mutations may help to explain variable outcomes in different studies and may serve as therapeutic targets. Expansion of our knowledge of mutations and altered signaling pathway offers hope for new targeted therapies in T-cell ALL.

The most common presenting features of ALL in adults include fatigue, dyspnea on exertion, fevers, ecchymosis, petechiae, bone pain, and headache. Bone pain is caused by expansion of the bone marrow with leukemic cells, leukemic infiltration of the periosteum or bone infarction. Affected bones include the long bones of the legs and arms. Renal involvement may manifest as nausea, vomiting, flank pain, or oliguria/anuria. Hepatic infiltration can cause icterus, dark urine, acholic stools, right upper quadrant fullness, or pain. Splenic involvement may be associated with left upper quadrant fullness, pain, or early satiety from splenic infiltration. Intracranial or subarachnoid hemorrhage may be a consequence of hyperleukocytosis syndrome or profound thrombocytopenia. Neutropenia may be associated with life-threatening bacterial or viral infection.

Clinical findings include nonbulky lymphadenopathy, hepatosplenomegaly, petechiae, or pallor. Hepatosplenomegaly due to organ infiltration is much more common in adults and is noted on imaging in 50% to 60% of adults presenting with ALL. Other presentations of ALL include CNS involvement, testicular involvement, and superior vena cava (SVC) syndrome. CNS involvement occurs in 8% of adults with ALL at presentation and should be suspected when the patient has headache, nausea, cranial nerve palsy, meningismus, or confusion. Testicular involvement may present as a firm testicular mass or hydrocele due to lymphatic stagnation. SVC syndrome occurs due to compression of the superior vena cava or brachiocephalic vein by a mediastinal mass. Bulky mediastinal disease is more often seen with T-cell ALL with an overall incidence of 10% to 15%. Other rare presentations include leukemia cutis, salivary gland involvement, and spinal cord compression from epidural infiltration or paraspinal mass.

Laboratory features seen in patients presenting with ALL include varying degrees of leukocytosis. Patients with t(4;11) with *MLL* gene fusion, t(1;19) with *E2A-PBX1* fusion, and t(9;22) with *BCR-ABL* fusion or patients with hypodiploidy often present with higher leukocyte count, whereas those with hyperdiploidy or t(12;21) with *TEL-AML* often present with lower WBC count. Thus the adverse risk associated with high WBC counts at presentation may be a reflection of the underlying genetic mutation. ALL patients may present with eosinophilia. For example, t(5;14) results in overactivation of interleukin-3 gene on chromosome 5 that in turn supports eosinophil proliferation. This is seen in patients with specific translocations resulting in overactivation of the interleukin-3 gene on chromosome 5 and eosinophil proliferation. Anemia (Hb< 8.0 g/dL) and thrombocytopenia (platelet count < 50,000/μL) are seen in 25% to 50% of adults at presentation.

Approximately 90% of patients have circulating blasts at presentation, and examination of Romanowsky stained peripheral blood films or bone marrow samples will confirm the diagnosis of ALL. Typically the B-cell precursor lymphoblasts are large with sparse cytoplasm and an enlarged nucleus, with fine chromatin and poorly defined nucleoli. Mature B-cell blasts (Burkitt lymphoma) are usually intermediate in size with intensely basophilic cytoplasm and prominent cytoplasmic vacuolation. ALL blasts do not stain with Myeloperoxidase or Sudan black; however, they often stain with Periodic acid-Schiff (PAS) reagent. TdT staining is frequently positive in early B lymphoblasts and can also be seen in early T-ALL. Bone marrow examination is recommended in patients with suspected leukemia since 8% to 10% of adults with ALL do not have circulating leukemic blasts. Some of these patients have significant pancytopenia, and the clinical diagnosis may be aplastic anemia before the discovery of ALL in the bone marrow. ALL patients may present with or develop tumor lysis during treatment resulting in hyperuricemia, hyperphosphatemia, hypocalcemia, and elevated creatinine associated with urate nephropathy.

The diagnosis of ALL was classically made by negative cytochemical staining for Myeloperoxidase and Sudan black with positive TdT and PAS staining along with morphologic features of the marrow lymphoblasts. Diagnosis now relies on flow cytometric determination of the immunophenotype of the marrow blasts (Immunologic Classification—Table 28.2). Characteristic patterns for B-cell ALL subtypes and T-cell ALL are shown in the table. AML blasts typically express CD34, CD13, and CD33. ALL blasts express a variety of B- and T-cell markers, but may also demonstrate aberrant expression of myeloid markers. In addition to flow cytometry studies, a bone marrow cytogenetic study should also be obtained. Demonstration of the Philadelphia chromosome, hyperdiploidy, and other translocations has prognostic significance and may determine whether patients are referred for transplantation in first or second remission. Specific genetic markers such as *BCR-ABL* are increasingly of interest as they provide prognostic information and may indicate targets for therapy.

Table 28.2 ALL: Immunological Classification of ALL

		Overall Percentage in Adults
B-Cell Lineage	CD19+, CD22+, CD79a+, HLA-DR +	
Pro-B	CD10−	11
Early pre-B	CD10+	52
Pre-B	CD10 +/−, cIg+	9
Mature-B	CD19+, CD22+, CD79a+, cIg+, sIg λ+ or sIgκ	4
T-Cell Lineage	CD7+, CD3+	
T cell	HLA-DR−, TdT+/−, CD2+, CD1+/−, CD4+/−	18
Pre-T cell	HLA-DR+/−, TdT+, CD2−, CD1−, CD4−	6

CASE SUMMARIES

Adolescent Young Adult B-cell Precursor ALL

D.N., a 19-year-old man, presented with fever, weight loss, knee pain, and petechiae. His WBC count at presentation was 8000/μL with 93% blasts and an absolute neutrophil count of 300/μL. His hemoglobin was 9.2 g/dL and platelet count was 120,000/μL. The uric acid was 11.6 mg/dL and serum creatinine was 1.4 mg/dL. Examination of a peripheral blood smear showed large cells with scant basophilic cytoplasm, and nuclei with fine chromatin and inconspicuous nucleoli. Flow cytometry of peripheral blood revealed a large population of cells that were CD10+, CD19+, CD22+, and CD79a+. Bone marrow examination revealed greater than 90% leukemic blasts; chromosome analysis demonstrated hyperdiploidy (>50 chromosomes). Fluorescence in-situ hybridization (FISH) for *BCR-ABL* transcript was negative.

Evidence-Based Case Discussion

This is a young adult with B-cell precursor ALL. The immunophenotype is consistent with CD10+ Early Pre-B-cell ALL that accounts for approximately 50% of all newly diagnosed ALL in adults. This patient has none of the usual adverse risk features in adults with B-cell precursor ALL, which include age > 60, leukocyte count > 100,000/μL, high-risk genotype (including *BCR-ABL*, *MLL-AF4*, other *MLL* translocations, hypodiploidy < 44 chromosomes, or complex cytogenetics ≥ 5 chromosomal abnormalities). Improved treatment has negated the prognostic significance of previously identified high-risk features such as male sex, African-American race, or the presence of the *E2A-PBX* fusion t(1;19). D.N. has hyperdiploidy, which has been associated with low leukocyte count, favorable responses to chemotherapy with >90% CR rates, and improved 5-year survival rates in the range of 70% to 80% (3).

Treatment strategies for B-cell precursor ALL focus on appropriate intensity antileukemic therapy, supportive care, and infection control (see Figure 28.1). Prognostic factors must be used to risk stratify adult and pediatric patients to determine the intensity of therapy, need for re-intensification, intensity and duration of CNS prophylaxis, and need for bone marrow transplant. In pediatric ALL, three risk groups are identified whereas in adults, due to the poorer outcomes, only standard risk or adverse risk are distinguished. Risk stratification tables for pediatric and adult populations are presented in Tables 28.3 and 28.4.

Standard antileukemic therapy for B precursor cell and T-cell ALL consists of three phases. Induction therapy is administered to induce a complete remission with acceptable toxicity followed by reconstitution of normal hematopoiesis, which enables administration of further intensive chemotherapy. A consolidation phase follows to weed out the drug-resistant residual leukemic cells and to eradicate minimal residual disease (MRD). This is followed by 2 to 3 years of maintenance therapy to reduce the risk of relapse. CNS prophylaxis is begun early during induction and given throughout the maintenance phase.

Induction regimens in adults traditionally include varying combinations and doses of corticosteroids, cyclophosphamide, vincristine, daunorubicin, asparaginase, and intrathecal methotrexate or cytarabine. The HyperCVAD regimen developed by the M. D. Anderson group (7) uses four alternating courses each of cyclophosphamide, vincristine, doxorubicin, and dexamethasone in conjunction with high-dose methotrexate/leucovorin and cytarabine for a total of eight cycles of combined induction and consolidation therapy. Maintenance therapy consists of 2 to 3 years of 6-mercaptopurine, methotrexate, vincristine, and steroids with intrathecal therapy. The CALGB 8811 regimen developed by Larson et al. (8) adds asparaginase to the standard induction regimen of prednisone, vincristine, anthracycline, and steroid. This is followed by an intensified postremission therapy comprising 6-mercaptopurine, 6-thioguanine, and L-asparaginase with cyclophosphamide, cytarabine, vincristine, methotrexate, and corticosteroids. Maintenance includes only methotrexate and 6-mercaptopurine. CNS irradiation is avoided because high-dose methotrexate/cytarabine penetrates the blood/brain barrier and provides CNS prophylaxis.

The goal of the maintenance therapy is to kill nascent, slow-growing ALL cells or suppress new clones that may arise. Reduction in the duration of maintenance therapy results in higher relapse rates. Most experts recommend

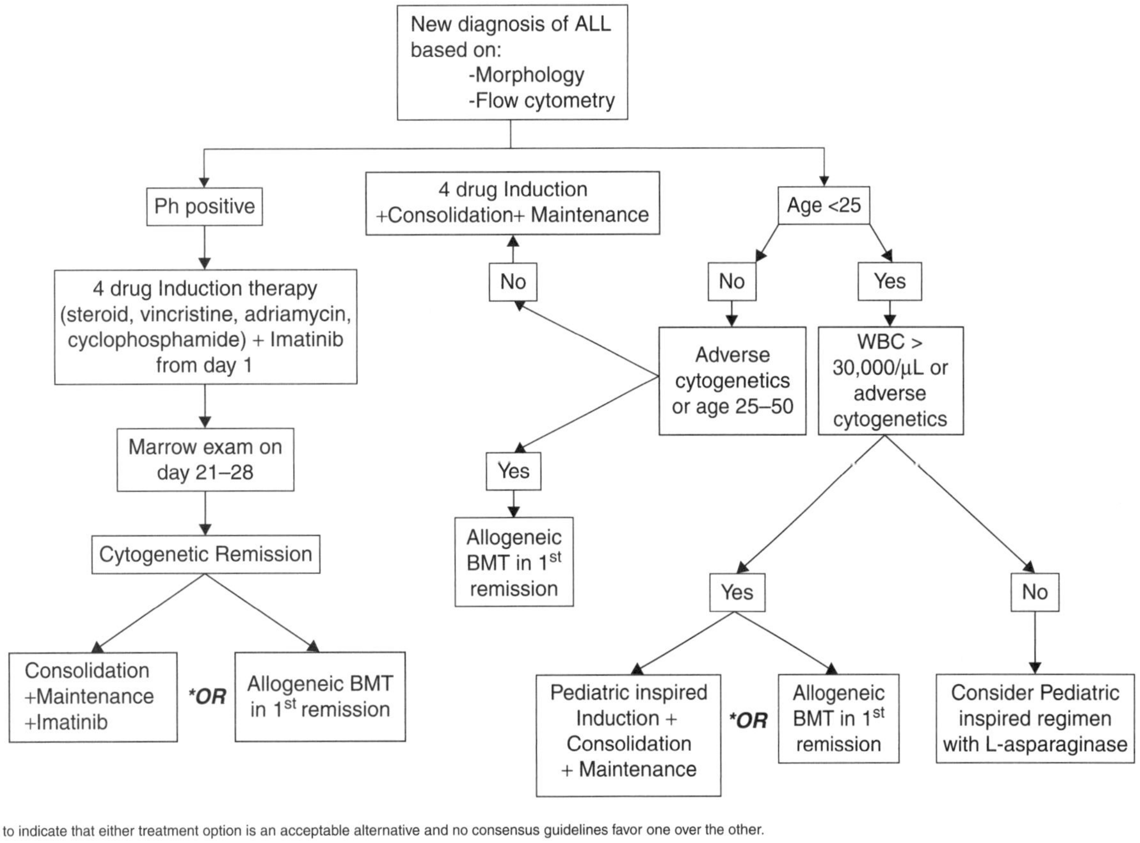

Figure 28.1

Treatment algorithm for the management of patients with ALL.

Table 28.3 Risk Classification in Pediatric ALL

Risk Group	Characteristics
High risk	–*BCR-ABL:* t (9;22); –Hypodiploidy (<44); –*MLL-AF4*/ or other *MLL:* {t(4;11); t(9;11); t(11;19)} –Minimal residual disease after induction > 1%
Standard risk	All others
Low risk	–B-cell precursor ALL –Age 1–10 years –WBC < 50 × 10^9/L –Minimal residual disease after induction < 0.01%

Table 28.4 Prognostic Factors in Adult and Adolescent Young Adult (AYA) ALL

	Standard Risk	Adverse Risk
Age (Years)	<35	>60
Immunophenotype	Mid T-cell	Early T-cell, Mature T-cell
Leukocyte count	<30,000/μL	>100,000/μL
Genotype	—	-complex (≥5); -Hypodiploidy (<44) -*BCR-ABL1*: t(9;22) -*MLL-AF4*/ other *MLL*:{t(4;11); t(9;11); t(11;19)}
Minimal residual disease after induction	<0.01%	>0.01%

continuing the maintenance for 2 to 3 years (9). Consensus guidelines from pediatric (but not adult literature) recommend escalating the doses of methotrexate and 6-mercaptopurine to achieve low leukocyte counts. Adequate dose intensity is an important factor associated with decreased relapse in maintenance phase (10). Adult ALL protocols have not been as stringent and aggressive with maintenance dose escalation, and this may be one of the factors resulting in poorer outcomes in adult ALL as compared to pediatric ALL. Another treatment strategy that has shown to be of benefit is the addition of one or two reinduction cycles shortly after achieving remission. The reinduction regimens use the same drugs that were initially used to achieve induction.

An approach for the adolescent young adult (AYA) patient gaining traction is to use a more intensive pediatric-inspired regimen, including higher doses of non-myelosuppressive "core" drugs such as L-asparaginase, vincristine, and steroids; early and frequent CNS prophylaxis with intrathecal chemotherapy, one or even two postremission re-intensification cycles, and long-term maintenance for 3 years. This is based on retrospective American and European trials (11,12) that showed significantly better 3- or 4-year event-free and overall survival (OS) with pediatric-inspired regimens in young adults between ages 16 to 21. The Spanish PETHEMA Protocol ALL-96 (13) was a prospective trial in which 35 adolescents (aged 15–18 years) and 46 young adults (aged 19–30 years) with standard risk ALL were treated with pediatric-inspired protocols. Patients received a standard five drug, 5-week induction; followed by two cycles of early consolidation, maintenance with monthly reinforcement for 1-year post-remission, and standard maintenance therapy for up to 2 years. The 6-year event-free survival of 61% and OS of 69% demonstrated the efficacy and tolerability of intensive pediatric regimens in AYA up to the age of 30.

D.N. received aggressive intravenous hydration with normal saline and oral allopurinol 300-mg daily starting on the day of admission. His creatinine and uric acid came down rapidly over the ensuing 24 hours and he underwent induction with five drug antileukemic chemotherapy (vincristine, anthracycline, cyclophosphamide, steroids, and L-asparaginase). Intrathecal chemotherapy with methotrexate was administered on day 3 of the induction regimen. He tolerated the chemotherapy relatively well with no serious infectious or metabolic complications. Frequent monitoring of uric acid, electrolytes, liver function, and coagulation profile was performed during the first 3 to 4 weeks of induction. Routine antiviral and PCP prophylaxis was initiated and supportive care included packed red blood cell transfusions for clinically significant anemia and platelet transfusions for platelet counts below 10,000/μL.

After recovering from the nadir of myelosuppression, bone marrow biopsy was performed on day 21 that revealed normocellular marrow with no identifiable blasts. Chromosome analysis revealed a normal male karyotype, confirming hematological, and cytogenetic remission. The absence of high-risk features discouraged the idea of proceeding with allogeneic stem cell transplantation, and a decision was made to continue with seven more cycles of the same chemotherapy used for induction along with intrathecal chemotherapy. This was followed by 3 years of maintenance with methotrexate, 6-mercaptopurine, steroids, and monthly vincristine. D.N. received intrathecal chemotherapy at 3 monthly intervals for the duration of maintenance therapy. He tolerated therapy well, except for an episode of transaminitis during year 2 of maintenance that resolved after reducing the 6-mercaptopurine dose by 25%. He is currently 4 years from initial diagnosis with no evidence of relapse. He continues to follow-up for bi-annual physical examinations and CBC checks.

Adult B-Cell Precursor ALL with Adverse Features

M.R., a 48-year-old man, presented with bilateral knee and shin pain worse at night for the last 3 months. Laboratory data revealed a WBC count of 73,000/μL. Flow cytometry demonstrated a large population of cells that were CD19+, CD20+, and CD10+. Bone marrow cytogenetics revealed t(4;11) with *MLL-AF4* fusion.

Evidence-Based Case Discussion

This is an adult patient with high-risk ALL based on his age (>35) and elevated WBC count (> 30,000/μL), which are poor prognostic factors. The presence of t(4;11) associated with the *MLL* gene transcript is linked with hyperleukocytosis and dismal outcome, and is more prevalent in infants and elderly patients. These features place M.R. in a high-risk group.

Although the basic approach to treatment of B-cell precursor ALL in adult patients remains the same, there are some important differences in the biology, tolerance to chemotherapy, postinduction approaches, and the role of transplant in older patients (see Figure 28.1). This patient should be treated using standard induction therapy with steroids, vincristine, anthracycline, and cyclophosphamide (7,8). High-dose cytarabine and methotrexate should be used with caution and may require dose reduction. The complications of L-asparaginase including hypersensitivity, coagulopathy, and pancreatitis increase with age. There is some evidence that CD20 positivity confers worse prognosis, and the use of anti-CD20 or anti-CD22 antibodies may improve outcome (14).

This patient should be evaluated early in his treatment for allogeneic stem cell transplant; autologous transplant has been shown to be inferior to maintenance therapy in the UK ALL XII/ECOG 2993 study (15). Initial studies showed survival benefit with allogeneic stem cell transplant in high-risk patients, consequently an evidence-based review panel recommended allogeneic transplant for adults with high-risk ALL in first remission (16). Although a recent MRC and ECOG trial showed a survival advantage for allotransplant in patients with standard risk (age < 35 and no adverse biological features), these patients usually receive maintenance therapy (15). M.R. underwent induction chemotherapy using the HyperCVAD regimen. He developed fever and was diagnosed with Pseudomonas pneumonia on day 10 of induction chemotherapy. He subsequently required ICU admission, intubation, intravenous pressors, and broad-spectrum antibiotics for a period of 5 days. His clinical course improved as his blood counts recovered. Bone marrow aspiration on day 24 revealed 40% cellularity with no discernible blasts on morphological examination. Cytogenetics revealed a normal male karyotype and a decision was made to proceed with allogeneic transplantation in first remission. The patient had a healthy HLA-matched sibling and underwent allogeneic transplantation approximately 2 months after initial diagnosis. He had mild acute and chronic graft versus host disease posttransplantation. Bone marrow biopsies on day 90 and day 365 posttransplant showed complete donor chimerism and no evidence of ALL.

Adult BCR-ABL Transcript Positive B-Cell Precursor ALL

W.L., a 46-year-old man, presented with headache, dyspnea on exertion, persistent low-grade fever with chills, and bleeding from the gums over the last 6 weeks. His white cell count on presentation was 180,000/μL and his platelet count was 8000/μL. Flow cytometry revealed a predominance of CD19+, CD79a+, CD10+ cells confirming a diagnosis of B-cell precursor ALL. Cytogenetics from the bone marrow specimen revealed t(9;22) in 6/20 metaphase cells and PCR demonstrated the p190 BCR-ABL variant.

Evidence-Based Case Discussion

W.L. is an "older" precursor B-cell ALL patient with the Philadelphia chromosome indicating the presence of the BCR-ABL fusion gene. BCR-ABL fusion transcripts are more common in elderly patients (30%), are often associated with leukocytosis, and confer a poor prognosis and high relapse rate (3).

Heretofore, allogeneic stem cell transplant in first remission was the only effective therapeutic option, with 5-year survival rates approaching 35% to 45% (17). The emergence of TKI therapy has changed the approach to such patients. Currently, induction chemotherapy for ALL is used in combination with imatinib (4) and preliminary data suggest CR rates > 90% (see Figure 28.1). Imatinib is usually started at a dose of 400-mg daily and continued through induction, consolidation, and maintenance phases. Newer data are emerging concerning the use of dasatinib, which may be a more potent drug as it inhibits multiple kinases and also seems to have higher CNS penetration (18).

W.L. received induction chemotherapy with Hyper CVAD. Imatinib was started on day 1 of induction and continued at 400-mg daily through the eight cycles of HyperCVAD chemotherapy. The patient achieved hematological and cytogenetic remission after cycle 1 of induction chemotherapy. After detailed discussion, W.L. opted to proceed with maintenance therapy over allogeneic transplantation. He is currently 18 months from initial diagnosis and continues to take 400 mg of imatinib daily in addition to maintenance therapy with oral methotrexate and 6-mercaptopurine. Imatinib will be continued indefinitely.

Adult T-cell ALL With Favorable Prognostic Features

A.A., a 27-year-old man, presented with fatigue, bone pain, petechiae and recent weight loss. He had a white count of 65,000/μL, a hemoglobin of 8.2 g/dL and a platelet count of 80,000/μL. His peripheral smear revealed many large cells with reduced cytoplasm, fine chromatin, and poorly defined nucleoli. Flow cytometry of peripheral blood demonstrated that the blasts were CD7+, CD3+, CD1a+, and CD13– confirming the diagnosis of T-cell ALL. No mediastinal mass was visible on chest x-ray. Cytogenetics from a bone marrow aspirate revealed a normal male karyotype.

Evidence-Based Case Discussion

A.A. has T-cell ALL; his age < 35 years and total WBC count < 100,000/µL are favorable factors (19). The UK ALL XII/ECOG 2993 study of 1927 ALL patients contained 356 subjects with T-cell ALL. A CR rate of 94% and 5-year OS of 48% was demonstrated for T-cell ALL patients using an aggressive chemotherapy regimen containing L-asparaginase. This study demonstrated that blast expression of CD1a, and lack of expression of CD13 in T-cell disease were associated with significantly better survival. Complex cytogenetics was also associated with poor survival, but CNS involvement at diagnosis did not seem to affect survival in T-cell disease (although it did in the overall cohort). The role of allogeneic stem cell transplant in T-cell ALL is still under investigation. Nelarabine has efficacy in the relapsed setting and is currently being tested in front-line regimens (20). On the basis of this study, the predicted OS at 5 years for this patient with favorable risk T-cell ALL is approximately 50%.

A.A. received standard antileukemic therapy and CNS prophylaxis with intrathecal therapy followed by consolidation and maintenance therapy for a total of 3 years. He remains in remission and has returned to work.

REFERENCES

1. Pui CH, Raimondi SC, Borowitz MJ, et al. Immunophenotypes and karyotypes of leukemic cells in children with Down syndrome and acute lymphoblastic leukemia. *J Clin Oncol.* 1993;11(7):1361–1367.
2. Liberzon E, Avigad S, Stark B, et al. Germ-line ATM gene alterations are associated with susceptibility to sporadic T-cell acute lymphoblastic leukemia in children. *Genes Chromosomes Cancer.* 2004;39(2):161–166.
3. Moorman AV, Chilton L, Wilkinson J, et al. A population-based cytogenetic study of adults with acute lymphoblastic leukemia. *Blood.* 2010;115(2):206–214.
4. Ribera JM, Oriol A, González M, et al. Concurrent intensive chemotherapy and imatinib before and after stem cell transplantation in newly diagnosed Philadelphia chromosome-positive acute lymphoblastic leukemia. Final results of the CSTIBES02 trial. *Haematologica.* 2010;95(1):87–95.
5. Harvey RC, Mullighan CG, Chen IM, et al. Rearrangement of CRLF2 is associated with mutation of JAK kinases, alteration of IKZF1, Hispanic/Latino ethnicity, and a poor outcome in pediatric B-progenitor acute lymphoblastic leukemia. *Blood.* 2010;115(26):5312–5321. Epub 2010 Feb 4.
6. Asnafi V, Buzyn A, Le Noir S, et al. NOTCH1/FBXW7 mutation identifies a large subgroup with favorable outcome in adult T-cell acute lymphoblastic leukemia (T-ALL): a Group for Research on Adult Acute Lymphoblastic Leukemia (GRAALL) study. *Blood.* 2009;113(17):3918–3924. Epub 2008 Dec 23.
7. Kantarjian HM, O'Brien S, Smith TL, et al. Results of treatment with hyper-CVAD, a dose-intensive regimen, in adult acute lymphocytic leukemia. *J Clin Oncol.* 2000;18(3):547–561.
8. Larson RA, Dodge RK, Burns CP, et al. A five-drug remission induction regimen with intensive consolidation for adults with acute lymphoblastic leukemia: cancer and leukemia group B study 8811. *Blood.* 1995;85(8):2025–2037.
9. Duration and intensity of maintenance chemotherapy in acute lymphoblastic leukemia: overview of 42 trials involving 12,000 randomised children. Childhood ALL Collaborative Group. *Lancet.* 1996;347(9018):1783–1788.
10. Relling MV, Hancock ML, Boyett JM,et al. Prognostic importance of 6-mercaptopurine dose intensity in acute lymphoblastic leukemia. *Blood.* 1999;93(9):2817–2823.
11. Stock W, La M, Sanford B, et al. Children's Cancer Group; Cancer and Leukemia Group B studies. What determines the outcomes for adolescents and young adults with acute lymphoblastic leukemia treated on cooperative group protocols? A comparison of Children's Cancer Group and Cancer and Leukemia Group B studies. *Blood.* 2008;112(5):1646–1654. Epub 2008 May 23.
12. Boissel N, Auclerc MF, Lhéritier V, et al. Should adolescents with acute lymphoblastic leukemia be treated as old children or young adults? Comparison of French FRALLE-93 and LALA-94 trials. *J Clin Oncol.* 2003;21(5):774–780. Epub 2003 Mar 1.
13. Ribera JM, Oriol A, Sanz MA, et al. Comparison of the results of the treatment of adolescents and young adults with standard-risk acute lymphoblastic leukemia with the Programa Español de Tratamiento en Hematología pediatric-based protocol ALL-96. *J Clin Oncol.* 2008;26(11):1843–1849.
14. Thomas DA, O'Brien S, Kantarjian HM. Monoclonal antibody therapy with rituximab for acute lymphoblastic leukemia. *Hematol Oncol Clin North Am.* 2009;23(5):949–971, v. Review.
15. Goldstone AH, Richards SM, Lazarus HM, et al. In adults with standard-risk acute lymphoblastic leukemia, the greatest benefit is achieved from a matched sibling allogeneic transplantation in first complete remission, and an autologous transplantation is less effective than conventional consolidation/maintenance chemotherapy in all patients: final results of the International ALL Trial (MRC UKALL XII/ECOG E2993). *Blood.* 2008;111(4):1827–1833.
16. Hahn T, Wall D, Camitta B, et al. The role of cytotoxic therapy with hematopoietic stem cell transplantation in the therapy of acute lymphoblastic leukemia in adults: an evidence-based review. *Biol Blood Marrow Transplant.* 2006;12(1):1–30.
17. Fielding AK, Rowe JM, Richards SM, et al. Prospective outcome data on 267 unselected adult patients with Philadelphia chromosome-positive acute lymphoblastic leukemia confirms superiority of allogeneic transplantation over chemotherapy in the pre-imatinib era: results from the International ALL Trial MRC UKALLXII/ECOG2993. *Blood.* 2009;113(19):4489–4496.
18. Ottmann O, Dombret H, Martinelli G, et al. Dasatinib induces rapid hematologic and cytogenetic responses in adult patients with Philadelphia chromosome positive acute lymphoblastic leukemia with resistance or intolerance to imatinib: interim results of a phase 2 study. *Blood.* 2007;110(7):2309–2315.
19. Marks DI, Paietta EM, Moorman AV, et al. T-cell acute lymphoblastic leukemia in adults: clinical features, immunophenotype, cytogenetics, and outcome from the large randomized prospective trial (UKALL XII/ECOG 2993). *Blood.* 2009;114(25): 5136–5145.
20. DeAngelo DJ. Nelarabine for the treatment of patients with relapsed or refractory T-cell acute lymphoblastic leukemia or lymphoblastic lymphoma. *Hematol Oncol Clin North Am.* 2009;23(5):1121–1135, vii-viii.

29

Acute Myelogenous Leukemia

MOHSEN ARANI AND SARVARI V. YELLAPRAGADA

EPIDEMIOLOGY, RISK FACTORS, NATURAL HISTORY, AND PATHOLOGY

Acute leukemias are clonal malignant disorders resulting from genetic alterations in normal hematopoietic stem cells. These changes limit normal differentiation and lead to proliferation of abnormal leukemic cells or blasts. Acute myelogenous leukemia (AML) is the most common variant of acute leukemia, accounting for about 80% of acute leukemia in adults. Approximately 13,000 people were diagnosed with AML in 2010, and around 9000 died of the disease. In general, the risk for developing AML increases with age with a 10-fold increase from age 30 (1 case per 100,000) to age 65 (1 case per 10,000), and a median age at diagnosis of 65 to 70. A notable exception to this escalating incidence with age is a rare (600–800 cases/year in the United States) subtype of AML called acute promyelocytic leukemia (APL) or M3 (see below). APL is very uncommon in children, but its incidence increases steadily during the teen years, reaches a plateau during early adulthood, and remains constant until it increases after age 60. Higher incidence of APL has been reported in persons from Mexico, Central and South America, Italy, and Spain, but this has not been reported in other forms of AML. AML is slightly more common in males than females.

AML can present de novo or can develop following another disorder (secondary AML). AML can evolve from a variety of bone marrow disorders including myelodysplastic syndrome (MDS), aplastic anemia, and inherited bone marrow failure syndromes, including Fanconi anemia, Dyskeratosis congenita, Diamond-Blackfan anemia, and Amegakaryoctic thrombocytopenia. Down syndrome and Bloom syndrome also predispose affected persons to develop AML. Exposure to benzene, pesticides, petroleum products, and radiation increase risk of developing leukemia. Chemotherapeutic drugs, particularly alkylating agents and topoisomerase inhibitors, can increase the risk of developing AML later in life ("therapy-related AML"). Acute leukemia resulting from exposure to alkylating agents usually has a latency period of 7 to 10 years, and it is frequently associated with MDS, monosomies or deletion of 5q and/or 7q and complex cytogenetics. AML following exposure to topoisomerase II inhibitors has a shorter latency period of 2 to 3 years, is not typically preceded by MDS, and usually shows monocytic differentiation with chromosomal translocations involving the MLL locus at 11q23. Therapy-related AML has a particularly poor prognosis (1).

Patients with AML present with fever and symptoms related to bone marrow failure including fatigue, infection, bruising, and bleeding. Some patients present with pain related to rapidly expanding disease in the marrow whereas those with elevated circulating blast count can have central nervous system (CNS) symptoms, retinal hemorrhage, or cardiopulmonary complications due to leukostasis. Patients with monocytic AML subtypes can present with infiltration of the gingiva or other tissues (chloroma). Disseminated intravascular coagulation (DIC) with abnormal clotting or bleeding is a common presentation in patients with AML, but it can also be seen in other forms of AML. Physical examination might reveal hepatosplenomegaly or lymphadenopathy.

In recent years, considerable progress has been made in deciphering the molecular, genetic, and epigenetic basis of AML and in defining new diagnostic and prognostic markers. AML must be distinguished from acute lymphoblastic leukemia (ALL), MDS, or AML arising in the setting of MDS, because therapeutic strategies and prognosis vary considerably for these diseases. AML can be distinguished from ALL by demonstrating definitive commitment to the myeloid lineage through judicious use of morphologic (e.g., presence of Auer rods), immunohistochemical, and immunologic methods. Diagnosis of AML requires identification of 20% leukemic blasts in the blood or bone marrow with a notable exception for AML with the recurrent genetic abnormalities t(8;21), inv(16), or t(16;16), t(15;17), and some cases of erythroleukemia, which are treated as AML regardless of blast counts. In order to make a diagnosis of AML, at least 200 leukocytes on blood smears and 500 nucleated cells in marrow smears should be counted, with the latter containing spicules. Myeloblasts, monoblasts, and megakaryoblasts are included in the blast count. In AML with monocytic or myelomonocytic differentiation, monoblasts, and promonocytes, but not abnormal monocytes, are counted as blast equivalents. Erythroblasts are not counted as blasts except in the rare instance of pure erythroid leukemia. Once a clinical diagnosis of AML is made, the morphologic and genetic subtype must be identified. AML is a heterogeneous disease caused by a variety of pathogenic mechanisms. At a morphologic level, this heterogeneity is manifested by variability in the degree of commitment and differentiation of the cell lineage. This variability has been used to define specific morphologic subgroups.

Immunophenotyping by flow cytometry is used to determine lineage involvement of a newly diagnosed acute leukemia. Quantifying expression of several surface and cytoplasmic antigens is necessary for lineage assignment, to diagnose mixed phenotype acute leukemia (MPAL), and to detect aberrant immunophenotypes allowing for measurement of minimal residual disease (MRD). Flow cytometric determination of blast count should not be used as a substitute for morphologic evaluation. Acute leukemias of ambiguous lineage are rare leukemias and comprise those cases that demonstrate no evidence of lineage differentiation (i.e., acute undifferentiated leukemia [AUL]) or those with blasts that express markers of more than one lineage (ie, MPAL). AULs often express HLA-DR, CD34, and/or CD38, but lack lineage-associated markers.

Conventional cytogenetic analysis is a mandatory component in the diagnostic evaluation of a patient with suspected acute leukemia. Chromosome abnormalities are detected in approximately 55% of adult AML. A minimum of 20 metaphase cells analyzed from bone marrow is considered mandatory to establish the diagnosis of a normal karyotype, and recommended to define an abnormal karyotype. A growing number of recurring genetic changes have been recognized in the new World Health Organization (WHO) classification of AML (Table 29.1) (2). Furthermore, novel therapies are being developed that target some of the genetic lesions. The recent WHO classification reflects the fact that an increasing number of acute leukemias can be categorized based on their underlying cytogenetic or molecular genetic abnormalities, and that these genetic changes form clinicopathologic genetic entities (see table). At presentation with the suspected diagnosis of acute leukemia, a marrow specimen should routinely be taken for molecular diagnostics. However, if this results in a "dry tap," the peripheral blood maybe obtained for cytogenetic and molecular diagnostics.

Table 29.1 Acute Myeloid Leukemia and Related Precursor Neoplasms, and Acute Leukemia of Ambiguous Lineage (WHO 2008)

Categories
Acute myeloid leukemia with recurrent genetic abnormalities
AML with t(8;21)(q22;q22); *RUNX1-RUNX1T1*
AML with inv(16)(p13.1q22) or t(16;16)(p13.1;q22); *CBFB-MYH11*
APL with t(15;17)(q22;q12); *PML-RARA*
AML with t(9;11)(p22;q23); *MLLT3-MLL*
AML with t(6;9)(p23;q34); *DEK-NUP214*
AML with inv(3)(q21q26.2) or t(3;3)(q21;q26.2); *RPN1-EVI1*
AML (megakaryoblastic) with t(1;22)(p13;q13); *RBM15-MKL1*
Provisional entity: AML with mutated NPM1
Provisional entity: AML with mutated CEBPA
Acute myeloid leukemia with myelodysplasia-related changes
Therapy-related myeloid neoplasms
Acute myeloid leukemia, not otherwise specified (NOS)
Acute myeloid leukemia with minimal differentiation
Acute myeloid leukemia without maturation
Acute myeloid leukemia with maturation
Acute myelomonocytic leukemia
Acute monoblastic/monocytic leukemia
Acute erythroid leukemia
Pure erythroid leukemia
Erythroleukemia, erythroid/myeloid
Acute megakaryoblastic leukemia
Acute basophilic leukemia
Acute panmyelosis with myelofibrosis (syn.: acute myelofibrosis; acute myelosclerosis)
Myeloid sarcoma (syn.: extramedullary myeloid tumor; granulocytic sarcoma; chloroma)
Myeloid proliferations related to Down syndrome
Transient abnormal myelopoiesis (syn.: transient myeloproliferative disorder)
Myeloid leukemia associated with Down syndrome
Blastic plasmacytoid dendritic cell neoplasm
Acute Leukemias of ambiguous lineage
Acute undifferentiated leukemia
Mixed phenotype acute leukemia with t(9;22)(q34;q11.2); *BCR-ABL1*
Mixed phenotype acute leukemia with t(v;11q23); *MLL* rearranged
Mixed phenotype acute leukemia, B/myeloid, NOS
Mixed phenotype acute leukemia, T/myeloid, NOS
Provisional entity: Natural killer (NK)–cell lymphoblastic leukemia/lymphoma

Unfavorable prognostic factors include white blood cell (WBC) count > 20,000/μL, prior MDS, previous cytotoxic therapy, and certain specific cytogenetic and molecular genetic changes in the leukemic cells at diagnosis. Various other factors, such as splenomegaly and elevated serum lactate dehydrogenase (LDH) levels, have been reported to confer some prognostic effect, but with variable consistency among studies. The cytogenetics of the leukemic cell is the strongest prognostic factor for response to induction therapy and for survival (1). The recurrent genetic abnormalities t(8;21), inv(16) or t(16;16), t(15;17) generally carry a favorable prognosis and are more commonly seen in younger adult patients. Monosomy 5 or 7, chromosome 3 abnormalities like inv 3(q21q26.2), 11q23 abnormalities other than t(9;11)(p22;q23), and complex karyotype, which occurs in 10% to 12% of patients, have consistently been associated with very poor outcomes. Complex karyotype has been defined as the presence of three or more chromosome abnormalities in the absence of t(8;21), inv(16) or t(16;16), or t(15;17). Complex karyotypes include a paucity of balanced rearrangements, and a predominance of chromosomal imbalances. Chromosomal losses most frequently affect 5q, 17p, and 7q, and gains affect 8q, 11q, and 21q. Normal cytogenetics, trisomy 8, and t(9;11)(p22;q23) are considered intermediate in risk.

Recently identified gene mutations and deregulated gene expression have helped to explain the diversity within defined cytogenetic groups, including the large and heterogeneous group of patients with cytogenetically normal (CN)AML (3). In this heterogeneous group, molecular studies have been useful in further risk stratification for establishing prognosis. In general, two classes of molecular mutations have been identified. Class I mutations activate signal-transduction pathways and increase proliferation and/or survival of progenitors. Mutations that activate the receptor tyrosine kinase FMS-like tyrosine kinase 3 *(FLT3),* particularly the Internal Tandem duplication (*FLT3*-ITD) or *N-RAS* (neuroblastoma RAS viral oncogene homolog) are good examples. Class II mutations affect transcription factors or components of the transcriptional coactivation complex and cause impaired differentiation. Mutations of this type include those in the *C/EBPα*(CCAAT/enhancer binding protein α) referred to as CEBPA, *MLL*(myeloid/lymphoid or mixed-lineage leukemia), and *NPM1* (nucleophosmin) genes.

Prognostic significance within younger adults with CN-AML has consistently been shown for mutations in the *NPM1, CEBPA,* and *FLT3* genes. CN-AML patients harboring internal tandem duplication (ITD) of the *FLT3* gene have an inferior outcome. The *NPM1* mutation in CN-AML has been associated with higher complete remission (CR) rates and better relapse-free and event-free survival especially if it occurs in the absence of *FLT3*-ITD. This observation also seems to hold among older patients. CN-AML with mutations in *CEBPA* is another AML subset associated with favorable prognosis and survival data, similar to AML patients with mutated NPM1 without *FLT3*-ITD. Although *FLT3* mutations are observed in APL and are associated with a higher WBC count at presentation, they do not add to the specific diagnosis of APL, influence management, or provide independent prognostic information. In the cytogenetically favorable core binding factor (CBF) AMLs—that is, AML with t(8;21) or inv(16)/t(16;16)—retrospective studies have demonstrated that several mutations in the *KIT* gene have an unfavorable influence on outcome. A growing list of genetic abnormalities in genes such as *WT1, RUNX1, MLL, KIT, RAS, TP53, TET2, IDH1* are being investigated for prognostic value in AML. Monitoring for MRD by reverse transcription polymerase chain reaction (RT-PCR) detecting leukemia-specific targets or by flow cytometry identifying leukemia-associated aberrant phenotypes remains an active field of investigation (4). Except for APL, there is a paucity of prospective trial data demonstrating the clinical utility of these strategies for detecting MRD. *NPM1* mutations likely provide one of the most promising new targets and studies are ongoing to evaluate the clinical utility of MRD monitoring in AML with *NPM1* mutation. AML with mutations in *NPM1* or *CEBPA* have been incorporated in the WHO classification as provisional entities in an effort to standardize the reporting system for molecular abnormalities. Screening for these two markers as well as for *FLT3* mutations should be done in clinical trials and is also recommended for patients undergoing intensive therapy for AML in routine practice. Table 29.2 provides

Table 29.2 Standardized Reporting of Cytogenetics, Incidence and Treatment Outcome in AML

Genetic Group	Subsets	Incidence	CR Rate	5 Year Survival
Favorable	t(8;21)(q22;q22); *RUNX1-RUNX1T1* inv(16)(p13.1q22) or t(16;16)(p13.1;q22); *CBFB-MYH11* Normal Karyotype with Mutated *NPM1* without *FLT3*-ITD Normal Karyotype with Mutated *CEBPA*	20%	85%	60%
Intermediate	Normal Karyotype with Mutated *NPM1* and *FLT3*-ITD Normal Karyotype with Wild-type *NPM1* and *FLT3*-ITD Normal Karyotype with Wild-type *NPM1* without *FLT3*-ITD t(9;11)(p22;q23); *MLLT3-MLL*	45%	76%	38%
Adverse	complex Karyotype, –5 or del(5q); –7; abnormal(17p); inv(3)(q21q26.2) or t(3;3)(q21;q26.2); *RPN1-EVI1* t(6;9), t(v;11)(v;q23); *MLL* rearrangement	30%	55%	12%

a summary of cytogenic features that are associated with a favorable, intermediate, or poor prognosis.

After conventional induction therapy, response assessment is commonly performed between days 14 and 28 after the start of therapy depending on the protocol. Definitions of response criteria are based primarily on those reported by Cheson et al. (5). A complete remission (CR) is defined as bone marrow blasts < 5%; absence of blasts with Auer rods; absence of extramedullary disease; absolute neutrophil count > 1.0 × 10^9/L (1000/µL); platelet count > 100 × 10^9/L (100,000/µL) and independence from red cell transfusions. All criteria need to be fulfilled. Just as in initial diagnosis, marrow evaluation should be based on a count of 500 nucleated cells in an aspirate with spicules; if ambiguous, a repeat examination should be done in 5 to 7 days. A marrow biopsy should be performed in cases of dry tap, or if no spicules are obtained. No minimum duration of response is required. In cases with low blast percentages (5–10%), a repeat marrow should be performed to confirm relapse. Cytogenetics should be tested to distinguish true relapse from therapy-related MDS/AML.

CASE SUMMARIES

Management of APL

Y.A., a 28-year-old woman with no significant past medical history, was brought to the emergency room by her sister with reports of generalized weakness, excessive bruising, and continuous vaginal bleeding for 1 week. Her physical examination did not reveal lymphadenopathy or hepatosplenomegaly. She had ecchymoses on her upper thighs, arms, and upper torso that were not associated with trauma. She had oozing from IV line sites and some vaginal bleeding observed on a gynecologic exam. A complete blood count showed a WBC of 1,800/µL, hemoglobin of 8.7 g/dL, and platelets of 13,000/µL. Examination of the peripheral smear showed large promyelocytes with a large nuclear:cytoplasmic ratio, prominent nucleoli, and several Auer Rods. Her coagulation parameters showed a PT of 18 s, PTT of 38 s, and fibrinogen of 80 mg/dL.

Evidence-Based Case Discussion

A presumptive diagnosis of APL should be made by review of the peripheral blood smear alone or with the bone marrow aspirate and core biopsy in the presence of the characteristic clinical findings. Immediate treatment must begin when the disease is suspected and confirmed by an experienced hematologist. As in the case of Y.A., the peripheral blood smear often shows leukopenia with circulating promyelocytes that usually have abundant, often irregular-appearing, primary azurophilic granules. Leukemic promyelocytes with multiple Auer rods may be found and are a distinctive feature of APL. Although often obscured by the granules, the nuclear contour is bilobed or reniform in appearance. The latter feature is important because patients with the M3 variant (M3V) may not have easily visible granules, but have the same predisposition toward catastrophic bleeding and the same excellent outcome with appropriate treatment.

APL maybe classified into three risk groups based on prognosis: (a) the low-risk group includes patients with WBC ≤10,000/µL and platelet count ≥40,000/µL with relapse-free survival (RFS) of 98%; (b) the intermediate-risk group includes patients with WBC ≤10,000/µL and platelets ≤ 40,000/µL with RFS of about 90%; and (c) the high-risk group includes patients with WBC >10,000/µL and an RFS of 70%.

Induction Therapy

On the basis of the examination of the peripheral smear and laboratory parameters, APL was suspected and risk stratification placed Y.A. in the intermediate group. After a negative pregnancy test, Y.A. was started immediately on all-*trans* retinoic acid (ATRA) and she was transfused with fresh frozen plasma, cryoprecipitate, and platelets. PCR for the *PML-RARα* transcript (performed on the peripheral blood) came back positive the following day. Subsequently, an analysis of the bone marrow aspirate and biopsy confirmed AML-M3 (APL) and t(15; 17). The introduction of ATRA (tretinoin) and arsenic trioxide (ATO) into APL therapy has completely revolutionized the management and outcome of this disease. Treatment strategies using these agents, usually in combination with chemotherapy, have provided excellent results with survival rates exceeding 70%. Cure of patients with APL depends not only on the effective use of combination therapy involving differentiating and classical cytotoxic agents, but also on supportive care measures that take into account the biology of the disease and the complications associated with molecularly targeted therapies. Once a diagnosis of APL is suspected, the disease should be managed as a medical emergency. Treatment with ATRA at 45 mg/m^2 per day in divided doses should be initiated without waiting for genetic confirmation of the diagnosis, preferably the same day the diagnosis is suspected. ATRA is unlikely to have deleterious effects should genetic assessment fail to confirm the diagnosis of APL (6). Diagnosis should be further confirmed by molecular detection of *PML-RARα* fusion (or rare molecular variants). In addition to conventional karyotyping, FISH, and RT-PCR can be used for rapid diagnosis of APL. Intracranial and pulmonary hemorrhages are relatively common life-threatening complications of APL coagulopathy. Central venous catheterization, lumbar puncture, and other invasive procedures (e.g., bronchoscopy) should be avoided before and during induction therapy due to high risk of hemorrhagic complications, but patients with APL may also have a higher incidence of thrombosis. Aggressive supportive care should include liberal transfusion with fresh frozen plasma, cryoprecipitate, and platelet transfusions to maintain the fibrinogen concentration above 100 to 150 mg/dL, platelet count above 30,000–50,000 /μL and INR < 1.5. Heparin, tranexamic acid, and other anticoagulant or antifibrinolytic therapy should not be used routinely outside the context of a clinical trial.

High-risk patients should begin chemotherapy without delay, *even if the molecular results are still pending.* Leukapheresis should be avoided due to risk of precipitating fatal hemorrhage. Early institution of anthracycline-based chemotherapy (idarubicin or daunorubicin +/– cytarabine [Ara C]) in combination with ATRA is the standard treatment approach in this life-threatening situation. Chemotherapy is generally started on day 1 within a few hours of the first dose of ATRA, aiming to control the coagulopathy and reduce the risk of APL differentiation syndrome (formerly retinoic acid syndrome), which is particularly high in these patients. The role of cytarabine in combination with the anthracycline is a topic of debate. The patients who are not candidates for anthracycline maybe treated upfront with a combination of ATRA and ATO.

APL differentiation syndrome associated with the administration of ATRA or ATO should be suspected clinically in the presence of dyspnea, unexplained fever, weight gain, peripheral edema, unexplained hypotension, acute renal failure, congestive heart failure, or a chest radiograph demonstrating pulmonary infiltrates, or pleural/pericardial effusion. Treatment with dexamethasone at a dose of 10-mg IV twice daily should be started at the very earliest symptom or sign. Discontinuation of ATRA or ATO is indicated in severe APL differentiation syndrome (i.e., patients developing renal failure or requiring admission to the intensive care unit due to respiratory distress). If a favorable response is obtained, dexamethasone should be maintained until complete disappearance of symptoms, and then ATRA or ATO should be resumed.

Virtually all *PML-RARα*-positive APLs are sensitive to ATRA and anthracycline-based chemotherapy leading to complete remission in 90% to 95% of patients and excellent long-term outcomes. Inclusion of cytarabine is somewhat more controversial, but data from the European Group suggests that there may be a benefit of adding standard-dose cytarabine both during induction and consolidation (7). Therefore, ATRA plus anthracyclines either alone or with cytarabine for induction is the standard of care. So long as the patient is tolerating therapy, ATRA is continued until CR is achieved (PCR negative for *PML-RARα* in the peripheral blood and bone marrow). No therapeutic modifications should be made on the basis of incomplete blast maturation (differentiation) detected up to 50 days or more after the start of treatment by morphology, cytogenetics, or molecular assessment (8).

Y.A. achieved complete hematologic and morphologic remission based on a bone marrow exam performed 4 weeks after treatment with ATRA and idarubicin. An important aspect of bone marrow assessment after induction is that it should not be done too early as the terminal differentiation of blasts may be delayed. Molecular remission need not be achieved at the end of induction and no change in therapy course should be made if PCR testing for PML-RARα is still positive.

Y.A. experienced no major complications during induction therapy. She used contraception throughout the duration of her treatment. Acute leukemia during pregnancy is a special challenge that should be managed jointly by the hematologist, obstetrician, and neonatologist in a tertiary care center. In a pregnant woman with APL, treatment should be started immediately because delays may compromise maternal outcome. The risk of teratogenicity is highest in first trimester, therefore, the crucial decision during this period is whether to continue with the pregnancy and receive chemotherapy or commit to terminate the pregnancy. Daunorubicin is the preferred anthracycline in pregnancy as idarubicin has a higher DNA affinity and is more lipophilic favoring an increased placental transfer. Chemotherapy delivered during the second and third trimester of pregnancy is safer for the fetus; however, delivery while the patient and fetus are cytopenic should be avoided. In APL, administration of ATRA is controversial in the second and third trimesters and should not be used in the first. ATO cannot be used in any stage of pregnancy.

Consolidation Therapy

Consolidation strategies depend on the risk classification for relapse at diagnosis. However, this is still an area of controversy and data continue to evolve on how to use the risk strata to help tailor consolidation. Three cycles of anthracycline-based chemotherapy are administered for low- and intermediate-risk patients in first complete remission (CR1). Many consolidation regimens incorporate ATRA in combination with chemotherapy whereas a few regimens do not incorporate ATRA. Although there is no consensus, there may be a benefit of adding cytarabine to the anthracycline in patients < 60 years old who are in the high-risk group. Consolidation regimens containing ATO and ATRA combined with anthracycline have also been effective. Molecular remission should be assessed at the end of consolidation therapy.

Y.A. received three cycles of consolidation therapy, the first cycle with ATRA and idarubicin followed by ATRA with mitoxantrone and a third cycle of ATRA and idarubicin again. At the end of consolidation therapy she attained a molecular remission.

Maintenance Therapy

Following consolidation, patients in complete molecular remission (*PMR-RARα* negative by PCR) are usually started on maintenance therapy. Although controversial, 1 to 2 years of consolidation with daily 6-mercaptopurine (6MP) and weekly methotrexate (MTX) given with a 2-week course of ATRA every 3 months is recommended. PCR monitoring should be performed every 3 months. Longer follow-up from the APL 93 trial demonstrated that maintenance treatment reduced the incidence of relapses (7). In patients presenting with WBC counts lower than 5,000/μL, the long-term benefit appeared less important. Recently updated Italian GIMEMA group results, using the same randomization design as in APL93 for maintenance treatment (i.e., no maintenance vs. 6MP+MTX vs. ATRA vs. both), found no difference in relapses among maintenance arms. Because early treatment intervention in patients with evidence of MRD affords a better outcome than treatment in full-blown relapse, every 3 months MRD monitoring of bone marrow or blood by PCR for *PML-RARα* should be offered to all patients for up to 3 years after completion of consolidation therapy. For patients testing PCR-positive at any stage after completion of consolidation, a bone marrow is repeated for MRD assessment within 2 weeks and samples are sent for confirmation. For patients with confirmed molecular relapse (defined as two successive PCR-positive assays with stable or rising *PML-RARα* transcript levels), preemptive therapy should be started promptly to prevent frank relapse. Although ATRA in combination with chemotherapy can be used as salvage therapy, ATO-based regimens are presently regarded as the first option for treatment of relapsed APL. Autologous hematopoietic stem cell transplant (HSCT) is considered the best option for patients without detectable MRD in the marrow (in second CR) and with an adequate PCR negative harvest. Allogeneic HSCT is recommended for patients failing to achieve a second molecular remission. For patients in whom HSCT is not feasible, the available options include repeated cycles of ATO with or without ATRA and with or without chemotherapy (7). The CNS is the most common site of extramedullary disease in APL and at least 10% of hematologic relapses are accompanied by CNS involvement. Because the majority of CNS relapses occur in patients presenting with hyperleukocytosis, some strategies include CNS prophylaxis for patients in this particular high-risk setting after the achievement of CR (lumbar puncture at presentation and during induction is extremely hazardous). Y.A. finished her consolidation therapy as outlined above. She declined maintenance therapy, but has continued PCR testing and has remained disease free for 3 years postconsolidation treatment. Figure 29.1 represents an algorithm for the management of patients with acute promyelocytic leukemia.

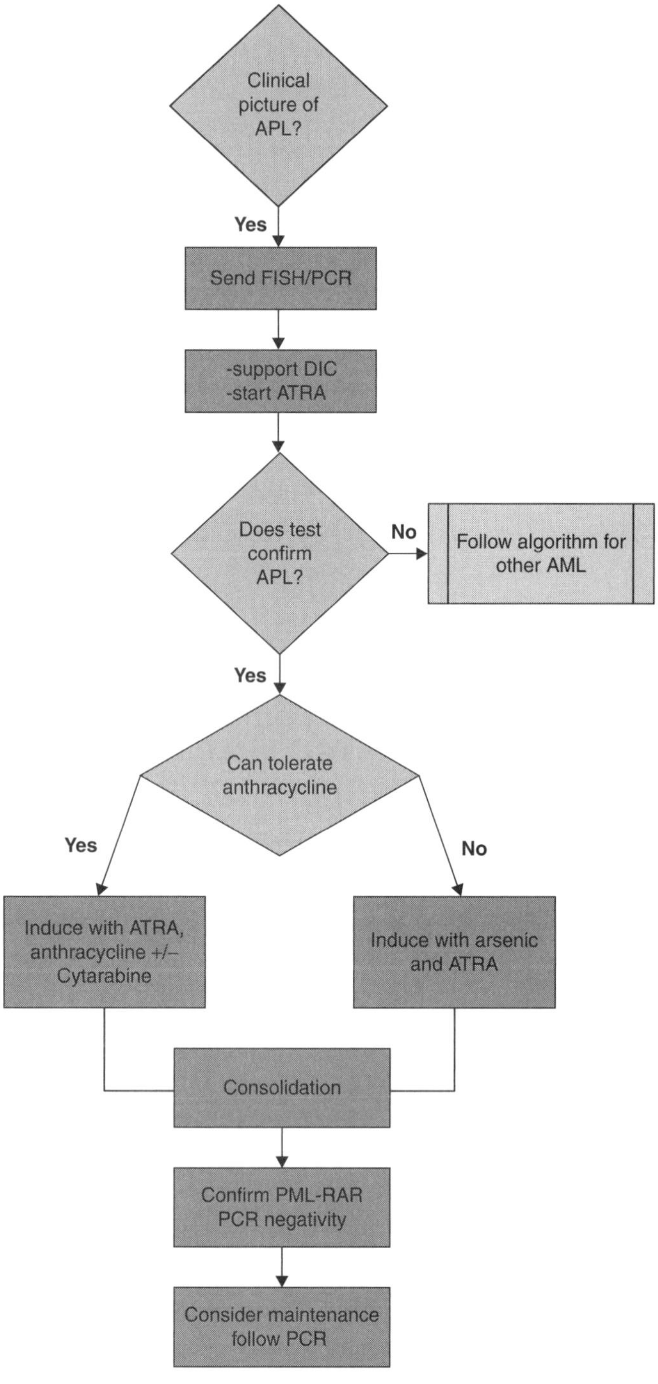

Figure 29.1

Algorithm for management of acute promyelocytic leukemia.

AML in Younger Adults (18 to 60 Years Old) With Favorable Risk Factors

A.M., a 48-year-old man with a history of hypertension, presented to his primary physician with a 1-month history of generalized weakness, fatigue, easy bruising, and intermittent epistaxis. He also reported a 1-week history of exertional dyspnea and chest pain. His physical examination revealed considerable pallor with no hepatosplenomegaly or lymphadenopathy. There was no evidence of bruising, but some petechiae were visible on his lower extremities. His CBC revealed a WBC count of 46,000/µL with a hemoglobin of 6.8 g/dL and a platelet count of 18,000/µL. A peripheral blood smear showed a large number of monocytoid appearing blasts and an increased number of eosinophils. A bone marrow aspirate and biopsy confirmed AML with cytogenetics showing inv(16). In this patient presenting with dyspnea and chest pain, a baseline EKG and chest x-ray were normal. He was transfused with packed red cells for symptomatic anemia and aggressively hydrated in preparation for treatment. An echocardiogram demonstrated a normal EF with no wall motion abnormalities.

Evidence-Based Case Discussion

Supportive care is an important part of induction therapy, including tumor lysis prophylaxis and management of hyperleukocytosis. A.M. has a WBC count less than 50,000/µL with no symptoms of hyperleukocytosis. Patients presenting with a WBC count of more than 100,000/µL, have increased induction mortality mainly due to hemorrhagic events, tumor lysis syndrome, and end-organ damage caused by leukostasis. Increased blood viscosity due to hyperleukocytosis and leukostasis can lead to respiratory distress from sludging in the pulmonary circulation or lead to retinal or cerebral hemorrhages that require immediate medical attention. This is considered a medical emergency. Hydroxyurea, given at dosages of up to 50 mg/kg/day until WBC count is less than 10,000–20,000 /µL should be initiated. Leukapheresis has been shown to reduce blast counts quickly and may improve early outcomes of induction therapy in AML; however, it has not been clearly shown to improve survival. There are no randomized trials comparing use of hydroxyurea alone versus the combination of hydroxyurea and leukapheresis in patients presenting with elevated white counts. Excessive red blood cell transfusions can lead to increased blood viscosity when white cell counts are elevated and should be avoided.

Induction Therapy

A.M. was started on allopurinol for tumor lysis prophylaxis and hydroxyurea for 2 days to reduce his WBC count while waiting to obtain bone marrow biopsy results, cardiac workup, and central line placement. Induction therapy was begun with 3 days of an anthracycline (e.g., daunorubicin, at least 60 mg/m^2; idarubicin, 10–12 mg/m^2; or mitoxantrone, 10–12 mg/m^2) and 7 days of cytarabine (100–200 mg/m^2 continuous IV infusion). This regimen, commonly known as "3 + 7" remains the standard for induction therapy in AML. With such regimens, CR is achieved in 70% to 80% of younger adults. No other intervention has been shown to be superior (8). Induction chemotherapy should be started only after the diagnostic workup has been completed, preferably within 5 days of diagnosis. Randomized studies comparing high-dose versus low-dose cytarabine have demonstrated higher toxicity with higher doses, but no improvement in remission rates or disease-free survival (9). Thus, higher doses of cytarabine are not recommended outside of clinical trials. Attempts to increase response rates by the use of additional cytotoxic agents (thioguanine, etoposide, fludarabine, topotecan) or modulators of multidrug resistance (MDR) in general have failed (9), and variable results have been obtained when attempting to sensitize leukemic cells with hematopoietic growth factors.

Consolidation Therapy

Various consolidation strategies have been evaluated including intensive conventional chemotherapy, and high-dose therapy followed by autologous or allogeneic HSCT. Patients with CBF AMLs (expressing the cytogenetic abnormalities t(8;21), inv(16), or t(16;16)) have a relatively good prognosis when consolidated with high-dose cytarabine without HSCT in first remission. A landmark study performed by Cancer and Leukemia Group B (CALGB) showed that four cycles of high-dose cytarabine (3 g/m^2 per q12h on days 1, 3, and 5) are superior to four courses of intermediate-dose (400 mg/m^2 continuous IV on days 1–5) or standard-dose (100 mg/m^2 continuous IV on days 1–5) cytarabine. The beneficial effect of cytarabine dose intensification was restricted to patients with good-risk AML and, to a lesser extent, to patients with CN-AML. The outcome of patients with other cytogenetic abnormalities was not affected by cytarabine dose (10).

Allogeneic HSCT as a postremission strategy is associated with the lowest rates of relapse. This benefit is attributable to both the high-dose therapy of standard conditioning regimens and potent graft versus leukemia (GVL) effect. However, benefits of allogeneic HSCT have been limited by the high treatment-related mortality (TRM). Single arm prospective trials have not shown a definitive survival advantage for allogeneic HSCT in patients with AML in first CR (CR1). A meta-analysis of clinical trials that prospectively assigned patients to allogeneic HSCT versus alternative consolidation therapies for AML in CR1 on an intent-to-treat donor versus no-donor basis showed that allogeneic HSCT offers significant OS benefit for patients with intermediate- and high-risk AML (11). For individual patients, disease risk as assessed by the cytogenetic and molecular profile of the leukemia and the risks associated with the transplant itself including comorbidities and other transplant-related risk indices must be weighed. In patients with favorable risk AML (Table 29.2) consolidation therapy with repetitive cycles of HiDAC (3 g/m^2 per q12h on days 1, 3, and 5) is considered a reasonable choice for younger adults especially those with CBF AML and for AML with mutated

NPM1 and wild-type *FLT3* or with mutated *CEBPA*. For *CBF* AML, retrospective studies by CALGB suggest that three or more cycles of high-dose cytarabine (cumulative dose: 54–72 g/m^2) are superior to one cycle (18 g/m^2). No advantage has been shown for autologous or allogeneic HSCT or CBF AML in CR1. Nonetheless, there are subsets of patients with CBF AML who do not fare well (e.g., t(8;21) with high WBCs, CBF AML with *KIT* mutations, or molecular disease persistence); allogeneic HSCT may be considered in these patients, especially for those with a low transplant risk.

A.M. achieved a CR with induction chemotherapy consisting of idarubicin, 12 mg/m^2, and 7 days of cytarabine (100 mg/m^2 continuous IV). He had a complicated course with prolonged cytopenias requiring frequent transfusion. He developed transfusion related acute lung injury (TRALI) and acute coronary syndrome that were medically managed. Subsequently, a bone marrow aspiration and biopsy showed that he was in cytogenetic and morphological remission. A cardiac evaluation was repeated to ensure his EF was still normal and his cardiac status was optimized. Based on his favorable risk AML, induction was followed by four courses of consolidation with HiDAC (high-dose cytarabine at dose 3 g/m^2 q12h on days 1, 3, and 5). He has remained disease free for 3 years. Figure 29.2 represents an algorithm for the management of patients who are younger than age 60 with AML.

AML in Younger Adults (18 to 60 Years) With Unfavorable Risk Factors

T.R., a 57-year-old businessman with a history of hypercholesterolemia and hypertension was brought to the hospital with an acute febrile illness and lethargy. On examination he had mild hepatosplenomegaly with no lymphadenopathy. Oral examination was significant for gingival hyperplasia and gum bleeding. Labs demonstrated a WBC of 60,000/µL with more that 50% blasts, a hemoglobin of 9 g/dL, and a platelet count of 44,000/µL. A bone marrow biopsy confirmed AML. The cytogenetics was as follows: 46XY,-7, +8, 21q-, and 11q- in all 20 of the analyzed cells.

Evidence-Based Case Discussion

Induction Therapy

T.R.'s AML displayed complex cytogenetics defined as greater than three cytogenetic abnormalities in the absence of *CBF* mutations, and he falls into the high-risk category with a poor prognosis. In choosing an induction strategy, several issues need to be considered including comorbid illnesses, performance status, ability to tolerate induction therapy, and existence of antecedent hematological disease. The standard induction regimen has continued to be 3 days of anthracycline with 7 days of infusional cytarabine commonly referred to as "3 + 7" (Figure 29.2).

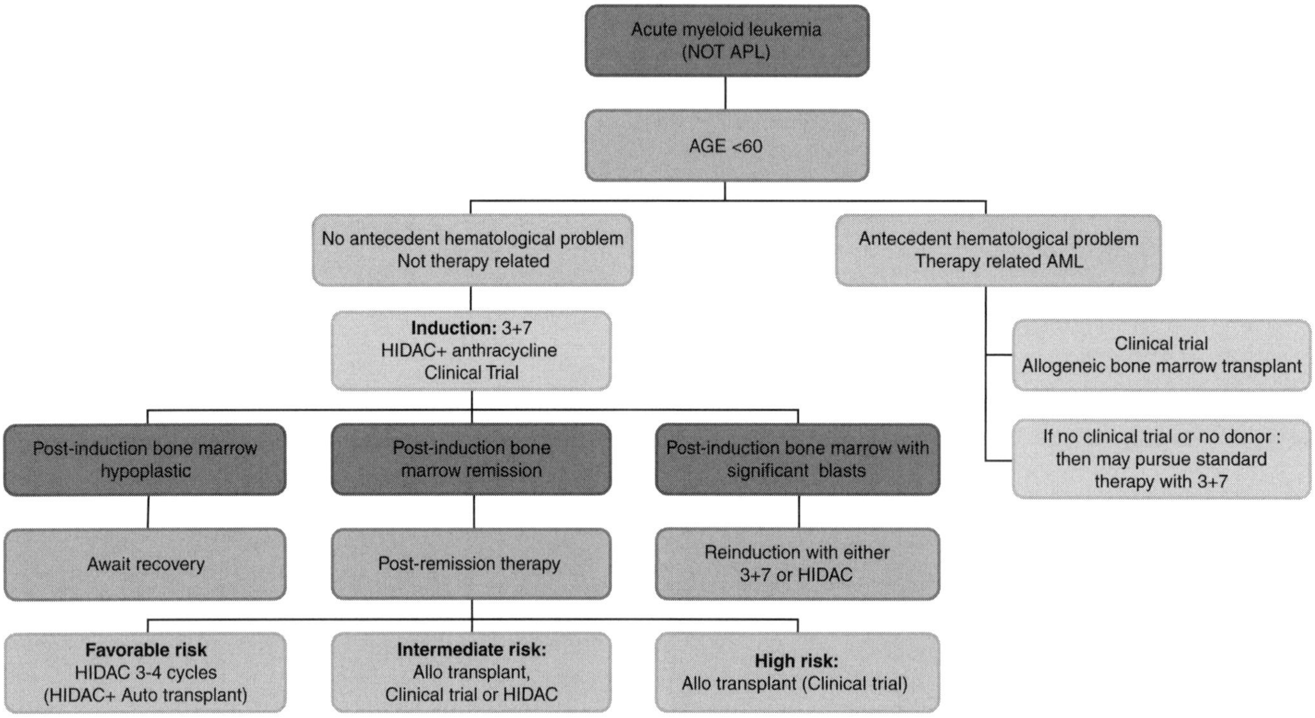

Figure 29.2

Algorithm for management of AML in patients younger than 60.

Moreover, there does not seem to be a clear benefit of adding additional chemotherapy agents such as etoposide to this regimen. Though a clear benefit of high-dose cytarabine in this high-risk population has not been established, multiple guidelines list HiDAC induction as an option. Patients who fall into the WHO adverse risk category typically have poor outcome with standard induction and consolidation. Hence a clinical trial is also always appropriate in this setting. In the case of antecedent hematological disease or treatment-related AML, there is accumulating evidence that induction therapy with an allogeneic HSCT is an attractive option for poor-risk patients with a donor. For those with no donor, either a clinical trial may be offered or standard chemotherapy regimens may be given.

At the end of induction therapy, risk stratification is once again performed by getting a bone marrow biopsy. Unlike APL where bone marrow biopsy assessment is not recommended until count recovery, it is reasonable to perform a bone marrow assessment 7 to 14 days after induction is completed. At this juncture if the bone marrow is hypoplastic, it is recommended that bone marrow be reassessed at count recovery. If the bone marrow examination shows significant reduction in blasts, consolidation can be pursued or delayed until count recovery has occurred. If there is significant residual disease, reinduction would be a reasonable course of action.

The most challenging patients are those with refractory disease. Several studies have shown that lack of early blast clearance or no response to the first induction cycle are major predictors of poor outcome, and conventional chemotherapy offers almost no chance of cure for these patients. In these patients, the only chance of cure is allogeneic HSCT with a dismal success rate of about 10%. Clinical trials should be considered for all patients with primary refractory disease. In patients with relapsed disease, that is, patients who achieved a CR with initial induction therapy, the rate of response will depend on duration of CR. Patients with a relapse of more than 12 months in CR have about a 50% chance of responding to cytarabine containing induction regimens. This should be followed with allogeneic HSCT. Patients with shorter duration of CR will not fare as well and are best treated in clinical trials.

Consolidation Therapy

Initial risk stratification can be useful in guiding consolidation therapy (Figure 29.2). For patients with intermediate- or poor-risk cytogenetics, a beneficial effect of allogeneic HSCT as consolidation therapy has been shown in CR1. This includes patients with unfavorable cytogenetics as well as CN-AML and unfavorable molecular markers, that is, those who lack the favorable genotypes of mutated *NPM1* without *FLT3*-ITD mutated *CEBPA*. In particular, allogeneic HSCT should be considered in patients whose leukemic cells have *FLT3*-ITD (12). An allogeneic HSCT from a matched related donor is currently considered the treatment of choice for patients with unfavorable cytogenetics in CR1. The outcome after allogeneic HSCT from fully matched and unrelated donor appears to be similar when compared to allogeneic HSCT from matched related donors. The Center for International Blood and Marrow Transplant Research (CIBMTR) recently reported a long-term survival probability of 30% for AML patients with adverse cytogenetics transplanted in CR1 from matched unrelated donors.

In general, there is no indication for intrathecal prophylaxis in AML patients without CNS symptoms although it may be considered in special situations (eg, hyperleukocytosis). In patients with CNS involvement, intrathecal chemotherapy with liposomal cytarabine or methotrexate should be administered. Intrathecal methotrexate is administered twice a week until two consecutive negative CSF cytologies are obtained and then weekly for 4 to 6 weeks. Liposomal cytarabine is typically administered every 2 weeks. Longer duration of intrathecal treatment (particularly more than 6 months) can cause CNS complications with no benefit and is discouraged. For prevention of arachnoiditis, oral dexamethasone (4-mg TID) may be considered on the days of intrathecal treatment. In patients with a CNS recurrence, craniospinal irradiation has also been shown to be effective; however, its impact on long-term outcome is unknown.

T.R. had seven siblings and a younger brother was an HLA identical match. After 3 + 7 standard induction, he attained a CR. Within 1 month, he proceeded to allogeneic stem cell transplant. Unfortunately, he had a prolonged period of neutropenia during which he developed a perirectal abscess and he succumbed to gram negative sepsis despite antibiotic therapy.

AML in the Older Adult (Age Over 60)

H.T., a 72-year-old man with excellent performance status and hypertension, presented to the emergency room with fatigue. His physical examination revealed pallor and petechiae on his lower extremities. He had no hepatosplenomegaly, no lymphadenopathy, and no other evidence of bleeding. Routine labs showed a WBC count of 500/µL, a hemoglobin of 6 g/dL, and a platelet count of 9,000/µL. Consultation with his primary physician revealed that his blood counts had been normal 2 months earlier. A peripheral smear showed normal red cell morphology, rare platelets, decreased WBC count, and a few circulating blasts with high nuclear:cytoplasmic ratio and several nucleoli. No Auer rods were observed in the blasts. The patient was admitted to the hospital and a platelet transfusion was begun followed by packed red cells. A bone marrow aspirate and biopsy was consistent with acute leukemia with 60% cellularity. The blasts constituted 50% of the bone marrow, and flow cytometry showed that they were positive for CD34, CD117, CD13, and CD33 consistent with myeloid blasts. Marrow cytogenetics was normal. *FLT*- ITD was negative and *NPM* mutation was positive. Cardiac evaluation showed a normal ejection fraction.

Evidence-Based Case Discussion

Induction Therapy

Patients older than 60 years of age with AML form a distinct subgroup, and "AML in the older adult" is an active area of research. There is wide variation in the way these patients are treated. This is especially so in adults older than 70 years who tend to have increased comorbidities and less tolerance to therapy. These older patients have a worse prognosis that is thought to be due to biologic differences including an increased frequency of secondary AML that is more resistant to therapy, adverse cytogenetic features, and overexpression of multidrug-resistant phenotypes. The decision to treat with intensive induction regimens versus less intensive treatments or supportive care alone needs to be individualized. Advanced age alone should not prohibit induction therapy. Recent studies have shown that older patients with good performance status can tolerate induction therapy reasonably well, and treatment with higher doses of daunorubicin at 90 mg/m^2 had a better outcome than a reduced dose of anthracycline at 45 mg/m^2 (13). On the other hand, investigators at MD Anderson Cancer Center recently published data showing that the majority of patients > 70 years at their institution did not benefit from intensive chemotherapy (14). A multivariate analysis of more than 900 elderly AML patients established that karyotype, age, *NPM1* mutation status, WBC count, LDH, and CD34 expression were independent predictors of prognosis. Patients were scored based on these variables and grouped into four prognostic risk groups: (a) favorable, (b) good intermediate risk, (c) adverse intermediate risk, and (d) high risk, and the corresponding 3-year OS rates were 39.5%, 30%, 10.6%, and 3.3% (15). Hence, induction regimens must be chosen keeping the patient's performance status and comorbidities in mind as well as the overall prognosis. In summary, the decision to give standard induction regimen has to be individualized. In fit patients with a favorable risk profile there is no benefit to reducing the dose of daunorubicin. Given his good performance status and relative lack of comorbidities, T.R. elected treatment with a standard induction regimen containing daunorubicin and cytarabine.

For patients who may not tolerate standard induction, therapy with a hypomethylating agent such as azacytidine is also an option and has been shown to prolong survival in a phase III study when compared to supportive care alone (16). Other agents such as clofarabine have also been used in this group with modest results.

Consolidation Therapy

Postremission therapy in older adults is also a topic of debate. The tolerability of high-dose cytarabine is poor, and core binding factor mutations, which traditionally are thought to have higher response rates with HIDAC, are less common in older adults. Postremission therapy with agents such as gemtuzumab has not been shown to be

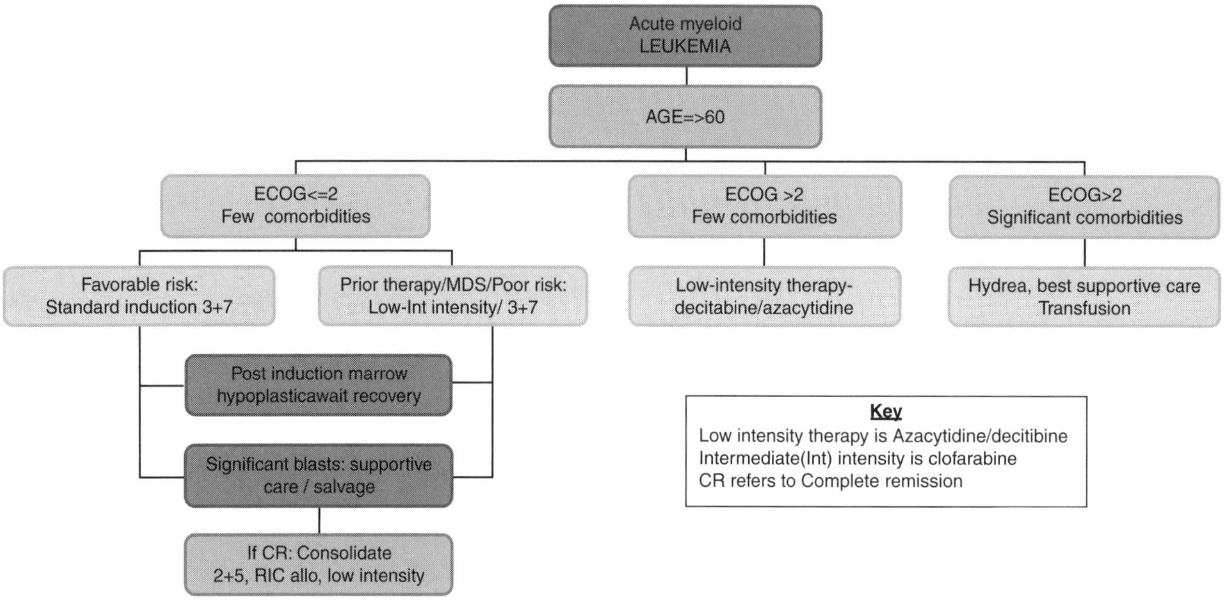

Figure 29.3

Algorithm for management of AML in older individuals (>age 60).

effective in a randomized phase III trial (17). Some studies have examined allogeneic HSCT with reduced intensity conditioning with varying response (18). These data point to the heterogeneity of the disease and the patient population and highlight again that age alone should not preclude consideration of HSCT. There is a paucity of randomized clinical trials addressing the question of HSCT in the older adult. Figure 29.3 demonstrates an algorithm for the treatment of older patients (> 60 years) with AML.

T.R. went into remission after receiving standard 3+7 induction with idarubicin and cytarabine therapy. Other options included low-intensity therapy with agents such as azacytidine. However, given his good performance status and his personal preference, he was induced with standard induction therapy that he tolerated well. For consolidation therapy he was given the option of 2+5 or reduced intensity conditioning and allogeneic transplant. Molecular studies revealed the leukemia to be *NPM1* positive and *FLT3*- ITD negative, which placed him in a relatively favorable risk group and he was not referred for transplant. He received two cycles of consolidation therapy with 2+5 (idarubicin at 12 mg/m^2 × 2 days and cytarabine 100 mg/m^2 × 5 days). Both cycles were complicated by neutropenic fever and requirement for multiple transfusions of blood products. After the second cycle, the patient declined further chemotherapy. He relapsed 6 months after completing therapy. At that point his performance status had declined considerably and he opted for supportive care alone with transfusion support. He succumbed to his disease 10 months after initial diagnosis.

REFERENCES

1. Lowenberg B, Downing JR, Burnett A. Acute Myeloid Leukemia. *N Eng J Med.* 1999;14:1051–1062.
2. Vardiman JW, Thiele J, Arber DA, et al. The 2008 revision of the WHO Classification of Myeloid Neoplasms and Acute Leukemia: rationale and important changes. *Blood.* 2009;114:937–951.
3. Dohner H, Estey EH, Amadori S, et al. Diagnosis and management of acute myeloid leukemia in adults: recommendations from an international expert panel, on behalf of the European LeukemiaNet. *Blood.* 2010;115:453–474.
4. Mrozek K. Cytogenetic, molecular genetic, and clinical characteristics of acute myeloid leukemia with a complex karyotype. *Semin Oncol.* 2008;358:365–377.
5. Cheson BD, Bennett JM, Kopecky KJ, et al. Revised recommendations of the International Working Group for diagnosis, standardization of response criteria, treatment outcomes, and reporting standards for therapeutic trials in acute myeloid leukemia. *J Clin Oncol.* 2003;21:4642–4649.
6. Tallman MS, Altman JK. How I treat acute promyelocytic leukemia. *Blood.* 2009;114:5126–5135.
7. Ades L, Guerci A, Raffoux E, et al. Very long-term outcome of acute promyelocytic leukemia after treatment with all-*trans* retinoic acid and chemotherapy: the European APL Group experience. *Blood.* 2010;115:1690–1696.
8. Sanz MA, Grimwade M, Tallman MS, et al. Management of acute promyelocytic leukemia: recommendations from an expert panel on behalf of the European LeukemiaNet. *Blood.* 2009;113:1875–1891.
9. Estey E, Dohner H. Acute myeloid leukaemia. *Lancet.* 2006;368: 1894–1907.
10. Bloomfield CD, Lawrence D, Byrd JC, et al. Frequency of prolonged remission duration after high-dose cytarabine intensification in acute myeloid leukemia varies by cytogenetic subtype. *Cancer Res.* 1998;58:4173–4179.
11. Meijer E, Cornelissen JJ. Allogeneic stem cell transplantation in acute myeloid leukemia in first or subsequent remission: weighing prognostic markers predicting relapse and risk factors for non-relapse mortality. *Semin Oncol.* 2008;35:449–457.
12. DeZern AE, Sung A, Kim S et al. Patients with FLT3/ITD AML may benefit from allogeneic transplant in first remission: outcomes from a consecutive series of patients at a single institution. *Oral and Poster Abstracts: ASH Conference* Dec 2010 Abstract No 2172:
13. Löwenberg B, Ossenkoppele G, van Putten W, et al. High-dose daunorubicin in older patients with acute myeloid leukemia. *N Engl J Med.* 2009;361:1235–1248.
14. Kantarjian H, Ravandi F, O'Brien S, et al. Intensive chemotherapy does not benefit most older patients (age 70 years or older) with acute myeloid leukemia. *Blood.* 2010;116:4422 –4429.
15. Röllig C, Thiede C,Gramatzki M, et al. A novel prognostic model in elderly patients with acute myeloid leukemia: results of 909 patients entered into the prospective AML96 trial. *Blood.* 2010;116:971–978.
16. Fenaux P, Mufti GJ, Hellstrom-Lindberg E, et al. Azacitidine prolongs overall survival compared with conventional care regimens in elderly patients with low bone marrow blast count acute myeloid leukemia. *J Clin Oncol.* 2010;28:562–569.
17. Löwenberg B, Beck J, Graux C, et al. Gemtuzumab ozogamicin as postremission treatment in AML at 60 years of age or more: results of a multicenter phase 3 study. *Blood.* 2010;115: 2586–2591.
18. McClune BL,Weisdorf DJ, Pedersen TL et al. Effect of age on outcome of reduced-intensity hematopoietic cell transplantation for older patients with acute myeloid leukemia in first complete remission or with myelodysplastic syndrome. *J Clin Oncol.* 2010;26:1878–1887.

30

Chronic Myeloid Leukemia

RAMI KHORIATY AND MOSHE TALPAZ

EPIDEMIOLOGY, RISK FACTORS, NATURAL HISTORY, AND PATHOLOGY

Chronic myeloid leukemia (CML) accounts for about 15% of all adult leukemias. The annual incidence rate of CML is about 1.5/100,000, and the lifetime risk of developing CML is 0.16%. In the United States, an estimated 4870 new cases of CML were diagnosed in 2010, and around 440 deaths occurred from the disease. CML can occur at any age, but it is essentially a disease of adulthood, with a median age at diagnosis of 66 years.

Established CML risk factors include older age, high-dose radiation exposure or high-dose radiation therapy used to treat other cancers, and male sex (male to female preponderance is about 1.5:1). Despite the fact that high-dose radiation is a risk factor for CML, most patients with CML do not have a history of radiation exposure, and most patients exposed to radiation do not develop CML. There are no known genetic factors associated with susceptibility to developing CML. A positive family history of CML is not a risk factor for the disease. There is no clear social or geographic predisposition for CML.

Without treatment, CML progresses from a chronic phase (CP) to an advanced phase (AP) and then to a blast phase (BP). In about 25% of cases, patients progress directly from CP to BP. The pace of the CP is highly variable; some patients stay in CP for more than a decade, whereas others progress to AP or BP within months. The median durations of the CP and AP in untreated patients are 3 to 5 years and 3 to 9 months, respectively. Prior to the development of tyrosine kinase inhibitors (TKI), CML patients who did not undergo allogeneic stem cell transplantation (ASCT) had a median survival of about 5 to 7 years.

Patients with CML could be classified into low-, intermediate-, and high-risk groups according to the Sokal formulation that is based on age, spleen size, platelet count, and percentage of circulating blasts (1). Although the Sokal risk stratification scheme was conceived prior to the advent of TKIs, it continues to be useful to stratify patients treated with imatinib. The 5-year rate of complete cytogenetic response in patients in the low-, intermediate-, and high-risk Sokal groups treated with imatinib is 89%, 82%, and 69%, respectively ($P < .001$), and the 5-year rate of disease progression in those patients is 3%, 8%, and 17%, respectively ($P = .002$) (2).

CML is thought to develop when the progeny of a hematopoietic stem cell transformed by the breakpoint cluster region (BCR) and Abelson kinase *(ABL)* fusion gene develop a proliferative advantage over normal hematopoietic stem cells. The t(9;22) (q34;q11.2) results in the fusion of *ABL* located on chromosome 9q34 and BCR located on chromosome 22q11.2. The *BCR-ABL* fusion gene, located on the shortened chromosome 22 (called Philadelphia chromosome), encodes the *BCR-ABL* oncoprotein that constitutively activates tyrosine kinase activity and is sufficient to cause CML. This kinase regulates downstream targets including c-Myc, Akt, and Jun, all of which are important in cell proliferation and survival. In addition, the fusion gene results in decreased DNA binding activity of *ABL* and increased binding of *ABL* to actin microfilaments, which affects differentiation and results in increased proliferation and decreased apoptosis. The fact that the t(9,22) is found in cells of myeloid, B-lymphoid, erythroid, and megakaryocytic lineages confirms that CML is a hematopoietic stem cell disease.

Depending on the specific location of the breakpoint in the *BCR* gene, the resulting fusion oncogene can have varying lengths. In CML, the *BCR* gene is typically disrupted at the e13 or e14 loci, and the resulting hybrid transcripts are e13a2 and e14a2, respectively, both resulting in the p210 *BCR-ABL* oncoprotein. Less commonly, the breakpoint in the *BCR* gene occurs either more upstream near the e1 locus or downstream near the e19 locus, resulting in the e1a2 or e19a2 transcript variants with the corresponding oncoproteins p190 and p230, respectively. The p190 oncoprotein is more common in Philadelphia positive acute lymphoblastic leukemia. The p230 oncoprotein is very rare in CML, but can be found in atypical CML cases and in cases characterized as chronic neutrophilic leukemia. Other fusion proteins are less common.

STAGING

There are multiple staging systems for CML, the most commonly used ones are the World Health Organization (WHO) and the MD Anderson staging systems.

Chronic Myeloid Leukemia

Phases of CML	WHO Criteria	MD Anderson Criteria
Chronic phase	CML diagnosis without features of accelerated or blastic phase	
Accelerated phase	PB or BM blasts 10–19%, PB basophils ≥ 20%, platelets < 100 × 10^9/L unrelated to therapy, or platelets > 1000 × 109/L unresponsive to therapy, cytogenetic evidence of clonal evolution, increasing spleen size, and WBC count unresponsive to therapy	PB blasts ≥ 15%, PB blasts + promyelocytes ≥ 30%, PB basophils ≥ 20%, platelets ≤ 100 × 10^9/L unrelated to therapy, cytogenetic clonal evolution
Blastic phase	PB or BM blasts ≥ 20%, extramedullary blasts, large foci or clusters of blasts in BM	PB or BM blasts ≥ 30%, extramedullary disease

PB, peripheral blood; BM, bone marrow; WBC, white blood cell count.

CASE SUMMARIES

Diagnosis of Chronic Phase CML

S.L. is a 61-year-old man who presented with generalized fatigue. His physical examination demonstrated palpable splenomegaly (about 5 cm below the left costal margin), and his complete blood count (CBC) revealed leukocytosis with a white blood cell (WBC) count of 52,000 /µL. The WBC differential showed a left shift; 52% neutrophils, 20% band forms, 10% myelocytes, 6% metamyelocytes, 1% blasts, 6% lymphocytes, 2% basophils, 3% eosinophils. His hemoglobin was 15 g/dL, and his platelet count was 355,000/µL. A bone marrow biopsy was performed and showed a hypercellular marrow with an increased myeloid to erythroid ratio and no significant dysplasia. Maturation was preserved in the myeloid series, but there was a left shift; reticulin stain was negative for fibrosis; and cytogenetics showed t(9;22) (q34;q11.2) in all 20 cells examined. Peripheral blood polymerase chain reaction (PCR) for *BCR-ABL* revealed the p210 BCR-ABL transcript.

Evidence-Based Case Discussion

S.L. has leukocytosis with a left shift, splenomegaly, t(9;22) (q34;q11.2) on metaphase cytogenetics, and p210 *BCR-ABL* transcript.

All myeloproliferative disorders (MPD) share some common features; however, the patient presented above fits the diagnostic criteria for CML. CML should be suspected in patients with persistent leukocytosis, especially in the presence of basophilia, after infectious etiologies have been ruled out. The absence of polycythemia, thrombocytosis, marrow reticulin fibrosis, and dysplasic features in the bone marrow rule out the following diagnoses in respective order: polycythemia vera, essential thrombocytosis, myelofibrosis, and myeloproliferative disease/myelodysplastic syndrome–overlap disorders. Nevertheless, there is significant clinical and laboratory test overlap among these syndromes (e.g., about 30% of patients with CML have thromobocytosis). Consequently, a specific diagnosis should be pursued in patients with similar blood count profiles through a bone marrow aspirate and biopsy, as well as cytogenetics and molecular testing.

Whenever CML is suspected, it is critical to obtain both a bone marrow biopsy with metaphase karyotyping and peripheral blood PCR for *BCR-ABL* to confirm or refute the diagnosis. The bone marrow biopsy is necessary, not only for diagnostic purposes, but also for staging of the disease as well as to serve as a baseline for follow-up monitoring. Moreover, metaphase karyotyping on the bone marrow aspirate may detect the unusual *BCR-ABL* translocations as well as additional cytogenetic abnormalities, which would otherwise not be detected by PCR. Approximately 90% to 95% of patients with CML have t(9;22) (q34;q11.2) by metaphase cytogenetics, which means that the absence of the Philadelphia chromosome does not completely rule out CML in the right clinical context. Peripheral blood PCR for *BCR-ABL* detects the p210 and p190 fusion transcripts, but not the p230 transcript. The absence of the Philadelphia chromosome and negative PCR testing for *BCR-ABL* should trigger an evaluation for diseases other than CML.

In the event that bone marrow metaphase cytogenetics analysis cannot be performed (secondary to inability to collect marrow or technical difficulties with the test), fluorescent in-situ hybridization (FISH) should be performed on the peripheral blood using a probe for *BCR* and another one for *ABL*. FISH should also be performed in the case of cytogenetically "silent" *BCR-ABL*, in order to rule out a falsely positive PCR for *BCR-ABL*, and thus to confirm or refute the diagnosis of CML. It is important to note that both PCR for *BCR-ABL* and FISH are equivalent if done on the bone marrow aspirate or peripheral blood. There is no role for screening for *BCR-ABL* mutations at baseline.

In our patient, metaphase karyotyping performed on the bone marrow aspirate showed t(9;22) (q34;q11.2), and peripheral blood PCR for *BCR-ABL* revealed the p210 *BCR-ABL* transcript—one of the typical transcript variants in CML—thus establishing the diagnosis of CML. On the basis of both the WHO and MD Anderson criteria, the stage of the patient's CML is chronic phase (CML-CP).

Treatment of Chronic Phase CML

T.S. is a 52-year-old man who presented with leukocytosis and splenomegaly and was diagnosed with CML-CP. He is otherwise healthy with no comorbidities, and has a good performance status.

Evidence-Based Case Discussion

In the past, the recommended first-line treatment strategy for a patient with newly diagnosed CML-CP was either ASCT if the patient was relatively young and had an appropriate stem cell donor, or interferon alpha with or without cytarabine if the patient was not a candidate for ASCT.

The treatment strategy for CP CML has completely changed since the advent of TKIs, which are now considered the preferred first-line treatment in CML-CP (see Figure 30.1). TKIs block the adenosine triphosphate (ATP) binding site of *BCR-ABL*, suppressing downstream signaling. Imatinib, dasatinib, and nilotinib are all TKIs approved by the Food and Drug Administration (FDA) for treatment of CML-CP. The response definitions are summarized in Table 30.1 (3).

First-Line Imatinib

After the promising results with imatinib in a phase II trial in patients with CML-CP who were resistant/refractory/intolerant to interferon alpha (96% complete hematologic response [CHR], 67% major cytogenetic response [McyR], 57% complete cytogentic response [CcyR]), the randomized phase III IRIS trial was conducted comparing first-line imatinib 400-mg daily with the standard of care then, interferon alfa plus low-dose cytarabine, in patients with CML-CP. Patients receiving imatinib had impressive outcomes with rates of CHR, McyR, and CCyR of 96%, 85%, and 69%, respectively at 12 months, and 98%, 92%, and 87%, respectively at 60 months (2). The rate of major molecular response (MMR) increased from 24% at 6 months to 39% at 12 months, and to a best of 86% with 8 years of follow-up. The response to imatinib was fairly durable and the majority of patients who had an event or who progressed to AP CML did so in the first 2 years of therapy. The rates of transformation to AP or BP were 1.5% at year 1, 2.8% at year 2, 1.8% at year 3, 0.9% at year 4, 0.5% at year 5, 0% at year 6, 0% at year 7, and 0.4% at year 8 (4,5). This translates to a remarkable 92% rate of freedom from progression to AP or BP after 8 years of imatinib. After 8-years of follow-up on the IRIS trial, patients who were randomized to imatinib had an estimated event-free survival (EFS) and overall survival (OS) of 81% and 86%, respectively. If only CML-related deaths and deaths prior to stem cell transplant were considered, the 8-year OS would be 93% (5). As discussed in detail below, CCyR and MMR are important milestones in patients with CML-CP. Among patients who achieved CCyR, only 3% progressed to AP or BP, the vast majority of whom progressed within 2 years of reaching CCyR. None of the 39% of patients who reached MMR at 12 months progressed to AP or BP. Despite the impressive results of the IRIS trial, an OS advantage of imatinib over interferon could not be established in this trial due to the high rate of crossover from the interferon alfa arm to the imatinib arm (about 90%). Nevertheless, a comparison between patients treated with imatinib and historical patients treated with interferon alfa +/− ara-c showed the anticipated survival advantage with imatinib (6,7).

It is important to note that in the IRIS trial, only patients who continued to receive imatinib were evaluated, and patients who stopped imatinib were censored. A single-center study examined a cohort of consecutively treated patients with CML-CP receiving first-line imatinib 400 mg/day, and aimed to estimate the outcomes by intention-to-treat analysis. In this study, CHR, MCyR, CcyR, and MMR were 97.1%, 71.1%, 57.4%, and 12.3% at 12 months and 98.5%, 85.1%, 82.7%, and 50.1% at 60 months, respectively. These numbers are slightly inferior (although fairly comparable) to those in the IRIS trial. Conversely, the 5-year EFS by intention-to-treat analysis was 62.7%, which is considerably lower than the 5-year EFS of 83% in the IRIS trial. However, the 5-year EFS was 81% in this trial when calculated using the IRIS trial definition. The 5-year progression-free survival (PFS) and OS by intention-to-treat analysis were 82.7% and 83.2%, respectively (8).

Imatinib is generally well tolerated; common side effects are neutropenia, thrombocytopenia, gastrointestinal symptoms, rash, edema, musculoskeletal symptoms, hypophosphatemia, and possibly congestive heart failure (CHF) (the rate of CHF is 1.7% in patients receiving imatinib, which is comparable to the rate of CHF in the general population).

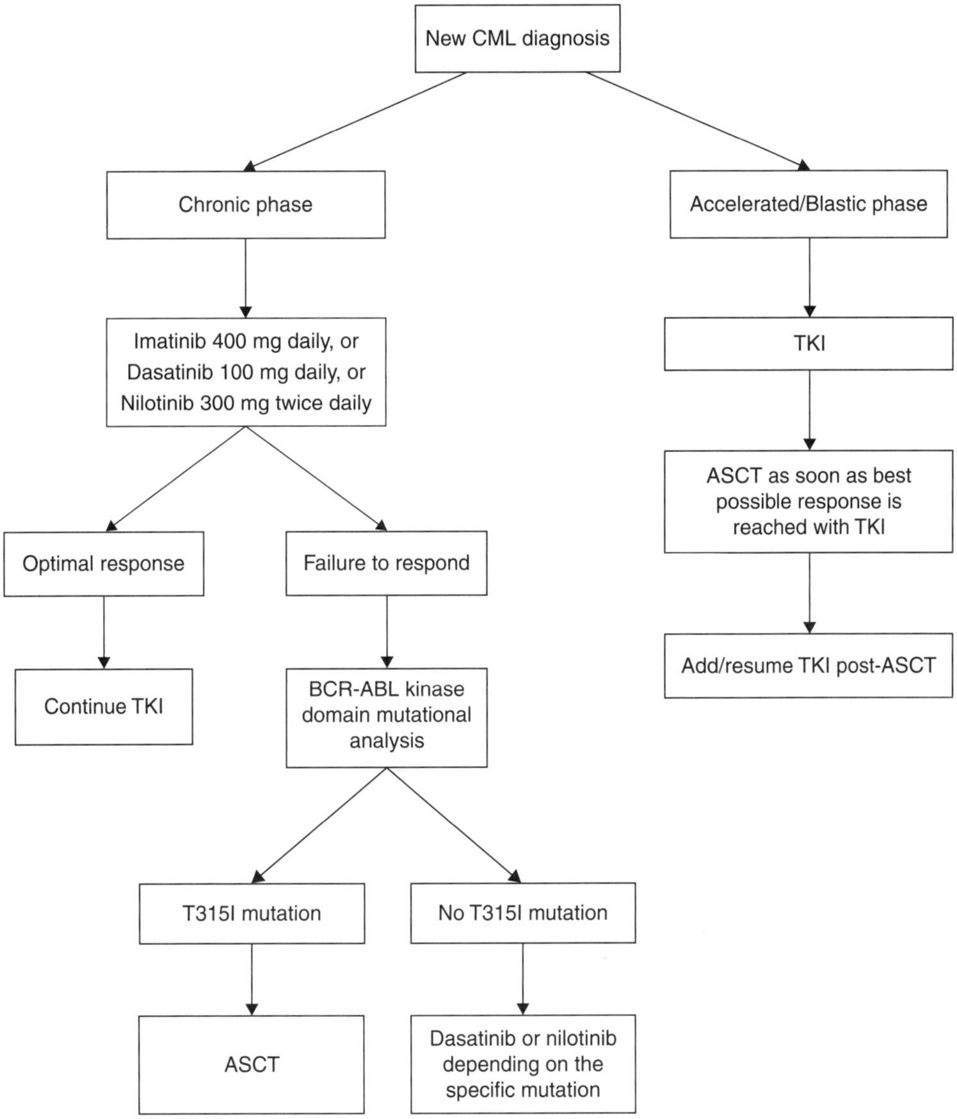

Figure 30.1

Treatment algorithm for chronic myeloid leukemia.

Table 30.1 Response Definition in CML

Hematologic Response	
Complete hematologic response (CHR)	Platelets < 450 × 10^9/L, WBC < 10 x10^9/L, basophils < 5%, no circulating immature granulocytes, no palpable spleen
Cytogenetic Response	
Major cytogenetic response (MCyR)	Ph positive metaphases: 0%
Complete cytogentic response (CCyR)	Ph positive metaphases: 1–35%
Partial cytogenetic response (PCyR)	
Minor cytogenetic response (mCyR)	Ph positive metaphases: 36–65%
Minimal cytogenetic response (minCyR)	Ph positive metaphases: 66–95%
No cytogenetic response	Ph positive metaphases > 95%
Molecular Response	
Complete molecular response (CMR)	No detectable *BCR-ABL* transcripts twice with PCR of sensitivity > 10^{-4}
Major molecular response (MMR)	Ratio of *BCR-ABL* / *ABL* (or other housekeeping genes) transcripts ≤0.1% on the international scale

Optimal Dose of Imatinib

After the IRIS trial established imatinib as the preferred first-line treatment in patients with CML-CP, the next important step was to determine the optimal initial dose of imatinib. Patients on the IRIS trial who achieved higher imatinib trough levels had improved responses and EFS. In addition, a phase II trial suggested that high-dose imatinib (800-mg daily) in first-line CML-CP results in earlier MMR as well as increased depth of molecular response. This observation triggered two randomized trials to address the optimal dose of imatinib in the first-line setting, and an additional trial to investigate the strategy of "induction therapy" with high-dose imatinib followed by standard-dose imatinib. In the phase III TOPS (Tyrosine Kinase Inhibitor Optimization and Selectivity) study, patients with CML-CP were randomized, according to their Sokal risk groups, to first-line standard-dose (400 mg/day) or high-dose (800 mg/day) imatinib (9). This trial showed a faster rate of MMR and CCyR in patients receiving the higher dose; however, the 12-month rate of MMR, which was the primary end point of the study (46.4% and 40.1% respectively, *P* = .2035), as well as the 12-month rate of CCyR (69.9% and 65,6% respectively, *P* = .347), were similar in both groups. There was no difference in MMR and CCyR at 24 months between the groups. Nevertheless, there was a correlation between the average dose-intensity received and the rate of MMR and CCyR at 12 months. Patients who actually received 600 to 800 mg/day of imatinib had higher 12-month rates of MMR and CCyR compared to patients who received <600 mg/day of imatinib (MMR 62.4% and 34.1%, respectively, *P* <.0001; CCyR 89.6% and 70.3%, respectively, *P* < .0001). There was no significant difference in the 24-month estimated EFS (95% and 95%, *P* = .71), PFS (98% and 97%, *P* = .64), or OS (98% and 97%, *P* =.70) between patients randomized to high-dose or standard-dose imatinib, respectively. Patients who received high-dose imatinib had an increased risk of grade 3/4 hematologic toxicities as well as slightly increased risk of grade 3/4 rash, diarrhea, and fatigue. The rate of discontinuation secondary to side effects was higher in patients on the 800 mg/day arm (10.7% vs. 4.5%). The second study, a randomized phase II trial from the European LeukemiaNet (ELN) group, compared high-dose (800 mg/day) with standard-dose (400 mg/day) imatinib in previously untreated (or treated with hydroxyurea only) patients with high Sokal risk CML-CP (10). There was no significant difference in CCyR or MMR between the two groups at any time point (3 months, 6 months, and 12 months) by intention to treat analysis; CCyR at 12 months, the primary end point of the trial, was 58% in patients receiving 400 mg of imatinib versus 64% in patients receiving 800 mg of imatinib (*P* = .435). It is important to note, however, that only a minority (28%) of patients randomized to receive high-dose imatinib received the full 800-mg daily dose. CCyR for these patients (96%) was higher than CCyR for patients who received less than 400 mg of imatinib (20%). There was no significant difference in 36-month OS (91% and 84%, *P* = .79), PFS (88% and 86%, *P* = .63), failure-free survival defined as time to failure or death (72% and 74%, *P* = .66), or EFS (62% and 66%, *P* = .89) between patients randomized to high-dose and standard-dose imatinib, respectively. The third study, the ISTAHIT phase III trial randomized CML-CP patients who were previously treated (but not with TKIs) to "induction" with imatinib 800 mg or 400 mg/day for 6 months, followed by "maintenance" with imatinib 400-mg daily in all patients (11). Patients who received induction with high-dose imatinib (800 mg) had higher MCyR and CCyR at 3 months, and higher MCyR, CCyR, and MMR at 6 months; however, the benefit of high-dose imatinib induction therapy did not persist during the maintenance phase of the study. Patients in both groups had similar 12-month rates of MCyR, which was the primary end point of the study (57% and 59%, respectively), and comparable 12-month rates of CCyR (48% and 37%, respectively, *P* = .29) and MMR (32% versus 25%, not statistically significant). At the time of the first planned interim analysis of this study, there was no difference in PFS or EFS between the groups. Patients randomized to "induction therapy" with high-dose imatinib had a higher rate of grade 3/4 hematologic toxicity, and were more likely to have reductions in the initial induction dose (54.4% vs. 34.9%). In patients who did not require drug interruption/dose reduction in the "induction" period, the cumulative rate of CCyR was higher in patients randomized to the higher-induction dose of imatinib (61% and 35.7% respectively, *P* = .014). In addition, patients who were not able to maintain the 800-mg induction dose of imatinib had similar cumulative rate of CCyR to patients who maintained the 400-mg induction dose of imatinib (34.9% and 35.7%, respectively).

In summary, there seems to be no significant benefit of high-dose imatinib (either given continuously or using an induction strategy) in the first-line setting in patients with CML-CP. This unexpected result could be secondary to dose interruptions/reductions that occurred in a significant proportion of patients randomized to high-dose imatinib. Nevertheless, the recommended dose of imatinib in the first-line setting in patients with CML-CP is 400 mg a day.

Imatinib in Combination With Other Active CML Drugs

The SPIRIT trial aimed to investigate whether the addition of cytarabine or interferon alfa, two active drugs in CML, to imatinib improves OS. Patients with CML-CP who had not received prior therapy (aside from hydroxyurea or anagrelide) were randomized into four groups after having received 400 mg of imatinib for 14 days: (a) continuing standard-dose imatinib (400 mg), (b) increasing the imatinib dose to 600 mg (intermediate dose), (c) adding cytarabine (20 mg/m^2/day from day 15 to day 28 of each 28-day cycle) to standard-dose imatinib, or (d) adding pegylated interferon alfa (90 µg/week) to standard-dose imatinib (12). Planned interim analysis at 1 year showed that in comparison to standard-dose imatinib, MMR was improved only in the group of patients who received imatinib + interferon. The rates of MMR for patients who received imatinib + interferon versus 400 mg of imatinib were 39% and 20% at 6 months ($P < .001$), and 57% and 38% at 12 months ($P < .001$), respectively. However, about 45% of patients receiving interferon alpha discontinued it within 1 year. Grade 3/4 nonhematologic toxicities were 31% in the imatinib + interferon arm and 19% in the standard-dose imatinib arm. Grade 3/4 neutropenia or thrombocytopenia occurred more commonly in the imatinib + interferon arm (40% and 8%, respectively). Thus there may be a role for interferon in the treatment armamentarium of CML, but more studies are needed before firm conclusions could be made.

First-Line Second-Generation TKIs

After dasatinib and nilotinib were approved as second-line therapies for patients with imatinib resistance or intolerance, there was interest in moving these agents to the first-line setting with the hope of improving outcomes. Phase II studies testing dasatinib or nilotinib in the front-line setting for CML-CP showed promising results and led to randomized phase III trials comparing these agents to imatinib.

The ENESTnd (Evaluating Nilotinib Efficacy and Safety in Clinical Trials of Newly Diagnosed Ph+ CML Patients) phase III trial randomized newly diagnosed CML-CP patients to nilotinib 300-mg twice daily, nilotinib 400-mg twice daily, or imatinib 400-mg daily (13). MMR at 12 months, the primary endpoint of the study, was 44% in patients receiving nilotinib 300-mg twice daily, 43% in patients receiving nilotinib 400-mg twice daily, and 22% in patients receiving imatinib ($P < .0001$ for each nilotinib group compared to imatinib). The rates of MMR at 3 months, 6 months, and 9 months were also higher in patients receiving either dose of nilotinib compared to imatinib. Cytogenetic responses were superior for nilotinib both at 6 and 12 months further indicating faster responses with nilotinib. Perhaps the most important finding of the study is that progression to AP or BP occurred less commonly in patients receiving nilotinib 300-mg twice daily (0.7%, $P = .0095$ compared to imatinib), and in patients receiving nilotinib 400-mg twice daily (0.4%, $P = .0037$ compared to imatinib) compared to patients receiving imatinib (3.9%). If sustained, this finding would suggest that nilotinib is a better first treatment option than imatinib. Both drugs were fairly well tolerated, and no patient developed $QT_C > 500$ ms or a decrease in the left ventricular ejection fraction. Muscle spasm, nausea, diarrhea, vomiting, and fluid overload were more common in patients receiving imatinib, whereas rash, alopecia, headache, elevations in transaminases, bilirubin, and lipase were more common in patients receiving nilotinib. Grades 3/4 neutropenia and anemia were more common with imatinib, whereas grade 3/4 thrombocytopenia was more common with nilotinib.

DASISION (Dasatinib versus Imatinib Study in Treatment-Naïve CML Patients), a phase III clinical trial, randomized newly diagnosed CML-CP patients to dasatinib 100-mg daily or imatinib 400-mg daily (14). The rate of confirmed CCyR by 12 months, the primary endpoint of the study, was 77% in patients receiving dasatinib compared to 66% in patients receiving imatinib ($P = .007$). Cytogenetic responses were attained more rapidly with dasatinib. Molecular responses were also improved with dasatinib at 3, 6, 9, and 12 months (12 months MMR of 46% and 28%, respectively). Progression to AP or BP occurred in 1.9% of patients receiving dasatinib compared to 3.5% of patients receiving imatinib. Both drugs were well tolerated and the majority of the adverse events were grade 1/2 in both arms. The rates of grade 3/4 neutropenia were comparable in both arms, but grade 3/4 thrombocytopenia and anemia were more common in patients receiving dasatinib. Nausea, vomiting, myalgias, muscle inflammation, rash, fluid retention, superficial edema, and grade 3 or 4 hypophosphatemia were more common in patients receiving imatinib. Pleural effusion (grade 1 or 2) occurred exclusively in patients receiving dasatinib at a frequency of about 10%. Only three patients (1.2%) required thoracentesis, and the rest of the patients with pleural effusions were treated with dasatinib dose modifications or medically (steroids and/or diuretics). The rates of discontinuation secondary to drug-related side effects were similar in both arms. Pending more mature results from the ENESTnd and DASISION trials, imatinib at 400 mg/day, nilotinib 300-mg twice daily, and dasatinib 100-mg daily are all acceptable first-line treatment options in CML-CP.

The choice of initial therapy should take into account a series of issues. Nilotinib requires twice daily dosage, whereas imatinib and dasatinib are given once daily. Nilotinib is the only TKI that must be taken on an empty stomach; patients cannot eat 2 hours before or 1 hour after taking nilotinib (food significantly increases the absorption of nilotinib). Proton pump inhibitors cannot be used with nilotinib because an acidic milieu is required for adequate absorption. Nilotinib has greater risk for causing QTc prolongation, thus caution is required in prescribing other medications that might increase QTc in patients receiving nilotinib. Dasatinib should not be used in patients with a history of pleural or pericardial effusions. Dasatinib should also be avoided in patients with bleeding tendencies, and in patients receiving antiplatelet agents or anticoagulants, because it can cause bleeding due to platelet dysfunction. Nilotinib should be avoided in patients with a history of pancreatitis. All three agents are substrates for CYP3A4; therefore, CYP3A4 inhibitors (macrolides, azoles, grapefruit juice, etc.) should be avoided in patients taking any one of the TKIs (particularly nilotinib) because they result in increased serum concentration and accentuated side effects, the most worrisome of which is QTc prolongation. CYP3A4 inducers (e.g., dexamethasone, phenytoin, St. John's wort, etc.) result in lower area under the curve of the TKIs, thus higher doses are required to attain the desired benefits. Patients on a CYP3A4 substrate (e.g. simvastatin) may need a reduction in the dose of this medication if a TKI is started.

T.S. was started on imatinib 400-mg daily.

CML-CP Follow-Up and Response Evaluation

M.P. is a 59-year-old man who was diagnosed with CML-CP 4 months ago when he presented with asymptomatic leukocytosis (WBC 46,000/μL) with a left shift (49% neutrophils, 17% band forms, 11% myelocytes, 8% metamyelocytes, 2% blasts, 8% lymphocytes, 2% basophils, 3% eosinophils) and splenomegaly. His hemoglobin was 13 g/dL, and his platelet count was 200,000/μL. His bone marrow biopsy at diagnosis showed t(9,22) in all 20 cells examined. He was started on imatinib 400-mg daily and was getting a CBC every 2 weeks. His blood counts completely normalized 6 weeks after starting imatinib, as did his splenomegaly. A bone marrow aspirate and biopsy performed after 3 months of treatment showed no morphologic evidence of CML, and cytogenetic analysis demonstrated 8 out of 20 cells examined with the t(9;22).

Evidence-Based Case Discussion

M.P. has been receiving imatinib for 3 months for his newly diagnosed CML-CP. Despite the multiple disadvantages for metaphase cytogenetics (including the need for a bone marrow biopsy, the necessity of timely processing of the bone marrow sample, the use of different marrow culture protocols in various labs, and the low sensitivity of this test [in the order of 5–10%]), it remains the gold standard to document CCyR given that it has been validated in large TKI clinical trials. Additional advantages of metaphase cytogenetics include the ability to detect cytogenetic abnormalities other than the Philadelphia chromosome, as well as the ability to detect clonal evolution that occurs in 5% to 10% of patients. Unlike metaphase cytogenetics, FISH analysis and qRT-PCR are equivalent whether done on the bone marrow aspirate or peripheral blood. Modern FISH probes have improved sensitivity for detecting *BCR-ABL* transcripts as low as 0.3% to 0.6%, and also allow for detection of der(9) deletions. FISH has not been adequately validated in large trials; thus its use in monitoring CML is limited to circumstances where a bone marrow aspirate and biopsy cannot be performed, in technical difficulties that prevent performance of conventional cytogenetic analysis (as a supplement to metaphase karyotyping if qRT-PCR for *BCR-ABL* is not available), and in resolving discrepancies between cytogenetic and molecular results. The most sensitive test for monitoring response to a TKI in CML-CP is qRT-PCR; the sensitivity of this test is on the order of 10^{-5} to 10^{-6}. PCR for *BCR-ABL* has been standardized by a National Institutes of Health Consensus Group, which set the baseline *BCR-ABL* (defined by the IRIS trial) as 100%, and the 3-log reduction as 0.1% representing MMR (15).

The important response milestones are summarized in Table 30.2 (3). It is critical to adequately monitor patients receiving treatment for CML-CP (as summarized below) and to initiate therapeutic changes immediately in patients who fail to respond, in patients who lose their responses, and potentially (although this is still somewhat debatable) in patients who achieve suboptimal responses. When a therapeutic change is necessary, immediate implementation results in better outcomes. For example, after switching to dasatinib, CCyR was achieved in 72% of patients who lost MCyR to imatinib compared to 42% in patients who lost both MCyR and CHR to imatinib. The 24-month EFS was 89% after loss of MCyR only, compared to 29% after loss of both MCyR and CHR on imatinib (16).

Table 30.2 Response Milestones in CP-CML Warnings*

	Optimal Response	Suboptimal Response	Failure to Respond
CHR	CHR at 3 M	CHR at 3 M	No CHR at 3 M
CyR	At least mCyR at 3 M	No mCyR at 3 M	No CyR at 6 M
	At least PCyR at 6 M	No PCyR at 6M	No PCyR at 12M
	CCyR at 12 M	PCyR at 12 M	No CCyR at 18 M
MR	MMR at 18 M	Less than MMR at 18 M	
		Loss of MMR; mutations	Loss of CHR or CCyR; clonal chromosomal abnormality

*These include high-risk disease, clonal chromosomal abnormalities at diagnosis; less than MMR at 12 M; increase in PCR transcript levels, or clonal chromosomal abnormalities in Ph- cells at any time during treatment.

Proper monitoring of response to imatinib includes performing a CBC twice a month until CHR is documented and confirmed. Subsequently, a CBC should be obtained at least every 3 months or as required. Cytogenetic monitoring should be performed at diagnosis (as mentioned earlier), then at month 6, and then every 6 months until CCyR is attained and confirmed. The European Leukemia Net group recommends obtaining a bone marrow biopsy at 3 months after starting therapy; however, this is not absolutely necessary because the results of this bone marrow biopsy do not necessarily alter the treatment. Subsequently, cytogenetic monitoring should be performed every 12 months if regular molecular monitoring cannot be obtained, in the presence of unexplained cytopenia(s), if treatment failure (primary or secondary resistance) occurs, and in the case of presence of myelodysplastic features. Molecular monitoring (qRT-PCR) should be done every 3 months until MMR is obtained and confirmed, then done at least every 6 months. BCR-ABL mutational analysis should be performed in patients who fail to respond or achieve a suboptimal response, and always before changing to second-generation TKIs or other therapies (3). Monitoring of patients on the second-generation TKIs includes the same tests; however, earlier and more frequent testing may be warranted as responses occur typically earlier with the second-generation TKIs.

The most important and best validated response endpoint in CML is CCyR. Whether prompt achievement of CCyR is important has been the matter of some debate. The IRIS study showed that there is no correlation between the time to achieving CCyR and outcome, as long as CCyR is reached (17). However, this analysis has been criticized because patients who received less than 12 months of imatinib were excluded from the analysis. Although not statistically significant, the duration of cytogenetic response was superior for patients who achieved CCyR at earlier time points. A recent study from M.D. Anderson Cancer Center showed that the likelihood of reaching CCyR decreases over time, whereas the risk of having an event increases (18). In this study, if CCyR is not reached at 12 months, the chance of achieving CCyR is 42%, whereas the chance of having an event is 38%. This highlights the importance of achieving early CCyR, especially within 12 months of therapy.

Monitoring the molecular responses may provide additional risk stratification for patients receiving imatinib therapy. Rapid achievement of MMR seems to correlate with a more durable response (19). Patients who achieve MMR by 6 months have fewer events (defined as loss of MMR or acquisition of *BCR-ABL* mutation), than patients who achieve MMR between 6 and 12 months, and patients who achieve MMR between 12 and 18 months (0%, 12%, and 19%, respectively). In addition, the probability of complete molecular response (CMR) is higher in patients who achieve MMR earlier rather than later (93%, 69%, and 37% in patients who achieve MMR by 6 months, 6–12 months, and 12–18 months, respectively). However, it is possible that faster MMR reflects better disease biology, rather than being the cause of a more lasting response and thus a desired goal of therapy.

It is not completely clear why some patients respond to imatinib better than others. Imatinib pharmacokinetics has been evaluated as a possible explanation. Imatinib trough levels were measured at day 29 in patients on the IRIS trial. Patients who had the highest quartile of trough levels had higher CCyR and MMR than the remaining patients (20). In addition, a Japanese study showed that 300 mg/day of imatinib was equivalent, in therapeutic efficacy, to 400 mg/day in patients with small body size because the plasma trough concentration of imatinib in these patients was higher than the therapeutic concentration. Imatinib trough levels correlated with response suggesting that the dose of imatinib is irrelevant as long as adequate trough plasma concentration is achieved (21). A third study showed that imatinib trough levels measured at or beyond 12 months of therapy were significantly higher in the group of patients who achieved CCyR compared to the group who did not, and in the group of patients who reached MMR compared to the group who did not (22). Nevertheless, the clinical utility of imatinib trough levels has not been validated prospectively, and it is not clear that increasing the imatinib dose to achieve a "desired" higher target will improve patient outcomes.

M.P. achieved a CHR and mCyR by 3 months after front-line imatinib therapy was started. His response is optimal and he should be continued on current therapy and followed up according to the above guidelines.

CML After Imatinib Failure

F.G. is a 72-year-old man who was diagnosed with CML-CP 18 months ago and started on imatinib 400-mg daily. He achieved a CHR at 3 months, but at 18 months had only achieved a partial cytogenetic response (PCyR).

Evidence-Based Case Discussion

F.G. failed to respond to first-line imatinib for CML-CP. The treatment strategy for patients who fail first-line standard-dose imatinib depends on two factors: the stage of the disease at the time of imatinib failure and the results of the mutation analysis of the *BCR-ABL* kinase domain. The therapeutic approach to patients in CP at relapse depends on the *BCR-ABL* kinase domain mutation. The T315I mutation accounts for 10% to 20% of all mutations detected after imatinib failure, and portends a poor response to higher doses of imatinib or to second-generation TKIs. The preferred treatment option in cases of T315I mutation is allogeneic stem cell transplantation; however, if the patient's disease status allows and while awaiting the pretransplant workup and a donor search, a clinical trial with a promising agent (e.g., the multikinase inhibitor AP24534) is an acceptable alternative. If the patient is not a candidate for stem cell transplantation or if an adequate donor cannot be found, then the treatment options in patients with T315I mutations include enrollment in a clinical trial with a "third-generation" TKI (AP24534 or others), omacetaxine (semisynthetic homoharringronine) given subcutaneously, or standard cytoreductive agents (interferon alpha +/− ara-c or hydrea). Treatment of patients with CML-CP who carry the T315I mutation with omacetaxine resulted in CHR of 80%, overall cytogenetic response of 20%, and CCyR of 13%. The *BCR-ABL* T315I clone was reduced to below detectable level in 60% of evaluable patients (23). The 2-year PFS with omacetaxine in patients with T315I mutation is 70%.

In patients without the T315I mutation, the treatment options include switching to an FDA approved second-generation TKI (as discussed below), increasing the dose of imatinib to 600- or 800-mg daily (if the patient was on 400 mg of imatinib), stem cell transplantation, or a clinical trial. Given that patients in this clinical setting invariably respond well to a second-generation TKI, stem cell transplantation should be reserved for a later stage; for example, in the situation where patients fail one of the second-generation TKIs. Some mutations have been shown to be more sensitive to one of the approved second-generation TKIs than the other, thus choice of agent should be based on the results of the mutational analysis (3).

Dasatinib and nilotinib are currently the only TKIs that are FDA approved after failure/intolerance to imatinib. The phase II START (*SRC/ABL* Tyrosine Kinase Inhibition Activity Research Trials of Dasatinib)–C study of dasatinib 70-mg twice daily in patients with resistance/intolerance to imatinib demonstrated 2-year CCyR of 53%, PFS of 80%, and OS of 94%. This study was followed by the START-R trial, which randomized patients with CML-CP resistant to imatinib to dasatinib 70-mg BID versus increasing the imatinib dose to 800 mg a day (24). The MCyR at 12 weeks was not statistically different in the two groups (36% for dasatanib patients and 29% for high-dose imatinib patients; P = .402). The CCyR at 12 weeks was higher in patients on dasatinib than patients on imatinib (22% and 8%, respectively; P = .041). At the 2-year follow-up, the rates of MCyR, CCyR, and MMR were significantly higher in patients receiving dasatinib than in patients receiving imatinib. It is important to mention that 80% of patients receiving imatinib and 20% of patients receiving dasatinib crossed over to the other treatment arm. Among patients who crossed over, MCyR was enhanced with dasatinib in comparison to high-dose imatinib (49% and 15%, respectively). The 24-month PFS was 86% in patients receiving dasatinib compared to 65% in patients receiving imatinib (P = .0012). The PFS advantage of switching to dasatinib was more noticeable in patients who were receiving 600 mg of imatinib at study entry. Grade 3/4 thrombocytopenia and neutropenia occurred in more patients on the dasatinib arm. Pleural effusions were exclusively reported in patients on dasatinib (grade 3/4 pleural effusion in 5%). These results provide support for switching to dasatinib in patients resistant to standard and particularly intermediate doses of imatinib instead of further intensifying the dose of imatinib, with the caveat of a worse side-effect profile.

The dose of dasatinib used in the START-R trial is not the currently recommended dose. A dose-optimization study of dasatinib in patients with CML-CP demonstrated that a dose of 100-mg daily had comparable MCyR and CCyR rates, as well as PFS and OS and an improved side-effect profile compared to multiple other doses tested. In particular, pleural effusions occurred in 14% of patients receiving 100 mg of dasatinib (2% grade 3/4) compared to 23% to 25% in patients receiving the other doses (4–5% grade 3/4) (P = .049). The risk of neutropenia, thrombocytopenia, and severe thrombocytopenia was also statistically lower at 100 mg of dasatanib daily, and there were fewer drug interruptions and discontinuations at that dose. Thus the preferred dasatinib dose is now 100-mg daily (25).

Nilotinib's activity in the setting of imatinib resistance or intolerance in CML-CP was demonstrated in a pivotal open label phase II trial where patients received nilotinib at a dose of 400-mg twice daily. At 24 months, CCyR was achieved in 46% of patients; 84% of patients who achieved CCyR maintained this response at 24 months. The overall MMR was 28% with a median time to MMR of 5.6 months. The rates of PFS and OS at 24 months were 64% and 87%, respectively.

For F.G., BCR-ABL kinase domain mutational analysis was performed, which was negative. The treatment options were discussed with him, and he was interested in switching therapy to dasatinib.

Advanced Phase CML

S.N. is a 57-year-old otherwise healthy man who presented with fatigue of several months duration. His CBC showed a WBC of 120,000/μL, a hemoglobin of 11 g/dL, and a platelet count of 88,000/μL. The WBC differential was as follows: 15% blasts, 15% promyelocytes, 11% myelocytes, 8% metamyelocytes, 20% neutrophils, 6% band forms, 3% lymphocytes, 20% basophils, 2% eosinophils). Physical examination showed splenomegaly (spleen palpated 8 cm below the left costal margin). Cytogenetic analysis of the bone marrow sample showed t(9,22) in all 20 examined cells. Peripheral blood PCR for *BCR-ABL* was positive for the p210 *BCR-ABL* transcript.

Evidence-Based Case Discussion

S.N. has a new diagnosis of AP-CML. Traditional cytotoxic therapies are essentially ineffective in patients with myeloid and undifferentiated blast crises; responses are infrequent, and when they occur, they tend to be short lived. The median OS of patients with myeloid BP CML who received cytotoxic chemotherapy ranged between 1.3 and 12 months. In lymphoid blast crisis, responses are somewhat more common, but are short lived as well. Decitabine has been studied in AP CML, but has not shown overwhelming overall improvement over cytotoxic chemotherapy (median OS of 4–13 months).

Although TKIs have revolutionized the treatment of CML-CP, their impact as single agents on CML-AP and CML-BP has not been dramatic. In imatinib naïve patients with AP or myeloid BP CML, single-agent imatinib resulted in rates of CHR and CCyR of 11% to 23% and 5% to 8%, respectively, and a median OS of 6.5 to 6.9 months. One study that combined imatinib with cytotoxic agents showed a significantly improved CHR at 81%; however, the median OS was only 6.4 months. In lymphoid blast crisis or Ph+ ALL, the rates of CHR and CCyR with imatinib are 10% to 20% and 10%, respectively, with a median OS of 7 months.

In CML-AP patients who are imatinib resistant/intolerant, dasatinib results in CHR and CCyR in 45% and 18% of patients, respectively. In myeloid BP, CHR is achieved in 24% to 35% and CCyR in 26% to 27% of patients with dasatanib. Similarly for CML-AP patients treated with nilotinib, CHR is achieved in 26% to 46% and CCyR in 13% to 19%. Nilotinib results in CHR in 8% and CCyR in 4% of patients in myeloid BP. Combining cytotoxic chemotherapy agents or decitabine with imatinib in patients with AP CML does not result in outcomes superior to those attained with single-agent dasatinib. In patients with lymphoid BP CML who are imatinib resistant/intolerant, dasatinib results in CHR and CCyR in about 70% and 30% respectively, whereas nilotinib results in even poorer responses (11% rate of CCyR). Thus the long-term outcome of patients with advanced CML when treated with TKIs is poor.

Unlike the majority of patients with CML-CP, patients with AP or BP CML require ASCT because TKIs do not provide long lasting responses in this setting (Figure 30.1). Timing of the ASCT is critical since the outcomes of patients with CML who undergo ASCT depend on the stage of the disease at the time of ASCT. The incidence of hematologic relapse at 3-years post-ASCT is 5.7% in patients who are transplanted in CP-CML, compared to 25.3% in patients transplanted at AP-CML, 27% in patients transplanted in second CP CML, and 26% in patients transplanted in BP CML (P = .0001). Imatinib pre-SCT does not result in unfavorable outcomes or increased transplant-related mortality. Imatinib can be safely given post-ASCT as well; and in fact, it may delay early relapses following reduced intensity ASCT. Patients treated with imatinib pre-SCT have inferior outcomes if they had a suboptimal response or loss of response at the time of transplant, further confirming the importance of achieving cytogenetic responses at the time of transplantation.

For our patient S.N., we recommend starting a TKI immediately in an attempt to control his disease to the best possible degree. Because even the patients with advanced CML who achieve an excellent response to a TKI relapse early, we also recommend HLA typing for the patient and his siblings and initiation of an immediate donor search through the national registry if none of his siblings is a good match. The patient should undergo an ASCT as soon as he has achieved the best possible benefit with the TKI. We recommend adding/resuming a TKI post-ASCT.

REFERENCES

1. Sokal JE, Cox EB, Baccarani M, et al. Prognostic discrimination in "Good-Risk" chronic granulocytic leukemia. *Blood.* 2003;63(4):789–799.
2. Druker BJ, Guilhot F, O'Brien SG, et al. Five-year follow-up of patients receiving imatinib for chronic myeloid leukemia. *N Engl J Med.* 2006;355(23):2408–2417.
3. Baccarani M, Cortes J, Pane F, et al. Chronic myeloid leukemia: an update of concepts and management recommendations of European LeukemiaNet. *J Clinl Oncol.* 2009;27(35): 6041–6151.
4. O'Brien SG, Guilhot F, Goldman JM, et al. International Randomized Study of Interferon versus STI571 (IRIS) 7-year follow-up: sustained survival, low rate of transformation and increased rate of major molecular response (MMR) in patients (pts) with newly diagnosed chronic myeloid leukemia in chronic phase (CML-CP) treated with Imatinib (Im). *Blood (ASH Annual Meeting Abstracts).* 2008;Abst 186.
5. Deininger M, O'Brien SG, Guilhot F, et al. International Randomized Study of Interferon versus STI571 (IRIS) 8-year follow-up: sustained survival and low risk for progression or events in patients with newly diagnosed chronic myeloid leukemia in chronic phase (CML-CP) treated with imatinib. *Blood (ASH Annual Meeting Abstracts).* 2009;Abst 1126.
6. Kantarjian HM, Talpaz M, O'Brien S, et al. Survival benefit with imatinib mesylate versus interferon-α-based regimens in newly diagnosed chronic-phase chronic myelogenous leukemia. *Blood.* 2006;108(6):1835–1840.
7. Roy L, Guilhot J, Krahnke T, et al. Survival benefit from imatinib compared with the combination interferon-α plus cytarabine in chronic-phase chronic myelogenous leukemia: historical comparison between two phase 3 trials. *Blood.* 2006;108(5):1478 –1484.
8. De Lavallade H, Apperley JF, Khorashad JS, et al. Imatinib for newly diagnosed patients with chronic myeloid leukemia: incidence of sustained responses in an intention-to-treat analysis. *J Clin Oncol.* 2008;26(20):3358–3363.
9. Cortes JE, Baccarani M, Guilhot F, et al. Phase III, randomized, open-label study of daily imatinib mesylate 400 mg versus 800 mg in patients with newly diagnosed, previously untreated chronic myeloid leukemia in chronic phase using molecular endpoints: Tyrosine kinase inhibitor optimization and selectivity study. *J Clin Oncol.* 2010;28(3):424–430.
10. Baccarani M, Rosti G, Castagnetti F, et al. Comparison of imatinib 400 mg and 800 mg daily in the front-line treatment of high-risk, Philadelphia-positive, chronic myeloid leukemia: a European LeukemiaNet study. *Blood.* 2009;113(19):4497–4504.
11. Petzer AL, Wolf D, Fong D, et al. High-dose imatinib improves cytogenetic and molecular remissions in patients with pretreated Philadelphia-positive, BCR-ABL-positive chronic phase chronic myeloid leukemia: first results of the randomized

CELSG phase III CML 11 "ISTAHIT" study. *Haematologica.* 2010;95(6):908–913.
12. Nicolini FE, Mahon FX, Guilhot J, et al. A phase III study exploring various doses of imatinib (Im) or Im in combination for newly diagnosed chronic phase (CP) chronic myeloid leukemia (CML) patients (pts): Results of an interim analysis of the SPIRIT trial of French CML group. *J Clin Oncol.* 2009;27(15s):(suppl; abstr 7058).
13. Saglio G, Kim D-W, Issaragrisil S, et al. Nilotinib versus imatinib for newly diagnosed chronic myeloid leukemia. *N Engl J Med*, 2010; 362(24), 2251–9.
14. Kantarjian H, Shah NP, Hochhaus A, et al. Dasatinib versus imatinib in newly diagnosed chronic-phase chronic myeloid leukemia. *N Engl J Med.* 2010;362(24):2260–2270.
15. Hughes T, Deininger M, Hochhaus A, et al. Monitoring CML patients responding to treatment with tyrosine kinase inhibitors: review and recommendations for harmonizing current methodology for detecting BCR-ABL transcripts and kinase domain mutations and for expressing results. *Blood.* 2006;108(1): 28–37.
16. Quintás-Cardama A, Cortes JE, O'Brien S, et al. Dasatinib early intervention after cytogenetic or hematologic resistance to imatinib in patients with chronic myeloid leukemia. *Cancer.* 2009;115(13):2912–2921.
17. Guilhot F, Larson RA, O'Brien SG, et al. Time to complete cytogenetic response (CCyR) does not affect long-term outcomes for patients on imatinib therapy. *Blood (ASH Annual Meeting Abstracts).* 2007;110:Abst 27.
18. Quintás-Cardama A, Kantarjian H, Jones D, et al. Delayed achievement of cytogenetic and molecular response is associated with increased risk of progression among patients with chronic myeloid leukemia in early chronic phase receiving high-dose or standard-dose imatinib therapy. *Blood.* 2009;113(25):6315–6321.
19. Branford S, Lawrence R, Grigg A, et al. Long term follow up of patients with CML in chronic phase treated with first-line imatinib suggests that earlier achievement of a major molecular response leads to a greater stability of response. *Blood (ASH annual meeting abstracts).* 2008;112:Abst 2113.
20. Larson RA, Druker BJ, Guilhot F, et al. Imatinib pharmacokinetics and its correlation with response and safety in chronic-phase chronic myeloid leukemia: a subanalysis of the IRIS study. *Blood.* 2008;111(8):4022–4028.
21. Kawaguchi T, Hamada A, Hirayama C, et al. Relationship between an effective dose of imatinib, body surface area, and trough drug levels in patients with chronic myeloid leukemia. *Int J Hematol.* 2009;89(5):642–648.
22. Picard S, Titier K, Etienne G, et al. Trough imatinib plasma levels are associated with both cytogenetic and molecular responses to standard-dose imatinib in chronic myeloid leukemia. *Blood.* 2007;109(8):3496–3499.
23. Cortes J, Khoury HJ, Corm S, et al. Safety and efficacy of subcutaneous (SC) omacetaxine mepesuccinate in imatinib (Im)-resistant chronic myeloid leukemia (CML) patients (pts) with the T315I mutation—results of an ongoing multicenter phase II study. *Blood (ASH Annual Meeting Abstracts).* 2008;112:Abst 3239.
24. Kantarjian H, Pasquini R, Lévy V, et al. Dasatinib or high-dose imatinib for chronic-phase chronic myeloid leukemia resistant to imatinib at a dose of 400 to 600 milligrams daily: two-year follow-up of a randomized phase 2 study (START-R). *Cancer.* 2009;115(18):4136–4147.
25. Shah N, Kim D-W, Kantarjian H, et al. Potent, transient inhibition of BCR-ABL with dasatinib 100 mg daily achieves rapid and durable cytogenetic responses and high transformation-free survival rates in chronic phase chronic myeloid leukemia patients with resistance, suboptimal response or intolerance to imatinib. *Haematologica.* 2010;95(2):232–240.

31

Chronic Lymphocytic Leukemia

RAMI KHORIATY AND SAMI N. MALEK

EPIDEMIOLOGY, NATURAL HISTORY, AND RISK FACTORS

The epidemiology of chronic lymphocytic leukemia (CLL) varies in different regions of the world. In the Western world, CLL is the most common hematologic malignancy (about 30% of all leukemias), whereas in Asia, CLL has a lower incidence (about 5% of all leukemias). In 2010, an estimated 15,000 new cases of CLL were diagnosed in the United States and about 4400 patients died of the disease. CLL is mainly a disease of the elderly, with a median age at diagnosis of 72 years.

The life expectancy of patients with CLL is significantly lower than that of matched controls, but it is also highly variable and influenced by multiple clinical and biological factors. Patients with Rai stage 0, for example, have a life expectancy of about 130 months, whereas patients with Rai stage III or IV have a life expectancy of about 60 to 70 months. Patients within the same Rai stage may display diverse clinical behavior. To address the limitation of the clinical CLL staging system (in particular Rai stages 0–2), multiple laboratory variables have been developed and were found to predict the outcomes of patients with CLL (this is discussed in detail in the first case summary and reviewed by Malek) (1).

Traditionally, CLL has been regarded as an accumulative disease, with defects in apoptosis. Recent evidence indicates that the CLL clone has a proliferative fraction that is primarily located in the lymph nodes and the bone marrow. It is not completely clear what the driving factors of CLL proliferation are, but it is thought that stimulation of the B-cell receptor by antigens is one of them. The exact etiology of CLL remains uncertain and no gene has been found to be mutated at a high frequency in this disease. CLL is an acquired disorder in the majority of cases; however, there are reports of familial CLL cases. A positive family history for CLL or other lymphoid malignancies is one of the strongest risk factors for developing the disease. Additional risk factors for the development of CLL include older age, male sex (with a male to female preponderance of approximately 2:1), and ethnicity. CLL is more common in Caucasians than African Americans, and is rare in Hispanics, Native Americans, and Asians. CLL is not associated with radiation exposure. There are no other clear environmental etiologic factors identified.

STAGING

There are two major staging systems in CLL; the Rai staging system and the Binet staging system. The original Rai staging system was modified to a simpler classification scheme. Both the Rai and Binet staging systems are easily implemented because they rely only on physical examination and a complete blood count (CBC). The Rai system is the most commonly used of these two staging systems in the United States.

Chronic Lymphocytic Leukemia

Rai Stage	Modified Rai Stage	Definition
0	Low-risk	Lymphocytosis only
I	Intermediate-risk	Lymphocytosis and lymphadenopathy
II	Intermediate-risk	Lymphocytosis with hepatomegaly or splenomegaly
III	High-risk	Lymphocytosis and anemia (Hb < 11 g/dL)
IV	High-risk	Lymphocytosis and thrombocytopenia (platelets < 100,000/μL)

(*continued*)

Binet Stage	Definition
A	Less than 3 nodal sites*
B	Three or more nodal sites*
C	Anemia (Hb < 10 g/dL) and/or thrombocytopenia (platelets < 100,000/μL)

*The 5 nodal sites for Binet staging are cervical (including the waldeyer ring), axillary (both axillae count as one area), inguinal (involvement of both groins is considered as one area), spleen, and liver.

From a clinical perspective, making the diagnosis of Rai stage III or IV and/or Binet stage C CLL requires that the bone marrow be packed with CLL cells. Otherwise, alternative causes of anemia/thrombocytopenia need to be investigated (discussed further in the last case summary).

CASE SUMMARIES

Early-Stage CLL

D.S. is a 73-year-old man referred to the hematology clinic because of incidental lymphocytosis. The patient is completely asymptomatic on review of systems; his energy level is good, and he does not have any fevers, night sweats, or weight loss. His physical examination is normal without any palpable lymphadenopathy or hepatosplenomegaly. His CBC shows a white blood cells (WBC) count of 25,000 /μL, hemoglobin of 15 g/dl, and a platelet count of 250,000/μL. The WBC differential is as follows: 90% lymphocytes, 7% neutrophils, and 3% monocytes. A peripheral blood smear shows small mature lymphocytes with a narrow border of cytoplasm and dense nuclei, as well as scattered smudge cells. Flow cytometry shows the following pattern: CD5+, CD10–, CD19+, CD20 (Dim), CD23+, surface immunoglobulin (sIg) Dim. The lymphocytes are lambda restricted. Fluorescent in-situ hybridization (FISH) testing shows del 13q14 as the sole abnormality in 68% of the nuclei. Zeta-associated protein of 70kDa (ZAP-70) expression by flow cytometry on the CD5+/CD19+ cells is negative (< 20%), IGVH mutation analysis discloses a mutated genotype (94.5% homology to germline), and CD38 expression by flow cytometry is negative (< 30%).

Evidence-Based Case Discussion

D.S. is an elderly patient with asymptomatic lymphocytosis. The most common presentation of CLL is incidental lymphocytosis or asymptomatic lymphadenopathy. Signs and symptoms related to CLL may include fatigue and malaise (most common); early satiety or abdominal discomfort secondary to splenomegaly; B symptoms: fevers, night sweats and weight loss (<10% incidence); recurrent infections (rare); and autoimmune cytopenias (~15% incidence).

The differential diagnosis of CLL includes various lymphomas (mantle cell lymphoma, marginal zone lymphoma, lymphoplasmacytic lymphoma, and follicular lymphoma), different leukemias (prolymphocytic leukemia, hairy cell leukemia, and large granular lymphocytic leukemia), reactive lymphocytosis, and monoclonal B-cell lymphocytosis (MBL). It is of paramount importance that the treating physicians confirm the diagnosis of CLL before making any therapeutic plans. In order for the diagnosis of CLL to be made, all the following criteria should be met (a) the peripheral blood monoclonal B-lymphocytes count needs to be ≥ 5000 /μL; (b) the immunophenotype of the peripheral blood lymphocytes ought to be characteristic of CLL; (c) the prolymphocytes should not comprise more than 55% of the lymphocytes. Flow cytometry is critical for making the diagnosis of CLL because it can provide evidence for clonality of the B cells by showing their restriction to either kappa or lambda immunoglobulin light chains and it shows the characteristic immunophenotype of the CLL cells. CLL cells typically express the T-cell antigen CD5, the B-cell markers CD19 and CD23, and have characteristically dim expression of CD20, CD79b, and surface immunoglobulins (sIg) (dimmer in the CLL cells compared to normal B cells). Based on the different immunophenotypic patterns, CLL can be distinguished from other lymphomas (Table 31.1). The pattern of positive expression of CD5, CD19, and CD20 is shared only by CLL and mantle cell lymphoma (very rarely in DLBCL or MZL), making the distinction between these two diseases crucial. Mantle cell lymphoma can be differentiated from CLL because the mantle cell lymphoma cells typically do not express CD23, and have the characteristic translocation t(11;14) resulting in aberrant cyclin D1 expression (this translocation is tested as part of the CLL FISH panel test). In rare cases, the mantle cell lymphoma cells may express CD23 or lack cyclin D1 expression, and the CLL cells may lack CD23 expression (atypical CLL). In those situations, the degree of expression of CD20 and sIg is helpful in making the distinction between these two diseases. CD20 and sIg are characteristically dimly expressed in CLL.

The following diseases: small lymphocytic lymphoma (SLL), monoclonal B-cell lymphocytosis (MBL), and prolymphocytic leukemia (PLL), may all have the same immunophenotype as CLL. The criteria in distinguishing CLL from these other diseases are summarized in Table 31.2. For practical clinical purposes, CLL and SLL are the same illness.

Our patient fulfills the diagnostic criteria of CLL. In addition, his peripheral smear is classic for CLL and shows small mature lymphocytes, with a narrow border of cytoplasm, and clumped nuclear chromatin. Smudge cells, seen on his smear as well, are characteristic of CLL. Our patient's CLL stage is Rai stage 0.

After the diagnosis of CLL is confirmed, the next step in management is to determine whether or not therapy is

Table 31.1 CLL Can Be Differentiated From Other Lymphomas Through Immunophenotyping by Flow Cytometry.

Malignancy	CD5	CD10	CD19	CD23	sIg	cIg	Cyclin D1
CLL	+	-	+	+	+ dim	+/-	-
MCL	+	-	+	-	+	-	+
FL	-	+	+	+/-	+	-	-
Splenic MZL	-	-	+	-	+	+/-	-
MZL	-	-	+	+/-	+	+/-	-
LPL	-	-	+	-	+	+	-

CLL, chronic lymphocytic leukemia; MCL, mantle cell lymphoma; FL, follicular lymphoma; MZL, marginal zone lymphoma; LPL, lymphoplasmacytic lymphoma; sIg, surface immunoglobulin; cIg, cytoplasmic immunoglobulin+ indicated more than 90% positive; - indicated more than 90% negative.

Table 31.2 Comparison Between CLL and Other Diseases That Have a Similar Immunophenotypic Pattern

	Clonal B Cells of CLL Phenotype	Peripheral B cell ≥ 5000 /μL	LN Enlargement or HSM	Prolymphocytes ≥ 55%
CLL	+	+	+/-	-
SLL	+	-	+	-
MBL*	+	-	-	-
PLL	+/-^	+	+/-	+

CLL, chronic lymphocytic leukemia; SLL, small lymphocytic lymphoma; MBL, monoclonal B-cell lymphocytosis; PLL, prolymphocytic leukemia.
*In order for a diagnosis of MBL to be made, patients should not have cytopenias or disease-related symptoms.
^It is important to mention that one half of patients with PLL are CD5-.

required. The initiation of treatment in early-stage asymptomatic CLL has not been shown to impact survival. Therefore, asymptomatic CLL patients with Rai stage 0 should be monitored closely without starting therapy. One of the following consensus criteria defined by the International Workshop on CLL (IWCLL) should be met in order to justify starting therapy in patients with CLL (2): (a) development of or worsening of anemia or thrombocytopenia from marrow failure (common cause of therapy initiation); (b) symptomatic, progressive, or massive lymphoid tissue enlargement (massive is defined as spleen > 6 cm below the left costal margin, or LN > 10 cm in longest diameter); (c) autoimmune hemolytic anemia (AIHA) or autoimmune thrombocytopenia that are poorly responsive to steroids or other standard therapy; (d) lymphocyte doubling time of less than 6 months or > 50% increase in absolute lymphocyte count (ALC) over a period of 2 months (this criteria should not be used in patients with ALC < 30,000; additionally infections as a cause of worsening lymphocytosis need to be ruled out); (e) fevers (> 100.5°F or > 38.0°C for more than 2 weeks with no proof of infection), night sweats (for > 1 month with no evidence of infection), unintentional weight loss (≥ 10% in the last 6 months), and fatigue (ECOG performance status of ≥ 2). An elevated WBC count, even if markedly elevated, is not a reason on its own to treat patients with CLL. The same is true for hypogammaglobulinemia and paraproteinemia.

Our patient has asymptomatic Rai stage 0 CLL and does not have any of the above criteria for treatment. Therefore, treatment is not indicated, and our patient should be monitored closely.

Commonly, physicians treating CLL are asked prognostic questions and the following guidelines can be provided. The median overall survival (OS) of patients with Rai stage 0, I, II, III, and IV CLL is 130, 106, 88, 58, and 69 months, respectively. In order to address the limitation of the CLL staging system, multiple biological variables have been found to predict the outcomes of patients with CLL (1). One of the most important and most robust of those tests is the clinically available CLL FISH test. FISH can identify abnormalities in more than 80% of patients with CLL. Del 13q (found in ~50% of the cases), del 11q (15%), trisomy 12 (20%), del 17p (~7–10%), and complex FISH (≥2 FISH findings found in ~10% of CLL) are the most common of these abnormalities and are prognostic for both OS as well as treatment-free survival. Compared to patients with normal karyotypes (median

OS >10 years), del 17p and del 11q portend a poor prognosis (median OS of ~ 3 years and 7 years respectively), trisomy 12 predicts an intermediate prognosis (median OS ~10 years), and isolated del 13q portends a "favorable" prognosis (median OS >10 years). Regarding complex FISH karyotype, it also predicts a poor prognosis (OS ~ 3–8 years). Importantly, all cases of del 17p CLL show loss of one copy and mutation of the second copy of *p53*. CLL patients with mutated *p53* have been found to have a poor prognosis regardless of the presence or absence of del 17p (rare isolated *p53* mutations). Other molecular/biologic factors that predict outcome in CLL are immunoglobulin heavy chain variable region genes *(IGVH)* mutation status, ZAP-70 expression, and CD38 protein expression.

About 60% of all CLL patients have mutated *IGVH (M-IGVH)* that is defined as less than 98% homology with the germline sequences. *M-IGVH* generally portends an excellent OS. There is one exception to this rule: patients expressing the *VH3-21* gene usually belong to the *M-IGVH* group; however, their survival is as poor as that of patients with unmutated *IGVH (U-IGVH)*. Positive ZAP-70 expression was initially thought to be a surrogate of *U-IGVH* CLL, but proved to be an independent predictor of short time to treatment (TTT). ZAP-70 is a flow cytometric test and should be measured in CD19+/CD5+ cells. ZAP-70 expression > 20% is considered positive; nonetheless, lower expression may also be associated with a short TTT. Regarding CD38, the optimal cutoff of positive expression is controversial (> 30% is considered positive by most investigators). Bimodal expression of CD38 could be seen in some patients. High CD38 expression predicts for short TTT.

In clinical practice, a combination of different molecular factors including FISH testing appears to be the most accurate way for prognostic classification. The CLL Research Consortium assessed the relative impacts of *IGVH*, ZAP-70, and CD38 in predicting TTT in CLL, and showed that patients can be grouped into three risk groups: low-, intermediate-, and high-risk groups (3). Patients who are ZAP-70 positive are at high risk for short TTT, while patients with ZAP-70 negative CLL can be classified into intermediate risk if IGVH is unmutated, and low risk if IGVH is mutated. CD38 has no added prognostic significance to ZAP-70 and IGVH. Based on the currently available data, the best use of ZAP-70 testing is in predicting TTT in patients with newly diagnosed Rai stage 0 to 2 CLL, and *IGVH* mutation analysis provides additional insight on TTT if ZAP-70 is negative.

Our patient has good prognostic features including del 13q as a sole abnormality on FISH, negative ZAP-70, mutated *IGVH*, and negative CD38. We predict that the patient will not require therapy for his CLL for many years.

First-Line Therapy in Advanced CLL

D.S. is a 61-year-old gentleman who was diagnosed with CLL 3 years ago. FISH testing at diagnosis showed del 11q as the sole abnormality. ZAP-70 testing, CD38 testing, and *IGVH* mutation analysis were not performed. He was observed closely with routine visits and physical examinations, as well as serial CBCs. Now, the patient is seen in follow-up. He is asymptomatic from his disease and his ECOG performance status is 0. On physical examination, he has three palpable cervical lymph nodes (all < 3 cm in size), and his spleen is palpated about 8 cm below the left costal margin. His ALC, which was 9000/μL at diagnosis, steadily increased over time, and reached 160,000/μL. The patient's hemoglobin is 9.5 g/dL, and his platelet count is 90,000/μL. LDH is 160 IU/L (normal 120–240 IU/L), and reticulocyte % is 0.5%. A bone marrow aspirate and biopsy shows that the majority of the marrow space is occupied by CLL cells.

Evidence-Based Case Discussion

D.S. is a patient with Rai stage IV CLL. He has multiple indications for instituting therapy for his CLL including massive splenomegaly, and importantly anemia and thrombocytopenia resulting from marrow failure.

Monotherapy with alkylating agents has long been used for front-line treatment of CLL. Chlorambucil (Clb) has been regarded as the "gold standard" first-line therapeutic option in CLL for many decades. More recently, fludarabine (F), bendamustine (B), and alemtuzumab (A) were each compared head to head to Clb in first-line CLL in phase III randomized control trials (reviewed in 4,5). These trials showed superiority of single-agent F, single-agent B, and single-agent A over Clb in terms of improved response rates and progression-free survival (PFS). F was also compared with other alkylator combination regimens, CAP (cyclophosphamide, doxorubicin, and prednisone) and CHOP (cyclophosphamide, doxoruvicin, vincristine, and prednisone) and the results were in favor of F. Other purine analogues, cladribine and pentostatin, are active in CLL as well.

Fludarabine and cyclophosphamide (FC) were found to have synergistic cytotoxicity in CLL cells. Three randomized control trials compared FC with F in first-line CLL and showed superiority of FC, with improved responses (both complete response [CR] and PFS) (4,5). FC did not seem to result in an increased rate of severe infections compared to F. Another purine analogue, Cla was also combined with cyclophosphamide (C) in clinical trials. One trial compared Cla alone versus Cla and Cyclophosphamide (C) versus Cla, C, and mitoxantrone (M), and showed superior CR with the three-drug combination, and a trend toward superior CR with the two-drug combination compared to Cla alone; however, the PFS was fairly similar among the three groups. The combination Cla and C was equally effective and safe as FC in first-line CLL.

Fludarabine and rituximab (FR) also showed synergistic activity in preclinical studies in CLL. The CALGB 9712 phase II randomized control trial compared concurrent FR followed by 4 weekly doses of R to single-agent F followed by 4 weekly R infusions (6). The response rates (CR and OR) were higher in the concurrent group. When the patients enrolled in this trial were compared retrospectively to patients enrolled in the previous CALGB trial (CALGB 9011) where therapy was with F only, patients receiving FR had a better PFS and OS than patients receiving F only (7).

The combination FCR, pioneered by Dr. Keating, showed very promising results in a large phase II study conducted at the MD Anderson Cancer Center (8). This led the German CLL Study Group (GCLLSG) to conduct a phase III randomized trial (CLL 8 trial) comparing FCR with FC in front-line CLL (9). This trial showed superiority of FCR in terms of response rates (OR and CR), PFS, as well as OS (although the OS benefit was modest). The benefit of FCR was at a cost of increased grade 3/4 neutropenia (34% vs. 21%), but there was no increase in treatment-related mortality (2% with FCR and 1.5% with FC). The benefit of FCR was evident in all the cytogenetic prognostic subgroups with the exception of patients with del 17p (see case #3 for treatment of CLL patients with del 17p). Specifically, in the subgroup of patients with del 11q (as in the case of our patient), the addition of R to FC resulted in a three-fold increase in the rate of CR from 15.5% to 53.2%, and in a marked improvement in PFS ($P < .001$) and OS ($P = .004$). The results of this study suggest that FCR may overcome the negative prognostic impact of del 11q, and that del 11q is likely a predictive marker for increased benefit from FCR therapy. It is important to note that 8 patients out of 300 enrolled in the MD Anderson phase II FCR study developed treatment-related MDS (8), a life-threatening complication.

Multiple variations have been made to the FCR regimen in an attempt to reduce its toxicity. The FCR-Lite regimen used a reduced dose of both F and C and an intensified R schedule instead, followed by R maintenance until disease progression (10). The results of the single arm FCR-Lite trial were promising, and the rate of grade 3/4 neutropenia was only 13%, which is lower than that observed with FCR.

Another variation in FCR was the substitution of pentostatin (P) for F with the hope of reducing the myelotoxicity of FCR. A phase II trial of PCR in previously untreated CLL patients showed promising results with a fairly low toxicity profile; grade 3/4 neutropenia only occurred in 16% of the cycles (41% of the patients). Patients older than 70 years had a similar benefit without excess morbidity or adverse outcomes compared to patients younger than 70 years (11). PCR was then compared to FCR in a phase III community-based randomized trial in untreated or minimally treated CLL patients. There was no difference in the overall response rates and OS between PCR and FCR. The infection rate—the primary endpoint of the trial—was not different between both arms of the study (12). However, it is important to note that the P dose was higher in this phase III trial (4 mg/m^2) compared to the P dose in one of the phase II PCR trial (2 mg/m^2), and the FCR schedule and dose was different from the traditional FCR regimen, making it difficult to make comparisons between the more traditional PCR and FCR regimens. Another promising CIT regimen in CLL is B + R (BR). BR showed encouraging results in a phase II CLL trial; this led to an ongoing phase III trial comparing it to FCR in previously untreated CLL patients conducted by the GCLLSG.

Attempts have been made to eliminate chemotherapy all together from first-line CLL therapy, particularly because some patients have many comorbidities and a poor performance status. A phase II trial of first-line high-dose methylprednisolone and weekly R (R-HDMP) in CLL showed encouraging results (even in patients with del 17p), but long-term follow-up data are not available (13). This regimen was fairly well tolerated and non-myelotoxic. It is a reasonable consideration in patients with baseline cytopenias, elderly patients with poor performance status, and patients with del 17p.

In summary, the three CIT regimens that are best studied in first-line CLL are FR, FCR, and PCR. There is growing evidence that FCR abrogates the poor prognostic impact of del 11q; we thus favor FCR in this setting. In all other circumstances, awaiting the results of the phase III randomized clinical trial conducted by the CALGB comparing FR and FCR, we favor using FR given its lower toxicity profile. This strategy allows FCR to be reserved for the relapsed setting.

Our patient is young (< 65 years of age) with a good performance status, and has del 11q without del 17 p. We recommend treating him with FCR. Vigilance should be given when administering R with the first cycle of therapy in patients who have an elevated WBC count, because of the reported risk of severe tumor lysis syndrome and death, likely secondary to a cytokine storm. We recommend splitting the R dose in the first cycle of therapy, and giving 100 mg on day 1 and the remaining of the R dose on day 2 (high-risk R protocol). Allopurinol should also be given to patients who have a high tumor burden and thus a high risk of tumor lysis syndrome. F is a lymphotoxic agent, and it decreases predominantly the CD4+ cells. Antipneumocystis prophylaxis with bactrim should be initiated at the start of therapy, and continued until the CD4 count increases to > 200, or alternatively for 1 year after completion of therapy. Herpes simplex virus prophylaxis is also recommended.

First-Line Therapy in Patients With Deletion 17p

B.P. is a 59-year-old man who was diagnosed with CLL 1 month ago. His presentation was low-grade fevers and night sweats for which he had an extensive negative infectious workup. On physical examination, he has no palpable lymphadenopathy and no hepatosplenomegaly. His CBC shows a WBC of 75,000/μL (ALC 69,000/μL), a hemoglobin of 9 g/dL, and platelet count of 80,000/μL. LDH, haptoglobin, and indirect bilirubin are normal. Bone marrow biopsy shows that the majority of the marrow space is occupied by CLL cells. CLL FISH panel shows del 17p together with del13q. CT scan of the chest, abdomen, and pelvis shows a few scattered mildly enlarged lymph nodes, none of which is > 3 cm in size.

Evidence-Based Case Discussion

B.P. is a relatively young patient with symptomatic Rai stage IV CLL characterized by del 17p and lack of bulky lymphadenopathy.

Symptomatic CLL patients with del 17p or *p53* mutation have a poor prognosis. A widely accepted standard of care in this setting is not available. The response rate of these patients to F or FC is poor. With FCR, the OR is higher (68%), with a 5% rate of CR; however, the duration of response remains fairly short (11.3 months). The OS of these patients is poor despite aggressive CIT regimens: the 3-year OS of patients with del 17p treated with FR is 33%, compared to 53% and 86% in patients with del 11q and normal cytogenetics respectively. In the GCLLSG randomized trial of first-line FC versus FCR, the 3-year survival of patients with del 17p was not improved with CIT (37% with FC vs. 38% with FCR) (9).

Agents that act independent of the DNA damage pathway and/or p53 have been studied in patients with del 17p CLL. Single-agent A, for example, results in OR of 64% and PFS of 10.7 months in the first-line setting (14). Allogeneic stem cell transplantation (ASCT) is currently the only treatment that may provide prolonged survival in this CLL group. There is mounting evidence that ASCT may mitigate the unfavorable prognostic impact of del 17p (15).

The treatment strategy of patients with del 17p is therefore distinct from other CLL patients (Figure 31.1). Even though a standard of care approach is not available, in the absence of a clinical trial, CLL patients with del 17p or *p53* mutation should be treated preferably with A or FCR followed by reduced-intensity ASCT (RI-ASCT) in first remission, if they are transplant eligible. Other combinations that could be used prior to ASCT on a study protocol include AR and R-HDMP.

RI-ASCT rather than myeloablative ASCT represents the standard ASCT modality in CLL (15). However, in young patients with a good performance status and poorly controlled disease, myeloablative ASCT may be the preferred option. A matched sibling donor is preferred over a matched unrelated donor (MUD) whenever possible, but MUD is an acceptable alternative in the event that a matched sibling is not available.

B.P. could be treated with either A or FCR, followed by RI-ASCT. The patient as well as his siblings should

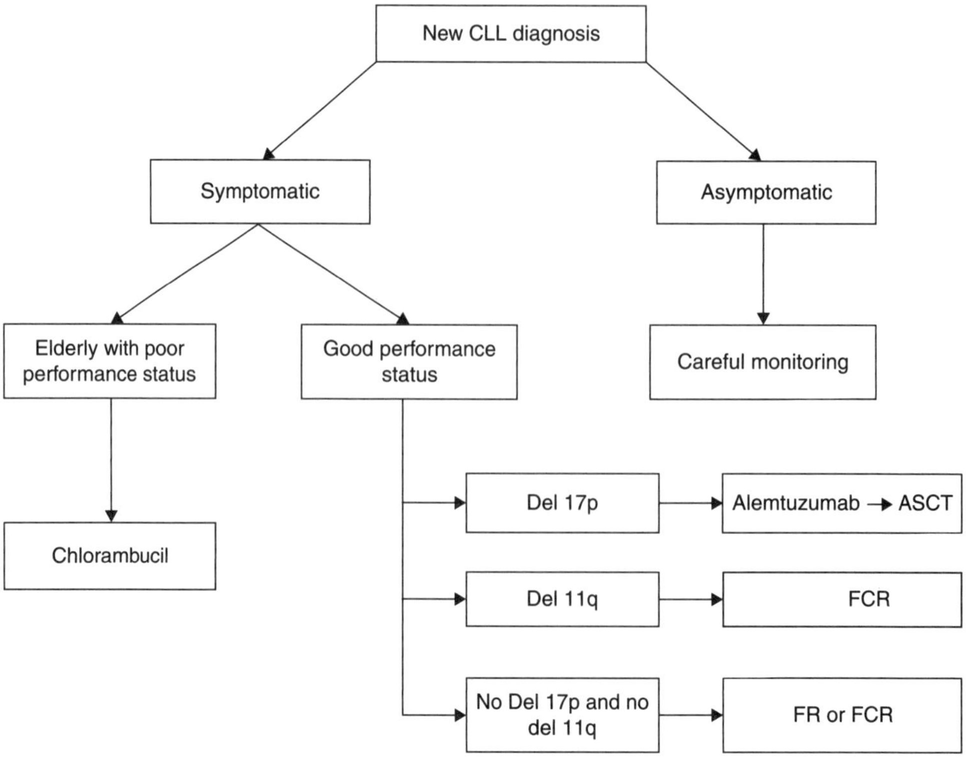

Figure 31.1

First-line treatment algorithm for chronic lymphocytic leukemia.

have HLA-typing performed. If none of his siblings is a match, an unrelated donor search should be initiated. It is important to note that significantly enlarged lymph nodes (particularly when > 3 cm) do not respond well to A. In those patients, FCR followed by ASCT is preferred over A followed by ASCT.

First-Line Therapy in Elderly CLL Patients

T.L. is a 79-year-old man with a recent diagnosis of CLL. He has early satiety resulting in decreased oral intake and weight loss. The patient's ECOG performance status is 2. On physical examination, he is found to have palpable lymphadenopathy and splenomegaly (spleen palpated about 8 cm below the left costal margin). The patient's CBC shows a WBC of 80,000/µL (ALC 71,000/µL), hemoglobin of 10.5 g/dL, and platelet count of 140,000/µL. His ALC was 30,000/µL 6 months ago. A CLL FISH panel was negative for all the chromosomal abnormalities tested in CLL.

Evidence-Based Case Discussion

T.L. has symptomatic Rai stage III CLL with a rapidly doubling ALC (less than 6 months doubling time), and requires therapy. He is different from the prior patients presented above in that he is elderly with a poorer performance status. This has important implications for the choice of therapy.

The majority of patients with CLL are elderly. The performance status of many of these elderly patients is poor enough that aggressive therapy, like FCR, could not be safely administered. In a single center cohort of 125 elderly patients (including untreated and relapsed patients) who received FC or FCR, the response rates were favorable; however, the toxicity profile was unacceptable (grade 3/4 myelotoxicity of 65–82%), resulting in a relatively elevated treatment discontinuation rate.

The majority of the CLL trials enrolled skewed samples of patients—younger patients—than the typical CLL population. Therefore, the results of these trials cannot be generalized to the elderly CLL patients. For example, the median age of patients enrolled on the CALGB 9011 trial, which showed superiority of F over Cbl, is 62 to 64 years (16). A similar randomized trial conducted by the GCLLSG targeted only patients who are older than 65 years. This trial, contrary to the CALGB trial, showed equivalence of F and Cbl in terms of PFS and OS (despite the higher response rates with F), suggesting that Cbl is still a valid first-line treatment option in elderly CLL patients who are not candidates for more intensive combination regimens (17). Other agents/regimens that may be considered in elderly CLL patients include the single agents: B, A (for patients with del 17p), and Cla and the combination BR.

It is important to note though that "physically fit" elderly patients without significant comorbidities may tolerate more intensive regimens. FR and PCR (with a P dose of 2 mg/m^2 and not 4 mg/m^2) are valid treatment options for these elderly "fit" patients (11). The treatment options were discussed with T.L., and the final decision was to treat him with single-agent Cbl.

Second-Line Therapy in CLL

S.C. is a 64-year-old man, who was diagnosed with CLL 10 years ago. He did not require treatment until 4 years ago, when he was treated with FCR. CLL FISH panel was performed before FCR was administered and showed trisomy 12 as the sole abnormality. The patient achieved CR after he was treated with FCR. The patient continued to be followed closely, and 9 months ago he showed signs of disease recurrence that manifested as an increase in the ALC to 12,000/µL and palpable lymphadenopathy in the cervical area. The patient was observed closely; his ALC steadily increased and reached just over 100,000/µL a week ago, and his cervical lymphadenopathy became cosmetically undesirable for him. Repeat CLL FISH showed trisomy 12 with no other abnormalities. The patient is physically fit, does not have significant comorbidities, and his ECOG performance status is 0.

Evidence-Based Case Discussion

S.C. has symptomatic relapsed CLL 3.5 years after FCR, and no del 17p and thus likely has a chemoresponsive disease.

Despite the major improvements in first-line therapy in CLL, the vast majority of the patients will relapse (median PFS is ~3.5–4 years after FCR). Asymptomatic patients at relapse should be monitored closely, and therapy should only be instituted at the time of development of one of the criteria for therapy defined by the IWCLL (criteria described in the first-line treatment section).

Treatment of relapsed CLL is not standardized, and depends on the duration of the first remission, the performance status of the patient, and the presence or absence of del 17p or del11q or complex FISH findings.

In general, if the duration of first remission is more than 12 months, it is reasonable to repeat the first-line treatment. In patients who are refractory to nucleoside analogues, defined as no response or response lasting < 1 year, the outlook is poor and therapy is individualized. Enrollment into a well-designed clinical trial is highly recommended. Physically fit patients with del 17p should be treated with A followed by ASCT. Physically fit patients who lack del 17p have a variety of treatment options if a clinical trial is not available but survival times are short. Some treatment options include CIT if prior therapy only comprised F, A (if LN < 3 cm), AR, BR, or ofatumumab and should be followed by ASCT.

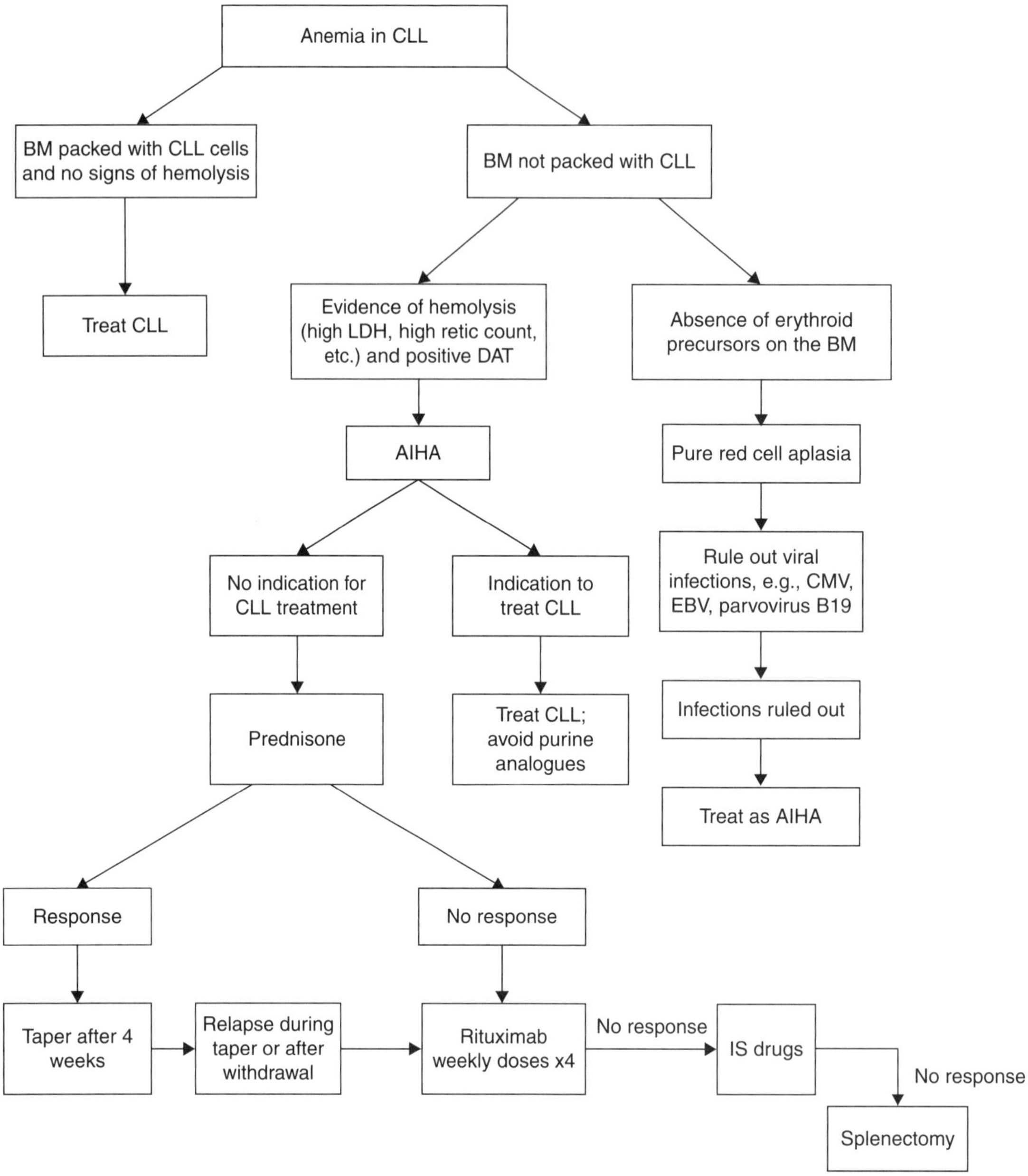

Figure 31.2

Treatment algorithm for anemia in chronic lymphocytic leukemia. AIHA, autoimmune hemolytic anemia; IS drugs, immunosuppressive drugs; CMV, cytomegalovirus; EBV, Epstein-Barr virus.

S.C. had recurrence of CLL > 1 year after FCR and lacks del 17p. He could be re-treated with FCR; other CIT regimens (like FR, BR) may be used as well.

Autoimmune Hemolytic Anemia in CLL

D.A. is a 63-year-old man diagnosed with CLL over a year ago. He was monitored closely, and is found to have new onset anemia. His hemoglobin that was 14 g/dL at diagnosis is currently 8 g/dL. His WBC is 17,000/μL and his platelet count is 255,000/μL. LDH is elevated at 650 IU/L (normal 120–240 IU/L), haptoglobin is undetectable (normal 22–239 mg/dL), unconjugated bilirubin is 2.5 mg/dL (normal 0–1 mg/dL), and the absolute reticulocyte count is 150,000/μL. The direct antiglobulin test (DAT) is positive (IgG). A bone marrow aspirate and biopsy shows 45% involvement of the marrow space with CLL cells, and expanded erythroid precursors. The patient is asymptomatic from the CLL standpoint, and his physical examination shows no enlarged lymphadenopathy or splenomegaly.

Evidence-Based Case Discussion

D.A. has CLL and anemia. His anemia is secondary to an autoimmune hemolysis. It is important to emphasize that not every CLL patient who has anemia or thrombocytopenia requires therapy for CLL. It is essential to identify the cause of the anemia or thrombocytopenia; if the cause is progressive marrow failure from CLL, then treatment of CLL should be instituted. On the other hand, if the anemia or thrombocytopenia is from an autoimmune process, then treating the autoimmune process should be done. Another rare cause of anemia in CLL is pure red cell aplasia. This diagnosis should be suspected in case of lack of reticulocyte response to the anemia, and is confirmed by finding absence of erythroid precursors in the bone marrow. If a diagnosis of pure red cell aplasia is made, it is important to rule out viral infections including Epstein-Barr virus, cytomegalovirus, and parvovirus before assuming that it is an autoimmune process (Figure 31.2).

The composite prevalence of autoimmune cytopenias (AIHA, ITP, and Evans syndrome) in CLL is ~15%. About half of these autoimmune cytopenias develop either during or after therapy. AIHA is the most common of the autoimmune cytopenias in CLL. The diagnosis of AIHA relies on a fall in hemoglobin, in association with a positive DAT and laboratory values suggestive of hemolysis: elevated LDH, low/undetected haptoglobin, increased reticulocyte count, and elevated unconjugated bilirubin. It is important to note that about 14% of CLL patients with AIHA have a negative DAT indicating that a positive DAT is not needed for the diagnosis of AIHA. In addition, about one third of patients with CLL have a positive DAT during the course of their disease, and most of them do not develop clinically evident AIHA.

There are no randomized controlled trials of treatment of AIHA in CLL. We follow the algorithm presented in Figure 31.2. Patients who have an indication for CLL treatment should have directed CLL therapy. In patients who do not have an indication for CLL therapy, the first-line treatment of AIHA is prednisone 1 mg/kg/day (capped usually at 80 mg) for 4 weeks together with folic acid, followed by a slow taper (fast tapers are a common cause of relapse). In patients who do not respond to steroids or who relapse during the steroid taper or after steroids withdrawal, the treatment options include rituximab, intravenous immunoglobulins, cyclosporine A, mycophenolate mofetil, azathioprine, daily low-dose oral cyclophosphamide, rituximab, alemtuzumab, and splenectomy. We generally recommend a trial of one immunosuppressive agent, and rituximab before consideration of splenectomy. Treatment-refractory AIHA is an indication for CIT directed at CLL.

In the early 1990s, multiple reports made the observation of severe (and sometimes fatal) AIHA in patients treated with purine analogues (mostly fludarabine). Even though the majority of these cases occurred in heavily pretreated patients and in the setting of active immune cytopenias, it is prudent to avoid fludarabine in patients with active AIHA, and in patients with a history of AIHA (particularly if purine analogue-induced). Otherwise, among patients who lack a history of AIHA, the latter does not develop more commonly in patients treated with F-containing regimens (4%) compared to patients treated with Cbl (5%) (18). Furthermore, the incidence of AIHA may be reduced with the addition of C to F (5%), compared to patients receiving F (12%) and patients receiving Cbl (12%) (19). In the GCLLSG trial, the incidence of AIHA was 1% with FC and < 1% with FCR.

D.A. has AIHA and lacks any indication for CLL therapy. Prednisone is the first-line treatment of choice for his AIHA. If the patient's CLL progresses to the point where it needs to be treated, consideration should be made to avoid fludarabine.

REFERENCES

1. Malek SN. Clinical utility of prognostic markers in chronic lymphocytic leukemia. In: *The American Society of Clinical Oncology education book*, 2010; 263–267.
2. Hallek M, Cheson BD, Catovsky D, et al. Guidelines for the diagnosis and treatment of chronic lymphocytic leukemia: a report from the International Workshop on Chronic Lymphocytic Leukemia updating the National Cancer Institute-Working Group 1996 guidelines. *Blood*. 2008;111(12):5446–5456.
3. Rassenti LZ, Jain S, Keating MJ, et al. Relative value of ZAP-70, CD38, and immunoglobulin mutation status in predicting aggressive disease in chronic lymphocytic leukemia. *Blood*. 2008;112(5):1923–1930.
4. Foon KA, Hallek MJ. Changing paradigms in the treatment of chronic lymphocytic leukemia. *Leukemia*. 2010;24(3):500–511.
5. Hallek M. State-of-the-art treatment of chronic lymphocytic leukemia. *Hematology Am Soc Hematol Educ Program*. 2009; 440–449.
6. Byrd JC, Peterson BL, Morrison VA, et al. Randomized phase 2 study of fludarabine with concurrent versus sequential rituximab in symptomatic, untreated patients with B-cell chronic lymphocytic leukemia: results from Cancer and Leukemia Group B 9712. *Blood*. 2003;101(1):6–14.
7. Byrd JC, Rai K, Peterson BL, et al. Addition of rituximab to fludarabine may prolong progression-free survival and overall survival in patients with previously untreated chronic lymphocytic leukemia: an updated retrospective comparative analysis of CALGB 9712 and CALGB 9011. *Blood*. 2005;105(1):49–53.
8. Tam CS, O'Brien S, Wierda W, et al. Long-term results of the fludarabine, cyclophosphamide, and rituximab regimen as initial therapy of chronic lymphocytic leukemia. *Blood*. 2008;112(4): 975–980.
9. Hallek M, Fischer K, Fingerle-Rowson G, et al. Addition of rituximab to fludarabine and cyclophosphamide in patients with chronic lymphocytic leukaemia: a randomized, open-label, phase 3 trial. *Lancet*. 2010;376(9747):1164–1174.
10. Foon KA, Boyiadzis M, Land SR, et al. Chemoimmunotherapy with low dose fludarabine and cyclophosphamide and high dose rituximab in previously untreated patients with chronic lymphocytic leukemia. *J Clin Oncol*. 2008;27(4):498–503.
11. Kay NE, Geyer SM, Call TG, et al. Combination chemoimmunotherapy with pentostatin, cyclophosphamide, and rituximab shows significant clinical activity with low accompanying toxicity in previously untreated B chronic lymphocytic leukemia. *Blood*. 2007;109(2):405–411.
12. Reynolds C, DiBella N, Lyons RM, et al. Phase III trial of fludarabine, cyclophosphamide, and rituximab vs. pentostatin,

cyclophosphamide and rituximab in B-cell chronic lymphocytic leukemia. *Blood (ASH Annual Meeting Abstracts).* 2008;112: Abst 327.

13. Castro JE, James DF, Sandoval-Sus JD, et al. Rituximab in combination with high-dose methylprednisolone for the treatment of chronic lymphocytic leukemia. *Leukemia.* 2009;23(10): 1779–1789.
14. Hillmen P, Skotnicki AB, Robak T, et al. Alemtuzumab compared with chlorambucil as first-line therapy for chronic lymphocytic leukemia. *J Clin Oncol.* 2007;25(35):5616–5623.
15. Dreger P. Allotransplantation for chronic lymphocytic leukemia. *Hematology Am Soc Hematol Educ Program.* 2009;602–609.
16. Rai KR, Peterson BL, Appelbaum FR, et al. Fludarabine compared with chlorambucil as primary therapy for chronic lymphocytic leukemia. *N Engl J Med.* 2000;343(24):1750–1757.
17. Eichhorst BF, Busch R, Stilgenbauer S, et al. First-line therapy with fludarabine compared with chlorambucil does not result in a major benefit for elderly patients with advanced chronic lymphocytic leukemia. *Blood.* 2009;114(16):3382–3391.
18. Moreno C, Hodgson K, Ferrer G, et al. Autoimmune cytopenia in chronic lymphocytic leukemia: prevalence, clinical associations, and prognostic significance. *Blood.* 2010; [Epub ahead of print].
19. Dearden C, Wade R, Else M, et al. The prognostic significance of a positive direct antiglobulin test in chronic lymphocytic leukemia: a beneficial effect of the combination of fludarabine and cyclophosphamide on the incidence of hemolytic anemia. *Blood.* 2008; 111(4):1820–1826.

32

Myelodysplastic Syndrome

JOHN MAGENAU AND DALE BIXBY

EPIDEMIOLOGY, RISK FACTORS, NATURAL HISTORY, AND PATHOLOGY

Myelodysplastic syndrome (MDS) represents a compilation of clonal myeloid neoplasms resulting in various degrees of ineffective hematopoiesis leading to neutropenia, anemia, and/or thrombocytopenia. Because of the asymptomatic nature of early-stage disease that can smolder for years, the reported incidence of approximately 10,000 to 15,000 cases per year in the United States likely under-represents the true frequency of the disease. The incidence rises exponentially with age, with a median age of 68 and a peak occurring in the ninth decade of life. There is a slight male predominance, but there is little evidence for a genetically inherited predisposition in the majority of patients. A number of rare congenital disorders can predispose younger patients for MDS, including Down syndrome, neurofibromatosis 1, congenital neutropenia disorders, and disorders of DNA damage repair, including Fanconi's anemia. Risk factors for the development of an acquired MDS include exposure to prior chemotherapeutic agents including alkylators and topoisomerase II inhibitors, high doses of radiation, and solvents such as benzene and carbon tetrachloride, as well as a prior diagnosis of aplastic anemia or paroxysmal nocturnal hemoglobinuria (PNH). However, more than 95% of patients have no identifiable risk factor other than advanced age.

The term MDS incorporates distinct pathological processes that carry a variable risk for disease progression, including worsening cytopenias and transformation into acute myeloid leukemia (AML). Our molecular understanding of the pathogenesis and evolution of the disease is poor. Pathologically, establishing the diagnosis of MDS requires both (a) cytopenias and (b) either evidence of morphological dysplasia or an increased myeloid blast count that equates to aberrant myeloid maturation. The minimal morphologic criteria for dysplasia change to indicate that at least 10% of the cells of at least one myeloid lineage (erythroid, granulocytic, and/or megakaryocytic) must show unequivocal dysplasia for the lineage to be considered dysplastic. If a patient presents with cytopenias consistent with MDS but has inconclusive morphologic changes, a presumptive diagnosis of MDS can be made if certain specific clonal chromosomal abnormalities are identified (1). Currently, asynchronous expression of maturation-associated antigens on myeloid cells detected by flow cytometry is not considered diagnostic of MDS when morphologic features are inconclusive.

Because of the recent Food and Drug Administration (FDA) approval of three chemotherapeutic agents, azacitidine (Vidaza; Celgene), decitabine (Dacogen; Eisai), and lenalidomide (Revlimid; Celgene) for this disease, understanding its diagnosis, prognosis, and treatment has become increasingly important. Nonetheless, an incomplete understanding of the predictive variables for treatment response to individual therapies, a lack of understanding as to the true mechanism of action of these medications, as well as a dearth of prospective randomized clinical trials create a continued challenge in optimally caring for patients with MDS.

STAGING

As with most myeloid and lymphoid leukemias, there is no formal staging system for MDS. There are several prognostic scoring systems that are used in treatment planning for patients with MDS, and these will be discussed in the relevant disease sections.

CASE SUMMARIES

Low-Risk Disease

L.S. is a 68-year-old woman with a prior history of hypertension and hyperlipidemia who presented to her physician for a health maintenance examination. She described some increasing fatigue and mild dyspnea on exertion. A complete blood count with differential was performed that demonstrated a WBC count of 3.3 K/mm^3 (absolute neutrophil count of 1.1 K/mm^3), a hemoglobin of 7.6 g/dL, and a platelet count of 111 K/mm^3. After receiving a red blood cell transfusion, a bone marrow biopsy demonstrated an overall cellularity of 80% with trilineage dysplasia in greater than 20% of the myeloid, erythroid, and megakaryocytic progenitor cells. A 500-cell differential of the aspirate smear contained 2.4% blasts. Cytogenetics demonstrated a normal female karyotype in all 20 cells examined: 46, XX [20]. The erythropoietin (EPO) level was 89 mU/mL.

Evidence-Based Case Discussion

The diagnosis of MDS is established by demonstrating cytologic dysplasia in one or more cell lineages together with cytopenias and/or an increase in myeloblasts. Two major classification systems have been developed for MDS, including the French American British (FAB) system and more recently the World Health Organization (WHO) scheme. The WHO scheme additionally recognized unilineage versus multilineage dysplasia, delineated sideroblastic anemias into those with and without multilineage dysplasia, incorporated cytogenetic information into subtyping (5q- Syndrome), further divided the distinction of refractory anemia with excess blasts based on blast percentage, and lowered the threshold for transformation into AML to the presence of 20% blasts in the peripheral blood or bone marrow (Table 32.1) (2,3).

Although both the FAB and WHO diagnostic categories stratify prognosis, they were not originally designed to aid in therapeutic decision making. The International MDS Risk Analysis Workshop collected data from seven prior studies on 816 patients and built a prognostic model based on the bone marrow blast percentage, bone marrow karyotype, and number of cytopenias—termed the International Prognostic Scoring System (IPSS) (Table 32.2) (4). The IPSS is currently the most widely used model for determining prognosis, estimating average

Table 32.1 WHO and FAB Classification Scheme of Myelodysplastic Syndrome

WHO Classification (12)		FAB Classification (2)	
Classification	**PB and BM Findings**	**Classification**	**PB and BM Findings**
Refractory anemia (RA)	Anemia, <5% blasts, <15% ringed sideroblasts	Refractory anemia (RA)	Anemia, <5% blasts, <15% ringed sideroblasts
Refractory anemia with ringed sideroblasts (RARS)	Anemia, <5% blasts, >15% ringed sideroblasts	Refractory anemia with ringed sideroblasts (RARS)	Anemia, <5% blasts, >15% ringed sideroblasts
Refractory cytopenia with multilineage dysplasia (RCMD)	Multiple cytopenias and multilineage dysplasia, <5% blasts, >15% ringed sideroblasts		
Refractory cytopenia with multilineage dysplasia and ringed sideroblasts (RCMD-RS)	Multiple cytopenias and multilineage dysplasia, <5% blasts, >15% ringed sideroblasts		
Refractory anemia with excess blasts—Type 1 (RAEB-I)	Multiple cytopenias and 5%–9% blasts in the BM	Refractory anemia with excess blasts (RAEB)	Multiple cytopenias and 5%–20% blasts in the BM
Refractory anemia with excess blasts—Type 2 (RAEB-II)	Multiple cytopenias and 10%–19% blasts in the BM		
Acute myeloid leukemia (AML)	≥20% blasts in the PB or BM	Refractory anemia with excess blasts in transformation (RAEB-t)	Multiple cytopenias with 21%-30% blasts
MDS—Unclassified (MDS-U)	Multiple cytopenias, but with findings not classifiable in other categories		
MDS Associated with Isolated del(5q)	Anemia, <5% blasts, normal to elevated platelet count, increased megakaryocytes with hypolobated nuclei, isolated del(5q) on karyotype		

PB, peripheral blood; BM, bone marrow.

time for transformation to AML, and guiding therapeutic decision making. The limitations of the IPSS include that it was originally designed for use only at the time of diagnosis and excluded patients with therapy-related MDS from the analysis. The WHO Prognostic Scoring System (WPSS) has been validated as a system that could be used throughout the disease course. It considers the WHO disease subtype rather than blast percentage and takes into account the number of transfusions received rather than just the number of cytopenias (5). However, few pathology centers report the WHO subtype of the biopsy, limiting the applicability of the system. Moreover, there appears to be a large variability in outcomes in patients designated "low-risk" by either the IPSS or the WPSS. More recently, a new MDS risk model was developed that further refines outcomes, segregating patients with traditionally low-risk disease into lower- and higher-risk populations, and it includes groups of patients that were excluded in prior models such as those with previously treated disease, secondary MDS, and chronic myelomonocytic leukemia (CMML) (Table 32.2) (6).

Patients identified as having lower-risk MDS, either by the IPSS or the new MDS risk model, have prolonged survival (median 5–10 years) and low rates of progression to AML (25% rate at 9.4 years). The focus of therapy in this patient population should be symptom control, including correction of transfusion-dependant anemia (Figure 32.1). Erythropoietin-stimulating agents (ESAs)—including epoetin alfa (Epogen; Amgen and Procrit; Ortho Biotech) and darbepoetin (Aranesp; Amgen)—can reduce red blood cell (RBC) transfusion dependency, especially in patients with low transfusion needs per month and a low endogenous EPO level of <500 mU/mL (Hellström-Lindberg Score—Figure 32.2) (7). Indeed, the Eastern Cooperative Oncology Group (ECOG) published a randomized phase III trial of ESAs with or without myeloid growth factor support compared to best supportive care (BSC) with transfusions alone (8). While there was no difference in progression-free survival (PFS) or overall survival (OS) on an intention-to-treat analysis, the erythroid response rates were higher in the patients receiving ESA support, and survival was longer in those patients responding to ESAs versus nonresponders (median, 5.5 vs. 2.3 years). Although ESAs are currently not FDA indicated for use in MDS, they are frequently employed off-label given the benefits noted above, and are currently recommended by the National Comprehensive Cancer Network (NCCN) guidelines. Iron overload may be associated with poorer survival in lower-risk MDS patients receiving significant RBC transfusion support. However, only retrospective

Table 32.2 Prognostic Scoring Systems in Myelodysplastic Syndrome (MDS)

International Prognostic Scoring System (IPSS) (4)

Entity	Score				
	0	0.5	1.0	1.5	2
Percentage of bone marrow blasts	<5	5–10	—	11–20	>20
Number of cytopenias	0 or 1	2 or 3			
Karyotypic risk	Good	Intermediate	Poor		

Cytopenias: Hemoglobin <10 g/dL, absolute neutrophil count <1800/µL, and/or platelet count <100,000/µL

Karyotype Risk: Good: Normal, -Y, del (5q), or del (20q)/Intermediate: all others/Poor: complex karyotype (≥3 abnormalities) or abnormal chromosome 7

Risk Groups: Low - 0 points; Intermediate-1 (Int-1)—0.5 to 1 points; Intermediate-2 (Int-2)—1.5 to 2 points; High—2.5 to 3.5 points

New Risk Model (6)

Entity	PS	Age	Plt Count	Hgb	BM Blasts	WBC Count	Karyotype	Transfusions
Variable (score)	<2 (0)	<60 (0)	≥200 (0)	<12 (0)	0–4 (0)	≤20 (0)	any other (0)	no (0)
	≥2 (2)	60–64 (1)	50–199 (1)	≥12 (2)	5–10 (1)	>20 (2)	Chromosome 7 abnormality or complex (≥3 changes) (score = 3)	Yes (1)
		≥65 (2)	30–49 (2) <30 (3)		11–29 (2)			

PS, performance status (as assessed per Eastern Cooperative Group criteria); Plt Count, platelet count (in thousands/mm^3); Hgb, hemoglobin (in g/dL); BM Blasts, bone marrow blasts (expressed as a percentage); WBC Count, total white blood cell count (in thousands/mm^3)

Risk Groups: Low—0 to 4 points; Intermediate -1 (Int-1)—5 to 6 points; Intermediate-2 (Int-2)—7 to 8 points; High—≥ 9 points

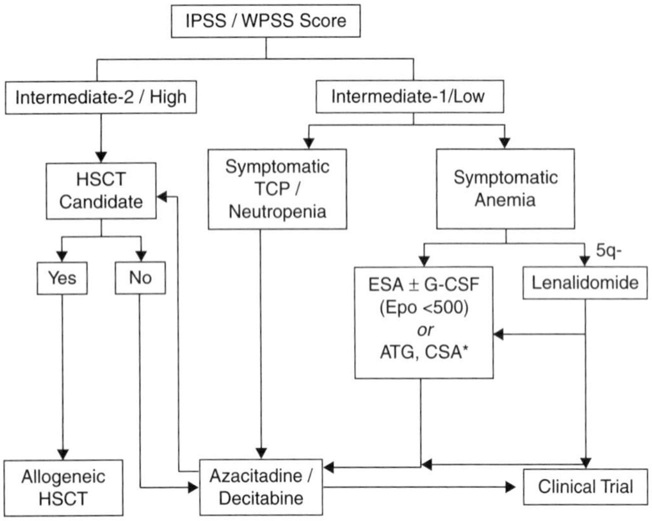

Abbreviations: IPSS = International prognostic scoring system; WPSS = WHO prognostic scoring system; TCP = thrombocytopenia; HSCT = Hematopoietic stem cell transplant; ESA = Erythropoiesis stimulating agent ; ATG = Anti-Thymocyte globulin; CSA = Cyclosporin A.

•Consider for patients ≤60 years, hypocellular marrow, HLA-DR 15, and / or demonstrating a PNH positive clone.

Figure 32.1

Treatment algorithm for myelodysplastic syndromes.

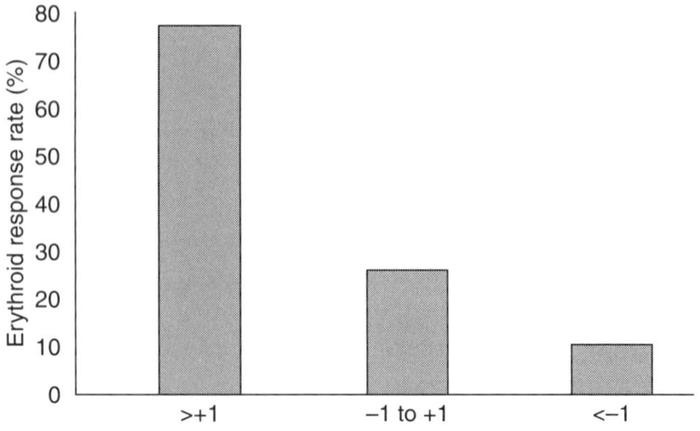

Total Hellström-Lindberg Score

Factor	Level	Score
Erythropoietin Level (mU/mL)	<100	+2
	100–500	+1
	>500	-3
Red Blood Cell Transfusions Per Month	<2	+2
	≥2	-2

Figure 32.2

Hellström-Lindberg predictive model (7). The graph represents the percentage of transfusion-dependent MDS patients responding to erythropoietin +/- granulocyte colony stimulating factor (G-CSF). A predictive model was developed based upon a score for the patients' endogenous erythropoietin level (measured in mU/mL) added to the score for the number of red blood cell transfusions received per month.

analyses are available describing improved OS in MDS patients receiving iron-chelation therapy (9). Nonetheless, chelation therapy is also recommended by the NCCN, especially in those patients receiving greater than 20 RBC transfusions and having elevated ferritin levels.

Although allogeneic hematopoietic stem cell transplantation (alloHSCT) remains the only curative option for patients with MDS, treatment-related toxicities make this approach challenging, particularly given the older age of MDS patients. Retrospective evaluation of allogeneic transplant in low-risk MDS patients (IPSS-low or Int-1) demonstrated a superior OS for those receiving BSC instead of transplant, likely secondary to the low rate of disease progression in those patients receiving supportive care alone (10). The Centers for Medicare and Medicaid Services (CMS) recently stated that there was insufficient evidence that the use of allogeneic BMT improves health outcomes in Medicare beneficiaries with MDS. They are currently restricting its use through the Act through Coverage with Evidence Development (CED) to patients participating in an approved clinical study addressing the long-term effectiveness of transplant in MDS. However, most private insurers continue to cover allogeneic transplant for patients with advanced MDS.

In summary, patients with MDS should have a prognosis calculated based on either the IPSS or the new MDS risk model. Those patients with lower-risk disease (Low- or Int-1 Risk) should be counseled about average survival and rates of transformation to AML, while understanding that each case is unique and medical observation is continuously required. In the lower-risk population, symptom control with transfusion support and/or the use of growth factors (ESAs) are common, but ESAs should be employed in the appropriate clinical setting (those with a low Hellström-Lindberg Score) (7). In this case, L.S. required a transfusion, had a low endogenous erythropoietin level, and had an IPSS score of 0.5 (0 for blast count, 0 for karyotype, and 0.5 for cytopenias). Given that her age is over 60, a median survival of 2.7 years is indicated. With a Hellström-Lindberg Score of +4, she would be predicted to have a 74% chance of an erythroid response to ESAs and can be counseled on their potential use to decrease transfusion needs, ensuring an understanding that there would likely be no OS advantage. In addition, an evaluation of her iron status (ferritin) would be appropriate, and iron chelation may be required if her transfusion needs continue despite ESAs.

5q-Syndrome

E.L. is a 78-year-old woman with osteoarthritis and hyperlipidemia who presented with complaints of increasing fatigue and dyspnea on minimal exertion. A complete blood count with differential was performed and demonstrated a WBC count of 5.2 K/mm^3 (absolute neutrophil count of 3.1 K/mm^3), a hemoglobin of 7.6 g/dL with mean corpuscular volume (MCV) of 102, and a platelet count of 525 K/mm^3. She was transfused, and an evaluation demonstrated no evidence of vitamin or mineral deficiency. Endoscopy failed to identify a source of GI blood loss. A bone marrow biopsy demonstrated an overall cellularity of 30%, with normal erythroid and granulocytic maturation. Increased numbers of small, unilobate megakaryocytes were seen. A 500-cell differential of the aspirate smear demonstrated 1.1% blasts. Cytogenetics demonstrated an abnormal female karyotype: 46,XX,del(5)(q13q33)[16]/46,XX[4]. The erythropoietin level was 510 mU/mL.

Evidence-Based Case Discussion

In 2000, the WHO began to recognize the central importance of cytogenetic abnormalities in the pathogenesis as well as the prognosis of patients with MDS. Therefore, a unique subgroup of MDS was defined, using the term 5q-Syndrome. The syndrome is characterized by an older female predominance (median age 65–70 years), with blood counts demonstrating an isolated macrocytic anemia along with a normal or elevated platelet count (11,12). The bone marrow typically displays micromegakaryocytes with monolobulated and bilobulated nuclei together with a low myeloid blast count. Cytogenetics demonstrate an isolated interstitial deletion of variable length on the long arm of chromosome 5, most often del(5)(q13q33), with nearly all cases lacking a 1.5-Mb segment extending from bands 5q31 to 5q32.3. Thus, the diagnosis is based on a compilation of morphological and cytogenetic information. Because of the normal neutrophil and platelet counts seen in most patients, there is a low incidence of infection and bleeding, but red cell transfusions are frequently needed. The disease typically has an indolent course, with few cases of progression to AML and a reported median survival of 63 months. Subsequent work identified RPS14, a protein required for the function of the 40S ribosomal complex, as a critical player in the pathogenesis of this syndrome, but haploinsufficiency of two micro-RNAs (miRNAs), miR-145 and miR-146a, may also participate (13).

During an early phase clinical trial with lenalidomide (Revlimid; Celgene) in patients with MDS who did not respond to ESAs, clinicians observed that 10 of 12 patients with the 5q deletion no longer needed red cell transfusions and had a complete or partial cytogenetic response. A subsequent phase II study (MDS-003) involving 148 low- or intermediate-1 risk transfusion dependent patients, demonstrating a chromosome 5q31 deletion that was either isolated or accompanied by additional cytogenetic abnormalities, showed that 67% became transfusion independent and 62% had a complete cytogenetic response (14). Moreover, the median time to transfusion independence was only 4.6 weeks, and the median duration of transfusion independence was not reached. Based on this data, the FDA approved lenalidomide for low- or intermediate-1 risk transfusion dependent MDS patients with a deletion 5q in isolation or accompanied by additional cytogenetic abnormalities (Figure 32.1). Additional trials in patients with MDS without del(5q) demonstrated an overall response rate of 26%, indicating lower response rates than with hypomethylating agents, and its use is typically restricted in patients without del(5q). To date, no studies have demonstrated a survival advantage for patients receiving lenalidomide versus other supportive measures, including patients with the 5q-Syndrome.

In summary, E.L. is a prototypical 5q-Syndrome patient having an isolated macrocytic anemia, elevated platelet count, low blast percentage, and karyotype displaying an isolated loss of the distal portion of the long arm of chromosome 5. Although this cytogenetic change is not a perfect predictive marker, therapy using lenalidomide may be optimal in this patient population. However, the goal would be to provide transfusion independence, with no evidence currently indicating an OS advantage.

High-Risk MDS

B.H. is a 78-year-old gentleman with a history of gout and coronary artery disease with a myocardial infarction 5 years ago, but without recurrent angina or heart failure symptoms. He presented to his primary care provider with increasing bruising and fatigue. A complete blood count with differential was performed and demonstrated a WBC count of 1.2 K/mm^3 (absolute neutrophil count of 0.2 K/mm^3), hemoglobin of 7.2 g/dL (MCV 98), and a platelet count of 25,000 K/mm^3. His EPO level was 922 mU/mL. He was transfused twice with red blood cells and platelets over the next month. A bone marrow biopsy demonstrated an overall cellularity of 70%, with trilineage dysplasia in a substantial number of myeloid, erythroid, and megakaryocytic precursors. There were 14% myeloid blasts on the aspirate. Cytogenetics demonstrated a complex male karyotype: 46,XY,del(13)(q12q22)[14]/50,sl,+8,+9,+13,del(13)(q12q22),+14[6].

Evidence-Based Case Discussion

Unlike their lower-risk counterparts, patients with higher-risk MDS (Int-2 and High-Risk IPSS scores) have shorter latency periods for transformation to AML and a median survival measured in months. Therefore, the focus of therapy is not only in improving symptoms but also in prolonging survival. As previously discussed, bone marrow transplantation remains the only curative option in MDS. Due to the increased risk of therapy-related morbidity and mortality with increased age, alloHSCT use has been restricted to those patients with higher-risk MDS under the age of 70 to 75 (Figure 32.1) (10). Because the average age of MDS patients is in the seventh decade of life, the majority of patients will not be transplant eligible due to underlying comorbidities and limited sibling donor options. Thus, alternative therapy options are desperately needed.

Both azacitidine (Vidaza; Celgene) and decitabine (Dacogen; Eisai) are agents that are thought to alter gene expression through inhibition of DNA methylation, although they may also demonstrate cytotoxic capacity through incorporation into DNA and RNA, resulting in strand cessation. Azacitidine was recently compared with conventional care options (transfusions alone, low-dose cytarabine, or induction chemotherapy) in a randomized phase III clinical trial (15). Restricted to those with Int-2 or High-Risk MDS and FAB-defined refractory anemia with excess blasts, refractory anemia with excess blasts in transformation (AML per WHO), or type II chronic myelomonocytic leukemia (CMML), patients randomized to receive azacitidine had an improved median survival of 24.5 months versus 15 months in the conventional care arms. The survival benefit held for most subgroups, including those with high-risk disease, age >75, poor-risk karyotype, as well as patients only achieving hematologic improvement rather than a morphologic remission. Notably, the median number of cycles of therapy received was nine and there was no limit on the total number of treatment cycles, as long as the patient was tolerating the therapy. Prior studies had reported that a median of four cycles of azacitidine were needed for a response, and 80% of responses occur by the eighth cycle. Cytopenias are common during the initial cycles of treatment, and patients should be counseled that transfusion support is often required during this time. Decitabine has also been evaluated in a number of phase II as well as a registration phase III clinical trial, but demonstrated no evidence of improved survival compared with best supportive care (BSC) (16). However, patients received on average only three cycles of therapy in the pivotal trial. The European Organization for Research and Treatment of Cancer (EORTC) also compared the outcome of patients receiving decitabine versus BSC (17). Importantly, patients could only receive two cycles past a complete remission and the maximum number of cycles was eight, with patients receiving on average only four cycles of therapy. Again, there was no survival difference between the decitabine-treated patients and those receiving BSC.

Alternatively, immunosuppressive therapy may be considered for a subgroup of patients with specific characteristics of their MDS, including younger patients with hypocellular bone marrows, low- or intermediate-1 risk disease (especially normal cytogenetics), a shorter duration of red cell transfusion dependence, presence of PNH-positive cells, and the presence of an HLA-DR15 (DR2) haplotype (Figure 32.1) (18). Prior therapies employing cyclosporine alone or in combination with antithymocyte globulin in these patients have demonstrated hematologic improvement in 30% to 70% of patients, with relatively good durability in those responding to therapy (19).

As previously noted, the only known curative option for MDS involves allogeneic bone marrow transplant. To date, there have been no prospective, randomized trials assessing medical therapy versus transplant options, and current recommendations are based largely on retrospective analysis of registry data. For low- and Int-1 risk MDS patients, delayed transplantation was associated with an improved OS, but for patients with Int-2 and High-Risk disease, transplantation at diagnosis was associated with an improved OS (10). Reduced-intensity conditioning (RIC) regimens may limit organ toxicities in older patients, but these benefits may be offset by higher relapse rates (20). However, as previously noted, CMS has restricted transplant to patients participating in an approved clinical study, although most private insurers continue to cover allogeneic transplant in this setting. There have been only single institution nonrandomized reports on the benefit of the use of the hypomethylating agents azacitidine or decitabine either prior to or after allogeneic transplant, and therefore, their associated use remains an active area of investigation (21).

In summary, B.H. presents with advanced MDS, with an IPSS score of 3 (1.5 for blast percentage, 1 for karyotype, and 0.5 for cytopenias), and thus has an anticipated median survival of only 0.4 months. His advanced age precludes the current use of alloHSCT, and his age in combination with the hypercellular marrow and the complex karyotype makes immunosuppressive therapy a poor choice. His elevated EPO level and transfusion requirements would predict only a 7% chance of responding to ESA. Options in this case should focus on supportive care, either alone or concurrent with the use of either azacitidine or decitabine, with the potential aim of decreasing transfusion dependency as well as delaying transformation to AML and improving OS. If he were younger without significant comorbidities, consideration for alloHSCT should be incorporated into his treatment plan as early as possible.

REFERENCES

1. Vardiman JW, Thiele J, Arber DA, et al. The 2008 revision of the World Health Organization (WHO) classification of myeloid neoplasms and acute leukemia: rationale and important changes. *Blood*. 2009;114(5):937–951.

2. Bennett JM, Catovsky D, Daniel MT, et al. Proposals for the classification of the myelodysplastic syndromes. *Br J Haematol.* 1982;51(2):189–199.
3. Vardiman JW, Harris NL, Brunning RD. The World Health Organization (WHO) classification of the myeloid neoplasms. *Blood.* 2002;100(7):2292–2302.
4. Greenberg P, Cox C, LeBeau MM, et al. International scoring system for evaluating prognosis in myelodysplastic syndromes. *Blood.* 1997;89(6):2079–2088.
5. Malcovati L, Germing U, Kuendgen A, et al. Time-dependent prognostic scoring system for predicting survival and leukemic evolution in myelodysplastic syndromes. *J Clin Oncol.* 2007;25(23):3503–3510.
6. Kantarjian H, O'Brien S, Ravandi F, et al. Proposal for a new risk model in myelodysplastic syndrome that accounts for events not considered in the original International Prognostic Scoring System. *Cancer.* 2008;113(6):1351–1361.
7. Hellstrom-Lindberg E, Negrin R, Stein R, et al. Erythroid response to treatment with G-CSF plus erythropoietin for the anaemia of patients with myelodysplastic syndromes: proposal for a predictive model. *Br J Haematol.* 1997;99(2):344–351.
8. Greenberg PL, Sun Z, Miller KB, et al. Treatment of myelodysplastic syndrome patients with erythropoietin with or without granulocyte colony-stimulating factor: results of a prospective randomized phase 3 trial by the Eastern Cooperative Oncology Group (E1996). *Blood.* 2009;114(12):2393–2400.
9. Leitch HA. Controversies surrounding iron chelation therapy for MDS. *Blood Rev.* 2011;25(1):17–31.
10. Cutler CS, Lee SJ, Greenberg P, et al. A decision analysis of allogeneic bone marrow transplantation for the myelodysplastic syndromes: delayed transplantation for low-risk myelodysplasia is associated with improved outcome. *Blood.* 2004;104(2):579–585.
11. Boultwood J, Lewis S, Wainscoat JS. The 5q-syndrome. *Blood.* 1994;84(10):3253–3260.
12. Bennett JM. World Health Organization classification of the acute leukemias and myelodysplastic syndrome. *Int J Hematol.* 2000;72(2):131–133.
13. Ebert BL, Pretz J, Bosco J, et al. Identification of RPS14 as a 5q-syndrome gene by RNA interference screen. *Nature.* 2008;451(7176):335–339.
14. List A, Dewald G, Bennett J, et al. Lenalidomide in the myelodysplastic syndrome with chromosome 5q deletion. *N Engl J Med.* 2006;355(14):1456–1465.
15. Fenaux P, Mufti GJ, Hellstrom-Lindberg E, et al. Efficacy of azacitidine compared with that of conventional care regimens in the treatment of higher-risk myelodysplastic syndromes: a randomised, open-label, phase III study. *Lancet Oncol.* 2009;10(3):223–232.
16. Kantarjian H, Issa JP, Rosenfeld CS, et al. Decitabine improves patient outcomes in myelodysplastic syndromes: results of a phase III randomized study. *Cancer.* 2006;106(8):1794–1803.
17. WijerMans P, Suciu S, Baila L, et al. Low dose decitabine versus best supportive care in elderly patients with intermediate or high risk MDS not eligible for intensive chemotherapy: final results of the randomized phase III study (06011) of the EORTC leukemia and german MDS study groups. *ASH Annual Meeting Abstracts.* 2008;112(11):226–.
18. Sloand EM, Wu CO, Greenberg P, et al. Factors affecting response and survival in patients with myelodysplasia treated with immunosuppressive therapy. *J Clin Oncol.* 2008;26(15):2505–2511.
19. Molldrem JJ, Leifer E, Bahceci E, et al. Antithymocyte globulin for treatment of the bone marrow failure associated with myelodysplastic syndromes. *Ann Intern Med.* 2002;137(3):156–163.
20. Martino R, Iacobelli S, Brand R, et al. Retrospective comparison of reduced-intensity conditioning and conventional high-dose conditioning for allogeneic hematopoietic stem cell transplantation using HLA-identical sibling donors in myelodysplastic syndromes. *Blood.* 2006;108(3):836–846.
21. de Lima M, Giralt S, Thall PF, et al. Maintenance therapy with low-dose azacitidine after allogeneic hematopoietic stem cell transplantation for recurrent acute myelogenous leukemia or myelodysplastic syndrome: a dose and schedule finding study. *Cancer.* 2010;116(23):5420–5431.

Index

Note: Page numbers followed by "*f*" and "*t*" denote figures and tables, respectively.